MAN AND MEDICINE

MAN AND MEDICINE
A History

FAROKH ERACH UDWADIA

MD, FCPS, FRCP (Edinburgh), FRCP (London), Master FCCP, FACP, FAMS
Emeritus Professor of Medicine, Grant Medical College and the J J Group of Hospital, Mumbai
Consultant Physician, Breach Candy Hospital, Mumbai
Consultant Physician, Parsee General Hospital, Mumbai

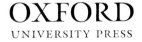

OXFORD
UNIVERSITY PRESS

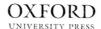

OXFORD
UNIVERSITY PRESS

YMCA Library Building, Jai Singh Road, New Delhi 110001

Oxford University Press is a department of the University of Oxford. It furthers the
University's objective of excellence in research, scholarship, and education
by publishing worldwide in

Oxford   New York
Athens   Auckland   Bangkok   Bogota   Buenos Aires   Cape Town
Chennai   Dar es Salaam   Delhi   Florence   Hong Kong   Istanbul Karachi
Kolkata Kuala Lumpur   Madrid   Melbourne   Mexico City   Mumbai Nairobi
Paris Sao Paolo   Singapore   Taipei   Tokyo   Toronto   Warsaw

with associated companies in

Berlin   Ibadan

Oxford is a registered trade mark of Oxford University Press
in the UK and in certain other countries

Published in India
By Oxford University Press, New Delhi

©Oxford University Press 2000
First published 2000
Second impression 2001

ISBN 0 19 565457 9

Typeset by InoSoft Systems, I. P. Extension, New Delhi 110092
Printed in India at Sahara India Mass Communication, Noida
and published by Manzar Khan, Oxford University Press
YMCA Library Building, Jai Singh Road, New Delhi 110 001

To Vera,
for her love, support and care.

Preface

There is no greater saga in the history of man than the epic of medicine. Medicine emerged out of the mists of magical and empirical beliefs of the shamans and priest physicians of ancient civilizations. The trail of medicine has witnessed several twists and turns, victories and defeats, scintillating light and sombre darkness. After over five thousand years of history, medicine has now evolved into a powerful force, an art, a science and a profession, poised to make a quantum leap into the twenty-first century.

A true appreciation of medicine is dependent on knowing the history of its evolution. It is as important to be aware of the mistakes and follies marking the path of medicine as it is to know the strides that have led to true progress. Unfortunately most people remain ignorant and unconcerned about the history of medicine and the great men that fashioned this history. This ignorance extends to many medical students, researchers and practising doctors whose acquaintance with medical history is generally confined to a vague notion of Hippocrates, Galen, Susruta, Fleming, and a few others. This book aims at fostering an interest in medical history among all people, especially in medical students and the medical profession.

The panorama of medicine through five millennia is not just a chronological sequence of events and discoveries. The romance of medicine lies in the dynamic cavalcade of men who walked its trail. It is embodied in the heroes and imposters, the caring and the uncaring who shaped its path. More than any other field of human endeavour, medicine through the ages has been influenced by the natural sciences, philosophy, religion, economics, sociology, geography, by art and culture, by war and natural calamities and by the rise and fall of mighty empires. The history of medicine therefore cannot be correctly viewed in a narrow "medical perspective". Its historical evolution can only be understood against the tapestry of the civilization of man. Man has influenced medicine through the ages as much as medicine has influenced man. It is for this reason that this book brings to life the story of medicine against the background of the history of man and of evolving civilizations.

The book has attempted the difficult task of giving a brief historical introduction, to each age or epoch of Man and Medicine. The story of medicine in this book begins with prehistory and then proceeds to the ancient civilizations of Mesopotamia, Egypt, India, China, Persia, and Greece. It then follows the fascinating chequered trail of history through Rome, the Dark Ages, the Renaissance, the Baroque, the Eighteenth century and culminates in Modern and Contemporary medicine. It also includes a special chapter on the impact of Western medicine in India, a subject generally ignored by western historians. The book ends by hazarding a peep into the future. The subsection on 'A Perspective of Contemporary Medicine' discusses the problems facing medicine today, its potential to do harm almost matching its ability to do good and the consequent tensions that have arisen between medicine and man. The comments in this subsection though more pertinent to prevailing conditions in India, would also have a general bearing on the rest of the world. The text has numerous illustrations, so that men, events, ideas and discoveries are brought to life not only by the magic of words but also by the beauty of art and the discerning eye of the camera.

Why should medical students and doctors study medical history? After all, it cannot be denied that a doctor does not need to know history to remove an inflamed appendix or treat typhoid fever. There are several reasons why the history of medicine is important. Medicine is not just knowing or treating a deranged organ or organ system. It encompasses a more holistic concept in caring for and treating not only man as a whole, but man in relation to the world he lives in and in the environment that surrounds him. A physician is better equipped to do so if he is familiar with the history of man and of medicine. He then adds wisdom to knowledge, art to science and humility to his prowess.

An awareness of history also helps to build character. Lives of distinguished physicians and surgeons of the past, their discoveries, achievements and humanity would be a source of inspiration and would help inculcate a modesty of being, which is the hallmark of almost all good and great men.

The lessons of history are indeed many but I shall dwell briefly on two important lessons in relation to medicine. The first and all-important lesson is that there are limits to medicine and that frustrations expressed towards medicine today, are because expectations of people from medicine have always been far more than what medicine can meet. The other important lesson of history is that truth is relative and never absolute. Many concepts and beliefs considered to be sanctified truths in the past were held to be utterly false at another time in the future. We should therefore be humble enough to realize that many aspects of contemporary medicine about which so many are so proud, may a hundred years from now prove to be false, and perhaps even harmful and dangerous. At the same time, history also teaches that discarded concepts of the past have been resuscitated and found useful in the future. Alternative forms of medicine therefore need our tolerance and even respect, not the disdain shown by practitioners of western medicine. Among all that is new and claiming to be used and all that is old yet still seeking recognition, we may adopt as our practice the wisdom expressed in the lines quoted below from Alexander Pope

"Be not the first when the new is tried.
Nor yet the last to lay the old aside"

'Man and Medicine' should be of as much or even greater interest to non-medical readers. After all, medicine deals with life and death, the preservation of health, the prevention and treatment of disease. These are surely of immediate interest and intimate concern to all men. The basis of medicine is the doctor-patient relationship—a symbolic bond of trust, faith and friendship between the physician and his patient. The more a patient knows about the trials and tribulations, the endeavours and achievements, the faults and virtues of physicians through the ages, the closer the bond with the physician, the greater the strength of medicine and the greater the benefit to man.

The goal of medicine is not only to improve the health of individual human beings but also to improve the health of all people, all nations, and thereby to add to the sum total of human happiness. Knowing the past could lead to a greater understanding of the present and help us to reach out to a healthier and happier future. I sincerely hope that this book goes a small way in achieving this distant goal.

I owe several people a great deal of gratitude for enabling me to complete this work. First and foremost, I am grateful to my wife Vera for her patience and forbearance and for the many hours spent in studying and summarizing the numerous references that were needed for this book. She is truly a part of this work. I wish to acknowledge my debt and gratitude to the Wellcome Trust, Medical Photographic Library, London, which has provided me with all the illustrations in this book and has permitted their publication without cost. I thank in particular Ms Michelle Minto of the Wellcome Trust, Medical Photographic Library for helping me to choose the illustrations and permitting me to make free use of the library.

I owe a great debt of gratitude to Mr Keki Dadiseth, the former Chairman of Hindustan Lever Limited, and Mr M.S. Banga, the present Chairman of Hindustan Liver Limited, who through their company generously provided a munificent subsidy towards the publication of the book. This has enabled the price of the book to be substantially reduced so that it is now within the reach of students, young doctors and most individuals.

I sincerely thank Mr Homi R. Khusrokhan, Managing Director of Glaxo and Burroughs Wellcome Limited for helping to establish a liaison with the Wellcome Trust Library. My friend Dr Hirji S. Adenwalla, a surgeon of class and distinction has been kind enough to read large portions of the manuscript, offering, encouragement, valuable criticism and suggestions. To him I express my grateful thanks. This work has drawn heavily from the publications of numerous historians and scholars of the past and present. To them I acknowledge my grateful debt. Any inadvertent omission of a work of reference in the bibliography is sincerely regretted. Dr Sameer Chowhan and Mr Neeraj Chawan have helped in the typing of the manuscript and in organizing my work. To them I am also very grateful. Finally I wish to thank Oxford University Press for their kindness, courtesy and cooperation in publishing this book.

Mumbai
July, 2000

Farokh Erach Udwadia

Contents

Roman Medicine

Medicine in the Dark Ages

Renaissance Medicine

Medicine in the Baroque Period

Medicine in the Age of
Enlightenment and Reason—Eighteenth Century

Modern Medicine

Western Medicine in India

Contemporary Medicine

75. The Future

List of Illustrations

The Prelude

Time present and time past
Are both perhaps present in time future
And time future contained in time past.

TS Eliot

In the late Palaeolithic period, between 25 to 40 thousand years ago, the fourth Glacial age mellowed into more temperate conditions and the first *Homo sapiens* appeared. The first men originated, in all probability in Africa, or South Asia, or in the lands now submerged in the Mediterranean basins, from some ape-like ancestor after hundreds of centuries of evolutionary struggle. During this long gestational period they learned to walk erect on their legs, acquired an increasing power of intellect and a larger sized brain. Century after century, they multiplied in numbers, and slowly spread into new realms that offered them food and plants to which they were accustomed. In this process *Homo sapiens* (the 'true men') exterminated their Neanderthal cousin the *Homo neanderthalensis* whose race had lasted for 2,00,000 years during the early Palaeolithic period.

Men of the late Palaeolithic age were hunters. In Europe, they appear to have hunted the mammoth, reindeer, bison and wild horse, using sharpened but crude stone implements as weapons. They led a precarious existence and were in turn hunted by the cave lion, the carnivorous bear, the hyenas and other wild denizens that roamed across the steppes of the continent. The animal world was however a source of sustenance for prehistoric man—the flesh of hunted animals provided food, the skin was used for clothing, and the bones for making implements.

The late Palaeolithic men moved naked or covered themselves with skins or fur-wraps, particularly in the winters. These hunters lived out in the open or in natural cave-dwellings for over 200 centuries—a period of time ten times the duration of our present Christian era. Savages they must have been, but they were artistic savages, and shared a common trait with civilized man—the inherent, perhaps genetic trait of artistic expression. They could draw incredibly well, better in fact than all their prehistoric successors till the dawn of history. They drew chiefly on the walls of caves they had wrested from the Neanderthal man and also on the walls of cliffs. They loved to draw animals, the artistic representation of beasts that shared their existence being astonishingly vivid. The artists of this period also sculpted, modelled figures in clay and scratched or engraved designs on ivory and bone. Their surviving drawings and works of art, meagre though they be, enable us to appreciate our ancient heritage and realize our common humanity. They form a beacon of light that illuminates the darkness of the prehistoric age.

Prehistoric men buried their dead, often with ornaments, weapons and food. They loved to paint, and painted the dead bodies before burial. They probably also painted their bodies during life. They used black, red, yellow, white and brown pigments, which have endured to this day in the caves of Spain and France.

The climate in Europe after over 20,000 years of the late Palaeolithic period underwent a further change. It became milder and damper, and mighty forests stretched across the continent. A new culture termed the Neolithic age dawned. Men had reached the Neolithic stage in south-west Asia, Persia, Africa, and Asia minor a few thousand years before the Neolithic age began in Europe, about ten to twelve thousand years ago. The new Neolithic culture had a more close-knit community life and a stronger social organization. It was characterized by the presence of polished stone implements, the use of a stone axe with a handle, javelins, and the use of bows and arrows with sharp arrow-heads. The age ushered in agriculture, with the use of plants and seeds, pottery and the cooking of food. Neolithic man domesticated animals. The dog was probably the first such animal, followed by cattle, sheep, goats and pigs. The huntsman of the Palaeolithic age became the herdsman of the Neolithic age. Neolithic man learnt to plait and to weave, and cover his body with clothes. He no longer lived out in the open or in caves but moved to the shores of the lakes left by glaciers. He built himself thatched roof shelters on stilts and often lived with his fellow-men in community settlements. He fashioned weirs, fish-hooks, and fish-traps and learned to build circular boats made of animal skins. The cave family grew into a clan or tribe, and each tribe evolved its own social codes, its rituals and its taboos. Clans and tribes viewed one another with suspicion and hostility, sowing the first seeds of internecine conflict in our world.

Speech, song and music made their appearance. Metal came into use. Gold, presumably the first known metal, began to adorn bone ornaments. Copper, followed by bronze, was discovered and used 7000 years ago. Man was now about to emerge from the dark shadows of prehistory and take his first faltering steps on a never-ending journey, leaving footprints on the sands of time.

The Evolution of Medicine

Medicine is as old as man and must have come into being with the first awakening of human consciousness. Disease existed among living creatures in the world long before the advent of man. What was the nature of disease in prehistoric times and how did man try and counter it? Our knowledge of prehistory is based on a study of anthropology, palaeontology, palaeopathology, sculpture and cave art. However, in the absence of documentary evidence, the evolution of medicine in the prehistoric period can at best remain a subject of reasoned conjecture. Folklore, the known medical practices of primitive races that have remained frozen in time, and the literature and archaeological findings of ancient historical civilizations help to give some indication of what preceded them. Even so, this information could well be misleading as ancient cultures were dynamic and must have undergone several changes over the centuries.

Palaeopathology is the study of the human and animal remnants of ancient times. A study of animal fossils has shown that prehistoric creatures were subject to many injuries and diseases. Fractures, periosteitis and osteomyelitis were common. Extensive callus formation with resulting bony deformities were also noted. Arthritis in dinosaurs and cave bears was frequent and was termed (by palaeontologists) 'cave-gout'. Studies of human remains of ancient times, particularly of mummies of ancient Egypt, have revealed the occurrence of many pathologies. Palaeopathologists have also reported on pathological abnormalities in the skeleton and teeth of prehistoric specimens available for study. Interestingly, the typical features of tuberculosis of the spine (Pott's disease), found in the skeletons of the mummified bodies of ancient Egypt have also been observed in a few

Neolithic skeletons. The exact aetiology of some of the pathologies discovered in the ancient specimens has been questioned. Pre-Columbian skeletons in the Americas have, for example, revealed changes suggestive of sphirocetal syphilis. It has been suggested that these changes could also perhaps be due to a different sphirocetal disease, or that the bones belonged to a later period of history than has been supposed.

Fossil teeth of both ancient history and of prehistoric times have shown evidence of erosion, caries, abscess and pyorrhoea. The first specimens of these fossils were studied in the nineteenth and early twentieth centuries. In this period of history, medical opinion erroneously linked septic foci in teeth to a number of diseases, including arthritis. Palaeopathologists were prompt in relating this erroneous prevailing concept to the historic and prehistoric past, and attributed the arthritis observed in prehistoric and ancient skeletons to changes observed in the teeth.

It is impossible to determine the incidence and nature of diseases of the soft parts of the human anatomy in prehistoric times, because no bodies or organs earlier than 4000 BC have been discovered. However, in the mummies of early Egypt there is ample evidence to show the prevalence of tuberculosis, urinary infections, urinary stones, parasitic infections and advanced atherosclerosis. Scientific proof that these were a continuum from the prehistoric past is unfortunately lacking.

How did prehistoric man treat disease and how did medicine evolve? One can surmise that, to start with, the patient must have been his own physician employing instinctive methods in self-healing similar to those observed in animals. Licking wounds, sucking, delousing one another, washing with water, reflexly rubbing an injured part, using heat to relieve discomfort, cold to deaden pain, and resting the sick or injured limb or body resemble instinctive activities of animals to relieve pain. Prehistoric and primitive men must very soon have appreciated the difference between the discomfort and anguish of disease from the well-being of good health. There must have been an overt or intuitive longing to preserve health and reverse or abolish disease. The need to heal and preserve health was perhaps second only to the urge to satiate hunger and thirst and to procreate. Hippocrates of Cos in the fifth century BC wrote:

> In the first place the science of medicine would never have been discovered nor indeed sought for were there no need for it. If sick men fared just as well eating and drinking and living exactly as healthy men do, and no better on some different regime, there would be little need for the science. But the reason why the art of medicine became necessary was because sick men did not get well on the same regime as the healthy, any more than they do now.

How was this need met and how did medicine advance beyond its early instinctive attempts at self-healing? How did medicine, as we know it today, originate in the history of man? Modern historical research and the evidence of palaeontology and anthropology affirm that medicine originated in magic and flourished as a priestly art. Primitive man must have led a precarious existence at the mercy of inexplicable events and occurrences. He must have wondered at the mystery of birth and life and at the inevitable finality of dissolution and death. The floods of mighty rivers, the violence of nature that often threatened his existence, would have been beyond his comprehension. Concerning his own immediate self, to start with, he must have made a distinction between what could be seen and explained and what could not. Thus pain or illness caused by wounds incurred in battle, or in fighting animals, or by foreign bodies was easily explicable, and the treatment empirical. On the other hand many life-threatening illnesses seemed to have no visible cause. Prehistoric or primitive man could never have understood an epileptic fit that seized a perfectly healthy man, or a sudden abdominal pain due to a perforated viscus, or the sudden loss of consciousness due to an intracerebral bleed. He was helpless and powerless when struck by what he considered unknown forces. His imagery now attributed illness, suffering, pain and death to be the work of invisible demons who unleashed evil forces against him. But then he needed an explanation for the pleasant occurrences in his personal life. He attributed these to kinder divinities. Thus, the concept of good and evil forces was born. This concept extended to include his environment. He became convinced that floods, storms and other natural disasters that threatened or harmed him were also the work of demons, or perhaps of angry spirits of the dead, or animals killed in the hunt. He conceived that the best way to counter these forces was by appeasing and placating them through worship, ritual and sacrifice. It was thus that magic came into being and magic medicine evolved. Magic offered an explanation to early man for the inexplicable. It enabled man in that period of time to cope with the adversities of his precarious existence.

The Practice of Medicine

The practitioner of magic medicine was the medicine man, variously called the sorcerer, the witch doctor, the shaman. He came to his profession in response to a call, a strange dream, an unusual experience, or on being convinced of possessing psychic powers that marked him from the rest. He professed to commune with spirits and conjured visions through fasting, solitude and hallucinogenic drugs. He claimed knowledge of the stars, of the herbs that healed, of poisons that killed and of the means to propitiate invisible demons around him. Women practitioners (witch doctors) also existed. They were usually herbal healers with a rank slightly lower than the medicine men. This was not always so, as many of the witch doctors were expert in the practice of magic medicine. Childbirth and the management of deliveries were the domain of witch doctors. Women delivered babies in the squatting or kneeling position, as they still do in many villages in India. Difficult deliveries were aided by rituals, chants, or by the witch doctor shaking the patient or massaging the abdomen. Expulsion of the placenta was eased by inducing the patient to sneeze.

The shaman mediated between the spirit world and man. Primitive man believed that demons or evil spirits inflicted disease if the victim had done some wrong, or committed an offence against the prevailing social code, or had violated a taboo. Perhaps the sufferer had excited the wrath of demons, or attracted evil spirits or allowed his soul to go astray. Disease was commonly thought to be produced by the intrusion of a stone chip, wood or bone-splinter shot into the body of the victim by an evil spirit or demon. The shaman would organize an elaborate ritual during which the foreign body was removed by sleight of hand. Another serious cause of illness was a separation and loss of the soul from the body. Professional soul-catchers could restore the soul and return the patient to good health. Illness could also be induced by a distant enemy through sympathetic magic. The shaman or sorcerer would model an effigy of the victim and mutilate it in the hope that the victim would fall ill and die, or he would cast a spell on the victim condemning him to suffering and death. Indeed, there are a number of reports from different parts of the world where exorcism and casting of spells had caused death. A psychophysiological mechanism lies behind such instances. The sorcerer's great power of hypnotic suggestion induced a strong death-wish in the victim who became thoroughly convinced that he had to die. In a primitive community the victim's friends and relatives shared this belief and he was looked upon and abandoned as being already dead. The terror and fear within the victim probably unleashed a severe disturbance in the autonomic nervous system that profoundly affected the heart and circulation, producing a state of shock leading to death.

When summoned to the help of an ill victim, the shaman first proceeded to divine the supernatural cause of his illness. He then proceeded to remove, nullify or counter this cause. Often this involved appeasement and propitiation of supernatural forces through a prolonged ritual. Hypnotic states were induced by hallucinogenic drugs and by elaborate ceremonies that could last for days and nights. Animal masks were worn during these rituals to frighten the demons away. A painting in the Trois Frères cave in France depicts a dancing figure wearing a deer-head mask. It dates back to 17,000 to 20,000 years and is believed, by some, to be the first representation of a shaman or a healing priest. Unquestionably, the effectiveness of many ancient medical practices depended on suggestion. The shaman believed deeply in the efficacy of his treatment; the patient or the victim believed in the shaman's power, as did the community to which the victim belonged.

The psychological effects of ritualistic therapy were further reinforced by the wearing of magic objects or talismans that warded off or countered evil spirits. These commonly took the form of amulets, rings, shells, stones and animal bones that were believed to be charged with magical energy. An 'evil eye' was believed to cause misfortune and primitive man devised various ritualistic objects that could thwart the 'evil glance'—a superstition still rampant in the world today.

Magical methods used by shamans or sorcerers also included empiricism. Empirical medicine thus flourished side by side with magic medicine. Magic rituals were occasionally accompanied by massage, application of poultices, and the use of medicinal plants and herbs. The explanation of their efficacy however may yet have been supernatural. The shamans or medicine men of some primitive societies understood the efficacy of several medicinal plants empirically effective for specific ailments. Laxatives, emetics, antispasmodics, local analgesics, sedatives derived from roots, plants and herbs came into use. Hallucinogenic drugs were popular in primitive societies, particularly the Omaha, Kiowa and Fox tribes of the American West. The shaman in tribal ritual ceremonies would at times smear his skin with plant substances which had a numbing effect, permitting him to bear severe heat and the pain of sharp implements. The use of mandrake to induce sleep and deaden pain, and that of antidotes to treat snake-bite, go far back into the dark and distant past.

We can only speculate on the knowledge of anatomy of prehistoric man. Battle wounds, cutting up animals killed in the hunt for food, cannibalism and human sacrifice must have given some idea of the visceral contents of the human body. Palaeolithic paintings recognize the heart as the best spot to strike a mortal blow. The Pindal cave in Spain treasures a remarkable drawing in red-ochre of a mammoth on which is depicted a dark leaf-shaped area where the heart should be. This is the work of Palaeolithic man and is probably the first representation of an anatomical illustration in our world.

The practice of surgery was empirical, being chiefly confined to the treatment of wounds and of injuries to bones. Wounds were cauterized, and sutured with strips of tendons using needles made of bone. Haemorrhage was controlled by pressure, cauterization and the application of styptic substances derived from plants. Foreign bodies such as arrow-heads and spear-points were removed with skill. Fractures were splinted with pieces of wood and casts of hide. Amputation was performed for ritualistic purposes—an amputation of the finger being commonly performed as part of puberty rites. The blood of animals and of humans was an important feature of the shaman's ritual of invoking spirits or exorcizing them from a victim. The origin of blood-letting, a practice that persisted well into the nineteenth and early twentieth centuries is shrouded in mystery. Perhaps it started as a ritual to release demons and evil spirits from a victim. The numbing effect on the sensorium produced by significant blood loss may have been found to be of therapeutic value, and so the practice might have been empirically perpetuated. In the first century of the Christian era, Pliny wrote on the virtues of blood-letting in animals, quoting the hippopotamus as an example. He wrote the rather improbable story that when ill, this animal would plunge its knee into a sharp reed to let out blood in order to heal itself. To stop the bleed the animal would then bury its forelimb in mud. This was indeed rather an absurd justification for the application of blood-letting as an effective treatment for almost every disease then known to man. Perhaps the most fascinating of the surgical procedures performed in prehistoric times was trepanation or the removal of a segment of the bone from the skull. Evidence of the practice of trepanation or trephining by Neolithic men has been found in France. A fair proportion of those operated upon must have survived the surgery, for examination of these skulls show signs of wounds having healed. Trepanation may have had several reasons. Almost certainly, the major reason was ritualistic—to release the demons or evil spirits afflicting the victim. The performance of trepanation, even on the dead, suggests that it could also have been a religious rite. Small, round pieces of bone (rondelles) removed from trephined skulls were used as magic charms in amulets or were strung together to form necklaces. Trepanation may also have been used for medical reasons, in the treatment of fracture of the skull or for the removal of a foreign body or bone splinters.

The shaman or medicine man was more than a healer. He became the protector of his tribe or community, interceding on its behalf to ward off evil and to summon good. He claimed to possess powers that could bring rain, arrest floods, ensure a good hunt and guarantee a bountiful harvest. When evil fell upon his community, he would determine its cause—whether due to a violated taboo, a breach of social code, or an insult to the spirit world. He would then ferret out the offender, pass judgement and execute it. He was feared for his awesome powers. Yet he was also revered as the one carrying the repository of faith, tradition, legend and folklore of his people. He combined within him magic and the seeds of religion. Magic resided in his personal powers, religion in the supernatural forces he could invoke. He represented the collective consciousness and conscience of generation after generation of his people. He soon came to embody the role of physician–priest–protector; and became the centre around which prehistoric and primitive man built a distinctive social fabric and culture.

In the forbidding hostile environment of the prehistoric age, it was the shaman who offered man the hope to cope with life and to come to terms with the strange powerful forces around him. The physician of today would consider the shaman a charlatan, his rites and rituals spurious and fake. But it cannot be denied that the ancient medicine man convincingly demonstrated the power of the mind in countering disease. His attempts to heal, to protect and to care were amongst the first milestones in the history of civilization. He played an important role in guiding prehistoric man through the darkness and mists of time into the dawn of the first civilizations of the ancient world. Medicine by then had become a priestly craft rooted in the temples and religious sanctuaries of antiquity.

Archaic Medicine

1 Archaic Medicine—Mesopotamia and Egypt

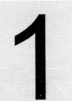

It was around 6,000 years ago that Man emerged from the shadows of the Stone Age into the first light of civilization and into recorded history. Mesopotamia was founded on the hot dusty plains of West Asia between the ancient rivers of the Euphrates and the Tigris. Egypt began to flourish on the verdant but marshy banks of the great river Nile, which rose from some unknown place in the middle of Africa and gushed on into the Mediterranean. There must be good reason why the book of civilization should have opened just along these hot and dusty strips of land rather than in any other part of the world. It is probably because these great river valleys provided just the right challenge to elicit the maximal creative response from man. This challenge did not overwhelm him into defeat, nor was it so mild as to lull him into a torpor of creative inactivity. It provided the right impetus so that a succession of challenges called forth a succession of responses culminating in the first great civilization of history.

There exists a fine controversy between those who would consider Mesopotamia before Egypt in the order of time and those who consider Egypt the mother of all civilizations. This is not of great importance; probably both flourished side by side. The difference between the two lay in the historical fact that for over 3,000 years, Mesopotamia existed as a succession of warring states. The earliest was the Sumerian civilization whose city states were united under Sargon I, a fierce warrior, a ruthless conqueror and one of the earliest empire-builders in Mesopotamia. The succeeding important civilization in Mesopotamia was the Babylonian–Assyrian state—Hammurabi being the king and founder of Babylon's might. Egypt, on the other hand, maintained an unbroken era of nationhood for a longer stretch of time. Each civilization achieved great wealth, and reached great heights, but ultimately, succumbed to disintegration and decay.

In both Mesopotamia and Egypt, the attitudes to life and living, to health and disease and to the practice of medicine, were conditioned by an overwhelming belief in the supernatural, magic, religion and the priestly craft.

2 Mesopotamia

If a doctor has treated a man with a metal knife for a severe wound, and has caused the man to die, or has opened a man's tumour with a metal knife and destroyed the man's eye his hand should be cut off.

from the Code of Hammurabi

The discovery of the ancient Mesopotamian civilization was made as late as 1929 by Sir Leonard Wooley, during his archaeological excavations in Ur in Mesopotamia. Towards the end of the excavation of the tombs of the Sumerian kings, he decided to dig deeper, against the advice of his colleagues, who maintained that the clay stratum under the tombs was the dried up bed of the old Euphrates river. Wooley's intuitive perseverance laid bare the treasured relics of a civilization whose remains were found buried beneath eleven feet of silt—obviously deposited by a great flood. There must have been a civilization here around 4000 BC, long before the birth of the biblical patriarch, Abraham. Wooley's discovery also corroborated the story of the Great Flood in the Book of Genesis—a flood so massive and horrendous that it would have appeared as if the whole earth had sunk below the waters. The biblical story of the flood was based on the legend of the Sumerians, the first civilized people of Mesopotamia. These people of the Euphrates–Tigris region contributed to some of the most significant and exciting inventions of the Archaic world. They invented writing, initiating into our world the annals of recorded history. They knew arithmetic, and thus began the science of numbers. They discovered the wheel, studied the stars and introduced the science of astronomy. They learnt to work with metals, becoming experienced in metallurgy and in the mining of ores. They established the power of man over nature by the control of river waters, by the irrigation of crops and by the reclaiming of marshy soil to build city states. Mesopotamia was the first civilization in the world to formulate a written code of law in which every man rich or poor had an equal right to theocratic justice.

The Mesopotamian man was Asiatic in origin, short in stature, had dark hair and spoke a language unrelated to any other. Intermarriage with Semitic and Aryan conquerors altered these traits in later centuries. For protection against the covetous nomads in the surrounding desert lands, Mesopotamians built large cities surrounded by massive high walls. Each city was a city-state. In its centre was the temple in which lived the king-priest and the local god. The ruler priest had great powers and combined the role of ruler, physician, astrologer, priest and manager of all affairs. In the religious centre of each city-state soared towers or ziggurats, over 80 feet high. The temples were encircled by an outer and an inner wall, within which the daily activities of the people were centred.

Other cardinal inventions of Mesopotamia included cloth, textiles, seals to identify property, astrological tables, weights and measures. They devised a solar calendar that enabled man to plan his work according to the season of the year. They also discovered that a circle divided into 360 degrees, an hour was divided into sixty minutes; a minute contained sixty seconds.

GOVERNMENT AND GODS

The priest king's rule was absolute, though he was guided by a council of elders. It is of interest that the earliest civilization was born with a social hierarchy. The priest and temple officials were at the upper rung of the ladder; below them came the freemen, artisans, husbandmen; and still lower were the slaves or those who had forfeited their freedom.

The most solemnly revered gods were the nature deities of the sky, sun, earth and water. These deities, enshrined in temples, were offered food and drink daily. Unlike the Egyptians, the Mesopotamians did not believe in life after death. Yet, when a king died, his wives, concubines, musicians, attendants and guards followed him to the tomb. The members of his household arranged themselves in the hierarchical order, and then drank a soporific to render their suffocation painless before following him to death. These immolations were meant to be a reflection of their loyalty to their sovereign.

THE CONCEPT OF SICKNESS AND DISEASE

Sickness and disease were equated with sin. The gods ordered the disease, the demons and the evil spirits carried out the diktat of the gods by stealthily possessing the body and playing havoc within it. Belief in evil spirits abounded. Dreaded demons of disease as those in the service of the powerful earth-goddess Ishtar, who was also the goddess of witchcraft and pestilence, lay waiting to invade men's bodies and spirits.

Sin was an act that displeased the gods, or contravened his commandments, or neglected his needs. The gods required more than homage and obeisance; they required food, money, gifts, even women. It was also considered a sin to spit or urinate into canals, eat out of a sick person's plate, or touch a menstruating woman with unclean hands. When the origin of sin was untraceable, the sick (sinner) became resigned to the judgement of the gods and accepted his punishment with fortitude. He sought the priest-physician's aid.

The Sumerian civilization declined in about 2000 BC and was replaced by the semitic Assyrians and Babylonians who conquered Mesopotamia. The political system was now dominated by kings, who were the intermediaries between the gods and the people. Astronomy and astrology assumed a greater importance to determine the will of the gods.

The Assyrio–Babylonian civilization of Mesopotamia was probably the most demon-conscious of all the ancient civilizations. There now appeared a hierarchy of fifteen divinities with the god Madruk, curer of all illnesses, presiding over medicine. The gods commanded their own specialties. Under the goddess Ninchursag there were eight other divinities, each curing a specific disease. The multiplication of so many gods and divinities was justified by the existence of a large number of demons which were supposed to infest the Assyrio–Babylonian world.

The king of the demons, and the god of destruction and death was Nergal. His visitation on earth caused devastation and despair. Nasutar was the dreaded demon of plague; he was the herald of Nergal and had a host of other lesser demons under his command. These included Axaxuzu who caused jaundice, and Asukku who caused consumption. It is of interest that in Babylonian mythology, Nergal appears also as an insect, suggesting that the role of insects in the causation of disease was appreciated even in this very early period.

THE PHYSICIAN

Medicine was a temple art and the most learned man in the city-state was the priest-physician or *âsû* (he who knows the waters). He could read and write, was learned in astrology, science, religion, literature and in the rituals of magic, charms, incantations and divinations. The *âsû* worshipped the healing deities Ninib, Gula, Ninazu and the son of Ninazu, whose emblem, interestingly enough, was a rod and serpent—an emblem which was taken over by the Greek Aesculapius and through him bequeathed to modern medicine.

The diagnosis of a disease was not performed by the *âsû*, but by the *barû*, who was the master of divination. Finally the exorcization of spirits in a sufferer was the duty of the *âshipu* (the incantation priest).

The physician was learned in magico-empiric medicine. Besides the use of ritualistic magic and charms, he would use drugs and could perform minor operations.

The art of diagnosis was chiefly centred around hepatoscopy—in the belief that the liver was the collecting centre of blood and thus the seat of life. The ritual of hepatoscopy was performed before the statue of a god. A sheep was sacrificed and its liver subjected to the minutest examination. Any real or imagined departure from the expected norm became the god's answer to specific questions. Thus when the right lobe was shaped like a purse, it portended disaster; if the common duct was to the right, it foretold recovery. The art of hepatoscopy was taught in temples with the aid of clay or bronze models of a liver.

Astronomy, the study of stars and the movement of stars, was used as a predictor of pestilence and outbreaks of diseases. Astrology also helped in the prognosis of individual illnesses. Soothsaying involved the examination of the entrails of killed animals, and the practice of casting horoscopes originated in the early Mesopotamian times. Physicians also used the dreams of the sick to interpret the outcome of an illness. They knew which gods to call upon for a specific disease—there was Nabu, the Assyrian god of the healing art, or Mabruk, the Babylonian god who had the power to overcome and cure all illnesses.

THERAPY

The magico-religious approach to treatment was of course paramount. Physicians also used medicated baths and drugs. They recognized tumors, abscesses, skin and venereal diseases, respiratory diseases and jaundice.

Drugs were given in anal suppositories or in enemas; they were also blown into the urethra through a tube. Commonly used remedies included garlic, onions, leeks, spices, condiments, resins and gums. The roots, leaves and fruit of the date palm were deemed efficacious for various maladies. Mandrake, opium and hemp were popular herbs in use. The minerals used as therapy were sulphur, arsenic, salt petre, antimony, mercury, alum, naphtha, and calcined lime. Potions prepared at night were ingested before sunrise; those prepared in the evening were ingested when the stars appeared. The Babylonians possessed an extensive pharmacopoeia—about 120 mineral drugs and around twice the number of drugs derived from the vegetable kingdom have been listed on their clay tablets. Colocynth, senna and castor oil were used as laxatives. Dressings for wounds consisted of wine dregs, oil, and juniper blended with alkali and herbs.

About a thousand of the 30,000 clay tablets covered with cuneiform writing in the library of Assurbanipal are related to medicine. They list the practice of medicine in the ancient period and contain material on diagnosis, prognosis, therapy and the ingredients used in therapy. These date from the seventh century BC, though the tradition of Mesopotamian medicine goes back to 3000 BC. The chief treatise on medicine is the *Treatise of Medical Diagnosis and Prognosis*. It comprises 3,000 entries on forty clay tablets and lists several ailments recognizable even today. Thus the entry stating—the patient coughs continuously; what he coughs up is thick and frequently bloody. His breathing sounds like a flute—suggests tuberculosis with obstruction to the airways.

Fumigation was a frequent practice. For chest ailments, fumigation was practised by spreading tar on a thorn fire and letting the smoke enter through the mouth and nose.

Physicians in Mesopotamia gained first hand experience in surgery during the many wars that afflicted the land. Phlebotomy, cupping were frequently used. The sand and the wind from the neighbouring deserts led to problems of the eyes. Operations on the eye were practised—and if this led to the loss of an eye, the physician's hands were cut off. If an aristocrat lost his life through the ministrations of the physician, the latter would lose his life. These draconian laws helped to prevent malpractice and ensured, as best as possible, the dexterity and knowledge of those professing the healing art.

One of the greatest contributions of Mesopotamia to medicine was the code of ethics laid down by Hammurabi (1728–1686 BC), the sixth king of the first dynasty of Babylon. Hammurabi was a great and mighty ruler who made Babylon supreme in his era. His reign was distinguished by the writing of mathematical and astrological treatises and dictionaries. His greatest contribution to civilization was a legal code comprising 282 laws which regulated society, family life and occupation. This code of Hammurabi was engraved on a 2 m. high stele found in 1901 in Susa, Iran, and now preserved in the Louvre. It clearly spells out instructions for the conduct of physicians. Professional fees were related to the social rank of the patient. Incompetence and negligence were punished by draconian laws.

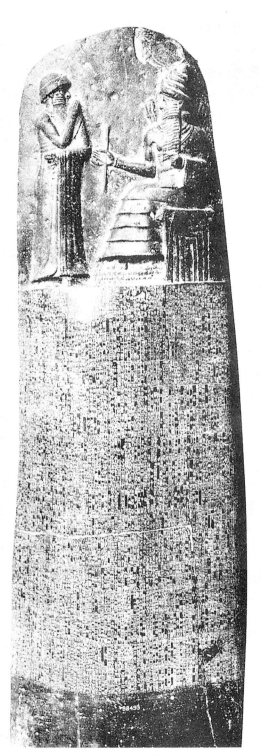

Fig. 2.1 The Hammurabic Code: A basaet stela inscribed with the code of laws of Hammurabi, King of Babylon.

If a physician has performed a major operation upon a lord with a bronze lancet and has saved his life, he shall receive ten shekels of silver, but if he caused the death of such a notable, his hand would be chopped off. A doctor causing the death of a slave would have to replace him.

The Mesopotamians were aware of public health measures. Large stone drains forming part of a sewage system, as also stone privies appear in the remains of Mesopotamian civilization. Awareness of public health and hygiene was present very early in the history of civilization.

The fertile triangle between the Euphrates and Tigris rivers saw both the birth of civilization and of medicine. Magico-religious beliefs and sorcery, which had earlier formed the basis of medicine, were now supplemented by the use of herbs and minerals and by simple practical methods for treating injuries and diseases. The duties and responsibilities of physicians and the rules for preserving public health and hygiene were codified and displayed for the first time in recorded history. Thus, Mesopotamia started Man and Medicine on the road to civilization—in a never-ending quest for health and happiness.

3 Egypt

Death is before me today.
Like the recovery of a sick man,
Like going forth into a garden after sickness.

Eulogy of Death in a scroll from the Middle Kingdom

In the mists of prehistory, neolithic man, more than 10,000 years ago, settled down along the banks of the Nile. The life-giving waters of this mighty river nourished these primitive settlements helping them to coalesce and grow. In the fourth millennium before Christ there blossomed a mighty civilization under the first of the Pharaohs or Kings of the land. This civilization shone with unbroken splendour for twenty-seven centuries!

A land of great antiquity, 'Egypt was ancient even to the ancients.' It flourished a thousand years before the Minoans built their palace at Knossos, 800 years before Moses led the Israelites from bondage into freedom, and about 2,500 years before the early beginnings of Rome. Sheltered by the desert sands and the sea, blessed by the abundance brought by the unfailing yearly floods of the Nile, Egypt passed century after century in peaceful existence weaving the threads of civilization into a splendid-textured tapestry, which remains the envy of the past and present. The great historian Herodotus who travelled through ancient Egypt in the fifth century BC, wrote of 'wonders more in number than those of any other land and works it has to show beyond any expression great'.

During its first thousand years of recorded history the king of Egypt, also called the Pharaoh, became identified as a god, the son of the sun-god, Re. Blessed with divinity, his rule was absolute and unquestioned. The day-to-day affairs of the country were managed by an organized system consisting of bureaucrats headed by the vizier who served as prime minister, treasurer and chief justice.

The people were slender, but robust, dark-haired and attractive. Men and women often shaved their heads; the nobility often wore elaborate wigs. The wealthier women rouged their faces, painted their lips and eyes, coloured their nails and perfumed themselves with creams, oils and scents. Social distinctions and classes prevailed from the beginning. There were five classes: the royal family, the priests, the nobles, a middle class (comprising merchants, artisans and scribes), and the farmers. In the period of the empire (*ca* 1500 BC) another class was added—they formed the professional soldiers and slaves captured during military campaigns against the neighbouring states.

Though society was governed by monogamy, an unusual custom of brother-sister marriages was practised. This was primarily introduced by the Pharaohs to preserve their property and wealth; this practice then spread to all classes of people.

As in all early civilizations, religion played a vital role in all aspects of life. The Egyptians believed in a multitude of gods and goddesses who could befriend man or be his deadly enemy. The sun-god Re (Ra, Amen or Amon) personified the beneficial deities. The gods of nature and of vegetation were fused into the one god Osiris, who was also god of the Nile. The official religion of the Pharaoh and the priests was the worship of Re, the god of righteousness and justice; the cult of Osiris grew among the common people of Egypt. While Re personified life, Osiris personified death and in the course of several centuries these two faiths were merged into one religion.

An attempt to change this ancient religion which had been degraded by corrupt priests practising ritual magic, was made by King Amenhotep IV (ca 1375 BC). He banished the priests, removed the traditional deities and proclaimed only one true god, Aten (the ancient sun-god). He changed his name to Akhenaten, founded a new city in honour of this deity and lived in happiness with his beautiful queen Nefertiti. Unfortunately his happiness was short-lived. His kingdom was attacked and he was forced to concede to the priests. After his death, his son-in-law Tutankhatan succeeded to the throne. The capital was shifted back to Thebes and Akhenaten's newly found city of Aten fell into ruins. Egypt returned to the original fold of the ancient god Amen Re. Tutankhatan changed his name to Tutankhamen, and the discovery of his tomb, sealed for over 2000 years, made a significant contribution to Egyptology.

After Tutankhamen, the power shifted back to the Hyskos dynasty. The enslavement of the Hebrews began from this period in the thirteenth century BC. Ramses II, the builder of the great temple of Abu Simbel, was probably the Pharaoh during the Exodus.

Egyptians strongly believed in the concept of life after death—for sustaining life after death, food and other essentials of life had to be provided in the tomb. They also believed that if the body were to be preserved, the soul and the Ka (the spiritual self, the small double of the body) would also be blessed with immortality. The desire to preserve the body led to the development of the art and science of embalming the dead. For this, the brain was first drawn out through the nostrils with a hook, and the cranial cavity washed out with salt water. The viscera were then removed through a 3½″ incision on both sides of the abdomen. The heart, believed to be the seat of life, was left in its place. The abdominal cavity was washed with wine and aromatic herbs, and stuffed with a combination of preservatives, the secret of which remains unfathomed to this day. The abdominal incisions were sutured and the body immersed for seventy days in a soda bath. It was then covered with wrappings smeared with gum and placed in a mummy case. This was, in turn, laid in a stone sarcophagus—the tomb. The degree of preservation that could be attained was incredible and the secret of the embalming techniques of the ancient Egyptians remains undiscovered.

Some of the magnificent architecture and remarkable feats of engineering were made possible by the desire of early Egyptians to protect and preserve their dead. The royal tombs grew increasingly impressive, culminating in the construction of the great pyramid at Giza, built by King Khufu (Cheops) in the second millennium BC.

The Egyptians invented the column and developed the concept of perspective. They used huge blocks of stone and developed engineering skills employing the lever and the ramp. Their massive sculptures of stone are awe-inspiring as are their enormous bas-reliefs. They made superb pottery, metalware, and jewellery, and left hieroglyphic accounts of their ancient history. There was a sense of massiveness and grandeur in Egyptian civilization and art, perhaps in the hope that their culture and works would last an eternity.

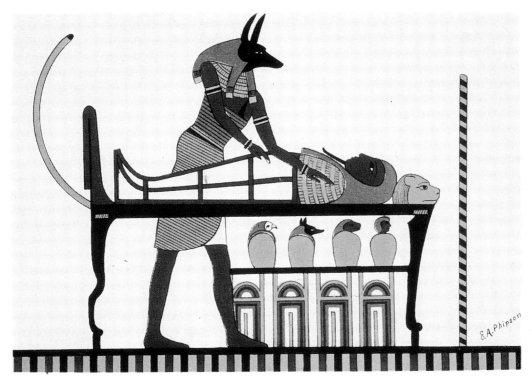

Fig. 3.1   Anubis tending a mummy. Tombs of the Kings, Thebes.

THE PRACTICE OF MEDICINE

In the early centuries of the Empire, medicine was a blend of magic and religion. The Egyptians believed that disease was caused by evil spirits, both supernatural and earthly, that entered through the body orifices wreaking havoc within the victim. The purpose of medicine was to rid the body of these demons. The gods would help, if correctly approached. This approach was in the form of supplication, incantations, spells and rituals. All cures revealed by the gods were believed to be categorized by Thoth, the ibis-headed god of wisdom (called Hermes by the Greeks and Mercury by the Romans), in secret books. These secret books were guarded in the medical school associated with the temples of Sais at Heliopolis. They formed the medical texts for the priest-physicians of Egypt. It was Thoth who knew the secrets of the gods, who invented all learning, science and art, and who could both cause and cure disease. Other popular gods to whom supplications were addressed or incantations recited were the falcon-headed sun-god Re and the goddess Isis with her son Horus, the god of health. The gods could cure, but also had magic that could kill an intended victim. Casting a curse through sympathetic magic is practised even today. Catherine de Medici of Austria who became the Queen of France in 1559 AD, was said to have been a devotee of this form of black magic. Hairs, threads of clothing, or nail parings from the intended victim were mixed with wax into a figurine that resembled the victim. When the figurine was cursed the victim succumbed to an illness and died.

Egypt over many centuries, was blessed with peace and plenty, and with the passage of time, empiric medicine came into being. There were now three kinds of healers. Physicians or *swnu* dealing with empiric medicine, the priests or *sekhmet* (surgeon and specialist), and the exorcist or sorcerer. While in the earlier dynasties the physician was a priest, in the later period he attained an independent professional status. He was now a man of wide learning and culture, possessed a sound

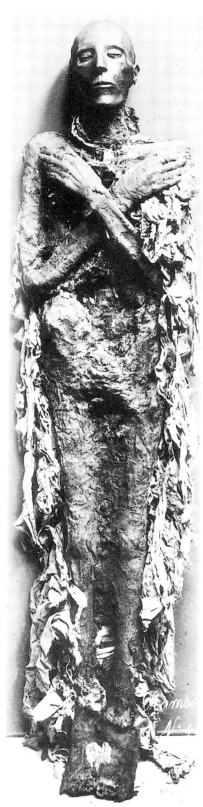

Fig. 3.2   Unwrapped mummy of Ramses II.

knowledge of empiric medicine, was steeped in the lore of centuries and had been trained under experienced senior colleagues. His learning and skills were admired even outside Egypt. He was even called to attend to royalty in other kingdoms, such as when Cyrus the Great of Persia sent for an Egyptian physician to treat his mother.

A study of ancient papyri suggests that medical practice to an extent was both organized and controlled by the state. At the lowest rung of the hierarchy were general physicians (those who did not specialize), followed in ascending order by a chief of physicians, an inspector and a superintendent. At the pinnacle of this medical hierarchy reigned the Greatest Physician of lower and upper Egypt. Physicians were appointed by the state to the army, the public works, the burial grounds and the Pharaoh's palace. The Egyptians, in a rather primitive way, anticipated some of the modern world's national health schemes. Diodorus Siculus, a Greek historian wrote thus:

In wartime and on journeys anywhere within Egypt, the sick are all treated free of charge, because doctors are paid by the state and scrupulous observance of the prescriptions drawn up by great doctors of the past is incumbent on them.

It is indeed amazing that in this age of antiquity, with medicine literally in a nascent phase, the physicians practising empiric medicine all tended to specialize. Just as their gods governed different organs, physicians specialized in special body parts and in the diseases afflicting them. The royal physicians, in particular, were all specialists. These included physicians of the eyes, teeth, nose, belly and even a 'shepherd of the anus'. Herodotus, in his history, describes the medicine of the people of the Nile thus:

The art of medicine is thus divided; each physician applies himself to one disease only and not more. All places abound in physicians; some are for the eye, others for the head, others for the teeth, others for intestines and others for internal disorders.

The inscriptions on gravestones of the doctors of the old Medical School of Heliopolis bear further witness to the penchant for specializing at a time when so little was known of medicine. The inscriptions make fascinating reading, as for example, 'the greatest of doctors' (the Dean of Sais who lived around 3000 BC), 'keeper of the king's right eye'. A doctor by the name Iri (who lived around 2500 BC) was entitled 'keeper of the king's rectum'.

Information on the content of Egyptian medicine is through inscriptions on hieroglyphics, Greek and Roman manuscripts, and most important of all from a study of medical papyri. The most important of these papyri are the Edwin Smith papyrus (1600 BC) found near Luxor, and the Georg Ebers papyrus (1550 BC) from Thebes. The Edwin Smith papyrus, though written around 1600 BC, describes medical practice of even earlier times. It gives instructions for the treatment of wounds, fractures and dislocations. Birch splints, held in place by bandages, were used to immobilize broken bones; the method of reducing a dislocated mandible was very similar to that employed today. The papyrus contains forty-seven detailed case records. It notes that lesions on the right or left side of the head are associated with a paralysis of the opposite side. The art of prognosis is introduced—'I will cure this disease,' if the outlook was favourable; 'He will die'—if the outcome appeared hopeless; 'nothing can be done in this case'—if the outcome was doubtful. The papyrus had writings on gynaecology and methods of detecting pregnancy. Methods of contraception included the use of pessaries made of cowdung, herbs and honey.

The Georg Ebers papyrus is a collection of medical texts which probably originated in the old empire (3300–2360 BC), during the time of the first eight dynasties whose Pharaohs expressed their might and glory by building the pyramids of Cheops, Chefren and Mycerinus. The Ebers papyrus is perhaps the oldest surviving treatise on medicine. Over twenty metres long, it deals with magic-cum-religious healing, as also with empiric medicine. The papyrus describes many diseases of the abdomen, and an even larger number of diseases of the eye and skin. It lists 700 drugs and numerous formulae chiefly herbs, but also includes mineral and animal remedies. It is of interest to quote an example of one of its formulae used to treat an inflammation of the eyes.

To drive away inflammation of the eye, grind the stems of the juniper of Byblos, steep them in water, apply to the eyes of the sick person and he will be quickly cured. To cure granulations of the eye, you will prepare a remedy of cyllyrium, verdigris, onions, blue vitriol, powdered wood. Mix and apply to the eyes.

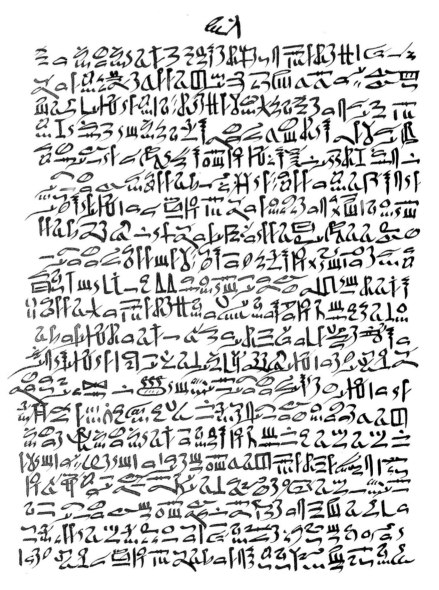

Fig. 3.3   A page from the Ebers Papyrus, written c. 1500 BC.

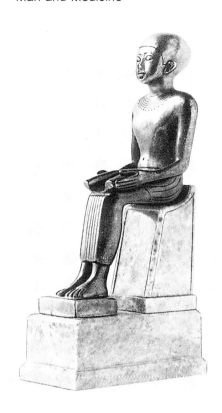

Fig. 3.4   Imhotep.

IMHOTEP

From the mists of antiquity, about 2,700 years before the birth of Christ, there emerged for the first time in recorded history, the vivid personality of a great physician. He was Imhotep (he who cometh in peace), the grand vizier to Pharaoh Zoser, also his architect and his high priest at Heliopolis. He must have been truly gifted for he was renowned as a sage, astronomer, scribe but above all was a great physician, wise, learned and kind. He built the first step pyramid at Sakkara, the oldest extant stone structure in the world. He designed the funerary temples of Zoser, introducing bas-relief and fluted shafts—features symbolizing Egyptian art and architecture for millennia to come. When he died, Egypt wept—people lined the banks of the Nile in grief as his body was taken up the river in a ceremonial barge. This was the first step to his glorification; within a few generations he was deified, and by the sixth century BC he had displaced Thoth as the god of healing in Egypt and had even been given a divine father, the god Ptah. The Greeks identified him with Asklepios, more commonly known today by his Latin name Aesculapius, their god of medicine. It is possible that Imhotep too was associated with healing temple shrines in ancient Egypt, just as Asklepios was to become associated with temple shrines in ancient Greece. The cult of Asklepios, the Greek god, in time fused with the Egyptian Imhotep to become the cult of Asklepios–Imhotep.

MEDICAL CONCEPTS

The Mesopotamians believed that the liver was the seat of life; the Egyptians believed the heart to be the centre of existence, with respiration being the breath of life. They imagined that the heart, at the centre, was connected to all parts of the body by numerous channels. The analogy was almost certainly related to the many intricate channels fanning out from the life-giving waters of the river Nile. The several channels connecting the heart to every part of the body carried air, blood, food and sperm. Obstruction to this transport or a 'flood' in one or more channels (again an analogy to the floods of the Nile) caused disease. Each organ was believed to have its own god and some demons specialized in producing disease in a particular organ. Demons caused disease, but prayers, incantation and magic could enlist the gods to drive the demons out and restore health.

The role of parasites in causing disease was first stressed in the history of medicine by Egypt. In Egyptian legend, the sun-god Re took ill from the bite of a worm, and Horus was said to have been stung by a scorpion. Parasites could be expelled by enemas and purgation. The Egyptians had a fascination for purgatives and enemas. Enemas were believed to be the invention and gift of the god Thoth. Their frequent use helped to guard against putrefaction within the gut which could destroy the body. Another bizarre concept held by the Egyptians was the belief in a close relationship between the anal region and the cardiovascular system. An additional benefit of retention enemas was that they were beneficial both to the anus and the heart.

PUBLIC HEALTH

Herodotus called Egyptians 'the healthiest of men'. Yet Pliny held the opposite view when he wrote that 'Egypt was the motherland of disease'.

The Egyptians were noted for frequent baths and cleanliness of attire. All social classes practised bathing morning and evening and washed before meals. Soap had not been then invented so a type of alkali was used in its place. As already mentioned, they were greatly fond of purges and enemas as a counter to the fear of putrefaction within the gut.

The waters of the Nile were clean and the regular abundant supply of water encouraged cleanliness. Though an elaborate system of canals, dams, and reservoirs fulfilled agricultural needs, the fertility of the land and the orderly flow of water through its sluices and canals were dependent on the yearly rise and fall of the great river. Ancient Egyptians almost certainly revered the waters of the Nile and it is unlikely that refuse was dumped into it. This was contrary to the practice of the Greeks, Romans and Moslems, who, in the centuries to come, converted the Nile into a cesspool of filth.

DISEASES

A large number of diseases prevalent in ancient Egypt can be identified from inscriptions and descriptive reports in medical papyri, pictorial representations and from the examination of mummies. Acute intestinal infections were common. Schistosomiasis and other worm infections have also been discovered in mummies. The dry desert air and sand were responsible for frequent eye problems, particularly trachoma. Epidemic diseases like smallpox and plague almost certainly existed; the vertebrae of some mummies demonstrated the presence of Pott's disease.

Atherosclerosis was certainly a common disease among ancient Egyptians, as judged from pathological findings in mummies. A few writings suggested the existence of gonorrhoea, but evidence of syphilitic infections of the bones is lacking. Leprosy may also well have existed but almost certainly was confused with other skin diseases. Acute illnesses causing death were known but their precise nature is undetermined. Muscle wasting suggestive of poliomyelitis is depicted in some temple reliefs. Cirrhosis of the liver almost certainly was prevalent, perhaps related to the consumption of beer and wine. Arthritis, gout, ovarian, bladder and kidney diseases have been identified by modern scholars in Egyptology.

MEDICATIONS

The Egyptians had a vast pharmacopoeia. Many of the medications, plants and minerals that were later incorporated into the works of the Greek, Dioscorides, and of the Romans, Pliny and Galen, came from Egyptian sources.

They administered their medications in many forms—pills, drops, cakes, ointments, suppositories, fumigations and baths. Enemas were the most popular route of administering drugs and for cleaning the bowels.

The Egyptians used a large number of medicinal plants. Castor oil from castor seed was effective as a cathartic and for the treatment of wounds. The soporific and analgesic use of the opium poppy was probably introduced in the second millennium BC. Scopolamus and hyoscyamus, both related to mandragora from the mandrake plant, were also used, though their time of introduction is undetermined. Rotten bread was an ingredient of several formulae—its efficacy for wounds may well have been due to the presence of antibacterial moulds (just as penicillin molds can be effective through penicillin). A thousand other prescriptions were included as therapy. They were compounds of fruits, spices, honey, portions of animals (fat, blood, excrement), organs of animals, myrrh, frankincense and manna.

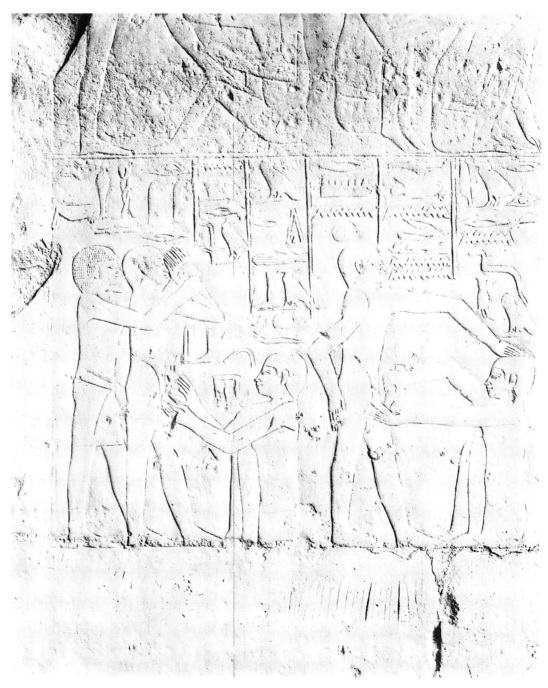

Fig. 3.5   The tomb of the physician, Saqqara, Egypt: Relief showing circumcision scene, operation on man's foot and an operation on back.

Minerals and metals in use included antimony, copper, salt and alum. Antimony was frequently used in beautifying a woman's eyes. Black eyelid linings were made of a combination of antimony and lead. The green colour in eye make-up was derived from the use of copper. These were all aesthetically appealing, but it is possible that they were inadvertently effective, through their antiseptic action, in preventing eye infections common in Egypt. Copper preparations, for example, were later shown to be useful in the treatment of trachoma, a frequent cause of blindness in ancient Egypt.

SURGERY

There is little mention of surgery in the medical papyri. Circumcision was a common practice in all social classes. Cauterization was indicated for the removal of cysts and tumours. Trepanation, though practised, was not as common as in other early civilizations. Treatment of injuries, wounds and fractures is mentioned. The Egyptians invented a type of adhesive tape by impregnating linen strips with resin or gum. These adhesive tapes helped to pull the edges of a wound into apposition. Though several kinds of blades were described—stone, metal, papyrus reed—no surgical instruments survived. The overall contribution of Egypt to surgery was poor.

THE DECLINE OF EGYPT

Egypt suffered a gradual decline after twenty-seven glorious centuries of civilization. The powers of the Pharaohs waned and the country came under the hegemony of Libya, Ethiopia, Assyria, and finally became the satrap of Persia. In 322 BC, Alexander the Great of Macedon and Greece defeated King Darius of Persia and placed his general Ptolemy on the throne of Egypt. He founded the city of Alexandria in Egypt which became the centre of medicine in the Mediterranean world. The last of the Ptolemies was Cleopatra who chose death through the bite of an asp clasped to her breast, rather than be the prisoner of Octavius Caesar of Rome. Egypt then fell under the hegemony of Rome.

Though magic and religion ruled medicine in Egypt, the seeds of empiric and scientific medicine had also taken root along the fertile banks of the mighty Nile. They were to soon germinate and flower in the craggy soil of Greece and the Hellenic islands. The epic of medicine was now about to witness an exciting and brilliant era of discovery.

4 Medicine in Ancient Persia

Of all the healers O Spitama Zarathustra, namely those who heal with the knife, with herbs and with sacred incantations, the last one is the most potent as he heals from the very source of diseases.

Ardibesht Yasht

Over a thousand years before Christ, the Indo-European Aryans moved from the shores of the Caspian Sea to the highlands of Western Asia, now known as Persia. By the sixth century BC, Persia had grown into a powerful, aggressive expanding empire. Cyrus the Great (c. 560–529 BC) of Persia who established the Achaemenid Dynasty, was one of the greatest kings of antiquity. Royal in spirit, noble in demeanour, wise in rule, ardent in conquest, yet magnanimous in victory he made Persia the master of the Middle and Near Eastern world. At the time of his death in 529 BC, the Persian Empire extended from the Aegean Sea in the west to the Indus in the east, from the Black Sea and Caspian Sea and the mountains of Central Asia in the north down to the Persian Gulf and Indian Ocean. Cambyses, the successor of Cyrus, added Egypt to the empire. The empire reached its zenith in the reign of Darius the Great (522–486 BC). It now also included among its twenty provinces or satrapies, Ionia, Cappadocia, Cilicia, Armenia, the Caucasus, Bactria, Sogdiana and parts of Central Asia. Never before had history recorded so powerful and vast an empire brought under one sovereign rule.

Darius now cast his covetous eyes on Greece. To the new fledgling city-states of Greece, the expansionist policy of Persia posed a life and death struggle. They buried their differences and defeated the might of Persia at the battle of Marathon. Then there followed the heroic stand of Leonidas and his 7,000 Spartans who defended the mountain pass of Thermopylae to the last man against the onslaught of the whole Persian army. Finally came the sea battle of Salamis where the Persian fleet suffered a humiliating defeat. These battles eternally symbolize man's quest for freedom and the burning urge to defend freedom. Thus, when Greece came under the yoke of the Ottomans in the early nineteenth century, the feelings evoked in the west by the battle of Marathon, even after two milleniums, remained fresh and strong. Lord Byron has expressed these feelings beautifully in verse:

> The mountains look on Marathon—
> And Marathon looks on the sea;
> And musing there an hour alone,
> I dreamed that Greece might still be free;
> For standing on the Persian's grave,
> I could not deem myself a slave.

The victory of Greece in the Greco-Persian wars which lasted for nearly half a century, led to the decline of Persia. The *coup de grace* was delivered by Alexander the Great of Macedon and Greece who defeated the Persian king Darius III in 331 BC at the battle of Arbela. Persia now became a subject province of the Greco–Macedonian Empire.

There are some who opine that the Persian civilization borrowed extensively from Egypt, Babylon and Assyria and had little to contribute to the world. This, however, is not true. Every civilization has elements that are borrowed from others and Persia was no exception. The Persians, like the Romans who came later, were more concerned with war, conquest and government than with philosophy, science, medicine, art or literature. Yet they were cultured, refined and enjoyed the luxuries of life. Again, like the Romans, they must have been expert in administration and in the art of government. Their system of roads and communications is unsurpassed in ancient history.

Persepolis, the capital of the 'great kings', is in utter ruins but even the ruins bespeak a splendid and unique architecture. Though grand in design, the palaces and halls of the great Achaemenid kings of Persia had a refined aristocratic elegance, a proportion and balance superior to that found in Egypt, Babylon or Assyria. The architectural heritage of Persia must have surely influenced and inspired the Greeks to greater heights. Persepolis, in the era of the 'great kings', was perhaps merely a step behind Athens at its full glory.

Unquestionably, the greatest gift of Persia to mankind was that it gave birth to the first great monotheistic religion in the world—Zoroastrianism. Before the seventh century BC and long after, the Persians believed in a pantheon of numerous gods, as did all members of the Indo-European race. Their priests were the Magi, who brought animal sacrifices to the gods, and like all primitive religions of contemporary and earlier civilizations, laid stress on magic, ritual and supernatural forces. Then there came a prophet, a reformer, an enlightened soul, Zoroaster or Zarathushtra. His birth is shrouded in mystery but he was believed to be of noble birth. According to Greek historians he preached in the seventh and sixth centuries BC. Modern oriental and Persian scholars however believe that he lived as far back as 1200 BC, attacking and denouncing the pantheon of old traditional gods. He preached that there was just one God, Ahura Mazda—the creator, the source of light, truth, purity and righteousness. He was opposed by an evil spirit or force, which Zarathushtra termed the Angra Mainyu, whose world was of darkness, falsehood and deceit. For the first time the world was introduced to the concept of a struggle between good and evil. Man was free to choose between the two. Zarathushtra urged Man to choose Ahura Mazda and to follow the true creed and the good path. 'For then, Right shall be strengthened; Evil shall be destroyed! I desire the union with the good will, I renounce every communion with the evil doer'. The good and righteous were promised happiness after death; the evil doer who sided with Angra Mainyu was condemned to eternal hell. In the present day, ritual has crept into Zoroastrianism, as is with every other great religion. But the tenets of Zoroastrianism remain amazingly simple and practical. They are embodied in the three words—*humata, hukata, havaraishta*—which mean 'good thoughts', 'good words', 'good deeds'. Righteousness is the essence of the religion, but it should be 'Righteousness for the sake of Righteousness'.

Zarathushtra wandered through Persia, teaching, preaching and being persecuted for his non-doctrinaire views. Greek historians suggest that Hystaspes, father of Darius the Great, gave him protection. When Darius at last embraced Zoroastrianism, the rest of Persia followed. Zoroastrianism spread all through the near east, middle east and further east up to India and even to China. It also prevailed, at one time, in vast areas of Central Asia.

The tenets of Zoroastrianism were embodied in the *Avesta*—the holy books or scriptures of the Persians. The *Avesta* was probably composed by different authors in different periods of time. The oldest scriptures are the *gathas*—hymns attributed to Zarathushtra himself. Written in the ancient

Avesta language, other books contain prayers, invocations, legends, and moral precepts. One such book is the *Vendidad* which, in its present form, was probably written in the Assacid period between 250 BC and AD 226, but which embodies material from earlier centuries. The *Vendidad* codifies law, stating what is permitted, what is forbidden and the penalties for transgressing the law. It also lays down the principles of hygiene and of good clean living.

There are many who believe that the Zoroastrian faith is too ancient and too esoteric to be of consequence. There are many who have never even heard of this religion. Yet Zoroastrianism is indeed the mother of all monotheistic religions that followed. The concept of one God, of good and evil and of man's obligation to choose between the two, of God and the Devil, heaven and hell, has found its way into all subsequent monotheistic religions—Judaism, Christianity and Islam.

It is of interest that besides archaeological findings, Zoroastrian scriptures (the *Avesta*, including the *Vendidad*) are the main source of our knowledge on the culture of Persia and of the practice of medicine in ancient Persia. Greek reports on Persia may well be prejudiced because Greece was an implacable enemy of Persia. This paucity of historical evidence is largely due to the plunder and pillage of Persepolis, which was razed to the ground by Alexander. Invaluable manuscripts and historical data housed in the library of Persepolis perished when the city was torched to cinders. Even less than a third of the holy scriptures of the Persians could be salvaged for posterity, and it is only parts of these that have remained extant. This desecration was indeed a crime against humanity. Even so, medicine in Persia never reached the level of Egyptian medicine, as practised in the late centuries of the New Kingdom, and was clearly inferior to the Hippocratic medicine of Greece. Historical anecdotes suggest that the great Persian kings called upon Egyptian or Greek physicians when a member of the royal family was taken ill. As in ancient Egypt and Babylon, priest-physicians dominated the scene. Persian society was divided into four classes—the nobility, clients, peasants, slaves. The priest-physicians belonged to the client class and were often trained in temple schools, the most famous of which was at Raga. The scriptures suggest that Persia had empirical medicine in the use of herbs by herb doctors, surgeons who practised surgery, and incantation-priests who healed through spells, incantation and prayers. The priest-physician who healed through incantation and prayer was considered the best of all.

> Of all the healers, O Spitama Zarathushtra, namely those who heal with the knife, with herbs and with sacred incantations, the last one is the most potent as he heals from the very source of disease.
>
> *(Ardibehest Yasht)*

Unfortunately, there are no extant medical writings or manuscripts from ancient Persia. The books of the *Avesta* remain our sole source of information. The *Vendidad* and other Avestan books list a number of diseases. Leprosy was known; as in ancient Mesopotamia, lepers were considered unclean and debarred from society. Epilepsy is described as also other nervous and mental diseases; they were treated chiefly through incantations and prayers. Fevers are frequently mentioned, the chill and rigor accompanying fever being of special note. There is also a mention of various skin ailments, including those that itch—perhaps scabies. The scriptures make note of the blind, the deaf, the deformed and those with the evil eye. Angra Mainyu, the evil force according to the *Avesta*, had harnessed man with a number of evils. He had created 9 and 90 and 900 and 9000 and 9 times of 10,000 diseases. These were to be fought by the holy words of the scriptures, by sacred incantations and prayers which had the power to heal and to cure. It would perhaps be appropriate to quote a part of one such prayer and incantation.

By their might may we smite down the *druj* (the evil spirit)! By their might may we smite the *Druj*! May they give us strength and power O Ahura!

I drive away sickness, I drive away death, I drive away pain and fever, I drive away the disease, rottenness and infection which Angra Mainyu has created by his witchcraft against the bodies of mortals.

Though priest-physicians who healed by incantations were the most favoured, the Persians also used herbs and medicinal plants. *Homa* (note the linguistic closeness to the Vedic word *soma*) was a form of wine which had medicinal properties. It was drunk as therapy for diseases and also for religious rites and rituals. The scriptures do not name the herbs, pills, potions and salves in use, but they were probably similar to those used in Egypt and Mesopotamia. The religious books obviously do not mention surgical procedures or operations, but surgery in some form must have surely been practised. There is no doubt that with a huge army and frequent wars, surgeons might have known how to treat battle wounds probably as competently as the ancient Egyptians, Babylonians or Greeks.

Physicians in both ancient Persia and Greece were itinerant, moving from one city to the other. The *Vendidad* mentions the tariff to be charged for the services rendered. The priest was to be treated free, the poor were charged a small amount in kind (an ox being a common fee in lieu of professional service), the wealthy and the nobility were charged a heavy fee—again in kind. "He shall heal the lord of a province for the value of a chariot and four."

As was in archaic Greece, a physician did not need a licence to practice. Any individual could thus claim to heal and practise for a fee. The surgeon was however treated differently, perhaps because lapses in surgery were more easily evident. The *Vendidad* mentions that a healer who claims to use the knife should first prove his professional skill on a worshipper of the Daevas (the evil spirit). Only if he is thrice successful in healing worshippers of the Daevas with the knife should he be allowed to use the knife on worshippers of Ahura Mazda.

The holy scriptures paid a great deal of attention to hygiene, purification regulations, purification ceremonies and rituals. Menstruating women and women after childbirth were considered unclean and at the appropriate time underwent a purification rite. Yet women were honoured and highly respected. Girls were to marry after the age of fifteen, abortion was a crime amounting to manslaughter, the abortionist, the woman and the man all being considered equally guilty. Fire, earth, water and the vegetable kingdom were venerated and were never to be defiled. Fire was the symbol through which the Zoroastrians worshipped the one and only creator, Ahura Mazda. The Sun was Ahura Mazda's great creation and the holy *Avesta* sings paens in its praise. It is of great significance that the preservation and respect for man's ecology was one of the prime tenets of the Zoroastrian faith.

The Persian Empire of Darius the Great barely lasted a century. As expected, the decay was due to the rot within. Only the records of Rome after Tiberius could rival the debauchery, deceit, crime, moral squalor and blood-stained magnificence of the royal court of Persia. It is remarkable that the strengths and weaknesses of ancient Persia were similar to those of the Roman Empire that came later. Both excelled in war and conquest. Both carried out the administration and governance of their far-flung empires with tact and wisdom. Both passed from stoicism to epicureanism; both died a moral death before being physically annihilated. The decline and fall of the Persian Empire anticipated in almost every detail the decline and fall of Rome.

Ancient Persia made no major contribution to philosophy, art, literature, science or medicine. However it did produce great rulers, who for many years offered good governance to its disparate people. Above all, ancient Persia should always be remembered for bringing into the world a great prophet who blazed an untrodden trail, opening a new religious vista in the history of Man.

After the fall of the Persian Empire, Persian culture and civilization sank into hibernation for several centuries. Persia awoke once again in the tenth and eleventh centuries of our era under the stimulus of Islam, a new vigorous religion that swept all before it. Her talents now blossomed and she made up for lost time by making worthy contributions to art and architecture, to science and medicine. Just as ancient Persia gifted the world a great prophet who preached a pure and ethical religion, the newly-awakened Persia gifted the world a great poet. He was Ferdowsi (also called Firdausi), whose epic poem the *Shah Nama* is comparable in beauty and rhyme to Homer's *Iliad* and *Odyssey*.

Indian Medicine

5 Ancient Indian Medicine

There are three kinds of physicians in the world. One wears a physician's disguise, another acquires sponsorship. But some do actually possess all the virtues of the true doctor.

Charakasamhita

The Indus valley civilization, which grew on the banks of the river Indus around 3000 BC, was an elaborate and highly-evolved civilization. The archaeological excavations of several cities, in particular, Mohenjodaro, Harappa and Lothal, suggest that there existed a complex social order, which also included occupational hierarchies. As with the contemporary civilization of Sumer and Egypt, the apex of this hierarchy was formed by the king or ruler, followed by the priest who often combined his priestly function with those of a healer or a physician. The medicine practised by priest-physicians of all ancient civilizations was similar—a mixture of magic, rites and ritual.

The invasion of northern India around 1500 BC by the Indo-European tribes from the Northwest saw an end to the Indus valley civilization and the start of the Vedic Period. The Vedas were written during this period. Though essentially treatises on philosophy, religion and knowledge, they gave a glimpse of the practice of medicine and of the prevailing belief in matters of health and disease in this period of history. Remarkably enough these views were comparable with those of Egypt and Sumer. The Atharvaveda suggests that there were two systems of medicine—magico-religious medicine and empirical medicine. The magico-religious medicine, as in Sumer and Egypt, attributed diseases to certain deities or wicked spirits. There were deities corresponding with specific healing powers for specific diseases. *Mantras,* charms, rites and rituals could help to propitiate the evil spirits, just as other *mantras* (incantations) could nudge the benevolent deities to exert their healing power. Vedic rites included animal sacrifice and even human sacrifice as a means to propitiate the gods. The empirical (and perhaps slightly rational) school of medicine as inferred from the Atharvaveda, used drugs to combat disease. Drugs were mainly plants and herbs. It is now believed that the knowledge of plants and herbs and their use in various forms of ailments in north India and in the foothills of the Himalayas almost certainly preceded the recorded systematization of Indian medicine by many centuries.

The birth of the Buddha and advent of Buddhism were a challenge to the Hindu religious and philosophical beliefs embodied in the *Vedas.* Almost certainly, Buddhism also gave birth to new medical practices. Buddhist religious books, such as the Vinaya pitaka, Deepavamsa, Mahavamsa, provide glimpses of these practices. Methods of making a patient sweat and the operation of blood-letting are described in the *Mahavamsa. Mahavagga* also gives an account on Jivaka, a famous physician of India in the sixth and fifth century BC. Jivaka was born to a courtesan of Rajagrita (near modern Patna), the capital of the Magadhan empire in the reign of Bimbisara. After birth, he was thrown on a dust heap. People noticed that the newborn child was still alive (*jivati*) and this was reported to prince Abhaya, son of Bimbisara. The prince named him Jivaka and brought him up under his care. Jivaka thus was also named Jivaka Kumarabhacca, meaning 'one brought up by the prince'. Jivaka studied medicine at Taxila, the famous centre of learning in India, for seven years. At his practical examination at the end of the term, his teacher asked him to go around Taxila with a spade and find him a plant with no medicinal value. Jivaka returned, saying that he could find none. The teacher was satisfied and gave him the licence to practice medicine. Many medical and surgical cures are attributed to him in that era. Perhaps some of these are legends, but there is enough in ancient writings to class him as a physician of ancient India who had exceptional talent and merit. He is credited among other feats, to have performed a successful abdominal operation of undoing a twist in the intestines of a young man. Jivaka was a contemporary of the Buddha, and was his devotee and is believed to have treated Buddha when the latter fell ill or was injured.

Buddhism spread far and wide down south of India to Sri Lanka, and to South-East Asia, including China. Buddhist monasteries sprang up first in India and then in other countries influenced by Buddhism. The monasteries were places of meditation but they often also included a sick-room. It is likely that these developed into hospitals serviced by monks, housing not only the sick but also offering shelter to the poor and destitute. It is remarkable that the first hospitals in the West emerged around the same time in the history of Man and served the same purpose.

6 Traditional Indian Medicine

India is an ancient land with a unique ancient culture. Religion, philosophy and tradition governed life and living. From time immemorial, the gods played a crucial role in shaping the destiny of the country. They bequeathed their wisdom through ancient scriptures that explained the meaning of life, the nature of man and man's relation to the universe around him. Medicine evolved in this milieu and for many centuries appeared as a canonical text handed down by the gods for the benefit of man. Science, art, philosophy, music and medicine were all clearly influenced by this milieu. The genesis and evolution of Indian medicine can only be understood against the cultural background in which medicine took root and flowered.

Archaeological excavations along the banks of the river Ravi (a tributary of the mighty Indus), have revealed the presence of the Indus Valley civilization which flourished 5,000 years ago. This was one of the most highly evolved civilizations of the ancient world, with superb town-planning (as in Mohenjodaro and Harrapa), two-to-three storey buildings, broad streets, an excellent system of drainage and sewage disposal and a huge communal bathing tank. Seals, pottery, and figurines demonstrate an interest in art. There was division of labour, commerce flourished and the people were prosperous. They knew how to write but unfortunately the writing so far has not been deciphered.

The Indus Valley civilization disintegrated in 1500 BC, with the invasion of the Aryans (an Indo-European race) into north India from the north and north-west. In the course of time, the Aryans moved from the Indus Valley region to the banks of the Ganga and Yamuna rivers. This was the start of the Vedic period of Indian history. It was during this period that religious, philosophical and socio-economic tenets were laid down—tenets that influence Indian culture very strongly to this day. The Vedic period saw the writing of the *Vedas*, supposedly dictated to the sages of the country by the gods. The *Rig-Veda* is the oldest, consisting of beautiful verses praising the various forces of nature as deities. The three other Vedas are the *Yajurveda*, the *Samaveda* and the *Atharwaveda*. They are all philosophical treatises expounding the nature of man, his spirituality and his oneness with Brahman, the all-pervading force in life. The *Atharwaveda* also listed solutions for day-to-day problems, anxieties, and difficulties, and listed the medicinal herbs and plants of use to man. The *Vedas* were written in Sanskrit, the root of several Indo-European languages, and laid down a philosophical-cum-religious doctrine, the beauty and wisdom of which is increasingly acknowledged by the world today.

The *Vedas* were followed by the *Brahmanas*, composed to illustrate the use of the *Vedas* in sacrificial rituals. The *Aranyahas* were composed in forests or *aranyas*. It was the Indian tradition that at a certain stage of life, a man would leave the joys and sorrows the world had to offer and meditate in some secluded spot in the forest. The *Aranyahas* originated from the sages who began this tradition. Finally came the writings of the *Upanishads* indicating knowledge acquired sitting around the teacher. The guru–disciple discussions were embodied in these *Upanishads*. The *Upanishads* constitute a philosophical treatise on Man and the Universe unsurpassed in the literature of the world. By this period of history, the communication of knowledge from teacher to students through discussion was firmly established. It pervaded and characterized the teaching of not only philosophy but also of music, dance, literature, poetry and medicine. The writings of the *Vedas, Brahmanas* and the *Upanishads* were spread out over a thousand years, starting from 1500 BC.

SOCIO-ECONOMY

The economy was chiefly agricultural. Currency had not come into use; cows were the medium of exchange. The division of labour had produced various professional occupations, with the skilled artisans of the same occupation coming together as guilds.

The family was the most important unit of society. Several families living together constituted a *gram* or a village. Several villages formed the *vish*, of which the Vishpati was the head. Several *vishas* formed a *jana*, the head of which was the king. The king offered protection to his people and ran an efficient administration.

THE *VARNA* (CASTE) SYSTEM

Over a period of time, Aryan society was divided into three sections—the *brahmins, kshatriyas* and *vaishyas*. Each division was called a *varna*, and the *varnas* were based on occupation. The *brahmins* studied the *Vedas* and instructed others on their teachings, the *kshatriyas* were administrators and warriors who defended their lands, and the *vaishyas* engaged in agriculture, trade and other occupations. The Aryans referred to the non-Aryans they had conquered as *das* or *dasyus*. The manual labour, as also the menial labour was done by the poor *dasyus*. Those engaged in manual labour were called the *shudras*, who were forbidden to study the *Vedas*—an inequity which is unforgivable by any standard. With the passage of time, the *varnas* came to be described on the basis of birth. The law now ordained that everyone had to take on his father's occupation. Marriages were permitted within people of the same occupation. Each occupation became identified by a caste and for several reasons these castes became subdivided into subcastes.

Towards the end of the Vedic period, around 600 BC, there must have been great discontent in society. The brahmins were all powerful. Religion, which in the early Vedic period was wedded to philosophy, now became complicated and ritualized, with animal sacrifices practised on a large scale. The *varna* system bred social discrimination as one could not choose the occupation of one's choice.

It was the right milieu for fresh religious ideas that could reform a society which had gone astray. The great religious leaders, Vardhaman Mahavir, who founded Jainism, and Siddhartha Gautama (later called Gautama Buddha—the enlightened one) showed India the true path.

Mahavir (born c. 550 BC) considered non-violence (*ahimsa*) as the highest principle. He advocated the practice of four other precepts—*satya* (truth), *asteya* (refraining from taking what belongs to others), *brahmacharya* (leading a chaste life), and *aprigraha* (not to hoard or accumulate worldly possessions). The five precepts of *ahimsa, satya, asteya, brahmacharya* and *aprigraha* were the five great vows of Jainism.

Gautama Buddha (563–483 BC) was born a prince named Siddhartha. He married Yashodhara at the age of sixteen and they had a son named Rahul. At the age of twenty-nine, deeply disturbed by the sorrow and misery he saw all around him, he felt an urge to help mankind free itself from sorrow. He renounced his princely life, left home, gave up his worldly possessions and with his five companions led a life of extreme penance and asceticism in his search for truth. In a jungle within the gorge of the

Vindhya mountains, enfeebled by starvation, he realized that illumination and wisdom could only come through a well-nourished brain in a healthy body. He demanded food, at which his shocked companions, disappointed and dejected, deserted him and returned to Varanasi. Gautama the Great, according to them had fallen from grace. Gautama wandered alone through thick forests and after several trials and tribulations seated himself under a banyan tree at a place now called Bodh Gaya. A sense of enlightenment now slowly dawned upon him—he saw life clearly and is said to have stayed day and night in profound meditation. He then rose to spread his message to the world.

He preached his eight-fold path. Right Views, insisting on truth as the keystone of life; Right Aspirations—which included service towards others and the desire to serve justice; Right Speech; Right Conduct; Right Livelihood; Right Effort; and Right Mindfulness. Finally came Right Rapture, probably directed against the pointless ecstasies of the devout *brahmins*. Buddha advocated the Buddhist doctrine of *karma* as the only explanation for the inequities of the world. The good or evil deeds of each life determine the happiness and sorrows of subsequent lives.

Gautama Buddha was one of the greatest souls that ever trod the earth. His influence spread far and wide in India and the Far East. The great religion he preached was different from any other religion that came into the world. It was a religion of conduct, not of observances. It had no temples and as it did not involve rituals and sacrifice, had no priests and advocated no theology. Buddha preached neither for nor against the reality of the numerous gods worshipped at that time in Hindu India. He passed them by and concentrated on the ethics of life and living. Buddhism enjoined above all, compassion and care. It is no small wonder that the roots of ancient Indian medicine became apparent at this point in the history of man.

The Influence of Indian Philosophy

In the Upanishadic period, sages concentrated their efforts on determining the nature of the self (*atman*) and the ultimate essence of the universe. Kanada, a sage living in the sixth century BC, proposed that all substances in the universe were made up of small indivisible *pramanus*. These were entities obtained when a substance was divided and repeatedly sub-divided till no further division was possible. The theory of *pramanus* came to be known as the *vaisesika* theory. It was the combination of various *pramanus* in different permutations and combinations that gave rise to the universe and its contents. According to the *vaisesika* philosophy, the universe could be divided into six categories. One of these six categories is substance (*dravvya*) which can be subdivided into nine entities, five of which are earth (*kshiti*), water (*apa*), fire (*teja*), air (*vayu*) and ether (*akasa*). It is these five entities which constitute matter and which also formed the basis for the Indian medical system. The *vaisesika* philosophy described the combination of different types of *pramanus*. This could take the form of a simple addition, or under the influence of *teja*, a chemical reaction (*paka*) could take place—the final product being different from each of the uniting constituents. The *paka* reaction was the basis of digestion and explained the formation of the *dosas* within the body (to be explained later).

Another sage around the fifth century AD, Gotama Aksapada systematized all knowledge in a philosophical treatise termed *Nyaya Sutra*. According to this text, there were four methods of establishing the true identity of a fact, phenomenon or object. They were perception, inference, comparison and testimony. These methods were used extensively in the study of drugs included in the Indian pharmacopoeia. Both the philosophical tenets stated above strongly influenced Indian medicine, giving an impetus to the spirit of scientific inquiry.

The political history of India after the Buddhist period was characterized by the rise and fall of empires. The Maghadha kingdom gave way to the Maurya period (321–185 BC). Alexander's invasion of India in 345 BC was the first prolonged contact between the West and India. The greatest king of the Maurya Empire and probably the greatest king of all time, was Ashoka the Great. This was the first and the only time when under Ashoka's suzerainty India (except for the kingdom of the Pandavas and Keralaputra in the extreme South) was united as one country. Convinced of the hopelessness and wanton destruction caused by war, Ashoka ruled through love and benevolence. He insisted that truth, non-violence, and compassion should be the features of daily life. He erected tall iron pillars with inscriptions to this effect in several parts of country. The *dharma chakra* (wheel on the pillar) he erected at Sarnath was later embodied in India's national flag. It was during Ashoka's reign that hospitals and *dharamsalas* were built for the care of the sick, poor and the destitute.

The period of history from AD 300–800 marked the rise of the Gupta dynasty. This period saw the rebirth of Hinduism with King Harsha at its head. There was a renaissance of sculpture, architecture, music, poetry, literature, science and medicine. The tenth century witnessed the barbaric invasions of the Muslims from the north-west. Mohammed of Ghazni, between 1001–1027, invaded India seventeen times, destroyed the rich temples of Somnath and Mathura, taking away all their wealth to Ghazni. Then came Mohammed of Gauri, who left his lieutenant to rule the large northern territory he had conquered. Now came the rule of the Sultanates in Delhi. In 1526, King Babar of Kabul Kandahar defeated Ibrahim Lodi of the Sultanate dynasty and founded the Mughal Empire. These events, in brief, describe the history of north India till the beginning of the sixteenth century.

The Deccan plateau, Western India, Eastern India and the South saw the rise and fall of many kingdoms. The country was divided and subdivided, with one faction warring with the other. The covetous eyes of the West on the riches of India and the Far East culminated in the unfortunate colonization of the country (discussed in a later chapter).

Art and Culture

The Vedas and Upanishads constitute a fount of philosophy, wisdom and knowledge. The beauty of their form and rhyme can be truly appreciated only by those familiar with Sanskrit.

The world famous epics, the *Mahabharata* and the *Ramayana* were composed between 300 BC and AD 300. Homeric in scope, the *Mahabharata*, composed by the sage Vyasa, relates, in beautiful verse, the conflict between the Kauravas and the Pandavas. The epic *Ramayana* was composed by the sage Valmiki and describes the conflict between Rama and Ravana—between the personification of good and evil. The *Bhagvat Gita*, a sacred text of the Hindus, is part of the *Mahabharata*. These epics explore the thoughts of man, his place in the universe, the role of destiny, fate and the importance of duty and righteousness. Noble in its thoughts, beautiful in expression and rhyme, sublime in philosophy, simple in its practicality, the *Gita* is a combination of poetry, literature, legend and philosophy, unsurpassed in the annals of the history of man.

Literature blossomed in the Gupta dynasty between AD 500 and 800. Kalidasa the great Sanskrit poet wrote *Shakuntala* and *Meghdoot*, now famous all over the world. The *Mudrarakshasa* of Visakhadatta and the *Mrichhakatika* of Shudraka also belong to this period.

Indian art and sculpture mirrored Indian philosophy. "The theme of Indian art in its essence is the universe in all its abundance and multiplicity of life and form." Yet within and behind these forms is the omnipotent, omniscient, transcendental spirit which is formless (*arupa*). Architecture, sculpture, art and music are paeans to the gods, singing their praise, devotional in form. The wall paintings of

Ajanta executed between the third and eight centuries depict the life of Gautama Buddha with beauty and religious adoration. The Kailas temple of Ellora is famous all over the world. It is carved out of a huge single rock and to many is one of the marvels of the world. Though sculpture, art, music and dance were chiefly devotional, Indian artists also depicted life in all its aesthetic splendour and sensuality, as was evinced by the highly erotic carvings of Khajuraho in Orissa, and by the treatise on erotica, *Kama Sutra,* written by Vatsyayana in the Gupta period.

Science

Ancient India, like ancient Greece, bequeathed to the world a rich legacy in the field of science. The earliest scientists of India were priests who, besides being physicians, also cultivated science in so far as it contributed to religion. Later, science became secular and divorced from priestly functions.

Astronomy grew out of the worship of heavenly bodies and the observation of their movements across the sky. The greatest Indian astronomer and mathematician was Aryabhatta (ca AD 499). He explained eclipses and equinoxes and proposed that the earth was a sphere and that it had a diurnal revolution on its axis. He anticipated Copernicus when he stated: "The sphere of the stars is stationary and the earth by its revolution produces the daily rising and setting of planets."

In mathematics, India was even superior to Greece. The so-called Arabic numerals were an Indian invention; these numerals have been found on the Rock Edicts of Ashoka (256 BC), a thousand years before their use in Arab literature. The decimal system was known to Aryabhata and Brahmagupta long before its appearance in Arabic and Syrian writings. It was adopted by China through Buddhist missionaries and probably introduced to the Arab world by Mohamed Ibn Musa (AD 830)—the great mathematician of his age. The 'zero' was another Indian discovery and it is generally accepted that the Arabs borrowed this concept from India.

Algebra developed independently in both Greece and India. Indian mathematicians found the square root of two, and in the eighth century AD solved indeterminate equations of the second degree—a thousand years before Euler did so in Europe. Aryabhata drew up a table of sines and calculated the value of π (pi) with remarkable accuracy. Bhaskara (b. 1114) is said to have anticipated the differential calculus. The Surya Siddantha expounded a system of trigonometry far more advanced than that known to Greece. The Indians wedded art to science for they discussed their observations in astronomy, mathematics and others sciences in beautiful verse.

Medicine in India from ancient times to the advent of the British in the seventeenth century was strongly influenced by religion, philosophy, legend, science, literature, socio-economic conditions, and even by climate and geography. It was a combination of these background factors that gave Indian medicine a rather unusual form and content.

Ayurveda

Ayurveda is the classical ancient Indian system of medicine, crystallized and systematically organized into a large corpus of writing in Sanskrit. Literally translated, Ayurveda means the knowledge (*veda* in sanskrit) of long life or longevity (*ayur*).

The origin of this ancient art and science of medicine is uncertain, controversial and clouded in legend. One legend recounts the miraculous birth of Dhanvantari (the god of medicine), who is to Indian medicine what Aesculapius was to Greek medicine. The god arose through the churning of the sea of milk together with the moon (Lakshmi), Surabhi (the sacred cow), Varuna (goddess of wine), Parijata (the tree of paradise), and a winged horse similar to Pegasus in Greek mythology. In years to come, he was so moved by the sufferings of Man that he wished to be reborn on earth as a prince of Varanasi. His wish was fulfilled; he then retired to live as a hermit in the forest, where he wrote the Ayurveda for the benefit of Man.

Another, more credible, legend is that at some time between the second and third millennium before the birth of Christ, the most enlightened sages, ascetics and teachers of India journeyed thousands of miles to meet in a remote Himalayan cave. They pooled their learning and experience on the nature of human suffering and went on to discuss ways and means to heal or alleviate this suffering. Their discussion led to the birth of Ayurveda. The first great ayurvedic teacher, Agnivesh, was a disciple of Atreya Punarvasu, one of the original body of sages who founded the science. Agnivesh was instructed by this sage to commit all discussions at the conference to memory. Agnivesh taught his disciples who in turn became *gurus* (teachers) to teach their own disciples. This oral tradition continued through centuries till the body of accumulated knowledge was systematized into a written text.

The first written evidence of Ayurveda was in the corpus of Sanskrit writing termed the *Charaka Samhita* and the *Susruta Samhita* (the Compendia of Charaka and Susruta). These two massive manuscripts form the twin pillars of Ayurveda. There is another early text that has survived as a single manuscript—the *Bhela manuscript.* The life and times of Charaka are uncertain. The name Charaka appears as a great medical authority in the fifth century AD in the Bower manuscript, discovered in eastern Turkistan in Central Asia on the caravan route to China. Originally, the manuscript was owned by a Buddhist monk, Yasomitra, who lived in a monastery near the old Silk Route trading station of Kuga. The manuscript contained medical-cum-religious texts and was written by scribes on birch bark in Sanskrit and Prakrit. After Yasomitra's death the manuscript lay buried in a stupa dedicated to the monk. It lay undisturbed for a thousand years before it was unearthed and discovered. In 1890, Lieutenant Hamilton Bower was

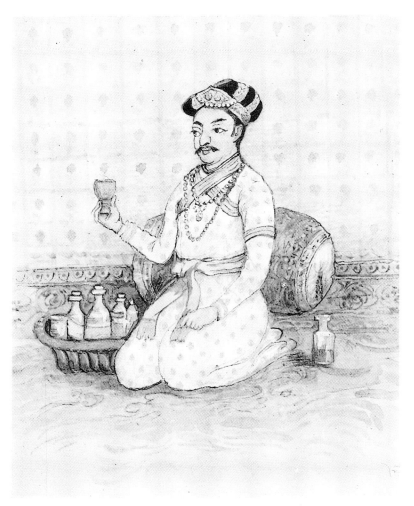

Fig. 6.1   Charaka (500 BC): Portrait of Charaka, Hindu physician.

appointed by the British government to track down the murder of a Scotsman Andrew Dalgliesh, who was murdered by an Afghan tribesman while camping in the Karakoram ranges. Bower was camping at Kuga, at the edge of the Gobi desert when a man offered to sell him old manuscripts. These manuscripts had been found by treasure-hunters excavating near a ruined stupa. Bower bought the manuscripts. The manuscript was forwarded to the President of the Asiatic Society of India, who sent it on to to be deciphered, translated and edited by A.J. Hoernle, an expert in oriental languages in Calcutta. Hoernle returned the manuscript to Bower, who later sold it to the Bodleian Library in Oxford.

Further historical evidence dates Charaka to an earlier date. The French orientalist, Sylvian Levy, discovered the Chinese translation of an old Buddhist manuscript written in Sanskrit, in the late fifth century AD. One of the chapters in this manuscript gives a description of the famous king, Kanishka. Kanishka, the manuscript says, had three close companions and friends—the famous physician, Charaka, Asvaghosa Bodhisatva, and his prime minister, Mathara. The date of Kanishka, though not absolutely certain, is considered by most historians to be around the first or second century AD. If written, scientific and historical evidence places Charaka in the first or second century AD, then how much further back in time do the roots of Ayurveda extend? When was this healing art and science born? Both the *Charaka Samhita* and the *Susruta Samhita* claim descent from the *Vedas*. This should not be taken literally. The claim that they are bequeathed by the gods might strongly serve to make them acceptable to those who learnt and practised Ayurveda and to those on whom this healing art was practised. Though the *Vedas* and, in particular, the *Atharwaveda*, contain references to medicine, they bear no resemblance to the classical texts of Charaka and Susruta. Zysk has provided evidence to suggest that Ayurveda as a system of medicine had its roots in the ascetic milieu of Buddhism that prevailed in India in the fifth and sixth century BC. Written evidence in the earliest manuscripts preserved by the Buddhist monks in that period of history bears a close similarity to the system of medicine in the early texts of Charaka and Susruta.

It is however possible that the birth of Ayurveda extends even further back into history, though concrete evidence to prove this might never be forthcoming. India, after all, is a land which, even today is characterized by oral tradition. It is, in fact, more than likely that the roots of Ayurveda and its early sproutings were passed on by numerous *gurus* to their *chelas* (disciples) through word of mouth. The same analogy is present in Indian music, which was never notated, and where the different *gharanas* in the country passed on their discoveries, their *ragas* and their variations through the *guru* to his disciples, who lived with him all their lives like his own sons and daughters. It is conceivable that the little trickles in the ancient science of Ayurveda, gathered through oral traditions, became visible streams in the Buddhist period, finally joining together to culminate in the systematized medicine treatises of Charaka and Susruta.

Interestingly enough, in the text of the *Samhita* (compendium), the name Charaka occurs only in a statement at the end of the chapter, which gives the name and number of the chapter just completed. Charaka's name does not appear anywhere in the text and neither is he termed the main author. It appears that the body of the work is by Agnivesh, who was taught this system of medicine by his guru and teacher Atreya. Charaka probably revised and edited this work. The dates of both Agnivesh and Atreya are lost in the mists of legend and time .

Finally, it needs to be mentioned that though Ayurveda has no direct connection with the *Vedas* written in the Vedic period, the thoughts and philosophy embodied in the prevailing literature must have certainly formed the background that influenced ayurvedic writings. This is proven by the fact that the knowledge of longevity, which Ayurveda stood for, was intertwined with the philosophy of life and living.

The Philosophy of Ayurveda

The fundamental philosophical tenet of Ayurveda was that suffering was disease and contentment was good health. Ayurveda recognized that suffering could be physical, mental and spiritual; good health necessitated a healthy body, a sound mind and a good soul. This philosophical concept transcended the medical texts, for it embodied a way of living based on the recognition of man's interdependence with all other forms of life. The spirit constitutes the intelligence of life, and matter its energy. Both are manifestations of Brahman, which constitutes the oneness of life. This concept stresses man's link with universal life. A realization of this link prevents him from being isolated from his own energies and from the energies of nature. As the highest form of life, man must be nature's guardian, realizing that his health and survival are dependent on nature and not unduly disturbing the fragile ecological balance within nature and its other living organisms. A corollary to this would be that man must prevent wanton destruction; he must not pollute the waters, nor poison the air, nor contaminate the soil. Ayurveda enjoins that just as a man's spiritual happiness lies in his ability to live in harmony with the external universe, his mental happiness depends on his ability to live in harmony with himself. It is this holistic view of life in which man is just a microcosm, as also a holistic view of the physical, emotional and spiritual aspects of man interacting with one another and with the world outside that make Ayurveda unique in the art and science of healing.

The Basic Tenets of Ayurveda

An in-depth analysis of the several ayurvedic texts is outside the scope of this book. There are, however, certain medical concepts underlying all these texts. The first major doctrine is that the state of the body is governed by the presence of humors (*dosa*), body tissues (*dhatu*), and by the relation between these humors, body tissues and waste matter (*mala*). The three humors (*tridosa-vidya*) that regulate the body are semi-fluid in consistency and are wind (*vat*), choler (*pitta*) and phlegm (*kapha*). This theory of humors is analogous to the Greek view, except that the latter includes a fourth humor 'blood', and that 'wind' is not included as a humor in Greek medicine. These three humors interact with the five basic constituents of the body—chyle, blood, flesh, bone-marrow and semen. They also interact with the waste products.

The next major concept is that of moderation and the avoidance of excess. This applies to diet, food, sleep, exercise, sex and to the medicines consumed. Almost certainly this view must have been influenced by the Buddhist teachings. An interesting ayurvedic concept is in relation to moderation of the natural urges of man—suppression of these urges was wrong as this could cause disease.

Ayurvedic diagnosis and treatment can only be understood in relation to the ayurvedic concept of the physiology and function of the body. These concepts have not been static, and have gradually evolved with the accretion of later texts. The central physiological process within the body is digestion. In Sanskrit, the process of digestion is considered similar to cooking (*pacana*) or burning. The digestive force is termed fire (*agni*). The first product of digestion is chyle (*rasa*). Through the heating influence of choler (*pita*), the chyle is transformed into the next body tissue—blood. Blood in turn is transformed into flesh, and so on, till all body tissues are formed. Ultimately, the highest product that finally evolves through this chain reaction is semen. Sarngadhora's compendium (a later ayurvedic text) describes the details of this digestive process and goes on to elaborate on the formation of waste products. Obviously a woman's physiology has no equivalent to semen. Ayurveda understood conception as the union of the male semen within the uterus with female blood.

Ayurvedic concepts include the presence of an energizing, ultimate force within the body responsible for health and normal function of organ systems. This energizing force is not abstract but a material substance described as cold and oily. The body is visualized as consisting of a network of tubes transporting energizing fluids from one place to the other. These tubes also carry the three humors, sensations and even the 'mind'. Diseases arise when the flow of these is obstructed, retarded, or channelized into the wrong locations. If the flow of air (one of the humors) is obstructed or incorrect, 'wind diseases' result. These include rheumatism, epilepsy, and paralysis. Insanity is said to result from blockage of tubes that transport the mind.

Man's relation and response to the changing environment and seasons is of great importance to health. Great emphasis is placed on diet and different qualities have been attributed to different foods. It may astonish many Indian readers to find that meat was considered a part of the diet and was recommended in certain conditions and diseases. Charaka gives this dietary advice without making any attempt to defend it. Later ayurvedic texts advocate benevolence to all living creatures, gently admonishing a doctor, as far as possible, from prescribing the meat of young animals to his patients. It is a remarkable fact that Ayurveda, while enunciating a great number of ethical norms on life and on the style of living, unhesitatingly advocated the use of meat and alcohol as 'therapy' in certain conditions.

A Brief Outline of Charaka Samhita

This earliest of the ayurvedic texts elaborates on anatomy, foetal development, and the *tridosa* theory of the three humors that govern function and malfunction of the body. It describes the classification of diseases, aetiology, diagnosis, prognosis and treatment. Thus it discusses the cause, nature and management of different fevers, of skin conditions, urinary problems, consumption, asthma, epilepsy, insanity, dropsy and several other pathologies. It deals with the science of rejuvenation and gives a detailed description of diseases of the eye, of the female genital organs, normal and abnormal deliveries, care of the newborn and diseases of children. The materia–medica within this compendium consists chiefly of numerous vegetable products, and also includes animal products and minerals. These are classified into fifty groups depending on their basis of action in the body. Treatment includes methods to induce sweating, cupping, bloodletting, the use of leeches, the use of enemas, ointments and the use of drugs from the vast array of plants, herbs, nuts and other drugs that comprised the ayurvedic pharmacopoeia.

The vast treatise gives an idea of doctors specializing in different medical subjects, offers a code of ethics, describes the centres of learning and the schools of philosophy which influenced medical theories, the classification of plants, medical botany, and the classification of the animal kingdom, with special reference to the properties of their flesh. It includes a description of customs, traditions, diets, exercise, the way of living, good and bad habits useful for the ordinary man.

By AD 1000 there were many commentaries in Sanskrit by renowned scholars on the *Charaka Samhita*. The work was translated from Sanskrit to Arabic in the eighth century and its name *Sharaka Indiana* occurs in the Latin translation of Avicenna and Razes.

Susruta Samhita

This vast compendium represents a treatise on surgery in Ayurveda. Susruta was an eminent surgeon of antiquity, just as Charaka was an eminent physician. It is difficult to determine when

Susruta lived and wrote his manuscript. Evidence from various sources suggests that he lived about two centuries before Christ, at which time the core of his manuscript on surgery was formed. This manuscript was then frequently revised and updated in the centuries before AD 500. It is in this revised and edited form that the world today sees this ancient manuscript.

The Susruta of antiquity was not only a great surgeon, but also a great teacher and a renowned author. He practised bedside teaching; he knew the aptitude of the students he taught, and had the wisdom to teach only as much as he felt his students could absorb and put into practice. He is

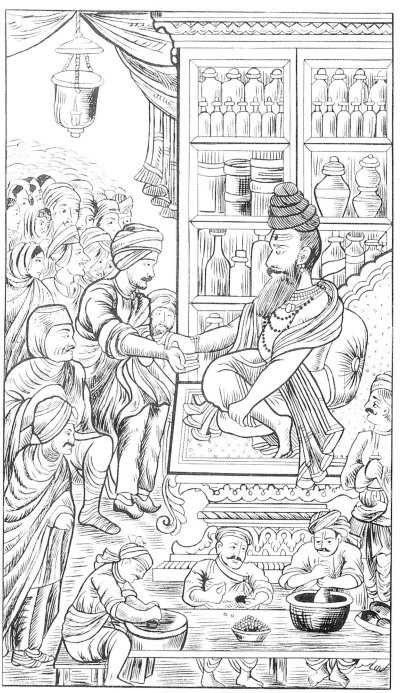

Fig. 6.2   Susruta (1000 BC): Portrait of Susruta.

believed to have innovated major operations and improved the general techniques of surgery. He also described a variety of surgical instruments. He taught his students surgical techniques first on dummies and then on dead bodies. His operations for the removal of cataract, for lithotomy, for removal of a dead foetus, and other abdominal operations, if true, could be classed as marvels of his time and age. Plastic surgery originated with Susruta. Cutting off the nose was a commonly practised punishment in females for adultery, and in males for a variety of offences. Plastic surgery to reconstruct the nose or torn ear lobes was innovated by this great surgeon.

Recent historical studies suggest that soon after Susruta, the practice of surgery by traditional trained ayurved physicians declined and that surgery came to be practised by barber-surgeons as in the west. To what extent this is true is difficult to ascertain, nor is the reason for this easily discernible. The caste system which steadily grew in the first millenium after Christ, might have created taboos concerning close physical contact with 'untouchables' or those of the lowest caste. Surgery, which involved such contact may have thus lost favour, and its practice by traditional ayurveds may have declined. Yet it was during this period of history that the importance of examination of the pulse, the urine and the value of body massage was emphasized in ayurvedic practice.

The famous surgical procedure of removal of the cataract described and practiced during Susruta's time reached China, probably through Buddhist pilgrim monks and not through ayurvedic Indian physicians. By the beginning of the twentieth century it was described again, but was more frequently carried out by barber-surgeons than by ayurvedic practitioners. Perhaps the practice of surgery either fell into disrepute or was disregarded by ayurveds, who preferred only to heal through medicine.

Even so, a documented performance of rhinoplasty (for which Susruta was famous) was witnessed and recorded in 1793 in Pune. A Parsee gentleman by the name of Cowasjee, living in Pune, had been a bullock-cart driver for the English army in the 1792 Mysore war. He was captured by the soldiers of Tipu Sultan and had his nose and one hand cut off. After a year, he and his four colleagues who had met the same fate sought help to reconstruct their noses from a man who was known to be an expert in this

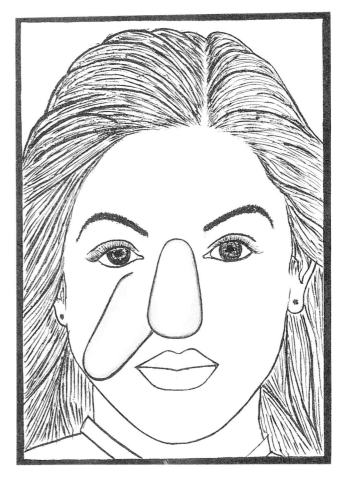

Fig. 6.3   Susruta's method of using a skin flap from the cheek for reconstruction of the nose.

field. It is believed that the person Cowasjee consulted was not trained in the practice of Ayurveda and was a bricklayer by profession. The bricklayer gave him a new nose.

The successful surgery performed by the bricklayer was witnessed by Thomas Cruso and James Findlay, senior British surgeons in the Bombay Presidency. They described and drew the skin graft procedure which was published in the *Madras Gazette.* It was subsequently reproduced in the October 1794 issue of the *Gentleman's Magazine* of London. The operation was described thus:

A thin plate of wax is fitted to the stump of the nose so as to make a nose of a good appearance; it is then flattened and laid on the forehead. A line is drawn around the wax which is then of no further use and the surgeon then dissects off as much skin as it had covered, leaving undivided a small slip between the eyes. This slip preserves the circulation till a union has taken place between the new and old parts.

The cicatrix of the stumps of the nose is next paired off and immediately behind the new part an incision is made through the skin which passes around both alae, and goes along the upper lip. The skin now brought down from the forehead and being twisted half around, is inserted into this incision, so that a nose is formed with a double hold above and with its alae and septum below fixed in the incision.

A little Terra Japanica (pale catechu) is softened with water and being spread on slips of cloth, five or six of these are placed over each other to secure the joining. No other dressing but this cement is used for four days. It is then removed and clothes dipped in ghee (clarified butter) are applied. The connecting slip of skin is divided about the twentieth day, when a little more dissection is necessary to improve the appearance of the new nose. Four, five or six days after the operation, the patient is made to lie on his back and on the tenth day bits of soft cloth are put into the nostrils to keep them sufficiently open.

This spectacular story caught the attention of J.C. Carpue, a thirty year old surgeon in London. Carpue successfully used the same skin-graft procedure for nose repair on a patient in 1814. He reported his successful results in 1816, introducing the 'Hindu surgical technique' and with it the 'Indian nose' to the West.

Further inquiries into the bricklayer's surgical prowess revealed that he was more an artist than a bricklayer and that he had also successfully reconstructed the noses of all four of Cowasjee's friends. He was also recognized as an expert in the repair of torn or split lips. He was considered the best in India and his art was hereditary in his family. Current research opines that even if the plastic surgery on the nose performed in Pune was a legacy of Susruta's times, the technique was passed down through centuries not through traditional ayurvedic doctors but through unconventional channels.

Interestingly enough, the technique of nose repair of the artist bricklayer was a little different from that described in Susruta's *Samhita*. In Susruta's technique, the surgeon repairing the mutilated nose first measured the portion of the nose to be covered on a leaf. This pattern was placed on the cheek and a suitable skin flap of the requisite size was raised from the cheek towards the cicatrix. The raised flap was kept attached to the cheek by a small pedicle; it was then half-turned, placed on the nose and sutured into position. A slender tubular reed was placed through each nostril till the graft took. The surgical area was dusted with a powder of sappan-wood, liquorice and barbery plant. It was then covered with cotton soaked in sesamum oil.

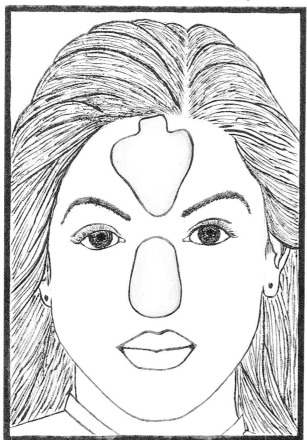

Fig. 6.4 A later Indian method using the forehead skin flap for reconstruction of the nose.

It is very likely that after Susruta, master surgeons of India perfected another technique in reconstruction of the nose, using the forehead flap method practised on Cowasjee. This innovation had two advantages—there was less tension in the pedicle of the forehead flap as compared to the facial flap and the scar on the forehead could be covered by a *tikka* in a woman and/or a *tilak* in a man. In Susruta's technique the facial scar could not be hidden.

It is of interest that Susruta also recommended the use of a facial skin flap for repair of a cleft lip. The first successful closure of a congenital cleft palate was performed by a French dentist Le Monnier of Rouen in 1764. Carl Ferdinand von Graefe (1747–1840) who popularized the 'Hindu surgical technique' in plastic reconstruction of the nose in Germany and Europe, devised in 1816 the first comprehensive surgical method for closing clefts of the velum. It is uncertain if cleft palates were reconstructed in ancient India, even though diseases of the palate have been described in ancient Indian medical texts.

The spread of Indian learning, including medicine, into Europe is of great interest. Sanskrit literature, particularly the scientific texts, were translated into Pahalvi in very early days. This was given a fresh impetus during the Sassanian regime in Persia and the Abbasid regime in Baghdad. Khusro I Naushiravan (AD 531–79) secretly sent his Zoroastrian physician-premier, Perzoes (c AD 579) to India. Perzoes known as Burzuya in Pahlavi and Burziachihar in Persian lived in India for many years and is believed to be none other than Varuchi, one of the esteemed ministers in the court of the legendary King Vikramaditya. On his return to Persia, Perzoes brought with him rare Sanskrit manuscripts on medicine and other sciences which were translated into Pahlavi.

The early Abbasid caliphs also promoted the translation of Hindu sciences into Arabic. In fact a number of Indians served as royal physicians and superintendents of hospitals in Baghdad. Indian sciences, including medicine, surgery and plastic surgery reached Italy and Spain through the Arabs. Techniques in plastic surgery practised in India must have almost certainly reached Sicily and Italy by the early fifteenth century. Then they remained forgotten for another 400 years. It fell to the good fortune of the English surgeon Carpue to reintroduce Indian plastic surgery to Europe in the early nineteenth century.

It is impossible to cover all the surgical procedures in Susruta's compendium in this book. A fascinating innovation, however, was the use of black ants for suturing. The technique was to bring the edges of a wound very close together and then have a black ant join the edges by biting through them with its mandibles. The ant's body was twisted off but the head remained, approximating the edges of the wound.

Of all the herbal and plant remedies used in ancient Ayurveda, the most mysterious was the use of the mystic *soma* plant. 'Ritual rites' were supposed to precede the use of the plant and the ingestion of its juice, leading to a fascinating mystical experience. The botanical identity of the *soma* plant has been a subject of endless debate. R. Gordon Wasson in his book *Soma–Divine Mushroom of Immortality* opined that the Soma plant was the poisonous hallucinogenic mushroom, *Amanita muscaria*. Recent research has gathered evidence that the plant is a member of the Ephedra family. It is a stimulant and was used for its stimulant effect by Vedic poets, who under its influence stayed awake the whole night, composing poetry.

Susruta's view of the use of the *soma* plant was totally different. He attributed to it rejuvenating properties, a magical formula which on ingestion changes one into a new individual with extraordinary beauty and health. There are very few references in ancient literature to the rejuvenating attributes of *soma* and the *soma* sacrifice. The Artareya–Brahmana (before 500 BC) describes the symbolic rebirth of a consecrated man at the start of the *soma* rite. Susruta's ritual for rejuvenation also employs the supposedly magical properties of this famous plant.

Did the practice of Ayurveda evolve after Charaka and Susruta or did it remain a canonical text, static and unchanged? Numerous Brahmanical texts followed those of Charaka and Susruta in the first millenium. The Bower manuscipt, also called the *Nava–Nitaka*, has already been discussed. According to Hoernle, this manuscript consists of at least six different sections. The first section is a monograph on garlic (*Lasuna or Rasuna*), considered the elixir of life. Its use in Ayurveda continues to be highly recommended even today. Another famous Brahmanical text is the *Astanghrdaya Samhita* of Vagbhata (c AD 700), which among new topics included midwifery and gynaecology. Then there was the *Sarangadhara Samhita* of Sarangadhara (fourteenth century AD), who introduced opium and metallic compounds into the ayurvedic pharmacopoeia under the influence of Islamic medicine and the *Bhavaprakasa* of Bhavamisra (sixteenth century). In the seventh century AD, Madhavakara's work titled *Rugviniscaya* established the new precedent of the pathological grouping of disease, which was followed by subsequent writers.

Ayurvedic writers often expressed dissenting opinions on old canonical ideas. New diseases were described—for example, syphilis known as the 'pharangi disease' (acquired through sexual contact with foreigners). The use of mercury in ointment form and taken orally in syphilis was learnt from Islamic physicians who practised their own system of medicine after the first millenium.

Examination of the pulse, its rate, rhythm, character and volume as an aid to diagnosis was established in the fourteenth century AD by Sarangadhara in the *Sarangadhara Samhita*. The art of feeling the pulse was termed *nadipriksha*. Sarangadhara made two notable advances in respiratory physiology. He mentions the lungs by the name of *puppusa,* and says that the *udana vayu* (one of the five *vayus*) dwells in the lungs. This is the first statement in Indian medicine connecting the lungs with *vayus* and thus with respiration.

> The *prana-vayu* after coursing through the interior of the lotus-like heart, goes out through the throat to drink the outside air, enters the body again to nourish the whole body and keep up the digestive fire.

In poetic language, Sarangadhara states that the function of respiration is to provide oxygen to the body for its metabolism. Examination of the urine soon became as important as the examination of the pulse. By the sixteenth century, diagnosis involved the following basic steps—the examination of the pulse, urine, faeces, tongue, eyes, general appearance, voice and skin.

After Islam entered India towards the end of the first millenium, Arabic medicine came into increasing prominence. It was termed Yunani medicine; its practitioners were called *hakims,* and they still practise their medicine in India. They introduced heavy metals in the materia medica of the country—a *practice* that influenced ayurvedic medicine in the second millenium.

In south India, the form of medicine, though akin to Ayurveda had some differences. It was termed Siddhi medicine and was strongly influenced by tantric ideas and the use of alchemy. The use of heavy metals was extremely popular and the Tamilians prized a substance termed *muppu* that had remarkable powers on the physical and spiritual aspects of man. The science of alchemy was believed to have been spread to China and the Far East and to Islam in the Middle East by the legendary founders of Siddhi medicine.

Ayurvedic medicine suffered an eclipse after the colonization of India by the British. By 1835, state-funded medical colleges in the country taught only Western medicine and the teaching of Ayurveda ceased. Following the independence of India in 1947, Ayurveda has gradually been re-established. Even so, large urban centres chiefly practise Western medicine. There are over one hundred approved ayurvedic training colleges recognized by the government—many are affiliated to the universities. Ayurvedic training now includes basic courses in anatomy, physiology, public health, and family planning. The practice of Ayurveda in this age has incorporated a number of features of Western medicine, including the use of antibiotics, injections and other drugs found in the Western pharmacopoeia. Its future lies in amalgamating the best in the old traditions with some of the invaluable modern methods and technology that characterize Western medicine.

Folk Medicine

The tribals in the many tribal belts that exist within and on the borders of India still practise folk medicine. So do the numerous villages that dot the large landscape of India. Even in urban centres, many of the poor and destitute take recourse to folk medicine. Folk medicine has its own concepts about the cause of disease—usually the wrath of gods, evil spirits, magic and witchcraft. The diagnostic tools rely basically on divination. Treatment is based on removal of the cause by propitiating the gods through incantations, exorcism and sacrificial procedures. It is indeed amazing that in tribal areas, even when the government opens clinics, dispensaries and hospitals, the tribals prefer their own indigenous system of medicine—of *vaids,* brahmins, herbalists, exorcists, snake-bite charmers and the village midwife or *dai*. These are specialists and healers who have the people's faith and confidence. It will require a great deal of education before true ayurvedic medicine, let alone Western medicine, becomes acceptable to these poor people. If the old order is to change, the new order, to begin with, must be so projected that it does not contradict or violate their ancient beliefs.

Yoga and Tantric Medicine

Yoga is an important school of Hindu philosophy, which influences other schools of Indian thought. Yoga and Tantra are not systems of medicine. However, they enunciate principles which aim at making a person both physically and mentally healthy with a constructive outlook on life and constant mental harmony. Its basic texts are the *Yoga Sutra* by Patanjali (*c* fifth century BC). Some Yoga practices are even seen in the Mohenjodaro seals, with a divinity sitting in a yogic posture. The *Rig Veda* and the *Upanishads* mention different yogic *asanas*. Yoga, in essence, is the joining of the individual soul to the universal soul or the union of the personal spirit with God.

There are eight stages of the Yoga process. The first two are preparatory stages of restraint and moral purification. The *asanas* are a series of exercises in which a single posture is held for a length of time, sometimes using breath control and without any distraction to achieve complete relaxation. The next stage demands withdrawal of the five senses from the world outside. With concentrated meditation, the *yogi* is aware of his own inner self and is able to attain a complete release from worldly bonds.

Different *kriyas* cleanse and refresh the body, while the *asanas,* by exercising every muscle through regulated exercises help to cure or relieve many diseases. Certain schools of Yoga have become an end in themselves, like Hatha Yoga with its various body postures and breathing exercises which are used for therapeutic purposes, mainly relaxation. Yoga is becoming more and more popular in the Western world, where it is being investigated scientifically. It is considered especially useful to help counteract and relieve the stress and strain of modern life.

A Tantric form of Yoga states that a latent power called the *kundalini* lives like a coiled snake at the base of the spine. Tantra aims at awakening the *kundalini* and bringing it up along the spine by yogic disciplines to a thousand-petalled lotus situated under the skull. When this succeeds, release and bliss are attained.

Tantra aims at making the human body immortal and undecayable through the use of the mystical or physical elixir the *amrita*. Practitioners of Tantra have experimented with metallic compounds, formulae and procedures, which were subsequently used in medicine. In Tantrism, the human body acquires an importance that it had never attained before in India. Tantric philosophy maintains that the human body is a manifestation of divine substances and energy. The practitioner of Tantra believes that he is the microcosm or the epitome of the universe. There is nothing in the universe which is not present in the human body. The physical processes of cosmic forces run parallel to the biological processes in man. Thus tantric processes are used for achieving both worldly and spiritual desires.

It does not require a great deal of contemplation to realize that Ayurveda, Yoga and Tantra all spring from the roots of Indian philosophy and religion.

7 Medical Education and Public Health

To learn and become proficient in Ayurveda, a student had three options. He could attach himself to a teacher (*guru*), in whose house he worked and lived. The teacher–disciple relationship was common not only in the sciences but also in the arts, in particular music and dance. The other option was to join a *gurkula*—a school in the forest, away from habitation, where the pupils and teachers lived together and where instructions were imparted on the art and science of healing. The last option was to enter one of the big centres of learning in India. These centres were located in larger cities, and were Taxila near Rawalpindi (now in Pakistan), Nalanda and Varanasi (Benares).

Taxila was the greatest centre of learning from the sixth century BC onwards. It was world-renowned and attracted students from all parts of India, as also from the Far East and the West. Vincent Smith in his *History of India,* writes:

> It was the leading seat of Hindu learning where crowds of people from all quarters were taught the Vedas and the eighteen accomplishments. It was the fashion to send princes and the sons of the well-to-do Brahmins on attaining the age of sixteen, to complete their education at Taxila, which may be properly called a university town. The medical school there enjoyed a special reputation, but all arts and science could be studied under the most eminent professors.

Some of the most learned men in ancient India graduated from Taxila or were teachers of this university. They included Chanakya (Kautilya), Panim, Jivaka, and Nāgarājuna.

Nalanda flourished from the fifth to the twelfth centuries AD. To be admitted to Nalanda and to study there was a mark of great distinction. Those who successfully went through its portals after completing their studies were dubbed the 'Nalanda Brothers' and were held in great respect. Two Chinese pilgrims Hiuen Tsang and I-Tsing, who came to India in the reign of Harsha and a little after, have left glowing accounts of Nalanda. Hiuen Tsang noted that students from China, Mongolia, Tibet, Korea and Japan came to study at Nalanda and returned home with the benefit of an excellent education.

Nalanda was a university town. The huge institute of learning was a mile long, half-a-mile wide and was completely enclosed by a huge wall. At its peak, it had 40,000 students and 1,500 teachers residing within or near the campus. It had probably the biggest library ever for its time and age, and was comprised of three buildings. Some of the buildings of the University were reported to be six storeys high. Amazingly, food, clothes and tuitions were free for the students—these being donated by the king, princes of the royal family and by affluent nobles.

Varanasi (Benares) was as ancient as Taxila and Nalanda and as famous. It remains today the oldest surviving active university in the whole world.

To be a teacher in these institutions required high qualifications and qualities. One had to be wise and learned, proficient in secular and spiritual knowledge, conversant with different aspects of medicine, and most of all, eager to continue to learn all one's life.

Students too were selected with great care. Only 20 per cent of those seeking admission to Nalanda were admitted. Besides good character, the candidates before starting the study of medicine had to be proficient in the study of the *Vedas,* the *Brahmanas,* the *Upanishads,* the *Sutras,* Sanskrit literature, *Dharma-sastras, artha-sastras,* as also the basics of arts and science, poetry, literature, philosophy, algebra, geometry, arithmetic and astronomy.

Admission into the university was solemnized by an initiation ceremony. Work was serious, hard and constantly supervised by the teachers. Practical training had three objectives—examination of the patient, training in surgery and preparation of medicines. The student was introduced to the various medical properties of herbs. He learnt the art of concocting herbal medicines, preparing combinations of minerals and herbs, combining and isolating minerals, reducing stones and minerals to ashes. He was taught botany and the care and preservation of plants.

For surgery, different techniques were taught on different inanimate objects before the student was permitted to try his skills on humans. Thus incisions were taught on gourds, watermelon, cucumber; excisions were taught by making openings in full water bags. Venesection was taught on the vein of a dead animal; probing was taught on worm-eaten wood; extracting by withdrawing seed from the kernel of jackfruit.

Equal importance was given to both theory and practice, and, as in modern times, discussions and seminars presided and moderated by teachers became a valuable and frequent method of imparting education.

The duration of a medical course at these universities was uncertain. At least in the case of Jivaka, the great Buddhist physician who studied at Taxila, it lasted seven years. On completion there was a theory-cum-practical examination. Successful candidates were given a degree at a special ceremony during which they took an oath to be exemplary in their conduct and behaviour. I quote relevant passages to point out that the Hippocratic oath in ancient Greece had an equally beautiful parallel in the oath embodying the ethical code of the medical profession in India. This ethical code is mentioned in the *Charaka Samhita.*

Day and night, however thou mayest be engaged, thou shalt endeavour for the relief of the patient with all thy heart and soul. Thou shalt not desert or injure thy patient even for the sake of thy life or living. Thou shalt not commit adultery even in thought. Thou shalt not covet other's possessions. Thou should be modest in thy attire or possessions. Thou should speak words that are pure, gentle and righteous, pleasing, worthy, true, wholesome, moderate. Thy behaviour must be in consideration of the time and place and heedful of past experience. . . . No persons who are hated by the king or who are haters of the King shall receive treatment.

While entering the patient's house thou shall be accompanied by a man who is known to the patient and who has his permission to enter, and thou shall be well clad, self possessed and conduct thyself with dignity. Having entered, thy speech, mind, intellect and senses shall be entirely devoted to no other thought than that of being helpful to the patient and of things concerning him only. The peculiar customs of the patient's house shall not be made public. Even knowing that the patient's span of life is coming to a close, it shall not be mentioned by thou there, where if so done, it could cause shock to the patient and to others. Though possessed of knowledge, one should not boast very much of one's knowledge. Most people are offended by the boastfulness of even those who are otherwise good and authoritative.

To the above charge in the *Charaka Samhita,* the *Susruta Samhita* adds:

The twice born Brahmin, the preceptor, the poor, the good and the destitute—these thou shall treat when they came to thou like thy own kith and kin and relieve their ailments with thy medications. Thus behaving, good will befall thee. Thus thy learning will attain popularity, fame, righteousness, wealth and fulfilment.

A qualified physician, before he started practice, needed the sanction of the King. This was to protect people from quacks. Charaka gave detailed descriptions and distinguishing features between trained ayurveds and quacks.

The brahmin, the preceptor, the poor, the friend, the recluse, the sage and the helpless were entitled to free treatment and medicine. Others paid the physicians for his services. Charaka emphasized that medical practice should be humanitarian. 'A medical teacher should be like a mango tree that gives all its fruits to others and retains none for itself.'

Public Health

Most ill patients were looked after in their own homes. Those who had none to look after them were admitted to hospitals. These were built and financed by the state.

The Edict number 11 of Ashoka (274–236 BC) reads:

> Everywhere in the kingdom of the King Piyadasi, beloved of the gods, and also of the nations who live in the frontiers such as the Cholas, the Pandyas, the realms of Satyaputra and Keralaputra, as far as Jambapani in the kingdom of Antiochus, King of the Greeks and of the Kings who are his neighbours, everywhere the King Piyadasi, beloved of the gods, has provided hospitals of two sorts; hospitals for men and hospitals for animals.

Fa-hein (AD 405–411), a contemporary of Chandragupta Vikramaditya, gave a description of charitable dispensaries in Pataliputra:

> The nobles and householders of the country have founded hospitals within the city to which the poor of all countries, the destitute, the crippled and the diseased may come. They receive every kind of help free *and freely*. Physicians inspect their diseases and according to their cases order them food and drink and medicine or decoctions, everything in fact that may contribute to their ease. When cured they depart at their own convenience . . . .

Hiuen Tsang (AD 629–645), who was in India during the reign of Harsha states:

> In all the highways of the towns and villages throughout India, the Emperor erected hospices (*punya-salas*) provided with food and drink and stationed there physicians with medicines for travellers and poor persons to be given without stint.

Thus hospitals and poor houses were spread out over the whole country. The poor houses were called *dharamsalas* and were the equivalent of western alms-houses, monasteries and infirmaries.

In the Deccan and the south, between the sixth and ninth centuries (in the Pallava period), there is evidence of village dispensaries often close to the temple complex. In the Chola period (AD 900–1200), dispensaries were termed *vaidyasalai*—*vaidya* meaning medicine and *salai* meaning a charitable institution. There were numerous such dispensaries manned by local physicians, whose posts were often of a hereditary nature. Physicians were often paid in kind, but many attended the physical needs of patients without expecting any returns.

Hospitals in the Chola period were also often attached to temples. This is proven by inscriptions on temple walls detailing the hospital built in the temple complex, the doctors attending it, and the salaries paid to them. Thus, for example an inscription in AD 1262, on a stone pillar of the Malakapur Temple in Andhra Pradesh commemorates the Kakatiya queen Rudramma and her father Ganpati, who donated several villages south of the Krishna to Vishweshwara. Vishweshwara used a third of the income accruing to him to build a maternity home, a third for a hospital and the remaining for a school.

The munificence of the kings, princes and the wealthy of the land funded these hospitals and dispensaries. The belief that an act of charity as magnanimous as this may open the doors of heaven might well have prompted this largesse.

8 Perspectives

There is an inescapable tinge of sadness when one reflects on the history of Ayurveda. An encouraging observation, however, is that this ancient art and science of healing, over 2,000 years old, is still acceptable to the millions who live in the villages of this country. Perhaps it is because the ethos of Ayurveda is close to the ethos and culture of India. Perhaps a rejuvenated Ayurveda may take its place side by side with Western medicine.

Till the eighteenth or even the nineteenth century, there was little to choose between Ayurveda and Western medicine except in surgery, where the West was clearly superior. Western medicine then started to gallop away, leaving Ayurveda far behind. One of the main features for this disparity is the spirit of scientific enquiry in the West, which led to the great advances in the natural sciences. It took a couple of hundred years for these advances to become relevant to patient care, but when this did happen, medicine in the West got increasingly transformed. This dedicated spirit of scientific inquiry was greatly lacking in India between the sixteenth and nineteenth centuries. There were of course a few brilliant stars in the Indian firmament, but by and large the landscape was bleak. There are probably several reasons for this. Once the British colonized the country, it was the Western system of medicine that was thrust upon the country. Ayurveda stagnated and continued to be taught through the guru-shishya oral tradition. Perhaps it was the sanctity of this oral tradition which hindered the progress of this art and science. The discovery of the printing press by Gutenberg in 1439 at Strasbourg made all knowledge, including medical doctrines, thoughts and practices available to most people in Europe. This was encouraged by a progressively increasing literacy rate in the West. In India, dissemination of knowledge was sparse and very limited. After all, among the millions in the country, how many could gain access to the few handwritten medical manuscripts inscribed on birch bark? On the other hand, the printed word was carried far and wide in the West. Ideas were disseminated not only to scholars but to all who could read. These ideas were like 'challenges' that were bound to elicit a 'response'. It was this basic fact that led to a quicker unravelling of scientific and medical truths in the West. In India, the oral tradition of imparting and spreading knowledge, coupled with the respect shown by a disciple (*shishya*) to his teacher (*guru*) were strong impediments to research and advance in science. There was thus no challenge to the old prevailing thoughts and therefore no response. All fields of human endeavour, in particular the natural sciences and medicine have advanced only through a series of challenges evoking responses, which in turn initiate further challenges and responses. Lacking this basic requisite, India fell far behind.

The history of India also influenced the history of Ayurveda. The roots of Ayurveda developed against the background of philosophy, religion and the realization of spiritual values. From the sixteenth century onwards, the socio-political history of India was disrupted beyond measure. The country became increasingly divided into warring kingdoms, the craving for power and pelf replaced the desire for knowledge and wisdom. The caste system alienated millions of poor destitute Indians, who would otherwise have surely contributed to the wealth of the country. The inequities of wealth, and the disparity in economies bred a feeling of resignation and despair rather than revolution, as it did in France in 1789, which changed the history of Europe. Into this maelstrom of confusion, the British, to serve their own ends, further damaged the fabric of civilization that was a heritage of milleniums. The natives were considered inferior, the white race superior—a scar on the psyche of India which has not healed to this day.

Let it not be said that natural sciences and medicine could have flourished in spite of this turmoil. No human endeavour succeeds in isolation; every endeavour is influenced by politics, political stability, religion, philosophy, economics and above all by the mental strength, ability and attitude to the emerging problems of the world. The ancient art and science of India stood handicapped at a crucial period in the history of man.

Chinese Medicine

9 Historical Background

The superior doctor prevents sickness;
the Mediocre doctor attends to impending sickness;
the inferior doctor treats actual sickness.

Chinese proverb

Chinese medicine is as old as Chinese civilization. It grew out of Chinese philosophy—for the basic thoughts that ruled Chinese philosophy almost since the birth of civilized time in that ancient country became promptly applicable also to the art and science of healing. Thus, the philosophy of the opposing forces of *yang* and *yin* that created and motivated the universe were the very same forces that operated in man, who was a universe unto himself. Medicine was also influenced by history, religion, customs, codes of ethics, the clash of arms, discoveries in science, by art, literature, by China's deliberate policy of isolating herself from the outside world and perhaps, to her feeling of innate superiority over other contemporary civilizations.

Traditional Chinese history begins 5,000 years ago in an era of legendary hero-kings, followed by the three dynasties of antiquity—the Hsia, the Shang and the Chou. It is from the Chou dynasty (1027–256 BC) onwards that we have a nearly perfect record of Chinese civilization and history. Kung Fu-Tsze or Confucius (551–479 BC) was the outstanding personality of this period. He was China's great reformer, a humanist, a colossus of his time who seemed to have inherited the wisdom of the ancients and who codified this wisdom into a set of rules and principles that governed life and society. Scholars revered him for editing the classics and for having written the *Spring and Autumn Annals*—a work of literature as influential as the *Bible*. Like Socrates, Aristotle and Plato of ancient Greece, Confucius too was concerned with the virtues of rulers and the features of an ideal society. His teachings were moralistic, benevolent, humanist, yet traditional and authoritarian in contrast to the dynamic and lively abstractions of the Greeks. Confucius exerted a tremendous influence on China in every field of human activity for several centuries. He gifted China the world's most efficient and stable bureaucratic power that helped to rule the country through many trials and tribulations with wisdom and efficiency.

The Chou dynasty was followed by the Ch'in dynasty and then by the great Han dynasty. It was the Han dynasty that established and consolidated China as a great sovereign power in the world. Starting out from the cradle of Chinese civilization along the banks of the Yellow river, military expansion extended the Han Empire to the land mass of what today constitutes modern China, including the region formerly termed Manchuria. The distant reaches of the Han Empire included North Vietnam, North Korea, Mongolia and many of the oasis cities along the Silk Route in Central Asia which the Han dynasty explored and established. The Han kingdom had a strong centralized government with the largest and probably the most powerful army in the world. The Hun nomadic tribes of the north were the kingdom's main enemies. There was no natural barrier to prevent their repeated incursions. China built the Great Wall as a barrier to these repeated invasions. The Great Wall snaked along the mountains and undulations of the north, proverbially like the Chinese dragon, keeping her enemies at bay. The wall began during the Ch'in rule and was continued during the Han dynasty till it stretched for over 3000 miles along the northern reaches of China.

Han rule lasted about 400 years from 206 BC to AD 220; its influence in East Asia was comparable to the influence in Europe of the partly contemporaneous Roman Empire. The expansionist goals of the Han Empire led to the conquest of China's fertile southern regions, gifting whole new fields of plants and herbs to the pharmacopoeia of Chinese medicine. Trade with India and the Persian Gulf area benefited both commerce and medicine.

Several dynasties rose and fell—there came the northern Wei, Sui and the Tang dynasties. The first two were short lived but prepared the ground for the long and glamorous rulers of the Tangs (AD 618–907). China entered into the golden age of domestic peace and prosperity and into a period of great imperial expansion. For once, there was a tolerance to all foreign people, to new ideas and images. Buddhism had reached China from India by the fifth century BC and was the main religion of the country. Other religions in small measure were also introduced. These were Zoroastrianism, Manichaeism, Nestorian Christianity, Judaism and Islam. They all contributed their own ideas and imagery to the exciting events within the country during the period of this Chinese Renaissance.

The capital of China in the Tang dynasty was Sian (Ch'ang-an). It was the seat of power of unquestionably the largest empire in the world, as also the world's most populous city of two million inhabitants. The capital was the richest, most carefully planned city of the world and expressed the highest achievements in organization, technology and art of the period.

The Tang dynasty disintegrated in 907, to be followed successively by the Sung (960–1279), the Yuan or Mongol (1279–1368) and the Ming dynasties (1368–1644). The last of the dynasties before the formation of the Chinese Republic in 1912 was the Ching or the Manchu dynasty (1644–1912).

Till the Ming period of China's history, Chinese civilization was, indeed, superior to any other civilization and the Chinese were firmly convinced of this. China remained unchallenged by any advanced civilization till modern times. Though often invaded by culturally inferior nomadic tribes, it ended by civilizing, absorbing and assimilating them within its teeming people. It had great discoveries in art, science, industry and agriculture to its credit. The Chinese were using water clocks 600 years before these were independently invented in Europe. Water processed armillarias were turning in China three hundred years before Copernicus. The Chinese invented paper and introduced the technique of paper-making to the rest of the world. China invented printing roughly five centuries before Gutenberg produced movable type. She invented gunpowder hundreds of years before the West, but unfortunately failed to utilize the firepower of this invention in time to avoid its prolonged humiliation by Western powers. China had evolved a system of medicine that was effective and appealing to the ethos and psyche of her people.

The beauty of China's art, her bronzes, the quality of her jade and the exquisite artistry with which jade was shaped and carved were the envy of the world. Chinese inventions in pottery and in porcelain—their shapes, colours, glazes and designs from ancient times—remain unsurpassed to this day. Chinese calligraphy was and continues to be like painting, and its paintings reflect the philosophy, the serenity and an exquisite artistry equal to the best in Western art. It is no wonder that China treated her neighbours as vassals and the rest of the world as barbarians. Westerners visiting China were treated with curiosity and as cultural inferiors. Said Emperor Ch'ien-lung of the Manchu dynasty to Lord Macartney, ambassador of Britain to China in 1793: 'Our celestial empire possesses all things in prolific abundance.'

It is a fact that China dominated the eastern half of the world for more than twenty centuries, up to 1839. The Chinese called their country *'the Middle Kingdom'* or *'All that is under Heaven'*. This was all to end in the middle of the nineteenth century. Events changed quickly in the west from the eighteenth century onwards. The Age of Reason and of Science led to a spate of scientific discoveries that changed the Western world. The Industrial Revolution was born, altering the face of Europe, but China lay asleep cocooned within its mesh of smug self-superiority and old traditions.

A clash of civilizations was inevitable. In the 1840s, Britain and France waged war on China to permit the import of opium into the country—a practice that was destroying the moral fibre of the Chinese people and was therefore strongly objected to by the Manchu king. The Manchu dynasty was repeatedly humiliated as the Western powers joined hands to seize and control the major ocean and river ports of the country. The corruption within the Manchu empire led to a decay within its internal politik. The great internal rebellion within China was the Taiping Rebellion—a titanic effort to overthrow the Manchu dynasty. After fourteen years of civil war and the loss of forty million lives, this peasant rebellion was finally crushed with the help of Western mercenaries.

In 1900, the smouldering hatred against the 'white devils' culminated in the Boxer Rebellion, which was defeated by an Allied invasion of Peking. The European powers, Japan and the United States imposed the most crushing and humiliating indemnities on China, robbing it of all prestige. Even the small countries of the west like Belgium, Holland, Portugal lined up like vultures to gobble up and share in the spoils of victory. The Manchu dynasty died and the Chinese Republic headed by Sun Yat-Sen was born. It was a short-lived republic.

China was now ravaged by war as never before in its long history. Famine stalked the land in 1929 and floods devastated it in 1939. The Japanese pounced on this benighted country in 1931 and resolved to conquer it. In the midst of the Sino-Japanese war rose the Nationalist Kuomintang under Chiang Kai-Shek and the peasant forces of the Communist Party of China led by Mao Tse Tung. A civil war to the death ensued. The armies of the Nationalist forces under Chiang-Kai Shek were large and trained, but the Communist forces under Mao Tse Tung were motivated and indomitable in their spirit. Mao and his troops followed by thousands of peasants broke through the Kuomintang ranks and began the historic Long March covering 6,000 miles and lasting 368 days till they reached the northern province of Yunan. It was from this northern redoubt that Mao waged his successful war against the forces of Chiang Kai-Shek. The Long March probably represents the greatest triumph of the spirit of man against every conceivable adversity. The feats of any other army in the world could be likened to picnics when compared to the exploits of the Red Army on the Long March under Mao Tse Tung. In the final analysis, the conflagration that enveloped China ended with the triumph of the Red Army under Mao Tse Tung and the defeat of Chiang Kai-Shek who fled China with his forces to Taiwan. Communist China under Mao Tse Tung was born in 1949. Chairman Mao was the modern icon that replaced Confucius. China, the rudely awakened giant was now astir, the world fears, and soon it may well begin to tremble.

The encounter with the West exposed China to its limitations and prompted it to draw level in the fields of science, technology and medicine. It is doing so, yet when one looks deep into its quickly-evolving modernity, the grip of ancient values and tradition can still be discerned. They are far too deeply buried in the Chinese psyche to be lost forever.

10 Traditional Chinese Medicine

An alchemy of legend and fact, of superstition and wisdom veil the roots and early growth of Chinese medicine. The history of Chinese medicine dates back to at least 5,000 years to the legendary Emperor Shen Nong (*c* 3400 BC) who is believed to have introduced agriculture to his country. Chinese historians consider him to be the discoverer of herbal medicine. A Han dynasty historian wrote—'Shen Nong tested a myriad of herbs and so the art of medicine was born.' Medicine in that era must have been the domain of tribal shamans and mountain recluses, very similar to what existed in ancient India. These 'hermits' or 'recluses' withdrew from community life and retreated deep into the forests and hills of ancient China to practise the 'Way of Long Life'. This included a herbal diet, the use through trial and error of herbal plants of medicinal value, kung-fu exercises, and the practice of special breathing techniques. The analogy to similar regimes followed by recluses and the *yogis* of ancient India is inescapable.

If Shen Nong is accepted as the founder of Chinese medicine, it took about another 2000 years before his observations and those who followed him were put down in writing. It was around the same time that the concept of 'medicine' in the Chinese written language first came into being— medicine as *yaa* and the doctor as *yi*.

By the time of the *Yin* dynasty (around 1500 BC), references to medicine were appearing on oracle bones. Archaeological excavations have unearthed 1,60,000 inscribed carapaces and bones briefly describing illnesses prevalent in that period of Chinese history. In about 500 BC the concept of herbal medicine came to be described in Chinese by the term *ben cao*—*ben* signifying a plant with a rigid stalk and *cao* any grass-like plant. The term soon included ingredients from the animal and mineral world, thus embracing the whole of the Chinese pharmacopoeia.

It was during this period of history that medicine and its further evolution became intrinsically and inseparably linked to Chinese philosophy. In fact it would be correct to state that medicine had its earliest origins in philosophy.

Philosophy and Medicine

The origins of Chinese philosophy are said to go back to the Emperor Shen Nong, 'who wrested from nature a knowledge of her opposing principles'. These opposing yet complementary and reciprocal forces were termed the *yin* and the *yang* forces of nature, and their concept is the core of Chinese philosophy and is central to the understanding of Chinese medicine. The *yin* and *yang* are the two primordial cosmic forces that pervade and control all life processes and all phenomena within the universe. It is the balance between the *yin* and *yang* and the interplay between the two that controls the universe and all life within it. *Yin* is the passive or the negative force—female in nature; dark, descending and is symbolized by water. *Yang* is the active positive force—male in nature; bright, ascending and is symbolized by fire. It is the relative balance between these two cosmic forces within the body and between the body and the environment that determines health and regulates life. An imbalance signifies a departure from health and when marked, leads to disease and death. To an extent the body adjusts the relative balance of the *yin* and *yang* automatically. When the imbalance is excessive, health is lost and medication is required to restore this balance. Chinese medicine con-centrates on avoiding this imbalance through preventive care involving proper diet, exercise and attention to changes in the external environment as with different seasons or changes in weather. Therapy in every aspect of Chinese medicine is aimed at redressing the imbalance between the *yin-yang* forces by supplementing the deficient force and attempting to reduce the excessive force.

From 600 BC onwards, two great Chinese philosophers incorporated the above concepts into rules and ethics of conduct and life. Confucius (551–479 BC), China's greatest sage propounded that right order and harmony within the universe were based on a delicate balance between the *yin* and the *yang* forces. Man must contribute positively to this balance by exerting an essentially moral force through the cultivation of the five virtues of benevolence, justice, propriety, wisdom and sincerity. Great as Confucius was, he not only upheld the values of

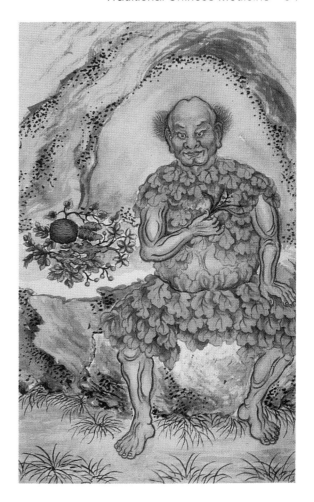

Fig. 10.1 Shen Nong seated at the mouth of a cave, dressed in traditional garb made from leaves, holding a branch with leaves and berries in his right hand.

old traditions, but also sanctified them as immutable and unchangeable. He thus maintained:

> Gather in the same places where our fathers before us have gathered; perform the same ceremonies which they before us have performed; play the same music which they before us have played; pay respect to those whom they honoured; love those who were dear to them.

Though this concept had an intrinsic value particularly in that time and age, it probably became an impediment to China's progress in the fast evolving, quickly-changing world of today.

The other great sage was Lao Tse, the father of Taoism. Tao became the 'path' to universal harmony and righteous order determined by the balance and the relation between the *yin* and the *yang*. The Neo-Confucian thinker Dong Zhongshu in 100 BC, considered man as a miniature universe, containing within him the locked forces of *yin* and *yang*. Physical health was thus integral and included within this all-pervasive Chinese philosophy. It followed that the Taoist principles of balance of opposing forces became applicable to diet and medicine. Food was not given for mere sustenance but to balance forces that regulated physical and mental health. They were classified thus into cold foods, such as fruits, vegetables, and fish to reduce heat in the body; hot foods such as fatty meals, fried foods, and spicy foods to provide heat to the system, and supplementary foods such as proteins, chiefly consisting of organs of animals, to strengthen the corresponding organs in the human system.

Medicinal diets were soon in practice. Only when these failed were drugs prescribed. Herbal tonics included garlic, ginseng or ginger. Herbal soups came to be used for minor ailments—for example, lotus root or watercress soup in a pork broth for colds and upper respiratory infections. Finally, medicinal foods were used for serious illnesses. These included various recipes of numerous medicinal herbs or plants in the Chinese pharmacopoeia. The purpose of this escalating assault on ill-health was to restore the disturbed balance between the opposing *yin* and *yang* within the body.

Influence of Other Medical Systems

China was perhaps one civilization in the world which literally blossomed in comparative isolation. There was however early contact with India and Tibet. Buddhism spread from India to China linking the two ancient civilizations. Medical practices and concepts were important aspects of Buddhist teachings. They were brought by Indian Buddhists who travelled to China. Famous Chinese scholars also visited India, studied its civilization and returned with ideas, precepts and valuable manuscripts that enriched Chinese civilization. The *kung fu* system of Chinese exercise as also the breathing exercises in Chinese medical mythology were closely related to the principle of Yoga and to aspects of Ayurveda.

As the might of the Chinese Empire increased, trade routes opened up to Persia, the Arabic world and the Mediterranean West, as also to other South-East Asian countries. In the second century BC, the Chinese ambassador Chang Chian spent many years in Egypt, Syria and Mesopotamia. He returned with knowledge on drugs and the practices of medicine in these countries. In the fifth century AD the Byzantine king expelled the Nestorian Christians from Constantinople on the ground of heresy. A portion of this diaspora travelled to China, bringing to the country the knowledge and wisdom of the Mediterranean world. It is of historical interest that the mother of Kublai Khan (1216–1294), the founder of the Mongol dynasty, was a Nestorian who arranged for European doctors to visit China.

Early Medical Writings

Ancient classical Chinese medicine was based on the wisdom of their legendary Chinese emperors. The most ancient was Fu Hsi who is believed to have originated the *pa kua*, a symbol composed of *yang* and *yin* lines combined in eight separate trigrams representing all *yin* and *yang* conditions. In the Han dynasty, the knowledge on herbs acquired by the legendary Shen Nong (said to have been transmitted orally for centuries) was recorded in a book called *Shen Nong ben Cao Jing*, the Pharmacopoeia of Shen Nong. In this book, herbal plants fell into three categories—the upper class which nurtured life, the middle group which nurtured vitality, and a lower group labelled poisons or medicines from toxic plants used only against dangerous life-threatening illnesses.

The wisdom and exploits of the Yellow Emperor Huang Ti (2600 BC) were recorded again during the Han dynasty in the *Nei Ching* (the Canon of Medicine). Transmitted orally for many centuries, this work was written in about the third century BC, but was subsequently revised to its present form in the eighth century AD. The section on Ling-Hsu (spiritual nucleus) deals with acupuncture. Huang Ti was also said to have been responsible for the *Discourses of the Yellow Emperor and the Plain Girl* which discussed the Taoist concept of sex in great detail.

Later works include those written by Sun Szu-Miao (AD 561–682) who summarized medical knowledge of that time and age into thirty volumes, and also, with the help of others, produced a fifty-volume collection on pathology. A treatise on forensic medicine titled *Hsi Yuan Lu* was written in the Sung dynasty. It remained an authoritative text on medical jurisprudence for centuries.

Great Ancient Physicians

China's first great physician renowned in Chinese history was Bian Que (407–310 BC). He was renowned for his skills, practised acupuncture and introduced the first gynaecological and paediatric treatments.

China's next most renowned physician was Zhang Zhongjing. Many consider him the Chinese Hippocrates. He wrote one of the most celebrated treatises in Chinese medicine titled *Discussion of Fevers*. It appears that many of the elders in his family succumbed to various fevers, and Zhang Zhongjing devoted his life to the study of fevers. His book contained over a hundred prescriptions based on as many medicines, most of which were herbal in nature. He classified diseases into six types—three of the *yin* types and three of the *yang* types. His prescription was designed to restore the balance between these two forces by inducing or reducing sweating, elimination or vomiting. Zhang contributed to the art and science of acupuncture by drawing the map of meridians along which the body's vital energy or *qi* was believed to flow.

One other great Han physician was Hua Tuo (AD 141–208) who introduced the use of 'narcotic soups' to dull the senses for the treatment of abscesses, superficial tumours and wounds. The herbal ingredients for these 'soups' were Datura metel, Rhododendron Sinense and Aconitum. History records his treatment of the Han general Guan Yu who had his arm badly injured by a poisoned arrow. Hua applied his anaesthetic successfully cutting the flesh and scraping the bone. The agony in spite of the supposed anaesthetic must have been fearful. The Taoist attitude towards pain was to bear it without emotion, and in true Tao tradition the general is supposed to have continued to play chess while Hua operated on his arm.

Hua Tuo was also a keen devotee of the martial arts developed by the mountain recluses and practised as one aspect of Chinese medicine. He developed a series of therapeutic *kungu fu* exercises based on the rhythmic activities of five animals—the deer, bear, tiger, monkey and crane. These exercises were invigorating for the circulation and respiration, helped digestion, prevented constipation, eliminated fatigue and preserved the strength and suppleness of muscles, joints and ligaments.

By the third century AD Chinese medicine had evolved in all aspects—its immense herbal pharmacopoeia, its philosophical science, its spiritual core, its sexual doctrine, the use of acupuncture, therapeutic exercises and its medicinal relation to diet. The Confucian doctrine that venerated tradition preserved these essential features of medicine with little or no change till the turn of the twentieth century when the West manoeuvred its first confrontation with China. However, modern China now stepping into the twenty-first century has not divorced herself from her ancient traditions.

Concept of Health and Disease—The Four Humors

Chinese medicine believes that there is an invisible life force or vital energy termed *Qi*, which permeates, animates and energizes all life in the universe. There is no equivalent to this 'humor' in the humoral theory of Western medicine, but there is a similarity to the Indian concept of *prana* meaning 'breath'. *Qi* is transferable; digestion extracts *qi* from food and drink and transfers it to the body. Breathing extracts *qi* from air and transfers it to the lungs. When these two forms of *qi* meet in the blood they form the human *qi*. Though *qi* is influenced by the external environment, it is largely influenced by the food and drink consumed, and the air that one breathes. This explains the great stress on the medicinal importance of diet and of breathing exercises in Chinese medicine.

The human *qi* has two forms—the 'nourishing *qi*' or the *ying qi* and the protecting *qi* or the *wei qi*. The nourishing *qi* is formed from the most nourishing essence of digested food; it nourishes organs, glands, bones and all tissues of the body. The protecting *qi* complements the nourishing *qi* and circulates on the surface of the body beneath the skin. It controls the opening and closing of the sweat pores and exerts a protective influence on the body. It is the harmonious balance between the vital energies within the body as well as the balance between those in the body and the external environment that determines the state of health. When the nourishing *qi* is deficient, the body succumbs to diseases afflicting vital organs. When the protecting *qi* is weak, the body is susceptible to environmental factors that can cause disease.

Taoist philosophy has an interesting concept of the *yuan qi* or 'primordial vital energy'. It is the original collective vital energy one is born with. From the time of birth it suffers a gradual progressive decay, deterioration and dissipation. The rate of decay determines life span. The secret of longevity in Taoism is to slow this decay of primordial vital energy, for which, Taoists advocate breathing exercises, *kung fu* exercises, diet and herbal tonics.

Human *qi* is the first and most important of the four humors of Chinese medicine. The others are blood (*xue*), vital essence (*jing*) and fluid (*jin-ye*). Blood, like the nourishing *qi* is formed from the most refined products of digestion. Its movement in the circulatory system is controlled by *qi*. Vital essence is also formed through the effects of *qi* on digested food and drink. It takes two forms—life-essence and semen-essence. Life-essence controls growth, development and well-being. Semen-essence is equivalent to the spermatozoa in the male and the ovum in the female. The embryo formed by the union of the male and female semen-essence is nourished by the life-essence formed by this union. The last of the body humors is a fluid (*jin-ye*) also extracted from digested food or drink and also acted upon by *qi* to assume a special quality of life. The quantity and balance of this fluid is a vital factor in health and is hence constantly regulated by all vital organs, in particular the kidneys. *Qi* and the three other body humors are closely associated with one another and a disturbance in one adversely affects the other. *Qi* may rightly be termed the master humor. It is the only one, which, besides being extracted through digestion, can also be extracted from air by the lungs.

The Five Elements

The world, according to Chinese philosophy is divided into five primeval forces represented by five symbolic elements—wood, fire, earth, metal and water. Each of these symbolically has its own sphere of influence and the interaction between these elements together with the *yin* and *yang* forces determines all activity in nature. The primeval forces represented by these five elements interact according to their relationship. Each force has a generative or suppressive action on the other. In turn it is influenced in the same manner by another force. This Chinese concept, like so many others, is purely symbolic. Man is a microcosmic representation of nature and the symbolism described above is also applied to man. Chinese medicine believes that each vital organ belongs to one of the five elements and the inter-reaction between the function of various organ-systems can be understood through the pattern of interaction that exists in nature between the five elements and the forces of *yin* and *yang* operating within the body.

The exact science of anatomy founded by Vesalius in the West was totally absent in China. Surgery on internal organs was not practised till the twentieth century. Traditional Chinese medicine was more concerned with establishing the functional relationship between organs to help in the diagnosis and treatment of disease. The symbolic, syncretic approach to health and disease involving the *yin* and *yang* and the five elements is indeed a unique feature of Chinese medicine. It combined art, science, and philosophy in the right proportions to create a system which the Chinese found effective both in the prevention and treatment of disease.

The Chinese Meridians

In addition to blood vessels carrying blood, lymphatics carrying lymph and nerve fibres carrying nervous impulses, the Chinese postulate the presence of an additional important connecting system which links various organ systems enabling them to influence one another. This additional system is termed the *jing luo* and is composed of 'meridians'. These meridians are of crucial importance because they circulate the body's singlemost vital essence '*qi*,' on which health and life depend. There are fifty-nine meridians within the body, of which twelve constitute the main or dominant meridians. Each main meridian constitutes an energy system centred around one of the vital organ-systems in the body. *Qi*·flows from one meridian to the other, covering the entire network and supplying energy to the body. Just as the Tantric Yogi in India can control the rise of the 'kundalini' coiled in the base of the lower spine, so can a Taoist sense and direct the flow of *qi* along this complexity of meridians. The main meridians directly connect coupled *yin–yang* organs. In addition to the main meridians there are fifteen 'connecting' meridians, twelve 'muscle' meridians, and eight extra meridians, all being branches of the twelve main meridians and serving to distribute *qi* to every single part of the body. The network of meridians forms a complex interconnecting grid. Stimulating one of the main meridians with acupuncture has a specific effect on the organs connected by that meridian as also a general effect on the body because of the intricate interconnection between the meridians. Chinese medicine acts not only by reaching a particular organ through the bloodstream but also by reaching it through the appropriate meridian. Disturbance or imbalance of vital energies from organs needs to be first diagnosed. It can then be corrected by stimulating the appropriate meridian through acupuncture or by the use of appropriate Chinese herbal medication.

Diseases

Smallpox was known since ancient times. In the eleventh century, prevention of smallpox was attempted by placing scales from smallpox pustules into the nostril. Wearing the clothes of a patient who had the disease was considered another method of protection. The relation of cow-pox as a protection from smallpox was perhaps vaguely realized, since ingesting powdered fleas from infected cows was thought to prevent the disease.

Pestilence, plagues and epidemics of various diseases swept the land from times immemorial. During the Han dynasty, an epidemic of what appears to have been typhoid decimated two-thirds of the population of one region.

Precise descriptions of leprosy and tuberculosis are given in Chinese medical literature. Venereal diseases were described and were given various therapies. The seventeenth century physicians used arsenic for syphilis.

Hospitals were established during the period of Buddhist influence in China, particularly in the Han and Tang dynasties. These hospitals were staffed by priest-physicians and they offered medical care for the poor and the sick. The rich or the upper classes preferred to be treated at home. In the ninth century, when anti-Buddhist sentiments prevailed, hospitals as well as temples were destroyed on a massive scale. However, by the twentieth century, hospitals had again become numerous and every district had a 'tax-supported' hospital.

Practitioners

The institutions of Chou, compiled hundreds of years before Christ, mentioned five categories of physicians. These were chief physicians (who collected drugs, and examined other physicians), food physicians (who prescribed food and drink), physicians for simple diseases, ulcer physicians (who probably included surgeons), and physicians for animals (veterinarians).

As early as during the Chou and Tang dynasties physicians had to submit their own medical audit—their successes and failures. This audit determined their professional rise or decline. An examination system was introduced by the seventh century AD. Only successful candidates were eligible to practice. This was four centuries earlier than the first licensing system in the West. Formal medical schools probably existed from the tenth century onward. These grew in number under royal patronage particularly in the fourteenth century during the Ming dynasty. Specialization started early in the Chou dynasty; there were nine specialties that grew into thirteen during the Mongol dynasty.

Obstetrics was practised by midwives for several centuries. However, it is not clear when women first practised medicine, but women were officially recognized as physicians by the fourteenth century.

Diagnosis and Treatment

The microbe hunters in the West revealed a host of micro-organisms causing disease. Even today, the Chinese physicians practising traditional Chinese medicine maintain that the true cause of disease is not the germs, but conditions which lower a patient's resistance or an imbalance of opposing forces which renders an organ susceptible to the onslaught of specific bacteria. Cure lies in not merely killing the micro-organisms; it lies in rectifying the relative imbalance of the *yin* and *yang* and restoring the normal energy flux of the weakened organ.

The diagnosis of ill-health or disease took the above concept into consideration. It involved a careful history, observing the tongue, the eyes, skin, voice and the rest of the body, feeling the pulse, and feeling the affected parts of the body. The history was crucial; the Chinese physician would want to know how his patient had violated the Tao and the reason for the imbalance of the *yin* and *yang*. This would involve a detailed study of his habits, lifestyle, temperament, household, economic position, type of work, recreation, sex, diet, sleep, dreams and his relations with his family and those with whom he was in frequent contact.

Feeling the pulse was an art and a science, and the most experienced and astute clinician trained in the West would consider the diagnostic claims made by Chinese physicians after feeling the pulse as either incredible or miraculous. The physician felt the pulse first at the right wrist and then at the left. Each pulse had three distinct divisions, each associated with a specific organ and each division had a separate quality. To confound Western minds, each quality also had a large number of varieties, and, again, each division of the pulse had a superficial and a deep projection. The hundreds of different characteristics of the pulses that both Chinese and Indian physicians claimed to recognize seem to be impossible to those trained in Western medicine. The treatise *Muo-Ching* required ten volumes to describe the intricacies and diagnostic possibilities on feeling the pulse. To what extent imagination influenced truth in this field of Indian or Chinese medicine would be impossible to determine.

Treatment was to direct attention to the cause of disharmony within the body forces and to restore this balance. This could involve first and foremost a change in habits and the approach to life. Food in China was medicinal and its medicinal importance has already been stressed. Exercise, breathing exercises, and the use of herbal tonics have already been mentioned.

Herbal medicine to cure disease was not just a form of medical treatment. It established itself as a philosophical concept central to the physical and spiritual well-being of man. The concept of herbal medicine included not only the use of herbs but also parts of trees, insects, stones and grains. The therapeutic minerals and metals included mercury (for venereal diseases), arsenic and magnetic stones. Animal-derived remedies included dragon teeth (powdered fossilized bone) and virtually any material obtainable from living creatures—parts or segments of organs, urine, dung. There were thousands of items and many more thousands of prescriptions to choose from.

A legendary medicinal herb, still in great use today is the *ginseng* (man-shaped root). This fabulous root in ancient China was famed for delaying old age, restoring sexual powers and increasing strength and vigour. It was also reported to improve diabetes and stabilize blood pressure. Its rejuvenating properties have come under scientific scrutiny today. Whatever the outcome of this scrutiny, millions in the East and many in the West are convinced of its efficacy and are prepared to pay fabulous prices to obtain the high-grade wild roots of *ginseng* obtained chiefly in China and Korea.

Another medicinal plant in existence in ancient China was *ephedra* (*ma huang*), described by the Red Emperor and used for thousands of years as a stimulant, to induce fever and perspiration and to treat asthma. *Ephedra* entered both the Indian and Greek pharmacopoeia and became known for its medicinal properties all over the world. Japanese investigators purified the active principle in *ephedra*, which was *ephedrine*. The scientific pharmacological *raison d' etre of ephedra* was thus established. There must be many such drugs in the oriental pharmacopoeia, which, though used empirically, may well have a scientific basis. Thus the seaweed used for centuries to treat enlargement of the thyroid is known to contain iodine. The willow bark used in China for fever contains salicylic acid, the mulberry flowers contain rutin, a treatment for hypertension. It is questionable whether opium was used in China in its early history or whether it was used only after the West began to export the drug into the country through India.

Acupuncture

The art and science of acupuncture is legendary, perhaps even antedating the introduction of Chinese herbal medicine. The aim of this treatment was to restore the balance between the *yin* and the *yang*. Needles are inserted in the skin at varying depths through any of the 365 points along the twelve meridians that carry the life force *qi* as detailed earlier. Each of these points is related to a specific

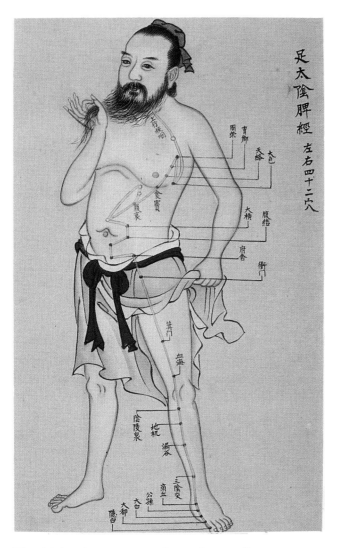

Fig. 10.2   Acupuncture chart of a standing man.

organ. The Chinese use acupuncture techniques to treat a vast array of illnesses and to relieve a number of symptoms, in particular pain. Its empiric use has now been shown to have a scientific basis as the insertion of needles (and twisting them about) within the skin has been shown to release endorphins—natural substances formed within the body known to cause relief of pain.

Acupuncture began to be used in Japan and Korea by the tenth century and spread to Europe by the seventeenth century. Today it is an important mode of alternative medicine in many countries outside China, especially for problems unrelieved by Western medicine.

Moxibustion is a form of treatment in which a powdered plant substance is fashioned into a small mound on the skin and burnt, producing a blister. The same meridian and points that govern the placement of acupuncture needles are also used in moxibustion.

Spread of Chinese Medicine to Korea, Japan

The influence of Chinese medicine in Korea was well established by the sixth century AD. In that era a dreadful epidemic ravaged Japan and the Korean physicians who were consulted to help combat this epidemic introduced Chinese medicine into the country. Soon Japanese doctors went across to China for greater experience. Late in the seventh century AD, a Chinese school of medicine was founded by the Japanese physician Wake Heroya. This school flourished in spite of initial opposition and aimed to bring back traditional Japanese medical practice. As in China, the Japanese insisted on intensive prolonged training in medicine followed by a difficult examination before granting a medical license to practise.

11 The Impact of the West

From the earliest period of recorded history extending into the golden period of the Ming dynasty of the 1600s, Chinese science and technology were perhaps a thousand years ahead of developments in the West. The art and science of healing, particularly when applied to patient care was also in no way inferior to that in Europe. But then the West changed—there came an age of reason and an age of scientific discoveries—and by the turn of the nineteenth century new vistas were being successfully explored in natural sciences and medicine. China, like India, was isolated and barred from the spirit of science by its ancient traditions, which had been almost sanctified with religious beliefs. Tradition preserved a sense of continuity, order and a graciousness of thought, manner and life, but it locked the door to change and progress in a rapidly evolving world. The impact of the West with China in the nineteenth century smashed this door open—awakening a giant which had gone into slumber for nearly three hundred years.

By the middle of the nineteenth century, Japan and the weak Manchu dynasty of China were confronted with the combined military, political and scientific strength of Western powers. There was arrogance and a sense of superiority behind this strength. The Meiji government in Japan adopted the German system of medical training and by the turn of the twentieth century had several medical schools modelled on the German style.

The weak Manchu dynasty was incapable of reforms. Western medicine was thrust upon the country by missionaries and by the Rockefeller-funded Chinese Medical Committee. The early decades of the twentieth century saw the establishment of medical schools in Beijing and in other cities of China.

Republican China (1911–1949) modelled the system of medical education and practice along Western lines. The plans looked good; medical institutions, hospitals and health centres from cities down to villages were organized, but their efficacy, when translated into actual health care, was poor for several reasons. The major drawback was the failure to realize that a system that was good for the West could not be easily transplanted into a land with an alien civilization and different values. Then again, war tore China apart. First there was the Sino-Japanese war and then the civil war between Nationalist China and Communist China. When Communist China was born in 1948, Chinese medicine made a comeback. Science began to be deified, traditions were purposely trampled upon and smashed, yet physicians trained in Western medicine were also required to train in traditional Chinese medicine. The success of the 'barefoot doctors' in attending to the basic medical needs and problems of the millions living in villages brought home to all the Third World countries the fact that health care was possible without resort to expensive technology.

Today, basic Western medicine and advanced medical technology are features of modern Chinese medicine. Yet, not only in China, but also in Japan and Korea, a familiarity with the ancient traditional Chinese medicine is necessary for all practitioners. An attempt to scientifically evaluate many of the empirical postulates of traditional medicine is under way and the science behind a number of empiricisms has indeed been proven.

Though modern China idolizes science and has made rapid advances to catch up with the West, amazingly, traditional medicine has survived. Perhaps this is because its philosophy remains deeply embedded in the collective consciousness of the Chinese people, because its concept of preventive care and holistic care are still valid even in the face of the 'miracles' that Western medicine has to offer. Thousands of traditional herbal medicine shops in China, Korea, Japan, Hong Kong, Singapore and in any large Chinese settlement in the Western world are witnesses to this survival. Medicine awaits a meeting ground between the East and the West where the best of each will enrich the future of Man.

Medicine in the Classical Age
of Greece

12 An Overview of the Greek World

Between wisdom and medicine there is no gulf fixed; in fact medicine possesses all the qualities that make for wisdom.

Hippocrates

During the thousand years before the birth of Christ, the heart of civilization moved from the heat and dust of the lands of Egypt and Mesopotamia to the craggy shores of the Greek peninsula, to the sunlit islands glistening like pearls afloat on the Aegean waters, and the coast of Asia Minor which had witnessed the ebb and flow of earlier civilizations.

Greece was not born along the banks of a river as were the civilizations in Egypt, Mesopotamia, India and China. She was born in a land of limestone mountains and valleys, lapped by the sparkling blue waters of the Aegean Sea, blessed by dazzling colours, a brilliant light and by a temperate climate. Nature posed a different kind of challenge, which evoked a different, and, even more brilliant response than the civilizations which preceded it. Classical Greece is rightly perceived as the mother of Western civilization and the cradle of the human spirit. No longer was man a pitiable plaything or pawn in the hands of tyrants. He was a being of great worth and honour, capable of great thoughts and great actions. Man was made in the image of their gods—only he was mortal. Freedom of the human spirit and respect for his individual worth, were at the very core of Greek civilization. In the words of the great Athenian statesman Pericles: "Each single one of our citizens in all the manifold aspects of life is able to show himself the rightful lord and owner of his own person and can do this moreover with exceptional grace and exceptional versatility."

Greece posed the eternal questions to the world. What is Nature and who is Man? Where does he come from and where does he go? Debate on these questions was free and fearless. From this debate and the curiosity of the human spirit to understand man and nature was born philosophy. The sixth and seventh centuries before Christ were unquestionably the most epochal 200 years in antiquity. It was during this short historical time-axis that by a strange coincidence, philosophy blossomed in Greece, Zoroaster preached the first monotheistic religion of the world in Persia, Isiah preached in Judea, Buddha taught in India, Confucius and Lao Tse appeared in China. Great philosophy and great religions were born into the world.

From the sixth century BC onwards the Hellenes (as the Greeks called their country) consisted of a number of city states—the greatest of which was Athens ruled by men who laid no claims to divinity. Greek civilization reached its apogee between 500 to 400 BC under Pericles, who presided over the destiny of Athens. These one hundred years witnessed the presence of Herodotus, Hippocrates, Aeschylus, Sophocles, Euripedes, Socrates, Plato and Aristotle. Science, literature, art and philosophy blossomed under their tutelage as never before. The concept of rational medicine and of medical ethics was born as a consequence of the spirit of scientific inquiry into man and nature.

The Greeks of the classic era, which dates from 750 BC, believed that they were the descendants of legendary heroes with splendid physiques, who performed feats of prodigious strength and valour. Archaeologists over the last century have unearthed evidence that this civilization of legendary heroes flourished between 1400 and 1200 BC and was centred around the city of Mycenae, the capital city of the king Agamemnon, who in legend led the Achaeans (the ancient Greeks) into the Trojan war. The heroic Mycenian civilization was in turn a development of an even more ancient world called the Minoan civilization which flourished from 1900 to 1400 BC and was centred in Knossos on the island of Crete in the Aegean sea.

Darkness fell over Greece from 1200 to 750 BC. Dorians, the barbaric Greeks from the north, came in waves to shatter the Mycenean world. Athens in the province of Attica was the only city that was able to resist the Dorians; it became the centre of the Greek revival. To escape the Dorian onslaught, Greeks from the mainland poured into Athens or emigrated across the Aegean Sea to make new homes on the many Aegean islands and on the western coast of Asia Minor. These Greek colonies came to be called Ionia, but they preserved their links with the mainland.

Three major factors were responsible for the unity and a sense of identity amongst the dispersed Greeks. The first was the beauty of their great epics, the *Iliad* and the *Odyssey,* sung and compiled by the blind bard Homer about a thousand years before Christ. Every Greek identified himself with these epics, and was proud of the strength, valour, beauty and magnificence of the heroes and their exploits Homer so beautifully extolled. These verses, written in hexameter, were the main-springs, the life-blood of the blossoming classical era, a source of inspiration and strength that bound the Greeks into unity. The second unifying factor was the Olympic Games held every four years from 776 BC. Strength, speed, agility and valour were tested between individual Greeks who arrived from far and near to compete for the victor's laurel wreath. Their marathon race commemorated the feat of Pheidippides—who, after the Greek victory over the Persians at Marathon, ran without pause from Marathon to Athens, gave news of the victory and then dropped dead. The third factor was the appearance of the Greek alphabet towards the end of the Dark Ages. The new alphabet included vowels to supplement the consonants of the Phoenician alphabet. The Greek alphabet led to the Etruscan alphabet, which in turn inspired the Roman alphabet—the alphabet of the Western world.

By 750 BC, darkness was replaced by a shimmering dawn and over the next 350 years the sunlight of Hellenism spread its glow of culture and beauty all over the Greek world. Commerce thrived, riches increased, releasing men to pursue art, science, literature, poetry, philosophy and politics. The freedom of thought and of speech encouraged a spirit of inquiry that contributed, as never before, towards every field of human endeavour.

In 336 BC, Alexander of Macedonia united Greece under his kingship. He carved out, with his heroic feat of arms, an empire that extended east as far as the Indus river in India and that included Eastern Europe, Egypt, Persia, the Middle East, and South Asia. After the death of Alexander, his empire split. For a while, Alexandria, which had been founded by Alexander, in Egypt, became the centre of learning and culture. The mantle of Greek civilization was now to be passed on to the rising star of Rome in Italy.

Politics

Democracy began as a Greek concept. There developed within Greece the concept of the city-state (*polis*) and there were many such city-states. Every free citizen of a city-state voted to elect men who would rule them. Yet slaves were not allowed to vote and the ratio of slaves to free men was generally ten to one. Each city-state jealously guarded its liberty and rights so that dissension and wars between city-states were common. Yet, by and large, these city-states were centres of order because the spirit of liberty was balanced by the enforcement of law. It was a democratic law made by the popular consent of people for the good of all people and not for a select group of priests or kings. Greek law was the fount of all legal systems that were to follow later in Western civilization.

The Greeks had an overriding passion for freedom and an abhorrence of tyranny. Aristophanes, the great playwright, castigated in a play an office-holder thus: "This public robber, this yawning gulf of plunder, this devouring Charybdis, this villain, this villain, this villain." And according to law "If anyone rise up against the people with a view to tyranny—whoever kills him—shall be blameless."

The Olympians

The gods worshipped and venerated by the Greeks were as close in their attributes to man as the ancient world had ever seen. They possessed all the ideal qualities of living man, only unlike man they were immortal. They frolicked, played, made merry, made love, made war and meddled constantly in human affairs. They could be afflicted by human frailties without loss of their godly state; they could conspire to mar, placate or destroy humankind, but they did not humiliate man nor did they demand his abject debasement. The Homeric heroes in spite of their legendary prowess had no illusions about immortality. The gods were for the strong; they did not succour the weak. They smiled on the brave and on those in whom great thoughts were matched by valorous action. Man's most grievous sin was 'hubris' when he claimed attributes that belonged not to mortals but to gods. Dreadful vengeance awaited such men.

Arts and Science

Classical Greece has bequeathed to the world some of the greatest treasures in art, literature, science and medicine. The greatness of this legacy is enhanced by the spirit they evoke—the spirit is centred in the belief that Man is unique, free and capable of great achievements. Periclean Athens was the centre of Greek culture.

Greek sculpture may have been equalled but has never been surpassed. The Greeks built temples, elegant in design and of pristine purity in form; they made monuments to commemorate victories and to honour gods, but what they sculpted most of all was man. The idealized human face, figure and form found its perfect expression in the sculpture of the classical Greek era. The stiff, stilted, statuesque art of Egypt gave way to a poetry of motion, to feeling.

Great playwrights wrote great works debating eternal questions on life and death, on love and hate, on retribution and revenge with unsurpassed splendour of speech. The great masters of Greek tragedy were Aeschylus, Sophocles, and Euripides. The great Attic comedian was Aristophenes.

The spirit of inquiry, and the freedom to think led to the founding of philosophy (literally love of knowledge) and science. Philosophers probed into the deeper meaning of life, and into the relationship between man and his environment. Pythagoras, Socrates and Plato were the great thinkers who gave expression to new thoughts, new ideas that are cherished with reverence to this day.

Investigations into the nature of the physical world led them to make important scientific hypothesis. The Egyptians, Babylonians and Indians had accomplished much in the fields of astronomy, mathematics and engineering. The Greeks used this knowledge as also the knowledge uncritically gathered through millennia by older cultures to establish a theoretic basis for applied sciences. Whereas the earlier civilizations observed facts, the Greeks went on to derive general principles from observing facts. They advanced the study of astronomy—a practical necessity for a sea-faring nation. They had a greater understanding of the weights and stresses for building, and derived general principles on the nature of space, matter and motion, which they expressed in mathematics and geometry. The foundation of western music was made in Classical Greece when Pythagoras discovered the numerical ratios of the length of string that would produce a seven-note scale.

Research into nature was combined with research into human actions and this made the Greeks the first historians. Amongst the intellectuals attracted to Periclean Athens was Herodotus, the father of history who wrote the history of the Persian wars. Herodotus' successor, Thucydides, wrote the history of the Peleponnesian wars.

To the Greeks, philosophy, science and medicine were closely related fields. Medicine, like science and philosophy, grew out of the curiosity to know more about man and his environment. Observation, argument and proof were used to postulate a hypothesis and to move from one hypothesis to another. Both philosophy and science influenced and shaped the study of medicine. Medicine was also naturally influenced by the spirit of the times, the spirit of the importance of man in the world, the spirit of inquiry, and the freedom to pursue and express this inquiry. People of Greece were at liberty to practice the art of healing as they chose. This must have led to debate, an exchange of thought, to diversity, and to a freshness in the approach to the growing art and science.

In the following chapters medicine in prehistoric Archaic Greece has been dealt with briefly, followed by the schools of medicine in Classical Greece. These include the cult of Aesculapius, the Italic school and, most important of all, the school of Hippocrates. We shall then briefly dwell on the relation between philosophy and medicine in Greece and finally on medicine in Alexandria.

13 Medicine in Archaic Greece—The Homeric Age

Little is known about the practice of medicine in ancient Greece before the advent of recorded history. Archaic Greece, by inference, must have been influenced to some extent by Egypt and therefore must have had priest-physicians using rituals, divinations, incantations and charms to ward off evil and restore health. But there were certain distinct features that characterized early Greek medicine. The Greeks even in the most ancient times were concerned, as no other earlier civilization had been with the cultivation of supreme physical fitness. The Olympic Games that began in 773 BC were a test of this fitness. Instructors in gymnastics, exercise, diet and massage were prominent at these games. Preservation of health and prevention of disease formed the basis of this rather unique philosophy of life. The human body in its strength, form and beauty was to be a reflection of the idealized immortal figures of their pantheon of gods.

The Homeric epics, the *Iliad* and the *Odyssey,* constitute the only written reference to medicine in Premycenean and Mycenean Greece. In that heroic age every warrior was a physician. Homer mentions how these warrior-physicians were adept at removing arrow-heads and javelin-points from wounds. They knew the use of pressure to stop bleeding, the importance of cleaning and washing wounds, the use of compresses, balms and salves to promote healing and of bandages to protect wounds. References are also found about medicines made of herbal extracts, of potions to relieve pain, and of wine to revive the injured.

Frolich in his impressive study noted that the *Iliad* described 147 wounds with an overall fatality of 77 per cent. Wounds from arrow-heads had the least mortality when compared to those inflicted by spears, javelins and sling-shots. Wounds from heavy iron swords were always fatal.

The warrior-physicians were aware of the rough anatomy and function of the muscles, tendons, joints and bones of the human body. They observed how an arrow that pierced the heart would quiver with each heart beat and how death occurred quickly from blood loss if the arrow was plucked from such a wound. They knew that the wounds in the forehead and through the windpipe were among the most dangerous of all, that a javelin thrust or an arrow piercing the breast could go through the lung, and that a thrust in the buttocks could pierce both the rectum and the bladder.

It is evident from a study of Homer's work that medicine even in the early years of Greek history followed a path distinct from that in Egypt. It remained empirical as it was in Egypt, but it divorced itself quickly from magic and priest-craft. It went on to become secular—being practised by laymen in times of peace and by warriors in times of war. The legendary hero and warrior Achilles himself was said to have been instructed in the art of healing by no less a teacher than the wine centaur Chiron.

A doctor commanded immense respect in ancient Greece. Homer wrote: "He is worth many lives, being unequalled in removing arrows from wounds and healing them with herb ointments." The doctor to whom Homer paid this fulsome tribute was Machaeon, son of Aesculapius, who with his brother Podalirius served as surgeon to the Greek army besieging Troy. Machaeon attended on king

Menelaus who had been wounded by an arrow. The surgeon removed the arrow-head, sucked the blood flowing from the wound, and then applied a healing salve—whose use had been taught by Chiron to his father Aesculapius. Legend had it that Chiron, the founder of Greek surgery was turned into a centaur, a creature half-horse and half-Man. He was so famous for his wisdom and excellence in surgery that on his death, he rose to heaven, taking the form of the constellation Sagittarius.

It is surprising that Homer, in his epics, does not deal with or recognize other diseases like plague, dysentery, tetanus, gangrene or other infections. But then, the ancient Greeks were cast in a heroic and often legendary mould. The Greek warrior fought as the gods would have him fight. If wounded he either died or he recovered with the medicines then available, to fight once again. Heroes of ancient Greece were made to die of wounds and not succumb to mundane illnesses that afflicted ordinary humankind.

14 The Cult of Aesculapius

The practical and pragmatic practice of medicine existed in the Homeric era side by side with a practice of medicine which used faith and religion as the means to heal. The pantheon of Greek gods delighted in meddling in human affairs. The *Iliad* contains references to Apollo and other Greek gods who could inflict infection and disease, and yet could also heed the prayers of the afflicted and grant succour if they so wished. This religio-magical medicine or healing through faith and through the intervention of gods is a legacy bequeathed to man from earliest antiquity. The Greeks did not escape it, nor have we, even as we stand at the threshold of the twenty-first century.

Many Greek gods came to be identified with the art of healing. The foremost of course, was Apollo, followed by Artemis, Aphrodite and Athene. The presiding deities of the underworld, Pluto, Prosperine, and Cerberus also had the power to cure or avert disease. The cult of Aesculapius or Asklepios perhaps originated from the worship of one of these underworld deities. The serpent on his winged staff is symbolic. On the one hand, the shedding of the serpent's skin could be construed as a renewal of life. On the other hand, the serpent was the ancient, well-accepted symbol of dark, mysterious, powerful, subterranean forces and was a sacred sign of the god of healing in ancient semitic tribes of Asia Minor.

Legendary powers of healing have been attributed to Aesculapius, but it is impossible to determine whether Aesculapius really lived and practised as a doctor, as did Imhotep of Egypt, or whether he was a legendary figure. He was mythically born of the god Apollo and the nymph Coronis. Her flirtation with a mortal aroused the ire of Apollo who killed the nymph with his arrow. But in death the god delivered her of an infant son Aesculapius. Aesculapius was taught the art of healing by the kind, wine centaur, Chiron. He grew up to be a great and kind doctor who had the supernatural power to raise the dead. Pluto, the prime deity of the underworld, felt that his domain would in time be underpopulated and complained to the gods. Thereupon, Jupiter struck Aesculapius dead with a thunderbolt and carried him up to the abode of the gods at Mount Olympus. Legend has it that Aesculapius then returned to earth as a hero among mortals. On earth, Aesculapius was father of a large family. There was Panacea who had the cure for all things; Hygiea who took care of public health; Telesphorus a surgeon and also a psychiatrist; Machaon the great surgeon who healed the arrow wound of king Menelaus at the seige of Troy and who died heroically in battle.

Aesculapius was worshipped in beautifully designed temples all over Greece. The temples were set in lovely pastoral surroundings with gardens, bathing pools, gymnasiums and often with spring-water acting as spas. Around his figure rose a cult of medicine which attracted the ill and the afflicted in thousands from all corners of Greece.

Artinos of Lesbos, one of the first known Greek poets, who lived around 770 BC, describes in verse the incredible healing powers of this figure. It was probably at this point in history that Aesculapian temples began to be constructed and that his cult began to spread. In the next few

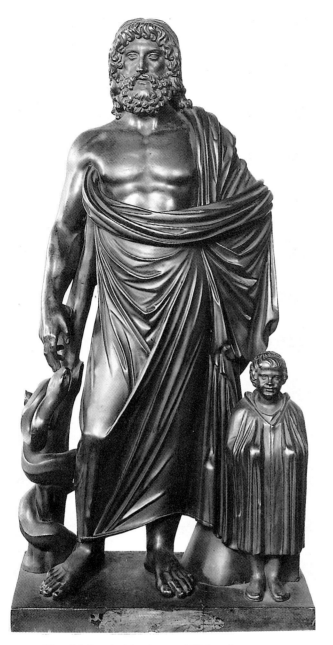

Fig. 14.1   Asklepios and Telesphoros.

centuries a number of these magnificent temples dotted the Greek landscape. Classical authors have identified at least 300 such sites—the most famous ones being at Epidaurus, Athens, Pergamon, Cnidus, Cyrene and on the islands of Rhodes, Delos and Lebera. Interestingly enough, Aesculapius was not recognized on the island of Cos, the birthplace of Hippocrates until the fourth century BC. This was well after the death of Hippocrates, so the cult of Aesculapius offered no rivalry to the Hippocratic methods on the island during the master's lifetime.

Those who flocked to these peaceful sanctuaries of healing went through a period of 'purification' through fasting and bathing. They were then made to approach the altar, and after a purification ceremony, were allowed to enter the sanctum sanctorum of the temple. Then wrapped in covers, they slept on sheep-skins, perhaps drugged by sleeping potions or draughts. They hoped to receive a vision or dream through Aesculapius who would either effect a cure himself or would offer a dream—which on awakening could be interpreted by a priest. If restored to health, the patient would raise a memorial plaque to the marvel of his recovery. These plaques hung outside the temple were a source of both awe and confidence, dispelling all doubts amongst the newcomers to the sanctum. The priests of course made a handsome living, being rewarded with gold by the numerous votaries.

Numerous miracles and cures were said to have been performed in Aesculapian temples—all attributed to Aesculapius the god of healing. Cures and miracles were recorded on tablets hung on the walls of the temple. A tablet recovered by an archaeologist in Epidaurus in 1883 reports of a miracle in a man seeking aid from the god of healing. He had only one eye, the other being an empty socket. He was thought to be a fool for believing that Aesculapius would restore his missing eye. He slept in the inner sanctum of the temple and in his sleep a face appeared. He dreamt that the god poured a special medicine into both his eyes. He awoke at daybreak and walked out of the temple with sight in both his eyes. Miraculous cures of the dumb speaking after a night's sojourn in an Aesculapian temple, of the paralysed walking out at daybreak, of women condemned to infertility, conceiving, are all recorded for posterity on votive tablets which were presented by grateful devotees.

There must, perhaps, have been some chicanery, hypocrisy or greed involved in the workings of these temples, but healing through faith is not to be scorned or laughed at. It persists to this day at many religious shrines, of which Lourdes in France is an outstanding example. The priests in Aesculapian temples did not go uncriticized. Aristophanes, the great playwright and master of satire, satirized with great irreverance the quackery, hypocrisy and greed of the practising priests in his comedy, *Plutus* first performed in 388 BC. The spirit of free thought which allowed intelligent criticism in all spheres of activity, be it religion or art or politics, was one of the basic tenets of Greek civilization. Independent minds saw through at least some of the chicanery that passed for Aesculapian healing in many of these temples. It needs to be remembered that Greek medicine, as practised by laymen, was even older than the Aesculapian cult. It graduated from the warrior-physicians of Homeric times into an art and science based on philosophy, observation and experience. The essence of Greek civilization was the free spirit of inquiry. A priestly religion or religio-magical cult involved supernatural forces and the Greek mind would not readily accept forces which could neither be observed nor measured. This is the reason why the objective and philosophical schools of lay medicine ultimately triumphed over the Aesculapian cult. Even so, the cult of Aesculapius continued into the fourth and fifth centuries AD. The belief in the importance of faith in the process of healing, which was so central to the Aesculapian cult, was borrowed by the Christian church for several centuries.

The pupils of the lay or non-priestly medical school were called Asclepiads—a name which had no connection with the Aesculapian temples. The term came from Podalarius and Machaon—famous doctors who were the sons of Aesculapius. To start with the art of medicine was handed down from father to son. But as time passed, students lived with and were taught by a master like his own adopted sons. By the sixth century BC medicine was recognized as a profession. The Asclepiads, after their study at school, could practice if granted a licence by a council. They charged professional fees for their service to patients. There were physicians in the army, and in the gymnasium (guiding and training athletes) and a number of midwives to supervise and help in deliveries.

Scientific medicine and philosophy were both born in the fifth century BC. The spread of Hellenic culture was not limited to the mainland of Greece, the Aegean islands and the coast of Asia Minor. It also included Greek colonies particularly those in southern Italy and Sicily, which came to be known as Magna Grecia. The school of Greek philosophy which spread its lustre over the Western world and gave birth to scientific medicine, originated in these Italian colonies. Aristotle named this great school of philosophy the Italic school.

15 The Italic School—The Birth of Rational Medicine

The founders of rational medicine in the west were early Greek philosophers of the Italic school. Rational medicine evolved from philosophy and philosophic discussions, and, in its early years, was inseparable from it. Philosophy in turn arose from the burning desire of the Greek mind to understand man and the world around him. Natural events were no longer considered to be miracles. The key to philosophy was reason and there had to be a rational explanation conforming to the laws of nature for all that transpired in the universe. Philosophy also demanded the study of man in his manifold aspects, with the express purpose of devising a healthy, satisfying and happy life. Pythagoras of Samos (580–489 BC) was the first to use the term 'philosophy' in the above context. Pythagoras left Samos because of the tyranny of its ruler Polycrates. He decided to live in Croton, a town in southern Italy already famous for its good medical school. Pythagoras fathered the Italic school of philosophy. He based his teachings on music, astronomy, geometry and mathematics. According to him 'things are numbers', meaning that the basic essence of an orderly universe, of life and living could be expressed in numbers. The universe, Pythagoras claimed, was the macrocosm, governed by the principle of harmony, balanced contrasts and a sense of proportion. Man was the microcosm, reflecting the same principles of harmony and balance.

Before Pythagoras, the concept of disease was shrouded in magical and supernatural beliefs. After his philosophical outlook and influence, disease required a rational explanation. He injected science and rational thinking into the medical school at Croton and instituted very strict rules for initiates wishing to join the school. Those joining the school swore an oath of allegiance to the leader promising never to divulge the knowledge gained within it to the uninitiated.

The most famous pupil of Pythagoras and the most famous doctor at Croton was Alcmaeon. He studied anatomy by dissecting animals. One of his important achievements was the separation of vessels into arteries and veins. He investigated the changes in the nervous function produced by injury to the brain and proposed a theoretic explanation for sleep and death. Sleep was related to the outflow of blood from the brain into the veins. Death ensued when this flow was complete and only in that one direction. Alcmaeon's famous treatise on Nature remained a fundamental medical text for many years. Unfortunately, most of this work has been lost, the only gleanings still extant are quotes from the treatise by later authors, particularly in Plato's *Phaedo*. Alcmaeon offered the Greeks a plausible explanation of disease based on the Pythagorean concept of numbers and on the theory of harmony. Health and ill-health were governed by the relation between elemental opposites—hot and cold, dry and wet, etc. A harmonious relationship between the two opposites resulted in health; disturbance or disharmony in their reciprocal relationship caused disease. The potential source of disturbed relationship or disharmony, according to Alcmaeon, was a natural predisposition, a poor diet and external factors such as climate and altitude. To the modern reader the above views might appear both meagre and elementary, yet at that time and age they were the beginnings of rational inquiry into the cause and prevention of disease.

Alcmaeon had many followers but none to equal him. Philolaus of Tarentum was one of his best students. He lived in the middle of the fifth century BC and taught that the world was the macrocosm and man the microcosm and there was a close analogy between the two. According to him, respiration allowed the coldness of the outside air to counter the heat within the body. This exchange of heat and air induced changes in blood, phlegm, yellow bile, and black bile. Abnormal changes in these humours resulted in disease. He accepted the Pythagorean concept of life as harmony related to a balance between opposing forces.

Another famous doctor of Croton and a contemporary of Alcmaeon was Democedes, considered by Herodotus to be the greatest and the best-paid surgeon of his time. He left Croton to practice in Aegina receiving the huge annual fee of one talent. From Aegina he went to Athens and then to Samos where, the tyrant Polycrates paid him a huge annual fee of two talents. After Polycrates was assassinated by the Persians, Democedes went into the service of the Persian king Darius. He showed his surgical skills by successfully setting right the king's dislocated ankle and healing an abscess in the queen's breast. Darius was happy to grant the physician any wish, except give him his freedom. But to a Greek, freedom was a birthright and cherished most of all. So Democedes persuaded Darius to let him lead a mission to win over the Greek rulers to the Persian cause. But no sooner did he set foot in Greece he deserted the Persians and went over to his compatriots. He was welcomed with open arms by the citizens of Croton, who made him the chief of their magistrature.

Other philosophic pioneers were Parmenides who believed that heat loss was the cause of death, Diogones of Apollonia who studied comparative anatomy, and Democritus of Abdera who showed interest in the cause of epidemic diseases and conceptualized the universe as consisting of space and atoms. Heracleides of Ephesus was the first to postulate that dreams were a retreat into the personal world and had no relation to supernatural causes.

A noteworthy contribution to medicine from the Italic school was Empedocles of Agrigentum who lived around 500–430 BC. He was a famous and majestic figure identified by a laurel wreath on his head, a purple tunic and a gold belt around his waist. A mystic poet, philosopher, physician and a great public speaker all rolled into one, he almost convinced himself that he was god on earth. Empedocles felt that the Universe was governed by the immutable laws of nature. The world was formed from four elements—earth, air, fire and water. He postulated that the heart was the centre of the circulatory system and the seat of the vital spirit *pneuma*. The *pneuma*, or the breath of life was distributed to all parts of the body through the blood vessels. Empedocles was interested in the epidemiology of disease. There is the story (though of dubious origin) that he was able to eradicate malaria completely from the city of Selinuntum by draining the surrounding marshes and that he rid his native city of a raging epidemic by purifying the air through fumigation. The Italic school of Pythagorean philosophy shaped the birth, growth and practicality of rational medicine in the west. This school propagated observation of nature and of Man, experimentation and investigation. It used reason and logic to explain natural phenomena in the universe and to investigate the cause and meaning of life. It introduced and elaborated upon the concept of four elements and their humors, a concept that dominated pathology and the theory of the causation of disease for many centuries. The Italic school was the immediate and necessary precursor to Hippocratic medicine.

Other schools flourished side by side with the Italic school of southern Italy and Sicily. The oldest school was that in Cnidus, off the southern tip of Asia Minor. It was influenced by Mesopotamian and Egyptian cultures and was famous for its *Cnidian maxims,* a collection of important medical prescriptions. Medical schools also developed at Cyrene in North Africa and on the islands of Rhodes and Cos. It was however the school at Cos that was to become the most famous of all the medical schools of antiquity. It was a school that concerned itself with the care of the sick, concentrating on observation of the features of illnesses afflicting man and arriving through rational thinking, at the diagnosis and prognosis of disease. The school at Cos must have been undoubtedly influenced by the winds of different neighbouring cultures—Egyptian, Assyro–Babylonian and Semitic. As mentioned earlier it was conditioned by the Italic Pythagorean School, but its everlasting fame was only possible because of the great teacher and a great humanist who taught at that school. That great man was Hippocrates—the Father of Medicine.

16 Hippocrates

In the fifth century BC, Greek medicine was epitomized by Hippocrates. His teachings have strongly influenced the philosophy and practice of medicine from that early period in history to the present day, and will perhaps continue to do so for centuries to come. Modern historians seem to be of the opinion that all we know about Hippocrates is legend. There is unquestionably no doubt that he did exist, that he was born around 460 BC on the island of Cos more than one thousand years after Imhotep, and died in Thessaly around 370 BC. It is also certain that he was famous as a great teacher, was an itinerant practitioner of medicine and the presumed author of a number of medical treatises. Antiquity has unfortunately cast a veil of uncertainty over his exploits, mixing fact with fiction and coating truth with legend. There were other prominent physicians of this time who were almost as well-known. Chrysippos (whose statue was for a long time mistaken to be that of Hippocrates) was a philosopher-physician of great repute. Euryphon of Cnidos was probably as famous and had contributed to the *Cnidian Maxims*. Praxagoras came after Hippocrates and made a great name as a physician and teacher. Yet, it was Hippocrates alone whose name shone as a star of increasing luminosity through the mists of time. Though he is surrounded by legend, there must have been more than a modicum of truth in his accomplishments and great fame. Aristotle called him 'the great', Appolonius spoke of him as 'divine', Plato likened him to Phidias, and Erotian to Homer. Galen wrote of him 'as the marvellous inventor of all that is beautiful'; authors in the medieval age were the first to describe him as the 'father of medicine'.

Hippocrates learnt the art of medicine from his father Heracleides, philosophy from his friend and patient Democritus, and the art of eloquence and public speaking from Gorgias Siculus. He lived in the golden age of Pericles with other great names of antiquity, including Sophocles and Aristophanes the playwrights, Plato the philosopher, Thucydides the historian, Phidias and Praxiteles. He taught (legend has it under a huge plane tree) for many years at Cos. Among his many students were his sons Thessalus and Draco and his son-in-law Polybus. He travelled a great deal as an itinerant physician to Thessaly, and Thrace, and according to legend, as far as Libya and Egypt. Two rather fascinating legends in his name are worth recounting here. The first is the story that he set fire to the archives of the Aesculapian temple in Cos, forcing him to flee to Thrace and Thessaly. Aesculapian temples did not exist in Cos in the fifth century BC—they came later. The other legend is that after his death his tomb was covered with a beehive—the honey from which had miraculous curative powers. His physical appearance till now was a subject of imagination—a handsome noble face had to accompany great attributes of the head and heart. Recent archaeological excavations have unearthed coins from Cos with profiles bearing the name of Hippocrates, which a sculpted head in a cemetery of Ostia closely resembles. Most authorities accept these archaeological findings as representative of the true likeness of this great man.

The writings of Hippocratic times have been collected together as the *Corpus Hippocraticum*. They number about seventy-two texts and over fifty treatises, documenting the medical history and medical knowledge of those times. These collections were assembled in the third century BC in the great library of Alexandria at the behest of Ptolemy, one of Alexander's generals who ruled Egypt after Alexander's death. It is certain that the *Corpus Hippocraticum* includes the writings of many authors from Cos, Cnidos, Sicily and other schools. Some are later additions, perhaps from the Sophist school. The authenticity of some of these works is doubtful and their authorship by and large undetermined. There are some who are of the opinion that Hippocrates, like Socrates and Christ, never wrote a word and the works so clearly attributed to him were perhaps written by his disciples who later jotted down his teachings. As far as can be judged, the medical texts originating from Hippocrates are—on art, diet, prognosis, the aphorisms, on wounds and ulcers, hemorrhoids, the fistula, on head injuries, fractures, reduction of dislocations, on airs, waters and places. Two of the seven books are on epidemics.

It is outside the scope of this book to dwell at length on the *Corpus Hippocraticum*. Some of the outstanding beliefs of the age of Hippocrates are perhaps best illustrated by memorable quotes—their wisdom and brilliance undiminished by the passage of over twenty centuries. Regarding the art of medicine he says: "I must first say what I believe its scope to be: to take away suffering or at least to alienate it. The fact that those who do not believe in it can be cured by it is strong proof of its existence and power." On the physician—"He must know how and when to be silent and to live an ordered life, as this greatly enhances his reputation. His bearing must be that of an honest man, for this he must be towards all honest people, and kindly and understanding. He must not act impulsively or hastily; he must look calm, serene, never cross; on the other hand it does not do for him to be too gay."

The Hippocratic concept of disease was arresting. He expelled the gods and their role in the causation of disease with one incisive statement: "I am about to discuss the disease called sacred (epilepsy). It is not in my opinion any more divine or more sacred than other disease, but has a natural cause, and its supposed divine origin is due to men's inexperience, and to their wonder at its peculiar character."

The natural cause of epilepsy, according to Hippocrates, was phlegm blocking the airways which thereby caused convulsions of the body in an attempt to free itself of the blocked phlegm. One of the basic concepts of Hippocratic medicine was that health was harmony (originally a Pythagorian teaching) and equilibrium; illness was disharmony and a loss of balance and equilibrium within the body. Balance, harmony, and equilibrium were related to the four humors' of the body—blood, phlegm, yellow bile and black bile, together with their four attributes—hot and cold, wet and dry. Hippocrates on the nature of man comments: "The body of man is composed of blood, phlegm, yellow bile, black bile; these are the humors which make up its nature and can lead to health and illness; man is essentially healthy when these elements are correctly adjusted to each other, both in strength and amount and are well mixed. Illness occurs when one of these principles is present in an inadequate or excessive amount or is isolated in the body and fails to combine with the rest."

The humor 'blood' was associated with life, yet the body expelled this humor when it was in excess as in menstruation or bleeding from other sites. It is possible that this concept was the basis for the practice of blood-letting which originated in Hippocratic times, was practised extensively by Galen and which remained a harmful therapeutic legacy upto the nineteenth century. The humors, white bile and phlegm were visible excretions in disease and were considered harmful. Black bile, the last of the four humors, was perhaps thought to contribute to the darkest part of clotted blood. Interestingly, the four humours (and their four attributes) constituting the body of man (microcosm) corresponded to the four elements, earth, air, fire and water (and their four attributes), making up the ordered structure of the universe (macrocosm).

The concept of humors and their pairs of opposite attributes controlling harmony and balance within the body allowed a rational (even if mistaken) explanation of the cause, effects and treatment of various forms of 'disequilibrium' or illnesses. Similar concepts were independently proposed in ancient Indian and Chinese medicine. Even though the above theory of health and disease may sound fantastic and far-fetched to modern man, it must have had an appealing inbuilt rationale and philosophy for it remained valid upto the middle of the nineteenth century. The role of constitution and other external factors in disease were elaborated upon for the first time in Western medicine in Hippocrates' treatise on airs, waters and places. Climate, ethnic features, diet, constitution and environment in different geographic locales all had a bearing on disease and disease patterns. An understanding of these aspects was central to the art of healing. Extensive and detailed medical-cum-geographic data in this treatise remained an invaluable store of information for over a thousand years.

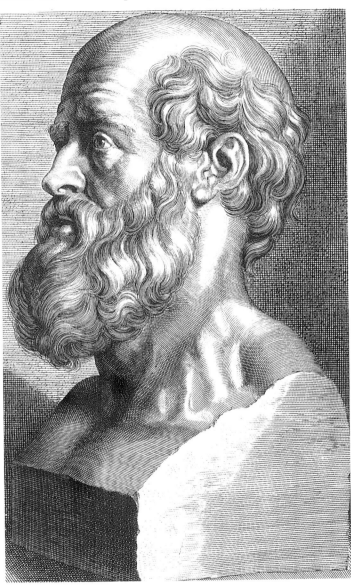

Fig. 16.1   Bust of Hippocrates.

One of the greatest attributes of Hippocrates and his teachings was on the practice of bedside medicine; and on the art of observation of the natural history of disease. The art of diagnosis was related to a holistic understanding of the patient's character, diet, habits, lifestyle, to a meticulous bedside history-taking and to an astute power of observation through the use of the eyes, ears and hands.

The clinical description of disease, considering the meagre facilities in that time and age, remain unsurpassed to this day and still make fascinating reading. One is amazed at the ability of the great healer to grasp the essentials and to ignore the rest. The descriptions of typhus, diphtheria, mumps, tuberculosis, and malaria are classic works of literature and medicine. His description of what is today called the Hippocratic facies in advanced peritonitis remains unequalled: "A prominent nose, hollow eyes, sunken temples, cold ears drawn in with their lobes turned outwards, the forehead's skin rough and tense like parchment and the face greenish or black or blue-gray or leaden." Even today the Hippocratic facies signifies certain death.

Even greater than the art of diagnosis was the ability to prognosticate in illness. This required experience, careful observation and sharp acuity. The art of prognosis often set the Hippocratic healer apart from the quacks and charlatans who practised side by side with Hippocrates in Greece. The desire to predict the outcome of an illness remains as great today as it was yesterday. Again, listen to Hippocrates: "I hold that it is an excellent thing for a physician to practise forecasting. For if he can discover and declare unaided, by the side of his patients, the present, the past and the future, and fill in the gaps in the account given by the sick, he will be the more believed to understand the cases, so that men will confidently entrust themselves to him for treatment."

Therapy in Hippocratic teaching was what we would consider nihilistic. But this great teacher had understood the healing power of nature and so in therapy was chiefly concerned with aiding nature and not hindering it. How pertinent and valid is his great dictum in medicine—*primum non nocere* (first of all, do no harm). Diet, fresh air, rest, exercise, baths, massage, and regulated bowel movements were the mainstays of treatment.

Perhaps the most thorough texts in the *Corpus Hippocraticum* are on surgery. Many surgical problems are treated conservatively; others are subjected to surgery or manipulation. Fractures and dislocations of all types are perfectly described, as are wounds of all kinds, in particular injuries to the skull. The injuries of war figure prominently: "He who desires to practise surgery must go to war."

Haemorrhage is to be controlled by compression, positioning the part when possible; cauterization is frequently mentioned. "What drugs fail to cure, that the knife cures; what the knife cures not, that the fire cures; but what fire fails to cure, this must be called incurable." This is a concept which is pre-Hippocratic, dating from ancient Indian medicine. In

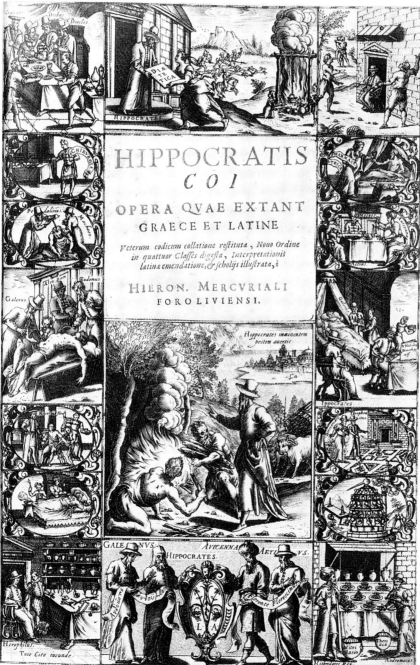

Fig. 16.2   Hippocrates curing the plague of Athens.

the Dark Ages it became an important feature of Islamic medicine and remained in practice in Western medicine till the coming of Ambroise Paré in the sixteenth century.

Operative techniques on tumours, ulcers, haemorrhoids and fistulae are described in detail. Operative techniques also included preparation of the patient, description of the operation table, importance of adequate light on the surgical field, surgical instruments and surgical assistants. Surgical writings in the *Corpus Hippocraticum* have been solely attributed to Hippocrates—they are concise, clear and pragmatic.

The vast experience of this great healer led him to coin 406 sayings in the famous book of Aphorisms. The first aphorism combines philosophy with the basic tenets of medicine: "Life is short; and art is long; and the right time an instant; and treatment precarious; and the crisis grievous. It is necessary for the physician not only to provide the needed treatment but to provide for the patient himself and for those beside him and to provide for his outside affairs." (translation by Dickinson Richards). Many other aphorisms are pearls of wisdom: "In jaundice, it is a bad sign if the liver hardens." "In acute cases, purgatives must not be used except at the start, and then with prudence after careful examination." "Those with hidden tumors should not be treated. If they are, they are liable to die quickly. If they are not then they may yet live a long time." The aphorisms were translated into Latin by the sixth century AD, and by about the mid-thirteenth century many of the aphorisms were assimilated into the popular rhymes of the medical school in Salerno.

Perhaps even greater than the medical texts of the *Corpus Hippocraticum* was the code of ethics laid down by Hippocrates. This Oath of Hippocrates was said to be recited under a great plane tree on the island of Cos by all young men who were formally initiated into the art of medicine. There are some who believe that the oath was not part of the teachings on the island of Cos or Cnidos. There is a view that it is Pythagorean in concept and that it was added to the *Corpus Hippocraticum* in the later years.

Hippocratic Oath

'I swear by Apollo the healer, by Aesculapius, by Health and all the powers of healing, and call to witness all the gods and goddesses that I may keep this oath and promise to the best of my ability and judgement.

'I will pay the same respect to my master in the science as to my parents and share my life with him and pay all my debts to him. I will regard his sons as my brothers and teach them the science, if they desire to learn it, without fee or contract. I will hand on precepts, lectures and all other learning to my sons, to those of my master and to those pupils duly appointed and sworn, and to none other.

'I will use my power to help the sick to the best of my ability and judgement; I will abstain from harming or wronging any Man by it.

'I will not give a fatal draught to anyone if I am asked, nor will I suggest any such thing. Neither will I give a woman means to procure an abortion.

'I will be chaste and religious in my life and in my practice.

'I will not cut, even for the stone, but I will leave such procedures to the practitioners of that craft.

'Whenever I go into a house, I will go to help the sick and never with the intention of doing harm or injury. I will not abuse my position to indulge in sexual contacts with the bodies of women or of men, whether they be freemen or slaves.

'Whatever I see or hear, whether professionally or privately, which ought not be divulged, I will keep secret and tell no one.

'If, therefore, I observe this oath and do not violate it, may I prosper both in my life and in my profession, earning good repute among all men for all time. If I transgress and forswear this oath, may my lot be otherwise.'

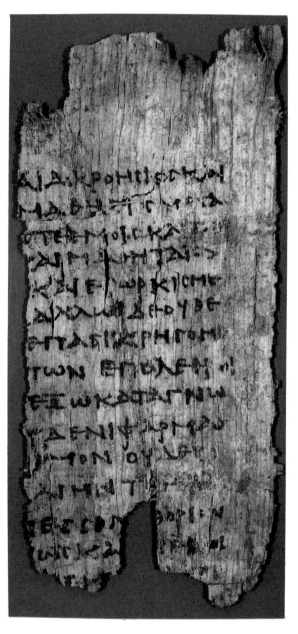

Fig. 16.3   Papyrus text: Fragment of Hippocratic oath, 3rd century AD.

The uncertainties of ancient history make it difficult to assess the exact truth. There are two inconsistencies in the oath when compared to Hippocratic writing. The oath prohibits abortion and contraception, yet the Hippocratic works contain a number of references to the methods of abortion and the use of pessaries. Again, the oath prohibits the use of the knife and yet, some of the most explicit treatises of Hippocrates advocate and explain the use of the knife in various surgical procedures. It is of interest that the main points of the Hippocratic oath are in consonance with the older Pythagorean interdictions against the use of the knife for any reason, the shedding of blood in which the soul was believed to reside, and the taking of life within or outside the body. Even if the oath might basically be a Pythagorean rather than Hippocratic document, it has remained the symbol of the physician's calling. Reference against abortion and contraceptives concurred with the beliefs and the dictat of the Catholic Church in later centuries. The earliest reference to the oath was in the first century AD and it may have thus been added on to the *Corpus Hippocraticum* in later centuries, as it reinforced the religious views of the early Christian era. But does it matter whether the oath is Hippocratic or non-Hippocratic in origin? What impresses one most in this ethical document is the importance of caring proficiently and selflessly for the sick, abjuring fame and gain; of doing no harm to the sick under one's care, of teaching the art of medicine freely to those who wish to learn; of acting with purity and conducting oneself in such a manner that generations in all time to come, in all corners of the world, cherish and value the physician's kindness, goodness and wisdom. Can one ask for a more fulsome code of ethics for Man and Medicine?

The Hippocratic Method

The rational attitudes expressed in Hippocratic writings represent a great advance in medical thinking. It would be tempting to think that these attitudes sprang suddenly and unexpectedly into the civilization of man. It would be more realistic to accept that reason and a rational attitude to life and medicine must have evolved slowly over centuries, or perhaps over millenniums. It is not that the earlier systems of medicine, steeped though they were in religion, magic and the supernatural, were totally devoid of reason and rationality. It is the consistency of the rational approach and the total exclusion of the other approaches that make Hippocratic medicine a great landmark in the history of Man and Medicine. The underlying principles of medical practice in the voluminous treatise of the *Corpus Hippocraticum* are recapitulated here.

1. Bedside Observation

   "A great part, I believe of the Art is to be able to observe." Hippocrates was the first to stress the importance of history-taking in medicine, an aspect of medicine as important as ever and yet often neglected in the mechanized medicine of today. Observation involved the cultivation of all the senses including taste and smell. They were collected without prejudice in a manner similar to the objectivity displayed by a natural scientist in collecting data. There was no attempt to fit observations into a recognized scheme of diagnosis. Hippocrates and those of the Hippocratic school thereby avoided the crime of Procrustes, so frequently committed in modern medicine.

2. The Patient is More Important Than The Disease

   The emphasis was more on the patient and on the care of the patient rather than on the disease. This constitutes the holistic Hippocratic approach comparable to that in ancient Indian medicine. Hippocratic writings have this to state: "Observe the nature of each country; diet; customs; the age of the patient; speech; manners; fashion; even his silence; his thoughts; if he sleeps or is suffering from lack of sleep; the contents and origin of his dreams. . . one has to study all these signs and to analyse what they portend." Listen also to Francis Adams, a nineteenth century physician and a renowned translator of Hippocrates: "The great superiority of the ancient savants (the Hippocratists) over the modern was that the former possessed a much greater talent for apprehending the general truth than the latter, who confine their attention to particular facts, and neglect too much the observations of general appearances."

3. Be Honest Unto Thyself

   Even today intellectual honesty is the trademark of the true physician. Hippocrates laid great emphasis on this attribute. In his collection of case histories more than half the patients died but the natural course of their illness and their lack of response to treatment was reported with the same objectivity as the case histories of those who survived.

4. Nature Heals—Assist It

   This is the essence of therapy in Hippocratic medicine—to help nature to restore a sense of harmony and balance within the body so that health returns. The physician must interfere when his learning and experience convince him that he can help. What he cannot help he must leave alone. "As to diseases, make a habit of two things; to help or at least not to harm."

5. Good Thoughts, Good Words, Good Deeds

   The character of a physician is all-important in the practice of medicine. His code of ethics towards his patients and to those all around him must be unblemished. Kind, caring, modest and attracted neither to fame nor money, he would be a beacon of light to Man through the ages.

Without doubt the Hippocratic method had its weaknesses. It lacked basic knowledge in human anatomy and physiology. This was largely due to the great Greek respect for the body of man which forbade the dissection of corpses. Yet the writings contain significant anatomical details on wounds, fractures, dislocations and on rectal diseases. Again, Hippocratic medicine focussed on the sick man and had little to do with the man in good health. A background knowledge of the physiology of the body was therefore absent, and this was an important lacuna in the interpretation of illness and disease.

The final important limitation was in the lack of specific diagnosis and the attitude of nihilism in treatment. Yet, his descriptions of a number of diseases we know are near perfect. To name a disease is a matter of semantics; the Hippocratic school recognized a particular disease even if they did not name it. Again, relying on the curative power of nature is to be considered praiseworthy. Perhaps many more deaths were caused by physicians in later centuries through meddlesome, dangerous interference, than cures attributed to them. At least the Hippocratic school believed "first of all do no harm". The physician of later years and the physician of modern medicine often forget this basic tenet. In spite of the weaknesses mentioned above, the Hippocratic method is as applicable today as it was in ancient Greece. There is an even greater need in the mechanized medicine of today to observe objectively, to avoid arrogance, to remain unswayed by doctrines and to return to a holistic approach to medicine.

COMPARISON BETWEEN GREEK HIPPOCRATIC MEDICINE AND MEDICINE OF EARLIER CIVILIZATIONS

Now we shall briefly point out the differences between Greek Hippocratic medicine and the medicine practised in earlier civilizations.

Greek medicine grew out of philosophy, which was the quest of the human mind to fathom the order of the universe and the nature of man. Medicine was not only born of but strongly influenced by these philosophic and metaphysical speculations. Hippocratic medicine was based on reason and discarded in its entirety the role of gods, magic, religion and supernatural powers in health and disease. In contrast, the path of medicine in ancient Egypt and Babylon was signposted by magic, rituals and religion, intrinsically and inseparably linked with bits and pieces of empiric medicine.

Politics and geography played a significant role in the development of medicine in Greece. Geographically, Greece consisted of a number of separate city-states on the mainland, in the islands of the Aegean Sea, on the coast of Asia Minor and in the colonies of North Africa. Though culturally united, these numerous and often disparate city-states bred a plurality of customs and methods in several fields of human activity. The diversity in thinking and in attitudes infused a sense of change and vitality in all Greek affairs, including the practice of medicine. Politically, the Greeks cherished freedom and despised tyranny. Free thought and speech led to free debate and discussions and the act of healing was related to other mental pursuits, notably philosophy. This interaction, which was open to public gaze and attention, unquestionably enriched medicine and set it on the path of reason and rationality. In contrast, this diversity, this dialogue between various fields of mental activity was noticeably absent in the Middle East civilizations. The imperial Hammurabic Code and Egyptian medicine laid down a strict code of instructions on health and disease admitting no controversy, no debate, no interaction with other disciplines, and, thus little scope for change. Thus medicine was severed from religion in Greece, but remained hopelessly wedded to religion in Egypt and Babylon; it relied on reason and on rational attitudes in Greece, but retained its irrationality through the belief in magic and supernatural forces in the Middle East; it gained knowledge, wisdom and strength through competition and debate in Greece but remained comparatively straitlaced and stagnant in Egypt and Babylon.

17 Medicine and Philosophy—The Centre in Alexandria

Though medicine was born of philosophy, the pragmatic, practical and rational teaching of Hippocrates had not only purged religion from medicine, but had also loosened the grip of philosophy on its practice. The post-Hippocratic era was characterized by a renewed and strong influence of philosophers and philosophical thoughts on the art of healing. Teachers and medical practitioners split up into a variety of separate sects or medical systems, depending on their philosophic leanings. Among the many philosophers the ideas of Plato and Aristotle exerted the greatest influence. It was Aristotle who pointed out that one could begin with philosophy and would end in medicine; or start with medicine and end in philosophy.

Plato (429–327 BC) was the student of Socrates, a contemporary of Hippocrates, and the teacher of Aristotle. His philosophy and thoughts have had a tremendous influence on Western civilization. Plato's heritage was Pythagorean, and so the science of numbers, mathematics, and geometry figured significantly in his philosophical system. His interest lay in unravelling the mysteries of the soul and of matter. His philosophical inquiries into the nature of man led him into theorizing on medicine. Plato's speculation in medicine was based on reason and logic, but it was divorced from Hippocratic traditions; it was reason at a distance, far away from the bedside and based neither on experimentation nor on direct observations of a patient's illness. Several of his opinions were erroneous but they persisted as staunchly held beliefs not only during his time but for centuries to come. Unfortunately, the method of using reason or logic divorced from the bedside was resurrected in the Middle Ages contributing to an accretion of faulty views in the practice of medicine. The physicians who had implicit belief in Plato were called 'dogmatists'. For them reasoning was more important than observation; logic superseded bedside examination. All diseases were classified according to the humors; therapy was aimed against an excess of a particular humor responsible for disease. Their therapy was as contrary to that of Hippocrates as was their methodology. Extreme therapeutic measures included purging, blood-letting and other dehydrating measures for the treatment of fevers.

Praxagoras, a dogmatist from Cos, will be remembered for being the first to separate the functions of arteries from veins, and for laying an emphasis on the examination of the pulse, whose characteristics could change with disease. However, he confused the prevailing medical concepts by increasing the humors to eleven, and must have inflicted great harm through his overemphasis on blood-letting.

Diocles who lived in the first half of the fourth century was another famous dogmatist who recognized fever as a symptom and not a disease. He distinguished inflammation of the pleura (pleurisy) from inflammation of the lung (pneumonia) and intestinal colic from intestinal obstruction.

Aristotle (384–322 BC), the son of a physician and a pupil of Plato, was a genius, with ideas far ahead of his time. Aristotle also had the distinction of being tutor to Alexander when he was the prince of Macedonia. He exerted a strong influence on his young pupil, and through him indirectly influenced the history of the world in that important epoch. Both master and pupil also directly influenced medicine—Aristotle by founding biology and Alexander by founding the city of Alexandria which was to soon become a centre of learning.

A man for all seasons, Aristotle had tremendous versatility, illuminating the fields of philosophy, logic, medicine, psychology, embryology, zoology, poetry and drama. His anatomical studies on vertebrates and pre-vertebrates were thorough; he could lay claims to be the father of comparative anatomy and of biology. In embryology, he described the *punctum saliens* (the first sign of the embryo), the development of the heart and the great vessels, and was the first to directly observe and describe the beating of the embryo's heart. It was Aristotle who named the large artery arising from the heart, the aorta. Aristotle, in spite of his wisdom, was unable to transcend the concept of humors. He believed in humors, placed the seat of intelligence in the heart, and could not distinguish between nerves, tendons and ligaments. He opined that the veins from the liver were connected to the right arm and those from the spleen to the left arm. A diseased organ situated to the left therefore merited blood-letting from the left upper limb, and that situated on the right merited bleeding from the right upper limb. In addition to the above accomplishments, Aristotle was a gifted teacher and was perhaps the first scholar to supervise and direct investigations carried out by his students. It is strange that though his teacher Plato was theoretical, mystical and metaphysical, Aristotle blossomed into an experimentalist, and a keen observer of nature and natural phenomena. Together, they strongly influenced science and medicine through the Dark and Middle Ages right upto the Renaissance.

The most talented student of Aristotle was Tirtanus from the island of Lesbos. His teacher renamed him Theophrastos, the divine orator, and he is known in history by this name. Theophrastos succeeded Aristotle as a teacher and had over 2000 students under his tutelage, including the playwright Menander. As a botanist he was unsurpassed, right upto the Renaissance. His *History of Plants* and *Cause of Plants* was a storehouse of the medicinal effects of herbs and plants. It was the standard handbook of treatment in Roman times.

There arose other systems in medicine besides the 'dogmatists'. They deserve only a mention just out of historical interest; their contribution was to merely add to a plethora of confused and erroneous theories, making it doubly difficult for future generations to sift the chaff from the grain and to unravel the truth. The group of physicians termed the 'empiricists' felt that nothing mattered more than the result of treatment as observed from experience. Heraclides who lived in the second century BC was a famous empiricist who wrote on symptomatology, and surgery and made contributions to pharmacy.

Methodism was one more system founded around 50 BC. It rejected the theory of humors substituting a far more inferior concept that disease was caused by the constriction or relaxation of the 'pores', as judged by evacuations, secretions and fever in the sick.

Another system was 'pneumatism', which was opposed to 'dogmatism, empiricism and methodism'. Man breathed in the vital spirit, *pneuma,* which first went to the heart and was then distributed by the vessels to all parts of the body. The concept of disease involved interrelation between *pneuma* and the warmth and moisture within the body. Abstruse and absurd as these views were, therapy of the pneumatists was not drastic, and was more in keeping with the Hippocratic practice.

A final sect was that of the 'eclectics'. They followed no single system and had different concepts to explain and treat different diseases. Galen considered himself an eclectic.

Two names need to be mentioned at this stage. Archigenes was an eclectic living and working around AD 100, chiefly in Rome. His contributions to surgery were outstanding. He ligated the vessels to a limb prior to amputation. He advocated amputation not only for gangrene but for injuries certain to lead to gangrene. He also advised against surgery in patients who were too feeble to withstand its trauma.

Aretaeus of Cappadocia (AD 120–180) was a Greek writer during the period of Roman hegemony over Greece. He described many diseases—notably diabetes, which he considered as the 'liquefaction of flesh and bones into urine to an extent that the kidneys and bladder do not stop emitting urine'. He also described diphtheria, epilepsy and mental disorders. He was probably the first to suggest that jaundice could be due to obstruction of the bile ducts. His description of tetanus is classic. "Tetanus consists of extremely painful spasms which are a peril to life and are very difficult to relieve. The attack begins in the jaw muscles and the tendons, but spreads to the whole body, because all bodily parts suffer in sympathy with the first one affected." Aretaeus used the word *opisthotonus* for seizures in tetanus causing hyperextension and an arching of the back; and *emprosthotonus* for a forward flexion of the body.

The tenets of the various schools or sects of medicine mentioned above held sway from the fourth century BC well into the Christian era. During this period of history the centre of learning and thought shifted to Alexandria, a city in Egypt founded by Alexander in 331 BC. Alexander, founder of a short-lived but glorious Greek empire, died in 323 BC, of malaria at the young age of thirty-five. Aristotle, his tutor, left Athens to live in Eubobia, as the political leadership in Athens was anti-Macedonian. He died a year later at the age of sixty-five. Egypt was now ruled by Ptolemy Soter, one of Alexander's generals. Ptolemy was a good soldier, an able statesman, and, above all, a true patron of the arts and sciences. He made Egypt the centre of Hellenic civilization with the city of Alexandria its hub. He built the famous library at Alexandria, gathered together and stored the *Corpus Hippocraticum* within it and collected thousands of manuscripts for the temple of learning. The Ptolemy dynasty was lavish in its financial support to all fields of science and art. These included the natural sciences, philosophy, medicine, mathematics, astronomy, history, music, poetry and other art forms. Ptolemy I Soter (305–284 BC) and Ptolemy II Philadelphos (285–246 BC) founded botanical and zoological gardens and also constructed two building complexes each, the Museum and the Serapeum, each with a huge library. Scholars from all parts of the world were attracted to Alexandria and were encouraged to study and research within its great library.

A contemporary rival centre to Alexandria after 250 BC was Pergamon under the reign of Eumenes I. The Ptolemaic rulers were keen to guard the ascendancy of Alexandria and they banned the export of the papyrus plant. The shortage of papyrus in Pergamon is believed to have stimulated the development of a material from animal skin called *pergamos* (parchment).

The hallowed library of Alexandria was graced by several great and learned men. They came from all over the civilized world. Amongst these were Euclid (*fl.c.* 300 BC), famous for his Euclidean geometry; Archimedes of Syracuse (287–212 BC), the great physicist; Heron (*fl.c* AD 62), the inventor of numerous mechanical devices including a primitive steam engine; Callimachos (305–240 BC) the poet and the great librarian who catalogued the huge collection of scrolls. Medical research flourished in the Museum of Alexandria, the greatest contribution to medicine being in the branches of anatomy and physiology, which had been left singularly undeveloped in Hippocratic times. The two great medical investigators were Herophilus of Chalcedon who lived around 300 BC and Erasistratus of Chios, a younger contemporary who lived around 250 BC. Our information on both these investigators is chiefly derived from the writings of Celsus and Galen in the Roman period. Herophilus was the pupil of Praxagoras of Cos; he concentrated on research in anatomy and physiology, and the study of the pulse. In contrast to Greece, Alexandria for the first time in history permitted the dissection of corpses; according to Galen, Herophilus was the first man to do so.

Celsus, the famous Roman believed that both Herophilus and Erasistratus also practised vivisection. In his foreword to *De Medicina* he wrote that subjects for vivisection were prisoners handed over to their keeping for the study of internal anatomy—shocking, barbaric, and a heinous violation of the Hippocratic code, if this indeed was true.

Herophilus studied the anatomy of the central nervous system, distinguished nerves from tendons and blood vessels, and described the anatomy of the liver, pancreas, intestines, the genital system, the eyes and the lymphatics. He also noted that arteries were six times the size of veins and contained blood and not air. Perhaps most important of all for clinical medicine, he was the first to make a systematic study of the pulse in Western medicine. He noted the various changes in the pulse with different diseases and measured the rate by means of a water-clock. In addition to his brilliant observations and discoveries in anatomy, Herophilus was a practising physician who believed in the humoral doctrine of health and disease using frequent blood-letting and purges to release an excess of humors.

Erasistratus, though more known for his experiments in physiology, also made original contributions to anatomy of the brain, the trachea, and of the nerves. He described the mitral and tricuspid valves in the heart and their functions. He described the epiglottis and noted that its function was to prevent food and liquid from going down the windpipe during swallowing. He also noted the association of fluid in the abdomen with a hard liver (probably a cirrhotic liver). Erasistratus disbelieved the theory of humors and believed that the body was made up of atoms. He opined that atoms required *pneuma* from inspired air to be activated and that they then circulated through arteries which did not contain blood. However bizarre his theories, in practice he was pragmatic, practical and used moderate measures such as diet, baths, and mild drugs, without recourse to blood-letting.

The post-Hippocratic era unfortunately suffered from a plethora of theories. Time has relegated most of these into the dustbin of history. The teachings and the rational attitudes of the Hippocratic era continue to shine with undimmed luminosity, emphasizing that the basic tenet of medicine is to care for the patient, to relieve suffering and to cure on the occasions when this is possible.

The school at Alexandria outlasted the Ptolemic dynasty. The successors of Herophilus and Erasistratus founded the empirical school in which the art of healing again focused on observation, on the natural history of disease and on therapeutics, giving little or no importance to the doctrines propagated by the previous medical sects. Outstanding figures at this time were Heracleides of Tarentum and Serapion of Alexandria. But there now commenced a steady decline in learning and the surreptitious return of occult practices, of mysticism and magic that Egypt and the rest of the Middle East had endured before being touched by the civilization of Greece. The school of Alexandria functioned till the death of Cleopatra in 30 BC. It then fell apart and slowly disappeared from history. By then it had succeeded in disseminating its learning and wisdom to most parts of the civilized world.

Athens and Sparta

The decline of Greece had started much earlier. A dreadful plague had decimated the population of Athens around 430 BC and the misfortunes of the country were compounded by the Peloponesian War between Athens and Sparta. The sun had begun to set over Greece by the second century BC, for Rome was now on the ascendant and becoming increasingly powerful. But a civilization such as that of Greece is never extinguished, it changes its locale and perhaps its garb, but it continues to breathe. The decline of Greece made room for the rise of Rome but not before Greece had passed on its great heritage to the West, and to the world at large. Greece had its follies, its internecine wars, its extreme individualism, its failure to reconcile individual liberty with public order and peace. But those who cherish freedom, love beauty and believe in reason, will ignore these blemishes.

We would rather dwell on Sophocles who sang in that age of antiquity an unheard of refrain, "The world is full of wonders, but nothing is more wonderful than man." Or perhaps smile and agree wistfully with the words of Pericles ruling Athens in all its glory: "Future ages will wonder at us as the present age wonders at us now." Or gaze through the haze of history at the figure of Hippocrates whose emphasis on patient care rather than on disease, and whose overwhelming stress on the ethics of medicine are even more relevant today than in ancient Greece. The beauty of the art and literature of Greece, the wisdom of its philosophy, medicine and science, and the concept of the freedom of man in this world are rich legacies that will nourish the fabric of all future civilizations.

Roman Medicine

18 An Overview of the Roman Age

Asclepiades said that it is the office of the practitioners to treat safely, speedily and pleasantly.

Celsus

Rome was founded around 750 BC and in less than a thousand years it had become the centre and hub of the greatest empire in the Western world. Like a wild and raging torrent carrying all before it, the Roman conquest swept over western Europe including Greece, Gaul, Spain, the British Isles and stretched far into the East to Asia Minor, Egypt, Persia and South-West Asia. Roman hegemony stemmed from force, valour, and a feeling of invincibility, all leading to an urge to conquer, subjugate and rule. The Roman historian Livy believed that Rome became an empire because the gods had ordained it so: "Go, proclaim to the Romans it is the heaven's will that my Rome shall be the capital of the world." Yet Rome's claim to greatness and fame is not solely related to the size and stability of its empire. A more enduring claim lies in the genius of Rome to absorb the cultural and intellectual achievements of Greece, to embellish these achievements and spread them far and wide among its conquered people.

Great though Rome's achievements were in law, administration, public works, technology and feats of arms, Rome lacked the graciousness, the spirit of freedom and the loftiness of thought and action displayed by Greece. Philosophy evolved no further; the spirit of scientific inquiry was feeble; medicine was stagnant, being only partially redeemed after the advent of Galen. Almost all that was great in the Roman civilization had its origin in the Greek world. Around this Greek core, Rome gave a stamp of force, authority, power and assurance. Horace's statement is indeed true—"Captive Greece took Rome captive."

The origin of Rome is shrouded in legend. The city was founded around 750 BC on the seven hills overlooking the river Tiber. The early Latin citizens of Rome were farmers tilling the soil in a hostile land, hardy, strong, with their roots fixed deeply in the soil they cultivated. It is probably from these forebears that the future generations of Rome inherited a respect for strength, discipline, industry and loyalty. The Romans defeated their Etruscan overlords around 506 BC and founded a republic that lasted for four centuries. The republic was first controlled by the aristocracy (*patricians*) who elected their consuls. The ordinary people (*plebians*) eventually exerted control over public affairs through the election of *tribunes.*

In these formative years, Roman armies engaged in ever-increasing foreign conquests. Her victories brought her into conflict with Carthage the mistress of the western Mediterranean. The three Punic wars, which began in 264 BC, represent a struggle unto death between two powerful nation states. Rome triumphed when Scipio Africanus defeated the great Carthaginian general Hannibal at the battle of Zama in 202 BC. Carthage died, never to recover. The history of the western world had hinged on this decisive battle.

The Roman republic gave way to the triumvirates and the world was now witness to the heroic character of Julius Caesar who epitomized the strength and character of Rome and who further extended the frontiers of Roman power. The assassination of Caesar in the Roman Senate by those he had trusted led to an internecine conflict, the chief characters of which were Octavius, Caesar's nephew, Mark Anthony, Caesar's best friend and Cleopatra, the queen of Egypt. Octavius triumphed when he defeated Anthony and Cleopatra at the sea battle of Actium, and as Augustus Caesar established the foundations of the Roman Empire. Perhaps a change to a new order was inevitable. The dominions of Rome which had grown from a village to a vast empire needed a central authority for good governance. Octavius personified that authority. The Roman empire reached its zenith of power in the first two centuries AD. Peace, prosperity, law and order permeated the entire realm. But then slowly over the next 150 years it fell apart, partly through corruption and corrosion within and to the onslaught of the hungry barbarian hordes knocking at its doors. The centre of Roman power shifted east to Byzantine where it was consolidated by Constantine the Great. The eastern empire died with the fall of Constantinople to the invading Turks in 1473.

Roman Life

Imperial Rome swarmed with over a million and a half people housed in thousands of insulae or apartment blocks, three to five storeys high erected of wood or brick. The rich tapped water from the city conduits or had private wells. The poor fetched water from the many public fountains in the city. Rome had a large slave population engaged in menial work. A rich patrician would own from 500 to 1,000 slaves; an emperor might have 20,000.

The free citizen had an easy and often langorous life. Roman men loved power, women, and money and were bloodthirsty in their leisurely pursuits. Public entertainment was often incredibly cruel to behold. The Colosseum would be packed with royalty and spectators to see gory battles between gladiators or between gladiators and wild animals. Public baths, sports and gladiatorial contests were free and open to the general public.

Rome from the days of the empire has been a city of monuments, massive public works, the symbols of imperial power contrasting starkly with crumbling tenements. Augustus restored eighty-two temples, Vespasian built the Colosseum seating 60,000 spectators. Trajan constructed a towering column to commemorate his greatness. The Forum Romanicun (Roman Forum) was the centre of Rome and the seat of government; its architecture was monumental. Roman architecture was a reflection of Roman character—proud, strong, imposing. Art and architecture were an eclectic confusion of the Attic, Asiatic and Alexandrian styles. Rome took over the Doric, Ionic and Corinthian columns of Greece and the arch of the Etruscans. Roman architects were the first to use concrete in order to achieve grandeur. They could then expand the Etruscan arch with mammoth domes as that of the Pantheon. The dome of the Pantheon was covered with gilded bronze, its visible shine reflecting the glory of the city. Yet for all its immensity, grandeur and strength the architecture of Rome could not match the organic unity, purity, elegance and beauty of that of Greece.

Technology

Technology was one field in which Rome was superior to Greece. Bridges, roads, aqueducts for water supply, sewage for drainage and public baths were constructed using advanced engineering skills. The baths of Caracalla in Rome covered twenty acres, and besides being a great engineering feat, were of great aesthetic beauty, providing every form of relaxation and luxury. The building of equipments for war and the technology of transport both on land and sea reached high standards. Communication was a necessity to administer a far-flung empire, and the Romans built more than 4,000 miles of highways to allow easy access to different parts of their empire. Difficult topographic obstacles were overcome with superb feats of engineering.

The paucity of great advances in medicine, science and in the realms of the mind must not detract from the merits of the Roman civilization. The Romans were too engrossed with conquest, in the worship of valour and strength, and in the art of government, to find the inclination and the time to indulge in great thinking or in scientific inquiry. They valued the physical aspects of life and the practical solutions to the problems of life far more than philosophical abstractions and thoughts that stimulated the Greeks to understand man and the universe. Rome in its chequered history may have committed a thousand crimes; yet for centuries it ruled with tolerance and justice, thereby winning the plaudits of future generations. It gave the vast Roman world the miracle of a lasting peace, the Pax Romana—an era yet to be repeated in the history of man.

19 The Practice of Medicine

Rome, though founded in 753 BC, was under the colonial rule of the Etruscans for about 140 years (750–510 BC). Little is known about the Etruscans. They were short and rather dark people and had probably migrated to the middle of Italy from Asia Minor. Though they had a fairly vigorous civilization, their script still remains undeciphered. The Etruscans undoubtedly possessed some knowledge of medicine, as is evinced by Theophrastus, in his book on the *History of Plants*. Pliny in the first century AD wrote: "The Roman people for more than six hundred years were not without medical art but were without physicians." Even so, early Rome must have almost certainly been touched by Etruscan medicine. This was primitive medicine practised by priest-physicians involving rituals, incantations, magic and the supernatural. The Etruscans, like ancient Egyptians and the Mesopotamians, placed great emphasis on the practice of divination from animal organs, especially the liver. The model of the liver in Etruscan bronze has been excavated by archaeologists in Piacenza. The organ is divided into compartments, each compartment representing an area of heaven and presided over by a special deity.

The early Romans invoked the assistance of gods and of supernatural forces when illness struck them. Different gods presided over different spheres of health. Those struck with fever invoked the assistance of Febris, women in childbirth called on Opigena. The cult of Aesculapius, so important in the civilization of Greece, reached the banks of the Tiber as late as 203 BC. The story of how Aesculapius reached Rome is part legend and part truth. Rome was struck by a devastating plague. The Romans, after consulting their sacred books, dispatched a mission to the Aesculapean temple in Epidaurus beseeching deliverance from the plague. The legend goes that a sacred serpent in Epidaurus left the temple, and of its own accord, took ship with the Romans. When the mission returned to Rome, the sacred serpent left the ship to reach an islet, where the Romans in gratitude for their deliverance built a temple to the Greek god.

The Lex Aquilia (Aquilian law) furnishes evidence to show that medical practice did exist in Rome in the fourth century BC. There appears to have been a law in that century imposing severe penalties on doctors who caused death by negligence. Even earlier, Numa Pompilius who was the legendary second king of Rome had decreed that Caesarian section was to be performed on women dying in childbirth.

By all accounts, the early Romans considered the practice of medicine to be below their dignity. Barring exceptions, medical ministration was reserved for family slaves, barbers, masseurs and priests. This lacuna in the practice of medicine in Rome was fortunately filled by Greek physicians voyaging across the seas to seek their fortune in what was then barbaric Rome. Almost certainly the best physicians stayed in Greece, and among those who sought greener pastures were quacks and charlatans who posed as physicians. The Romans would be none the wiser. The first Greek doctor arrived from the Peleponnese in 219 BC. His name was Archagathus, which means 'the one who makes a good start'. He became a Roman citizen and to start with his work was well thought of—

but not for long! His patients called him at first *vulnerarius* (healer of wounds), but very soon dubbed him *carnifex* (the slaughterer).

The patrician Romans frowned on Greek doctors. An example was Cato (234–149 BC) who raved against Greeks and Greek doctors in the Roman senate calling them effete and useless. In fact, he went so far as to state that the Greek doctors were a menace to Roman health. Said Cato in a letter to his son, "If that pack passes on to us what they know, it will mean the end of Rome, especially if their doctors come. For they have sworn death by medicine to barbarians and the Romans are barbarians to them. Beware of doctors!" But then Cato, the senator of Rome perhaps raved even more than the *graeculi delirantes* (raving Greeks)! Cato proclaimed that cabbages (cooked and raw) were the panacea for all illnesses. A nasal polyp would go away if one smelt a cabbage and an extract of cabbage in wine could cure deafness. Stoic as he was, he advocated incantation as the next best treatment to cabbages. Here is an example of this nonsense, guaranteed to set a dislocated shoulder: "*huat hana ista pista sista domina damnaustra luxato*".

Asclepiades

A great impetus to the acceptance of Greek doctors in Rome was given by Asclepiades of Prusa, who arrived in Rome in 91 BC from Bithynia. He was of humble birth, but had studied oratory in Athens and medicine in Alexandria before coming to Rome. He must obviously have been a man of great charm for he captivated the patrician clientele of Rome. Cicero, Mark Antony, Crassus and other great names of the day became his patients, friends and patrons. He was probably one of the most famous and fashionable doctors of ancient times and was even credited with a miraculous cure. The story goes that on his way back home, he met a funeral procession. The pall-bearers tired of the weight they carried, set down the body to rest. Asclepiades on not receiving a satisfactory answer as to the cause of death went up to inspect the corpse for himself. Asclepiades persuaded the pall-bearers to delay the final rites and carry it to a nearby house. There he revived the man taken for dead. The story of this miraculous cure spread like wildfire in Rome. Asclepiades the famous had worked a miracle!

Asclepiadus was influenced by the teachings of Erasistratus who lived in the third century BC; he deliberately repudiated Hippocrates. It was not nature that effected a cure, it was the good and clever physician that did so: "*cito, tute et jucunde*" (safely, quickly and pleasantly). He also disregarded the Hippocratic theory of the four humors. He regarded the body as consisting of an infinite number of moving atoms between which flowed the body fluids. A smooth motion of the atoms conferred health; disease resulted from a disorderly motion of the atoms. Themison, a pupil of Asclepiades, developed this theory further to found the system or sect of 'methodism', which influenced medical thinking for several centuries.

Yet in spite of his antipathy to Hippocrates, his therapy was moderate. Perhaps he was shrewd enough to realize that the wealthy epicureans of Rome would never accept foul-tasting medicines prescribed by other Greek physicians. Perhaps he did not believe in the nostrums of the day. Instead, he prescribed diet, exercise, baths, massage, enemas, soothing medications, music and singing. His principle was to avoid drastic and weakening procedures—in fact he practised the Hippocratic method even while criticizing him!

Though Rome was all for Asclepiades, both Pliny and Galen were against him. Galen wrote of him, "He had no respect for the great thinkers or the truth, but was guided by a boasting spirit, arrogance, false reasoning and bare obstinacy to behave in a shameful manner." Galen particularly disliked his repudiation of the theory of humors. Perhaps Galen being a contemporary may not have been objective in his views of a famous colleague. History judged Asclepiades differently from Galen. According to Celsus, "He was in the forefront of doctors and apart from Hippocrates, the foremost."

Asclepiades made a number of contributions to medicine. He described malarial fevers accurately, observed the periodicity of some diseases and distinguished between acute and chronic diseases. Perhaps his most significant contribution was establishing the procedure of tracheostomy (making an opening in the trachea or windpipe), probably for diphtheritic obstruction to breathing. He employed the term *phrenitis* for mental illness and treated the mentally deranged with kindness and humanity. Posterity continues to respect him. Besides Themison, his other famous student was Antony Musa, who became the personal physician to Emperor Augustus and who also treated Maecenas, the patron of the arts and of the great Roman poets, Horace and Virgil.

One of the great younger Roman contemporaries of Asclepiades was the poet and philosopher Lucretius Carus, who was born in 95 BC and died in 55 BC. His great work was *De rerum natura* (the Nature of the Universe). It is the greatest scientific treatise in Latin. The universe, according to Lucretius, was composed of invisible atoms in continuous motion. Life was a continuous cycle without beginning or end, a strange echo in a far distant land of one of the basic tenets of Indian philosophy. Though Lucretius was not a doctor, *De rerum natura* contains a number of excellent observations on anatomy, physiology and the influence of environment. It was a great Latin contribution to the history of science and medicine.

Soranus of Ephesus

Just as Asclepiades was one of the most famous practising physicians in the Roman era, Soranus of Ephesus was a great obstetrician. He was, in fact, the father of obstetrics and gynaecology. He lived in the first century AD of the Christian era, belonged to the methodist school of medicine and initially practised in Alexandria before settling in Rome in the reign of the Emperor Trajan. His magnum opus was *On the Diseases of Women*, which remained the standard text for fifteen centuries. Soranus made notable contributions to his subject. The anatomy of the female genital tract was poorly understood in Hippocratic times. Hippocratic medicine believed that the position of the uterus in the body varied, and was unaware of the existence of the fallopian tubes. Soranus described the female genital organs in detail and wrote extensively on menstruation, amenorrhoea and conception. He noted that amenorrhoea could be physiological as in pregnancy and breast-feeding, or could be caused by inflammation of the genital tract or by debilitating systemic illnesses. He wrote on contraception by the insertion of cotton, or ointments, but advised against abortion by mechanical means. He paid great attention to difficulties attending childbirth. These could be due to maternal deformities like a contracted pelvis or to problems involving foetal size and position. He was probably the first to advocate support and protection of the perineum during labour.

Soranus described various abnormalities in foetal positions and wrote extensively on manual methods to correct them. If these were of no avail he advocated the use of hooks or forceps to extract the foetus. He also wrote extensively on the care of the newborn child. Breast-feeding was to start only after two days, the child being fed with boiled, diluted honey before this period. He completed his monumental treatise with advice on weaning, on the management of teething problems, and on the description and management of common childhood illnesses.

A contemporary of Soranus was Dioscorides who was born about 40 AD in Cilicia. He rose to become the most famous and respected army surgeon during the reign of Emperor Nero. Posterity remembers him for writing his *Materia Medica* in five volumes. It remained the standard textbook in pharmacology upto the Renaissance, containing all available information on the subject upto that period in time and also including an appendix on poisons and antidotes. The original text was in Greek but was soon translated into Latin incorporating excellent illustrations. Dioscorides joined the Roman legions as a surgeon, so that he could visit many countries and thereby indulge his love of botany and pharmacology.

The Encyclopaedists

Aulus Cornelius Celsus and Caius Plinius Secundus (AD 23–79), Pliny the elder, were the two greatest writers and encyclopaedists of the Roman era.

Celsus lived at the start of the Christian era and remains the most celebrated Roman writer in medicine. Amazingly enough, Celsus in all probability was not even a practising doctor; he was a rich patrician, a man of leisure, with a great thirst for all existing knowledge. He succeeded in recording all knowledge available at that time into an encyclopaedic work which he termed *De Artibus*. This work included agriculture, law, philosophy, military science, rhetoric and medicine. Only the eight books comprising *De Medicina* and fragments on a few other subjects have survived. Perhaps the encyclopaedic work might have been read in his day and time but was forgotten during the Dark and Middle Ages. The Renaissance brought a renewed interest in ancient Rome and classical Greece, leading to the discovery of this great work by Pope Nicholas V in 1443. The *De re medica* of Celsus was the first medical book to be printed in 1478 in movable type after Gutenberg's invention. His medical treatise was the first comprehensive, well-organized medical text in history. He was faithful to Hippocrates but refrained from discussing doctrinal disputes. He systematically arranged and divided known diseases not by causes but by treatment. Therapy could be by diet, drugs or surgery.

Celsus wrote extensively on the care of wounds and discussed methods of arresting bleeding through compresses, exerting pressure on and tying vessels. He recognized the importance of cleaning the wound and of gently removing congealed blood within it to avoid infection. He advocated suturing of the wound edges with thread and holding the edges together with clips. It was Celsus who summarized the four famous and cardinal signs of inflammation taught to medical students to this day: *"rubor, calor, dolor, tumor"* (redness, heat, pain, swelling).

The management of fractures was clearly discussed in *De re medica*. He stressed the importance of immobilization of the fractured limb by splints and bandages stiffened by wax, flour and paste. The bandages were to be changed after a week by which time the swelling of the fractured limb would subside. For compound fractures Celsus advised excision of the protruding bone segment.

Descriptions of surgical procedures were in some instances notably advanced and precise. Celsus described plastic surgical procedures on the nose, lips and ears. This was further developed fourteen centuries later by the Sicilian Branca and perfected by the Bolognese surgeon Tagliacozzi in the sixteenth century. His description of plastic surgery included restoration of the prepuce in the circumcised male. Obviously this operation must have been devised for the few Jews in Rome who wanted to hide their racial origin in order to gain social acceptance or aspire for lucrative positions. Numerous surgical instruments have been described in his medical treatise. These include scalpels, sounds, probes, hooks and forceps of various kinds. He described a lithotome to surgically remove stones from the bladder and special bone forceps to remove fragments of bone after trephining the skull. Many of the instruments described were astonishingly new to surgical practice in that era. Amazingly enough, surgical instruments found by archaeologists during the excavation of Pompeii fit exactly the description given by Celsus in his medical treatise. Celsus gave a remarkable description of the qualification of a surgeon in Roman times: "A surgeon ought to be young, or at any rate not very old; his hand should be firm and steady, and never shake, he should be able to use his left hand with as much dexterity as the right; his eyesight should be acute and clear; his mind intrepid and so far subject to pity as to make him desirous of the recovery of his patient, but not so far as to suffer himself to be moved by his cures; he should neither hurry the operation more than the case requires, nor cut less than is necessary, but do everything just as if the other's screams made no impression on him."

Pliny was perhaps an even greater encyclopaedist than Celsus. He possessed an insatiable intellectual curiosity. His monumental *Historia Naturalis,* dedicated to Titus, the son of Emperor Vespasian, contained as much information as possible on any and every subject. He is said to have spent every waking hour for two years collecting and recording data and information. He wrote extensively on physics, chemistry, history, geography, magic, folklore, plants and medicine. In relation to medicine, his main interest was in drugs obtainable from vegetable, animal and mineral sources. He devoted thirteen of his thirty-seven volumes to drugs, listing a barbaric polypharmacopoeia of remedies, from human excrement, blood, woman's milk and spittle, the dead, and various animals in particular the turtle and the crocodile. He was the first scholar to cite references and to list a large number of physicians of antiquity.

Pliny paid greater attention to public health than to the practice of medicine. In fact he disliked doctors, in particular Greek doctors. Venting his ire on them he said. "And there is no doubt that they all busy themselves with our lives, in order by the discovery of some new thing or another to win reputations for themselves." "There is also no law against incompetency; no striking example is made. They learn by our bodily jeopardy and make experiments until the death of the patients, and the doctor is the only patient not punished for murder."

Curiosity in the end killed Pliny. He was a naval commander in AD 79 when the disastrous eruption of Mount Vesuvius buried the cities of Pompeii and Herculaneum. He was curious to see these effects at close quarters. He braved dangerous seas to come ashore at Stabiae, close to the site of the disaster. His nephew, in a letter to Tacitus described Pliny's last day on earth—after a bath, a meal and a night's rest Pliny went on to the beach just below the smouldering volcano. He suffocated and died through the inhalation of the sulphurous fumes.

Public Health and Hygiene

Roman medicine may have lacked the spirit of scientific inquiry that characterized Greece but it was unquestionably superior in the field of public health and hygiene, particularly with reference to water supply and sanitation. By the end of the first century AD Rome was being supplied water through nine aqueducts. Water was purified by allowing for settling basins and reservoirs along the route; drinking water was kept separate from the rest. The distribution of water was to the baths and public fountains, which were open for public use, either free or for a small fee.

Rome in the Christian era had a fairly efficient system of draining used water and sewage into the Tiber. The famous Cloaca Maxima was just one part of a complex of sewers running beneath the buildings and streets of imperial Rome. As mentioned earlier, people in ancient Rome emptied their sewage onto the streets, but with time, the streets were clean and wide, abundant water was available, and stagnant water and marshy land were drained to satisfaction. The association of disease and death from undrained marshland was known to Romans in very early times. However, institutional care of the sick and wounded was neglected till late in the Roman era. Earlier in Roman history the sick were perhaps looked after in the homes or offices of their physicians. Better facilities were available for the military legions. Military medicine was efficiently organized during the early period of the Roman Empire. A corps of twenty-four surgeons accompanied every legion for the prompt treatment of the wounded. The wounded soldiers were first looked after in field tents, then in well-stocked infirmaries and hospitals set up in all the garrison towns of the empire. It was only in the fourth century AD that hospitals for civilians first came into existence. The first civilian hospital in Rome was founded around the year AD 394 by the Christian benefactress, Fabiola.

The Practitioner

There was no regulation of medical practice in Rome. Trained physicians had thus to compete with quacks and charlatans. Augustus in AD 10 granted physicians exemption from paying taxes in gratitude for the successful cure of his rheumatism by his physician, Antonius Musa. Yet there were no rules and regulations to determine who could practise. Privileges to physicians were further extended by Vespasian (AD 69–79) and Hadrian (AD 117–138) who exempted doctors from medical service and other public duties. Comprehensive regulations in the training and certification of physicians were finally brought about by Emperor Severus Alexander (AD 222–233).

Strangely enough, as the Roman empire declined, the physicians assumed an increasing status and respectability in society. They became the most important members of the court and the most trusted friends of the reigning emperor. A few physicians were accomplices in palace intrigue and murder. Stertinius Xenophon provided poisoned mushrooms which killed Emperor Claudius, Vetius Valens was the confidante and counsellor of the evil Messalina.

In imperial Rome, therapy was a strange mixture of rational procedures, physiotherapy (baths, massage) and barbaric polypharmacy. A popular anti-epileptic remedy was a compound of camel's brain, turtle's blood and crocodile dung. Antonius Musa claimed to cure Emperor Augustus of rheumatism by prescribing cold water, lettuce, celery and endives in his diet. It is not surprising that the profession came in for a valid share of insults at the hands of sceptics who had little faith in these nostrums.

20 Galen

The great Greek physician Claudius Galen (AD 138–201) was a towering figure who ranked next only to Hippocrates in the history of medicine. Galen was the most influential writer of all time, his views on medicine being fossilized as gospel truth for almost 1,500 years. He wrote voluminously; the *Editio Princeps* of his work extended into twenty-two massive volumes being equivalent to more than half the sum total of all extant Greek and Roman medical literature. He was both a great thinker and an accurate observer, yet he was authoritarian, dogmatic and uncritical in his beliefs. He was the first great physician of antiquity who combined within himself the attributes of an excellent bedside clinician in the mould of Hippocrates, and a medical scientist attempting to unravel the secrets of man through observation and experiment.

Galen was born about AD 140 at Pergamon, an important centre in Roman Asia Minor. His father was a wealthy architect who took keen interest in his son's education. At the age of fourteen he received instructions in philosophy, natural science and was introduced to anatomy and the doctrines of Hippocrates. Galen reports that his father guided him with an unerring hand to medicine, on advice from Aesculapius in a dream. After his father's death, Galen travelled widely. He studied philosophy at Smyrna, where he was a pupil of Pelopides, and medicine at Alexandria, where he came under the influence of several good teachers in anatomy. It was in Alexandria that he sowed the seeds that led him to greatness. Physicians from all over the Roman world gathered there to study, teach and practise. Galen had a chance to observe different illnesses, different medical philosophies and different forms of treatments. He also gathered information on the pharmacology of plants and minerals both in Alexandria and during his other travels.

After years of travel when he returned to Pergamon he was appointed physician-in-charge of the gladiators. He learnt the importance of diet, exercise and other hygienic methods necessary to keep his gladiators fighting fit. He also had the great opportunity to study living anatomy while treating severe injuries sustained by his gladiators during combat. He became particularly familiar with the anatomy of bones, joints and muscles and gained great experience in treating fractures as well as dreadful abdominal and chest wounds. Though Pergamon was a cultural centre, it was still provincial in character. Claudius Galen set his eyes on Rome—the glittering centre of the Roman Empire. And so in the Rome of Marcus Aurelius in AD 162, there came from Pergamon a brilliant, young physician seeking fame and fortune. Little must he have realized that his fame would outstrip his wildest imagination and that he was destined to go down as one of the immortals in the history of Man and Medicine.

Galen rapidly won attention in Rome. His brilliance, wit, logic, oratorial skills in debate and above all his astute bedside diagnosis captivated the glitterati of Rome. The capital's patrician elite were soon crowding into the public theatres where he gave lectures, debated against the views of the methodist school and performed demonstrations in experimental anatomy and physiology with a flair and showmanship that won him acclaim. An outstanding example of one of his public anatomical demonstrations was when he cut one nerve after another in the neck of a pig; the pig would continue to squeal till the exact nerve to the voice box was cut, when the pig would fall silent.

His clientele was impressive and included the rich and famous of Rome. Unaccountably, after four successful years in the capital, he suddenly left Rome, in his view to escape an attempt on his life by rivals, but according to others, to escape a threatening epidemic. He was called back in a year but evaded summons from Marcus Aurelius to accompany him on his campaigns, on a plea that he had a dream in which Aesculapius had prophesied that his services would be required for the royal children. This indeed did transpire, and he was to become the physician and confidante of the emperors Marcus Aurelius and Lucius Veris.

In spite of his busy practice and his experimenting, studying, debating and accumulation of the sum total of medical knowledge of antiquity, Galen wrote extensively in his native Greek. A dozen scribes wrote down his treatises dictated with incredible speed. Anatomy, physiology, pharmacology, pathology, therapy, hygiene, dietetics and philosophy were all subjects for his penetrating mind and facile pen. He wrote about 400 treatises, most of which were lost in a fire. Only eighty-three remain and the genuineness of these works has been proved as Galen was methodical enough to catalogue all his works.

It is of interest and value to briefly consider his achievements in anatomy, physiology and clinical diagnosis. His views on anatomy are chiefly contained in sixteen volumes of his works on anatomical preparations. They were based on his experience in Pergamon as a physician to the gladiatorial school, on studies of the human skeleton and, most of all those from the dissection of animals (chiefly apes). Some of Galen's anatomical work was pioneering. His description of bones and muscles was accurate. He showed that the veins were connected to the heart and that the nerves arose from the central nervous system. He described the nerve to the larynx and the anatomy of the spinal cord. Yet great thinker and experimenter that he was, he also made grievous mistakes in his anatomical conceptions because he equated what he saw in the internal anatomy of the animals he dissected to the internal anatomy of man. Thus, he wrongly assumed that the *rete mirabilis,* a plexus of blood vessels found at the base of the brain in ungulates was also present at the base of the brain in man. He also, at times, postulated a theory and assumed the presence of structures to fit his preformed theory. Thus he postulated that blood had to pass from the right

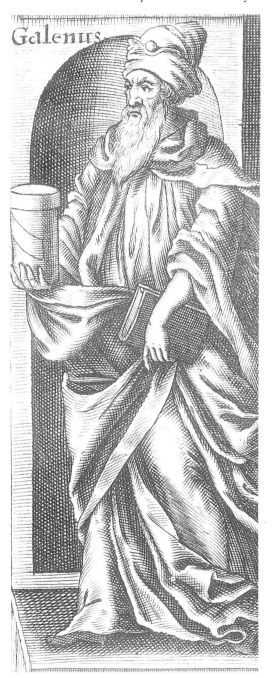

Fig. 20.1   Portrait of Galen holding a book and ointment jar.

ventricle to the left ventricle and he invented minute pores in the interventricular septum to allow his theory to stand. Perhaps if the direct dissection of human bodies had been permitted, as they had once been in Alexandria, Galen would have been more discerning in his views.

His work on physiology was based on animal experiments and is embodied in his treatise on the use of the parts of the human body comprising seventeen volumes. He studied the function of the nerves by cutting them and observing the effects so produced. He distinguished between sensory and motor nerves, and studied the effects of transection of the spinal cord. To study the function of kidneys in producing urine he tied the ureters and demonstrated a swelling of the kidneys. He proved that the heart could continue to beat even if denervated and showed for the first time, that arteries contained blood and not air. He believed, with Hippocrates, that the four fundamental humors—phlegm, blood, white bile, black bile—were responsible for health and disease, and, on this basis, classified all personalities into the four types—phlegmatic, sanguine, choleric and melancholic—terms in use to the present day.

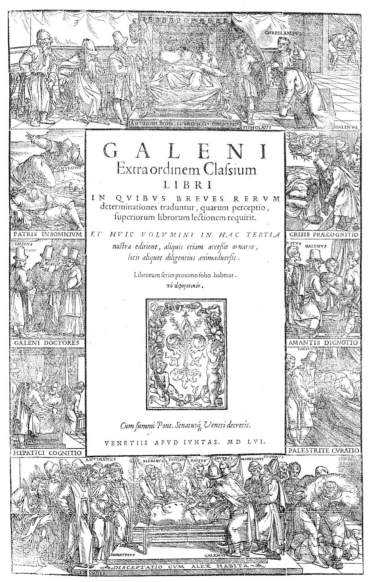

Fig. 20.2   Opera omnia.

Galen formulated a remarkably facile theoretical concept on the physiology of the human body. He postulated that the fundamental principle of life was *pneuma*, which existed in three forms and had three types of actions. They were—animal spirit (*pneuma psychicon*) in the brain, responsible for sensory perception and movement; vital spirit (*pneuma zoticon*) centred in the heart and regulating blood flow and temperatures; natural spirit (*pneuma physicon*) residing in the liver and responsible for nutrition and metabolism. *Pneuma* entered the lung through the trachea, and passed through the pulmonary vein into the left ventricle where it came in contact with the blood from the liver. In the liver blood was imbued with the natural spirit (*pneuma physicon*), and received through the portal vein, nutritive products of digestion transformed into chyle. Blood from the liver was now distributed by veins arising from it to all body tissues supplying them with nutrition. The blood entered the right side of the heart through the vena cava, the impurities within the blood being expelled from the lungs via the breath. Blood then passed from the right to the left ventricle through small invisible pores in the septum. The vital spirit was now distributed to the whole body by the heart through the arteries. Some of it reached the brain where it was split by the *rete mirabilis*. In the brain the vital spirit was transformed into the animal spirit, which was distributed by the nerves arising from the brain to all parts of the body. Galen postulated that nerves, like arteries and veins, were hollow structures.

There were cardinal grievous mistakes both in anatomy and physiology in Galen's postulate of the circulatory system, which, unfortunately remained sacrosanct till the time of Vesalius in the Renaissance, and of Harvey's discovery of the circulation in the seventeenth century.

Galen's writing on clinical medicine were as voluminous as those on anatomy and physiology. His treatise on *Prognosis from the Pulse* was a detailed study of the pulse with its numerous variations in different diseases. His clinical acumen was unequalled in his time. When Emperor Marcus Aurelius fell ill, his physician diagnosed an acute impending febrile illness. Galen after feeling the Emperor's pulse diagnosed it as a 'stomach upset' due to overindulgence in food. The emperor seemed mighty impressed and probably preferred Galen's simple explanation which required as treatment the mere application of wool soaked in a salve to the abdomen. Another good diagnosis which brought him fame needs to be recounted. A Persian philosopher lost his sensation in the last three fingers of one of his hands. He had been to many physicians, but without much relief. Galen elicited the history that he had a bad fall and had injured himself between the shoulder blades. Galen diagnosed trauma to the spinal cord with injury to the sensory nerve root arising from the cord and supplying the affected fingers. He prescribed rest with application of soothing salves; recovery ensued.

The therapy employed by Galen often followed the Hippocratic doctrine, i.e., reliance on the healing power of nature. Though, unlike Hippocrates he believed a great deal in blood-letting and was fond of using medications. He often prepared his own prescriptions containing several ingredients. An extraordinary medication which Galen elaborated was *theriac*. This was an extremely ancient antidote to snake bite, and with time numerous fresh ingredients were added to its prescription, so that it became the antidote to all poisons as also to pestilences like the Black Death. Legend has it that Mithridates, the King of Pontus (132–65 BC) experimented on slaves to find antidotes to various poisons of which he had a tremendous fear. He ultimately found a combination which he called *mithridatium*. In the first century AD, Nero's physician added viper's flesh to the formula of this antidote and designated it *theriac,* a word derived from the Greek for a 'wild beast'.

Though Galen personally practised very little surgery in Rome, he made excellent observations on surgical techniques and made a number of suggestions on the use of surgical instruments.

In the final analysis, Galen was one of the great figures of medicine who combined within himself the qualities of a thinker, a physician and experimental scientist. It was a combination unsurpassed in antiquity and for that alone he deserves our homage. He was, unfortunately, an extreme egoist who made out that there was no other true path than the one he walked; those who were not with him aroused his ire and vitriolic contempt. The only seeker of truth other than himself whom he acknowledged was Hippocrates. "It is I, and I alone, who have revealed the true path of medicine. It must be admitted that Hippocrates already staked out this path... he prepared the way, but I have made it possible."

Galen made many mistakes as most men do. The tragedy of his mistakes is unique in that they were perpetuated for over 1,500 years after his death. There must indeed be few mistakes in any other field of human endeavour which would equal this unenviable record. Although it is unfair to sit in judgement over ideas and events that prevailed several centuries ago, two basic questions need to be asked—why did a man with his brilliance commit such fundamental mistakes, and why was it that these mistakes went uncorrected for so many years? Galen believed strongly with Plato and Aristotle, that philosophy was linked to medicine. There is truth in the link between philosophy and medicine; yet his errors were partly because many of his theories in medicine were based on and built around philosophical doctrines. His entire work was imbued with teleological explanations for structure and function within the body. Thus a view that the purpose of all anatomical and physiological functions was predetermined deluded him into seeing what did not exist or distorting what he saw, or presuming a function in an organ because nature must have determined for it a clear purpose. Galen thus unfortunately committed the crime of Procrustes—a crime that has plagued medicine from the time it was born to this modern day and age. Procrustes was a robber and an innkeeper who allowed the weary traveller to rest at night on a particular bed. If he found the traveller's legs too long for the bed he would chop them off so that they fitted the bed exactly. If too short he would stretch them so that they did likewise. Medicine has invariably suffered from the attempt to squeeze or stretch it to fit preconceived ideas.

Galen's mistakes stood the test of time. Why was this so? The Dark and Middle Ages were characterized by uncertainty, turmoil and strife; there was a longing desire for certainty and authority that would put an end to unsettled conditions. Galen provided that certainty and authority in his writings. He gave clear cogent answers to even the most uncertain questions; he wrote with authority, as if he knew everything there was to know. His teleological reasoning and explanations had an underlying moral theme acceptable both to the Christian church and to Islam. Again, since both these religions frowned upon and forbade dissection of the human body, Galen's errors remained conveniently hidden for a long time. Galen's systematic arrangement and encyclopaedic codification of all ancient knowledge made his work a ready source of reference. An important reason for their influence was that eighty-three of his five hundred known works survived and continued to be read and believed by posterity. Even the great names who came after him, as for example, Alexander of Tralles, and Paul of Aegina, perpetuated the belief that the works of Galen embodied all that was to be known in medicine. It took a free spirit like Andreas Vesalius of the Renaissance, and a great thinker and experimenter like William Harvey of the Baroque period to separate fact from fiction in the works of Galen and to set the record right.

Galen lived and wrote at a time when the Roman Empire was at its zenith. The next 200 years saw its decline and disintegration, ushering in the Dark Ages. The causes of the decline and fall of the Roman Empire are briefly discussed in the introduction to Chapter 21. It is easier to explain Rome's fall than to explain her long survival. She began with a ruthless conquest of the Mediterranean world and then expanded further west and east. Yet she embraced the culture of Greece, gave it order, peace and prosperity for 200 years, held back the barbarian hordes for 200 years more, and even as she died bequeathed its classic legacy to the West. This was indeed a great achievement.

Rome's forte was the art of government, the establishment of law and authority, the enrichment of the world through commerce moving across secure seas and over a brilliantly engineered network of enduring roads. Rome stood for force and action, but not for the realm of great thoughts nor for the spirit of dedicated inquiry. Rome made no great advances in medicine, science or philosophy. Asclepiades, Soranus, Dioscorides and Galen all contributed to medicine in the Roman era, but they were Greeks from subjugated Greek colonies. The Roman era provided tolerance, justice, security and prosperity to keep the torch of medicine burning bright.

Medicine in the Dark Ages

21 Decline and Fall of Rome— Medicine and Faith

Nothing in life is more wonderful than faith—the one great moving force which we can neither weigh in the balance, nor test in the crucible.

Sir William Osler

The Dark Ages is a term employed to denote an era during which there was an eclipse in the civilization of the West. It was ushered in by the fall of Rome in AD 476 and includes the early medieval period of Western European history to the time when there was no emperor in the West (AD 800). More generally, it includes the period between AD 470 and 1000. Many historians of today find the value judgement implicit in this term unacceptable and prefer not to use it. Yet, it is an incontrovertible fact that this period of the history of the West was marked by strife, disorder, pestilence and war, by intellectual darkness and barbarity. The Dark Ages began to see the light of day after AD 1000, but for convenience in narration, I have included within this era the time span extending to the birth of the Renaissance. The history of Man and Medicine in this period starts with the Decline and Fall of Rome–Medicine and Faith. It goes on successively to Byzantine Medicine, Islam and Medicine, and Medicine in the Medieval West.

Rome reached the zenith of its glory by the end of the first century AD. A free citizen of Rome living in that era would have probably considered the Roman Empire to be eternal. But the seeds of decadence had already been sown and by the end of the second century AD, there began a gradual decline and fall of the Roman Empire. Barbarians had scented their prey and made repeated incursions from the east and the north. Aleric, the Goth, delivered the *coup de grâce* when he pillaged and sacked Rome in AD 410. Rome now was in its death throes; the official death knell of Rome and the Western Roman Empire was tolled in AD 476, when Emperor Romulus Augustulus was deposed by Odoacer, king of the barbaric Herulians. In AD 336, Constantine had already shifted his capital from Rome to Constantinople strategically situated on the Bosphorus, and by AD 395, Byzantine, the eastern Roman Empire under Constantine was separated from the Western Roman Empire. When the last Roman Emperor Odoacer was deposed by the barbarians, Byzantine remained the sole bastion of civilization through more than six centuries of the so-called Dark Ages.

No great civilization has ever been conquered from without before having first destroyed itself within. The most important cause of the decline and fall of the Roman Empire was the corruption and increasing rot within its body politic. It lay in the crimes committed by the Roman state, the sadistic cruelty and the unabashed hedonism of its many emperors, the stifling taxes, decadent morals, the exploitation of its conquests and the impoverishment of its colonies to feed a selfish oligarchy in Rome and Italy.

Gibbons in his *Decline and Fall of the Roman Empire* blames Christianity as the chief cause of the fall of Rome. There may be a modicum of truth in this view. Christianity destroyed the old faith which had nurtured the moral character of the Roman citizens and had lent stability to the Roman state. It divided loyalties. Rome was great when its undivided loyalty was to the state and what it stood for; Rome declined and fell when its loyalties were divided between religion and state, with religion taking an obvious precedence over the state. Christianity abjured violence at all costs, and preached the ethic of love, charity and peace, even as the survival of the empire demanded the will to war. Indeed, the coming of Christ had sounded the death-knell of Rome.

Yet, it has been endlessly argued that Christianity flourished and grew because Rome already lay decadent and dying. Men had already lost faith in a state which committed a thousand crimes, worshipped the cult of force and violence, practised barbaric cruelty, trampled upon the poor, taxed the impoverished to support the luxury of the rich, and failed to protect its citizens from famine, disease and death. They were ready to abandon Caesar and embrace Christ, to choose a faith which gave dignity to their poverty, recognized their humanity, and which considered the poor the chosen children of God. Therefore, a more balanced view would be that the barbarian onslaught from without and Christianity from within were not the root causes of Rome's fall, but hastened its decline and death.

Wars, famines, disorder and unrest spread, increasing anarchy in the Roman Empire. This was further aggravated by epidemics of disease and of plague, that ravaged the country. Pestilences were an important contributory internal factor that hastened Rome's demise. A number of these epidemics have been well recorded. An epidemic ravaged the province of Campania in AD 79 after the eruption of Mount Vesuvius had destroyed the cities of Pompeii and Herculaneum. Tens of thousands of citizens were reported to have died everyday. In AD 125 Carthage and Numidia in North Africa were reported to have been hit by a plague of locusts which destroyed all crops and also by a dreadful epidemic disease that took a toll of millions. Two other epidemics struck the Roman Empire in AD 251 and AD 312; they were thought to be of smallpox.

Plague has played an important role in the history of man from ancient times. Modern medicine recognizes that plague is an epidemic disease caused by an organism called *Pasteurella pestis*. Ancient physicians were unaware of the nature or cause of the disease, so 'plague' was used as a term for any epidemic disease that resulted in high mortality. The clinical features of plague have been described by both Thucydides and Galen. Thucydides recorded the great disastrous outbreak of plague that decimated Periclean Athens in 430 BC at the height of its glory. Galen described the epidemic that hit Rome in AD 164; he had fled the city in fear to escape this epidemic, returning only when the epidemic had ceased.

Many other authors give a description of epidemics of plague all through antiquity. Their chief common denomination was a high death rate. The clinical descriptions of these epidemics called 'plague' were seen to include a number of different diseases. There appear to be descriptions of what were presumably small-pox, diphtheria, bubonic plague, scarlet fever and cholera, all described under the generic term 'plague'. The ancients were aware of the clinical features of bubonic plague—painful swelling of the lymph nodes in the groin or axilla discharging pus and blood, leading to toxaemia and death. They also knew that it was a disease of rodents which spread plague to man. They were, however, unaware that it was the flea that spread the disease from rodent to man.

It is conceivable that some of the clinical manifestations of fulminant epidemic diseases may have been different in antiquity from what we observe today. The alternative possibility is that the ancients were exposed to certain diseases which are now extinct and have ceased to afflict man. Thus, the devastating epidemic of plague that killed thousands in Athens was reported by Thucydides to cause among other features, gangrene of the hands, feet, genital organs and eyeballs—a description which does not fit into a single pattern of disease in modern medicine.

The link between history and medicine is perfectly illustrated in the era of the decline and fall of the Roman Empire. The fall of Rome signalled the demise of civilization in the West. Europe now sank into the 'Dark Ages', into a prolonged painful night from which it would awake after many centuries. This winter of discontent was marked by chaos, despair, lawlessness and a blatant lack of human decency and values. Each man was a law unto himself; life was cheap and security nonexistent. The light of learning was extinguished; medicine, philosophy, science and the liberal arts declined to a point where they almost never existed. The uselessness of medicine against the pestilences that swept the west further demoralized man, so he turned to supernatural power for aid. Magic, incantations, rituals, charms, all used by prehistoric man and in very early civilizations, were reborn.

In this dark, chaotic and savage era there was, however, a glimmer of light. This glimmer was the birth of Christianity. The birth of Christianity was preceded by the coming of Jesus Christ. There would have been no Christianity without the advent of Jesus, yet Jesus did not found the Christian religion. He merely preached a message, a doctrine. It was his apostles, in particular Paul, who founded Christianity and the theology of the Christian church.

Jesus was a young man of thirty (around AD 28–30), when he entered history and began to teach and spread his message. He must have possessed a strange, powerful, personal magnetism for he attracted followers wherever he went and filled them with love, devotion and courage. He preached from place to place within Judea for three years and finally came to Jerusalem. He was accused of trying to foment rebellion; he was convicted of this charge and crucified along with two thieves. He died on the cross within six to eight hours, and according to Christian belief, sacrificed himself for the salvation of Man.

His message, in essence, was of universal love and brotherhood. Above all, he preached the doctrine of the Kingdom of Heaven, one of the most revolutionary doctrines that influenced human thought. The Kingdom of Heaven, he claimed was within us, only it required a complete change of heart, a cleansing of individual lives and of the whole struggling human race. Thereby, in the same measure we would be revolutionizing the outside world. Jesus preached no religion, no ritual, no sacrifice; he preached a code of ethics that few could understand and fewer still could follow. "To take him seriously was to enter upon a strange and alarming life, to abandon habits, to control instincts and impulses, to assay an incredible happiness. Is it any wonder that to this day this Galilean is too much for our small hearts!"

Like most great religions of the world, Christianity was born in the Near East. It imbibed a fair degree of mysticism of the orient, and, as Christian theology took shape one could unravel the theocracies of earlier religions that went into its doctrines. Christianity became the anchor that steadied a disordered, disintegrating West. It had an inherent appeal, for it preached brotherhood and charity. The poor, the humble and the afflicted were offered a consummate meaning to their earthly life. They were to receive a glorious after-life if they followed the path of righteousness, love and the other tenets of Christianity. How could the dispossessed in the western world resist a promise and a vision as glorious as that proclaimed by the founders of the Catholic Church? It is not sufficiently realized that it was Emperor Constantine who played a great role in the acceptance and spread of Christianity in the early Christian era. He made Christianity the official religion of the Empire after he moved the capital from Rome to Byzantine in AD 326. Incredible as this may sound, this great man knew neither to read nor write, yet he succeeded in settling the theological disputes between the early sects that threatened to cause a rift in the Catholic church. He remained a pagan all his life, being baptized as a Christian just before his death. He was shrewd enough to grasp the fact that though Christians were a small minority of only 20 per cent in the Eastern Empire, they had the moral courage and the intellectual strength that the pagans could not equal. So he took their side and used the Cross of the Christian God as his banner when he led his armies into battle. His attitude to Christianity facilitated its acceptance within the western world.

It is of interest here to briefly consider the outlook of Christianity on disease and the art of healing. Christianity considered man to have a body which was temporary and a soul which was eternal. Its doctrine was the salvation of the soul. The priest ministered to the eternal soul and was thus superior to the physician who ministered to the physical body. The 'eternal' obviously took precedence over the 'temporary', though the borders between the two were at times indistinct. Even so the physician and the priest over a period of centuries learnt to respect each other and lived in happy symbiosis.

The concept of disease in Christianity was partly influenced by earlier religions, like the Egyptian religion and the Old Testament of the Jews, and was partly original in its flavour. Disease was thus considered as a punishment for sins as in the Old Testament or as a visitation of the wrath of God. Egyptian and Mesopotamian beliefs were similar except that these civilizations believed in many gods whilst both the Jewish and Christian religions were monotheistic. An unusual concept of disease in Christianity was that disease could be a God-given trial for those whom He loved and who after death would reap the bounty of perpetual bliss in paradise. This concept was not as original as it appears. It invoked supernatural powers and phenomena exactly as the earlier Egyptian, Mesopotamian and Greco-Roman civilizations had done. However, the Christian concept was more refined and in the Dark Ages had a great human appeal. Christianity's attitude towards medicine was embodied in the tenet that healing was its mission. It regarded medicine and the care of the poor, the sick and the afflicted as a work of charity. The religion reaped a tremendous advantage and unmeasurable goodwill when it proclaimed that helping the sick was a bounden duty for both the individual and the community. It was not an empty proclamation; it was put to effect with zeal and devotion. Healing, however, was not through the naturalistic methods of Hippocrates and Galen. Medicine in the Dark Ages was usurped by the church and given a strongly religious flavour. Healing was through faith, through inviting the help of God, the Father. The use of holy oil, prayer and the laying of hands helped to heal better than the medicaments of the Egyptian or the Greco-Roman age.

The healing power of faith was demonstrated in the gospel. Jesus Christ performed miracles in healing by invoking the help of God, the Father—the blind could see, the lame could walk and the leper became free of his dreadful scourge. There are more than thirty miraculous cures recorded in the Bible; healing was considered by the apostles of Christ as 'a gift of the spirit'. It is understandable that the numerous sick, diseased individuals in the Dark Ages turned to Christianity both for a physical cure and for eternal salvation. Men, women, children and even infants in arms would wait patiently for baptism, annointment with holy oil or the use of some holy relic to bring relief to their suffering bodies. Christian shrines, where the act of healing through faith and prayer became popular were established—often on the ruins of old pagan temples. Two of the first Christian doctors who practised healing by faith were Cosmas and Damian. A brief account of these twin brothers who were martyred and later beatified is given in the chapter on Byzantine Medicine.

Christianity may well be considered as an important cause of the decline of medicine and of a temporary end to the spirit of scientific inquiry. But then a religion is more concerned with the promotion of its religious doctrines than speculation on natural science. Perhaps, a more appropriate view is that medicine, natural science and the liberal arts all declined through default in an age riven by disorder and strife. Even so, Christianity did a great deal to relieve suffering in difficult times.

Hospices called *xenodochia* were built at different sites, affording food and shelter to the poor and to pilgrims; in later years these were converted to hospitals. Christian charity was institutionalized first in the eastern Empire as a sequel to Constantine's recognition of Christianity as the official religion of the state. The bishop of Antioch, in the middle of the fourth century, set up hostels in his see. The first great Christian hospital was built in the Eastern Empire by St Basil at Caesarea in the year AD 370. The hospital was like a township with as many wards as there were diseases. Charity, love, care and compassion were also extended to lepers who from time immemorial had been kept in isolation. St Basil's hospital also included a leper colony, where the inmates were cared for with true dedication.

It has already been mentioned that the first hospital in the western world was built by the Roman Lady Fabiola in AD 394. She suffered two unhappy marriages, became the follower of St Jerome and did penitence in the Chalcis desert from where she returned in AD 381. She devoted herself to the sick and poor, spending her wealth on charity.

The role of Christianity in the decline of the Roman Empire will always remain a matter of debate. Its stabilizing influence in the immediate phase of turmoil that followed is however accepted by all. It was the solitary pillar of strength, a bastion that resisted the forces of disintegration both without and within. When Hippocratic and Galenic medicine well-nigh perished, Christianity substituted the practice of medicine with the power of faith. It helped preserve and perpetuate the Hippocratic tenet of care and devotion to the sick and afflicted. It provided first for 'retreats', and then for hospitals all over Christendom. It also woke up to the fact that in the strife and turmoil of the age, in the wars and pestilences that raged, the treasure house of learning and wisdom of past civilizations would be lost to the world forever. Having withstood and triumphed over the turbulence of this unsettled age, the realization dawned that it owed a duty to itself and to the world to preserve the achievements of the Greco-Roman past, and to save them from being annihilated forever. This was achieved within the confines of the churches and monasteries all over Christendom.

22 Byzantine Medicine

The physician should look upon the patient as a besieged city and try to rescue him with every means that art and science place at his command.

Alexander of Tralles

Historical Background

The Byzantine Empire founded by Constantine the Great survived as a fortress of civilization and the centre of culture for over a thousand years before being engulfed and destroyed by the Ottoman Turks in 1453. The heart of the Empire consisted of the Balkan Peninsula embracing the Greece of today, parts of Yugoslavia and Asia Minor. It withstood the onslaught of the Visigoths, Persians, Arabs, Venetians and Christian crusaders; the capital city of Constantinople seemed impregnable.

Christianity, as mentioned earlier, had a strong ally in Constantine. Although pagan all through his life, being baptised only on his deathbed, he considered Christianity as the official religion of his empire and dedicated his capital Constantinople to the Virgin. Pagan religions were soon banned. The church gained ascendancy; Christian culture mixed with the mysticism of the Orient gained increasing influence in every aspect of Byzantine society. Byzantine society all through its thousand years of civilization produced no outstanding figures in science, medicine, literature or philosophy. Yet it preserved a wealth of classical learning which would have otherwise perished after the fall of Rome. It encouraged scholarship and education and produced some of the most brilliant art works and handicrafts the world has seeen.

CONSTANTINOPLE

The capital city and the heart of the Byzantine Empire was at the crossroads of the world—where the East met the West. It was strategically situated—guarded by nature with sea-walls and water on three sides and fortified by man-made thick stone walls that were deemed impregnable. It was dubbed as 'the city guarded by God'. At the height of its glory in the eleventh century it was populated by more than a million people, representing a mixture of a dozen races. Constantinople outshone Rome and Alexandria at their pinnacle of fame in wealth and trade. It was resplendent with its marble, its collonades, frescoes, mosaics, sculptures, gold, jewellery and silk. It was an amalgam of the East and the West—devout and sensuous, civilized, yet corrupt and cruel. It surpassed all the previous civilizations in the rigour of its religious rituals and in the splendour of its decorative arts.

The city possessed palaces, churches, schools, pavilions and great libraries. The Imperial Palace had ostentation and luxury befitting an eastern potentate. On one of the seven hills stood the university founded by Thedosius II in the fifth century. In an old basilica converted into a library, the walls were lined with over 150,000 books. Scholars from all over the world worshipped at this temple of learning.

A harbour along the six mile long bay, the Golden Horn, swarmed with ships from East and West. Trade flourished; the city grew richer over the years. A popular sport all over the Empire was chariot-racing. Constantinople's hippodrome could hold 100,000 spectators who frequently turned violent over their favourite charioteers. The hippodrome also served to hold battles between men and beasts, acrobatic displays and circuses.

The crowning glory of Constantinople was the Basilica of Haga Sophia (St Sophia) built by Emperor Justinian in the sixth century. A mixture of oriental and Roman design, it is, even today a fascinating masterpiece of blue and gold, mosaic and marble, arches and cupolas, with a dome exquisitely proportioned as if suspended from the sky. Yet the city was not all riches and luxury. The poor quarter of the city was incredibly overcrowded with dark filthy alleys into which the light of the sun barely penetrated.

The inhabitants of Byzantine were a mixture of several races. There were Greeks, Latins, Gauls, Semites, Phrygians, Hittites, Persians, Armenians, Slavs. As in the medieval West a feudal system also existed in Byzantine. It grew out of the need of the poor to seek protection from the rich and powerful in times of trouble. At the head of the social ladder stood the senatorial aristocracy and the mercantile princes. The Patriarch was the head of the Eastern church; there was frequent conflict with the Papacy of Rome. Amazingly the Patriarch was often a eunuch. Castration was not a stigma but was deemed an opportunity. Eunuchs swelled the ranks of the bureaucracy; they were not employed as guardians of the harem, as was the custom in the Moslem world.

THE STATE

Byzantium had developed a strong central authority and power. The Emperor was an absolute monarch, the Chosen one of God, the Anointed of the Lord, the Vicar of God on earth. He was considered a prince equal to the apostles. Remarkably enough, power was not hereditary, nor were the emperors always of noble blood. The office of the basileus was open to the one who gained the vote of the Senate, the approval of the army and the consent of the populace. The commonest of common people, including a butcher, a swine-herd and a horse-trader rose to wear the diadem. Three women too had risen to the throne—a circus girl, a cook, and a tavern-keeper's daughter.

The Byzantine army and navy did the empire proud. The army had an excellent cavalry arm. Each army unit was provided with a surgeon and stretcher-bearers. The Byzantines enjoyed complete naval superiority, dominating the seas for centuries before the Arabs appeared. The day-to-day running of the state was in the hands of officials who, though often corrupt, were efficient with good administrative skills.

CULTURE

The four great centres of learning were Alexandria, Antioch, Athens and Constantinople. These cities and their libraries became the repository of Hellenic culture and preserved for posterity a vast treasure of Greek poetry, philosophy, drama and literature, as also the works of Hellenic scientists and historians. Scholars in Byzantine remained secular; they studied, translated and annotated Greek classics of Sophocles, Aristophanes, Plato, Aristotle and Thucydides.

Byzantine's original literary output was poor, being limited to essays, chronicles and devotional poems. The only impressive work was the eleventh century epic poem *Digenis Akritas*. Byzantine art was a mixture of Hellenist traditions and oriental art forms, producing an ornate, ostentatious, ornamentative effect enhanced further by the use of brilliant colours. All art forms breathed an atmosphere of pomp and splendour—yet they could not compare with the elegance and grace of Greek art. The golden age of Byzantine was between the ninth and eleventh centuries. It was an era where the ornamentation and ornateness of the east were suppressed, so that churches and public buildings became more refined and elegant in design, with beautiful works in mosaic and ivory, and beautifully illustrated manuscripts.

The Practice of Medicine

Byzantine medicine was based on faith—faith in Christianity and the Christian church. The poor, the dispossessed, the downtrodden, the sick and the afflicted were offered healing through the grace of God mediated by His church and by His vicars on earth. In any case they were guaranteed redemption and the blessings of heaven in the after-life.

The earliest Christian physicians were believed to be the twins Cosmas and Damian who became the patron saints of medicine. They lived in Asia Minor around the close of the third century and became famous because of their extraordinary healing powers. They were martyred by the Emperor Diocletian. The story goes that despite being burnt, stoned, crucified and sawed in half they survived, dying only after they were decapitated. They were later beatified and honoured by a shrine erected in Constantinople. Cosmas and Damian appear in the heraldry of barber surgeon's companies. Churches were dedicated to their memory; many claimed to house their remains and became places of pilgrimage for the sick. A legend credits Cosmas and Damian with performing a miracle by carrying out the first transplant. They were said to have amputated the gangrenous leg of a white man and transplanted, in its place, that of a dead Moor. Paintings describe the scene graphically, the patient supine, one leg black, the other white and spectators staring wonderstruck at this miracle.

Specific saints were believed to have the power to cure specific diseases, very much like specialists relating to their specialities. Thus St Artemis was for general afflictions, St Sebastian against pestilence, St Job against leprosy. St Michael and St Luke were comparable to the general physicians and could be called upon to help, relieve or cure a wide variety of illnesses. In addition to saints, other reputed healers were the Stylite hermits who spent their lives on platforms atop pillars.

The strong religious affiliations of Byzantine society prevented the frequent use of drugs or the development of practising physicians. Sickness and death were considered a divine visitation. Outside of the church there flourished sorcerers, poisoners, dealers in magic, charms, and amulets and those specializing in the casting of spells.

Though starved of Hippocratic medicine, the Byzantine state founded a number of welfare institutions and hospitals to care for the sick. An outstanding example was Constantinople's combined military hospital, orphanage and home for the blind, housing 7,000 patients. By the fifth and sixth centuries, hospitals in the East grew large and complex. Jerusalem, Constantinople, Antioch, and Edessa, could all boast of hospitals with 200 or more beds. The Pantokratos in Constantinople had a medical faculty, and medical and surgical wards; beyond its walls was a colony for lepers. Charity and care in the spirit of true Christianity was thus extended to the poorest of the poor and even to those considered as outcasts of society.

Oribasius of Byzantine, Alexander of Tralles and Paul of Aegina were amongst the few who prevented the lamp of learning in medicine from being totally extinguished.

Oribasius (AD 325–403) was the son of a nobleman from Pergamon; he had studied in Alexandria and became the physician and friend of Emperor Julian, who in history is known as Julian the Apostate because he was opposed to the religious beliefs of his uncle Constantine. Oribasius made no original contribution to medicine. His claim to fame lies in his collection of excerpts from the best medical authorities. His anthology *Synagogae Medicae* gives the medical historian a glimpse of many ancient and eminent medical authors who would otherwise have remained unknown and lost to us. His *Euporista* was a manual of practical instructions on accidents and diseases that might afflict travellers who had no easy access to a physician's aid. His major contribution to medicine was in summarizing, simplifying and arranging the works of past masters, particularly of Galen. His systematic, summarized arrangements of Galen's works went a long way in preserving the sanctity of the master's works for several centuries.

Alexander of Tralles (sixth century) was the brother of the architect who designed the Hagia Sophia church in Constantinople. Though a devout follower of Galen he occasionally differed from the master. When reminded that he had once departed from Galen's principles in one of his works, he retorted: "I love Galen, but I also love the truth and if a choice be made between them, I give preference to the truth." He is famous for his *Twelve Books on Medicine,* which were translated into Arabic and Latin. He travelled widely in Greece, Italy, Gaul and Spain but finally settled to practise in Rome. He suggested bleeding for plethoric patients; rest, vinegar potions and cold compresses to the chest for haemoptysis. He was the first physician in the West to advocate the use of rhubarb as a laxative. He found that *henbane,* a poisonous hairy plant with an unpleasant smell, was effective as a medicine only if held between the thumb and index finger, and used while the moon was in Pisces or Aquarius. Other exotic remedies and the use of unusual magical charms served to efface the picture of rational medicine advocated and practised by the Hippocratic school of medicine.

The last of the well-known Byzantine physicians was the surgeon and gynaecologist-obstetrician, Paul of Aegina. His works on medicine appeared in seven volumes, all of which were also translated into Arabic. Paul's description of the radical operation for inguinal hernia was considered a classic till the seventeenth century—"An incision is made three fingers long on the tumour of the inguinal region. Skin and fat are laid aside to reveal the peritoneum, and the intestines are pushed down with the end of a sound. Bulging bits of the peritoneum on either side of the sound are sutured together and the sound is then extracted; the peritoneum is not cut, nor is the testicle touched in any way. The procedure is simply to treat the wound thereafter." Amongst other surgical descriptions are those on nasal polyps, excision of tonsils, the procedure for tracheostomy, irrigation of the bladder with an ox bladder attached to a catheter, resection of the ribs for an empyema, and expanding rectal and vaginal speculums. The last of his seven books is on drugs and includes the use of colchicine for gout.

The main achievement of these Byzantine physicians was to preserve the medical knowledge of the ancients, to systematize and present this knowledge as a learning text for future generations. By AD 500 medical texts in Alexandria comprised not only the works of Hippocrates but also those of Galen. The latter ran into sixteen books and were studied in a stated order beginning with *On Sects and The Art of Medicine.* Alexandrian scholars further summarized these Galenic texts to allow for easier study. Galenic doctrines were thus launched into the Western world and the great deal of dogma mixed with some degree of truth, remained unchallenged till the Renaissance.

Byzantium stood for a thousand years, bridging the gap between the fall of Rome and the modern world. In 1453, the Ottomans under Sultan Mohammed II attacked Constantinople from the European side with a great force of artillery. Constantinople fell; Constantine XI, the last of the

Byzantine emperors was killed in battle; there was looting and massacre. The great church of St Sophia built by Justinian in AD 532 was pillaged and converted into a mosque. A tremor went through Europe at the fall of this great ancient citadel and an attempt was made to organize a crusade—but the days of crusades were over.

Sultan Mohammed II tried his best to preserve the ethos and glory of Constantinople as it once was—the city of Emperors. But this was not to be. According to Mark Sykes: "Constantinople as the City of Sultans was Constantinople no more; the markets died away; the culture and civilization fled; the complex finance faded from sight; and the Turks had lost their governors and support. On the other hand, the corruptions of Byzantium remained, the bureaucracy, the eunuchs, the palace guards, the spies, the bribers, the go-betweeners—all these the Ottomans took over, and all these survived in luxuriant life. The Turks, in taking Constantinople (presently called Istanbul), let slip a treasure and gained a pestilence."

By the time the Byzantine Empire crumbled, the West was in the sunshine of the Renaissance. Medicine preserved by the Byzantines had been passed on to the medical schools in Europe. The schools of Salerno, Bologna, Padua, Paris, Montepellier and Oxford had by now flowered and were in full bloom.

Byzantine, besides preserving the intellectual treasures of the Greco-Roman world, had also unwittingly planted the seeds of medicine in what was to become the Arab world. It did so a thousand years before it fell, through Nestorius the patriarch of Constantinople who was evicted with his followers for the crime of heresy. The seeds planted by these heretic Byzantines on foreign soil grew into a school that lent lustre to medicine. Strangely enough, a heresy furthered the cause of Man and Medicine.

23 Islam and Medicine

The truth in medicine is an unattainable goal and the art as described in books is far beneath the knowledge of an experienced and thoughtful physician.

Rhazes

Historical Background

The dawn of the seventh century saw Europe engulfed in strife or crumbling in decay. Even the Byzantine Empire, the sole heir to Greco-Roman culture and the only pillar of political strength in a disintegrating West, was fighting for its survival against the Persians and the Avars.

Jesus of Nazareth had held forth a grand vision which promised to usher in a new order in the history of Man. Yet within five centuries after his crucifixion his simple, new, revolutionary doctrine of universal love, and of the coming of the Kingdom of Heaven lay buried under and encrusted by old familiar concepts of temples and altars, of consecrated priests and elaborate rituals. Theological controversies caused a rift in Christianity, and threatened its unity. Italy lay prostrate with the Papacy under Pope Gregory trying hard to gain a semblance of control. Gaul witnessed the fratricidal feud between two Frankish chieftains; England was split under the warring kingdoms of Angles, Saxons and Jutes; Egypt lay crushed under Persian rule and suzerainty.

Towns were depopulated and in ruins, precious libraries burnt or ransacked, scholars killed or in hiding. Famine, pestilence and wars ruled the West. The heritage of the Greco-Roman world was about to perish.

Into this bleak and dark night now appeared a ray of light. From the sands of the Arabian desert arose an ever-increasing force that gathered a large mass of humanity under one new religious banner—Islam. Islam and the civilization that came in its wake were great counters to Christianity and the West. Islam brooked no opposition to its religious beliefs; yet it served as a cultural bridge that linked the classical age with the modern world.

From times immemorial the Arabian peninsula has been the land of origin of the ancient nomadic Semitic race. At various times in history these nomadic Semites migrated east, west and north into the early civilizations of Mesopotamia, Egypt and the Mediterranean. Semitic hordes had swamped the Sumerians, established their power in the Eastern Mediterranean as Phoenicians, founded the Babylonian and Assyrian Empires and established themselves in Syria with Damascus as the capital city. As the Hyskos they had conquered Egypt and as the Hebrews they had conquered the greater part of their promised land. There seemed to be an inexhaustible self-rejuvenating tribal Semetic core in the sands of Arabia that gave birth to one invasion after another. History was to record yet another of these invasions, whose cataclysmic force the West as yet had not witnessed.

The majority of these nomadic tribes were pagan and believed in a pantheon of some 300 gods. Medina and Mecca were the two main towns in the region. Mecca, even then, was a place of pilgrimage for the pagan nomads who worshipped in its sanctuary, the Kaaba. This was a small square temple of black stones which had for its cornerstone, a black meteorite, the main object of devout worship. But the paganism of the Arabian peninsula was being influenced and assailed from many sides. There had been a period of proselytizing of the Arabs during the reign of the Herods in Judea. The southernmost strip of Arabia called Yemen, had been in succession under the rule of the Jews, Christians and Zoroastrians. Medina had neighbouring Jewish settlements and had obvious Jewish proclivities. There was a sizeable Nestorian Christian community in the north-east and a sprinkling of Zoroastrians in the north. Christianity, Judaism, Zoroastrianism and the pagan beliefs of the Bedouin nomads rubbed shoulders with one another. The Arabian peninsula was ripe for a religious and political upheaval.

PRE-ISLAMIC MEDICINE

Pre-Islamic medicine was primitive and possessed very few features of the Hippocratic school. Knowledge of plants and herbs and their medicinal use was however akin to Greek medicine. Dates were prized from antiquity for their nutritive value during desert travel and were prescribed as therapy for various maladies. The camel was an Arab's treasure—its urine was considered as cure for several illnesses. Ophthalmic disorders were rampant in the heat and the stinging sands of the Arabian desert. Various medicaments made from herbs and vegetables were used for ophthalmic complaints. Blood-letting through venesection, cupping and the application of leeches were as commonly practised in the Arabian peninsula as in the Mediterranean West. Beliefs in supernatural phenomena were rampant. The *jinn* was a supernatural spirit that influenced human affairs both for better or worse. They were held responsible for a number of illnesses including fevers and insanity. The 'evil eye' was to be warded off by the use of supernatural phenomena in the form of special talismans or charms. A glance from the 'evil eye' could bring harm and bad luck on those upon whom it fell. This ancient belief remains very strong even today in modern Turkey. Medicine and magic remained closely interwoven as in most ancient civilizations.

ISLAM

Into this melting pot of different religions and races within the Arabian peninsula was born about the year AD 570, a man with prophetic vision—Mohammed, the founder of Islam. He was born in poverty, a shepherd's boy who probably never learnt to write. He became the servant of Kadija, the widow of a rich merchant, who married him when he was twenty-five years old. He lived an undistinguished life in Mecca till he was forty years of age. He then had a prophetic vision that he was the prophet of the one true God. He believed that Jesus and Abraham were also divine teachers, but that he was the last and supreme prophet and the world must follow his teachings. Mecca disowned him and he fled to Medina. The details of his trials and tribulations are beyond the scope of this book. Mohammed became the fighting Prophet. He believed in the sword as much as in prayer. The unfaithful should be destroyed if they did not embrace Islam. He practised this with single-minded fierceness and passed this tenet on to those who followed in his footsteps. Mohammed died at the age of sixty-two in AD 632. Before his death he succeeded in the political and religious unification of Arabia under Islam which proclaimed one God, Allah, and his one and only prophet, Mohammed. He produced certain verses which he declared had been divinely revealed, and these verses constituted the holy book of Islam—the *Koran*. Under the unifying and menacing banner of Islam, the next three centuries witnessed one of the most powerful and rapidly-expanding empires known to history. The feat of Arab arms was stupendous, none could withstand their force and fury. It would appear that faith in Allah and Islam could move mountains; the Arab armies, small though they were, appeared invincible. Starting from the small town of Medina in the centre of Arabia, Islamic rule extended over 4000 miles to the West—over Egypt, North Africa, Spain and Southern France. It was at the battle of Poitier in AD 731 that the Frankish infantry led by Charles Martel finally withstood and defeated for the first time in history, the hitherto unvanquished Arab cavalry. This was a crucial battle in world history; as an Arab victory could perhaps have spelt Moslem domination over the heart of Europe. To the north, Moslem rule spread to Syria, Armenia, the Caucasus; the northeast Arab conquests included Mesopotamia, Persia, Afghanistan; and further east the empire extended to the northwest of India. The spiritual centre of the empire was the holy city of Mecca, which even today is the place of pilgrimage that every devout Muslim hopes to visit at least once in his lifetime. The religion which suffered most at the hands of Islam was Zoroastrianism. It was the main counter to Islam in the Near and Middle East; Islam made sure that this religion was completely destroyed. A diaspora of Zoroastrians refused to relinquish their ancient beliefs and set sail from Persia to escape persecution. They landed on the western coast of India and exist to this day as a dwindling Zoroastrian community called the Parsees.

THE JUNDISHAPUR SCHOOL

The conquering Moslems, however, did not destroy all; they preserved the centres of learning they encountered during their victorious expansion. One such centre of learning in the Dark Ages was Jundishapur founded in Persia by the Persian King Shapur in the fourth century. It was an academy that attracted physicians and philosophers from far and near. The history of Jundishapur now becomes closely related to the Nestorian sect of the Catholic Church. Nestorius was the patriarch of Constantinople who was deposed in AD 431 for proposing the doctrine that the Virgin Mary could not be considered the mother of God and that the divine and human aspects of Jesus were separate. He was branded a heretic and had to flee with his followers to Syria and Mesopotamia where they founded a medical school at Edessa which was second only to Alexandria. In AD 489, the church prevailed upon Emperor Zeno to expel the heretic Nestorians from the empire. They fled to Persia and settled at Jundishapur. There are some who believe that it was the Nestorians, who, with their physicians and scholars, founded the academy at Jundishapur. It is more likely that the centre had already been established by King Shapur of Persia and the Nestorians added to its fame and lustre.

There was now a great mingling at Jundishapur of Nestorian scholars, Platonic philosophers who had left Athens when Emperor Justinian closed their schools, Persian scholars, Hebrew scholars who had a command over several languages, Syrian scribes and translators, and Indian and Chinese sages from South and South-East Asia.

When Khalid one of the great generals of history (and the general of Abu Bakr, successor of Mohammed and the first Caliph) destroyed the army of Heraclius, the Emperor of the Eastern Roman Empire, the scholars of Jundishapur feared an end to their academy of learning. But the Moslems preserved and encouraged learning at Jundishapur as also the learning and culture of other conquered nations and civilizations. In fact they made Jundishapur the centre of Islamic learning, and, according to some, the cradle of the Arabian school of medicine. Sergius, a Christian physician, translated Greek manuscripts of medicine into Syriac; this was then translated into Arabic by the Persian Jew Masawayh. Arabic blossomed into a flexible virile language and slowly, in this period of history, supplanted all other languages of learning.

At Jundishapur the Nestorians had built a large hospital staffed by famous physicians. The most famous of these physicians belonged to the family of Bukht-Yishu (servants of Jesus). One of them, Jurjis was summoned in AD 785 to the capital Baghdad, to attend to Caliph al-Mansur who had an obscure abdominal problem. The Caliph took a great liking to Jurjis and kept him in his court as his personal physician for four years. When Jurjis fell ill and lay dying, al-Mansur tried to convert him to the Moslem faith, promising him eternal paradise. Jurjis pleaded that he would rather join his own ancestors even if they were in hell. Al-Mansur allowed Jurjis to return to Jundishapur. It is of interest that the grandson of Jurjis became the personal physician to the great Harun-al-Rashid.

It was not just medicine which held Moslem interest. The Moslem invaders were considerably influenced by Greek learning in all spheres. Euclid, Plato, Aristotle, Hippocrates and Dioscorides held a special influence over Arab culture and the works of these great men were avidly translated into Arabic.

MEDICINE AND THE KORAN

Allah was the prime cause of all things big and small. Disease resulted from transgressing his tenets as laid down in the *Koran*. The wrath of Allah could manifest in the form of catastrophes and epidemics which could demolish kingdoms as the wages of sin.

The *Koran* accepted the ancient concept that the *pneuma* supplied the breath of life reaching the heart via the nostrils and the respiratory passages. The soul resided in the heart, and, on dying, returned to Allah via the dying breath. The Koranic view of physiology was primitive. The coarse elements of food were removed through the urine via the kidneys and through faeces via the rectum. The finer elements were converted to milk and the very finest to blood. Procreation resulted from the encounter of the male seed with female blood in the uterus. A clot was thereby formed from which came the skeleton clothed by a covering of muscles and flesh. The seminal fluid originated in the head reaching the testicles through the spinal column.

The *Koran* is notable for its rules on personal hygiene. Water was regarded as both a spiritual and physical cleanser. Frequent washing of the body and wearing clean clothes were strict Koranic commands. All food was permitted except the flesh of pigs. Both honey and milk were valuable; alcohol was forbidden as were drugs that produced a loss of mental control. There is no reference to surgery in the *Koran;* circumcision was however an obligatory ritual at birth. The religion expressively disallowed the study of human anatomy through the dissection of human bodies.

THE ARAB WORLD

It is of interest to take a bird's eye view of the Arab world at the peak of its grandeur and power. The picture of medicine in this era would be better appreciated if viewed against this backdrop. The first two caliphs after the death of Mohammed were Abu-Bakr and Omar. They were deeply religious, devout, fanatical followers of Islam. Clad in home-spun clothes, living on camel's milk, dates, meat and cheese, they and their hardy followers were simple incorruptible soldiers of Allah who began to carve out a vast Islamic Empire. A ninth century Muslim scholar writes thus: "As for the desert Arabs, they have never been merchants, tradesmen, or physicians nor had they aptitude for mathematics and agriculture. On the other hand, when they gave their minds to poetry and oratory, to horses, weapons, and implements of war, or to the recording of tradition and annals, they were unexcelled." Slowly and steadily the simplicity, frugality, piety and justice of the earlier caliphs began to be replaced by deviousness, luxury, debauchery and cruelty of the later rulers of the Arab world.

The early poet-warriors of the desert found themselves masters of vast territories which they had to rule and administer. They borrowed from their Persian enemies the systems of taxation, the art of local and central government and the need to vest absolute power in the hands of the ruler (the caliph). Within a few years, the softness and luxury of Persian life replaced the austerity and frugality of their desert existence. The home-spun shirt of the desert warriors thus gave way to brocaded silk; the desert fare of milk, dates, honey and meat was replaced by exotic Persian delicacies; gargantuan banquets replaced the communal kuskus bowl. Persian customs began to be adopted; wine consumed (against the *Koran's* injunction), and Persian feast days began to be celebrated.

Islamic culture and civilization were centred around two great cities—Baghdad and Cordoba. Baghdad existed, from Sumerian times, as a small town squeezed between the Euphrates and the Tigris. In AD 762, the Caliph al-Mansur of the Abbasid dynasty ordered some 1,00,000 labourers to build him a new capital for his Moslem empire. There emerged in four years a splendid city a mile and a half in diameter, ringed by three lines of walls. In the centre arose the palace of the Caliph resplendent with domes, arches and dotted by fountains and by courtyards enclosing beautiful gardens.

Caliph al-Mansur lured many scholars from various centres, in particular from Jundishapur. He established schools of medicine, chemistry, astrology and mathematics. Qifto was a contemporary scholar who gave a good description of medicine in Baghdad. There was progress in science, and the development of new methods in the treatment of disease along pharmacologic lines. Furthermore, their physicians adopted the scientific methods of the Greeks and the Hindus, and modified them by their own discoveries. They elaborated medical laws and recorded the work they had done.

Vizier Abud al-Daula founded Baghdad's best known and most famous hospital in AD 970. It had wards as also an outpatient department, a system of interns and externs, a teaching faculty, a pharmacy stocked with drugs from all parts of the world and even a basic though primitive nursing system.

Under Caliph al-Mamun, the son of Harun al-Rashid, Baghdad was next only to Constantinople as the most opulent city West of the Indus. The city was termed the Abode of Peace and had within its centre a great academy of learning aptly called the House of Wisdom.

CORDOBA

This city became the centre of civilization at the western end of the Islamic Empire. With Rome in ruins, London and Paris a miserable collection of mud houses, Cordoba was the most splendid and most civilized city of Europe. In the tenth century, Cordoba had a million citizens, over 300 mosques (each with an attached school), seventy libraries, 900 public baths, fifty hospitals and a university that was renowned throughout Europe. The city was dominated by its great mosque with its nineteen bronze gateways, thousands of glittering lamps fed by perfumed oil, a roof supported by over a thousand columns of porphyry, marble and jasper, double arches that gave the impression of infinite space and perfect geometry. Cordoba did not possess the opulence of Baghdad but it was an important trading centre acting as the terminus for caravans arriving from places as far as China. Moslems brought civilization to Spain—arts and crafts which they had acquired in their path of conquest, the construction of roads and canals, the manufacture of ceramics and the introduction of plants from Asia and Africa. China invented paper; the Moslems learnt this art and passed it on to the West. Spanish Moslems produced some of the most beautiful books the world had yet to see.

Moslem culture merged with the indigenous local Spanish culture to produce great centres of Hispano-Arabic civilization in Seville, Granada and Toledo. Toledo became a great centre of learning and culture after Cordoba fell to the invading Berbers in the eleventh century.

Art, literature, crafts, science, medicine flourished between Baghdad in the Middle East and Cordoba in the west. The crumbling West was ringed by a civilized belt of Islam. Though Islam never compromised on its religious beliefs it encouraged medicine and science, preserved ancient centres of learning and saved the classic Greco-Roman heritage from being lost to the modern world.

Medicine in the Arab World

One of the earliest Arabian physicians of the sixth century was Al-Harith who studied medicine in Jundishapur and then worked as a practitioner in Persia. He, then, went on to Mecca and became a friend of Mohammed the Prophet. Medicine, together with science, philosophy and art flourished in the Arab world from the seventh to the tenth centuries. This period marked the spring and summer of a vigorous Arab culture. The leaders of medicine were members of the Bakht-Yishu family. The cause of medicine was also furthered by translators in various centres of learning all over the Arab world who considered it their duty to render into Arabic the great works of Hippocrates, Galen and other physicians. Hellenic culture, extinguished with the fall of Rome, was like a phoenix reborn from its ashes. Harun al-Rashid (AD 763–809) the first Abbasid Caliph and his son al-Ma'mun (AD 813–833) were great patrons of Arab learning.

Al-Ma'mun had a passion for collecting valuable Greek manuscripts from every possible source. His huge collection was stored in the great Baghdad library which he founded. Al-Ma'mun also established the Bryt al Hikma (AD 832), a school of translators under the direction of his personal physician Yuhanna ibn Masawahy (latinized as, Mesue or Johannes Damascenus). Scholars gathered in this great centre translating several important non-Islamic works into Arabic. The initial translators were chiefly Christian because of their knowledge of Greek, Latin and Syriac. Mesue, the older, was a Nestorian and the student of Gabriel Bukht-Yishu; he translated many Greek manuscripts into Arabic and also authored original writings. His work on dietetics and gynaecology was famous not only in the Arab world but even in the West until the early Renaissance.

Mesue's most distinguished student was Hunain ibn Ishaq, a Nestorian Christian born at Hira in Mesopotamia in 809. He was known in Europe as Johannitius. He rendered into Arabic the entire works of Hippocrates (*Hippocratic Corpus*), the works of Galen, Oribasius and Paul of Aegina; he also translated the *Materia Medica* of Dioscorides. Hunain was extremely prolific. He was a linguist who was as familiar with Greek as he was with Arabic, and was known to recite Homer in the streets of Baghdad. Galen was his particular favourite and the translations of about 130 of his texts ensured that the world today has more Galenic texts in Arabic than in Greek. It is of interest that Galen was given a greater importance than Hippocrates in the Arab world. Hunain's important original works include the *Quaestiones Medicenae* (a question and answer manual in medicine) and the ten dissertations on the eye, which is the oldest treatise on ophthalmology. Hunain ferreted out ancient priceless manuscripts with the zest and zeal of an avid hunter. He described how he was obsessed in tracking down a particular work of Galen. He hunted for it in Mesopotamia, Palestine, Syria and Egypt, finally locating half of this work in Damascus. This zeal to preserve knowledge for posterity was one of the most endearing features of Islam. When the Moslems defeated the Byzantine Emperor Michael III in battle, they insisted on the surrender and transfer of a large number of precious manuscripts from the libraries of Constantinople to the library of Baghdad.

Hunain also contributed to the formulation of a scientific vocabulary and language in Arabic by coining new words or creating the Arabic equivalent of Greek and Syriac terms. Thus many Arabic scientific words have Greek or Syriac roots. At the same time, English words like alcohol, aldehyde, alembic, alchemy, alkaloid, are derived from Arabic terms. The Arab Jabir ibn Hayan lived in the ninth century and was the first to devise the alembic or retort; he founded the science of chemistry. He is also reported to be the first to examine the blood and faeces.

RHAZES

One of Islam's greatest physicians and one of the Arab world's best known authors was Abu Bakr Muhammad ibn Zakaria, known as al-Rhazes (865–965), a Persian born near Tehran. He studied medicine in Baghdad and became chief physician at the Baghdad hospital. He was widely travelled, visiting Africa, Jerusalem and the academies of learning at Cordoba. He was soon acclaimed as the greatest physician of the Islamic world. Rhazes epitomized the finest elements of Islamic learning and culture. He was interested in mathematics, astronomy, religion, and philosophy, in addition to his devotion to medicine. He wrote 237 works, over half of which were on medicine.

His monumental masterpiece was the twenty-volume work called *al-Hawi* (meaning 'Comprehensive Book'), known in the West as the *Liber Continens*. This book was an encyclopaedia of medical practice and treatment, assembling medical knowledge up to his time and incorporating his own experiences as also the views of Greek, Persian, Syrian and Indian authors. Another great work was the *Liber Medicinalis* and *Almansorem*, a collection of ten medical treatises. These were compiled from various sources, but mainly from Hippocrates, Galen, Oribasius and Paul of Aegina. The ninth volume on general medicine was widely used for many years in Western universities. This volume contained some striking aphorisms, a few examples of which are worth quoting:

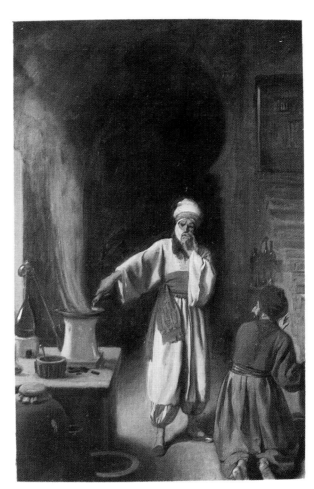

Fig. 23.1   Rhazes.

Ask many doctors, make many mistakes.
Truth in medicine is an unattainable goal and the healing art described in books is much inferior to the experience of a thoughtful physician.
When Galen and Aristotle agree about something, then it is easy for doctors to make a decision, but when they differ it is very difficult to arrive at agreement.

Rhazes wrote many other medical treatises dealing with renal and vesical calculi, a description of spina bifida, the use of animal gut in sutures and the introduction of a mercurial ointment. He also wrote on the anatomy of the recurrent laryngeal nerve. But his most celebrated work, which was reprinted several times even as late as the nineteenth century was his treatise on smallpox and chickenpox, the *Liber de Pestilentia*. This book contained his own experiences and observations giving a beautiful clinical description of these infectious diseases, the differential diagnosis and views on management. A quote from the clinical description is given below:

> The eruption of smallpox is preceded by continuous fever, pains in the back, itching in the nose and delirium in sleep. . . . When the pustules appear care must be taken first of the eyes, then the nose and ears; very small white pustules coming up in contact with each other, hard and without fluid are dangerous; and if the patient remains ill even after the eruption it is a fatal sign. When fever increases after the appearance of greenish or blackish pustules, and there is palpitation of the heart, it is a very bad sign, indeed.

His treatment was simple, based on proper diet, rest and the use of nature's healing power—principles stressed by the Hippocratic school. For fever he advised cold water sponges, for inflammation he recommended wine, for phthisis milk and sugar. Indigestion was to be treated by a diet of buttermilk and cold water, constipation could be corrected by mercury. He advocated music and chess for melancholia and stressed on the Koranic teaching of frequent washing and bathing as a hygienic measure of great importance.

Rhazes also wrote a book on the art of alchemy. This great book was discovered less than seventy years ago. He classified all substances into vegetable, animal and mineral, and distinguished between volatile and non-volatile substances.

Rhazes could be counted as a follower of the Hippocratic School both in the practice of medicine and in his code of ethics. He commanded a huge practice in Baghdad and charged high professional fees, but he impoverished himself by spending what he earned on the poor. He was blind towards the end of his long and illustrious life. It is believed that he refused an eye operation saying that he felt repugnance at the sights the world had to offer. His blindness is believed to have resulted from the blows to his head received on the command of al-Mansur, the Persian prince, who was incensed at Rhazes' inability to convert a base metal to pure gold. He was ordered to be beaten on his head by his own book till either one or the other broke! The authenticity of this story is however questionable

AVICENNA

Abu Ali al-Hussain ibn Abdallah ibn Sina, known as Avicenna was a shining star in the Arab world of learning whose influence extended far and wide for many centuries to come. Avicenna was born in AD 980 near Bukhara in Persia, the son of a tax collector. He was a precocious boy, for at the age of ten he could recite the entire *Koran*. He went on to study logic, philosophy, geometry, and astronomy. At sixteen, he started his medical studies and at eighteen, he was a reputed practitioner. When summoned to treat Prince Nuh ibn Mansur, he asked as his reward the freedom to browse through the rare manuscripts in the prince's library. He was fascinated with Aristotle, read his *Metaphysics* several times, but admitted to not understanding the work at all.

Avicenna was a remarkable man for he combined high scholastic application and ability with a passion for life, and a love for wine, woman and song. He composed poetry, wrote on mathematics, chemistry and theology. When at last he began to understand Aristotle's *Metaphysics* he turned his full attention to the study of philosophy. Avicenna's masterpiece was called *al-Quanun* (the Canon). It attempted to combine and coordinate the medical doctrines of Hippocrates and Galen with the biological doctrine of Aristotle. The Canon consisted of five books. The first one dealt with diseases and their symptoms, their treatment and the general rules of health and hygiene. The second book was based on Dioscorides—it listed a pharmacopoeia largely unknown to the Greeks. The third book dealt with pathology and contained accounts of various disease states, such as jaundice, pleurisy, duodenal ulcer, pyloric stenosis, venereal diseases. The fourth book dealt with surgery and various contagious diseases; the fifth and final book dealt with the preparation of drugs and was the accepted text on materia medica till the Renaissance. *The Canon* was translated into Latin by Gerard of Cremona in the twelfth century. It became the standard medical text of Western universities for centuries, and was used as late as 1650 in the medical schools of Lovain and Montpellier. The works of Avicenna and Galen became the gospel of the medical world till well into the Renaissance.

It was Paracelsus who pronounced a war on both these hitherto unquestioned authorities when he burned their works in a public square in 1527. As with Galen the main drawback of Avicenna's work was the poverty of knowledge in both anatomy and physiology.

It is of interest even today that the impact

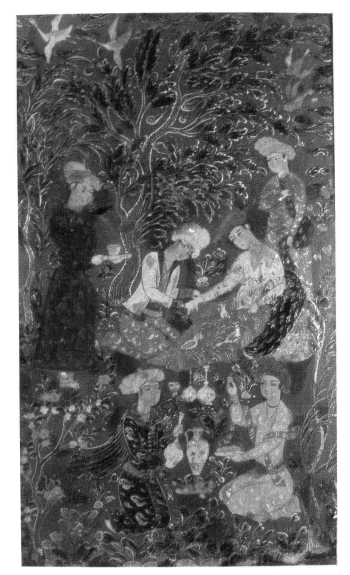

Fig. 23.2   Physician taking patient's pulse.

of Avicenna's great work was due to the ideology and the philosophy that attempted to reconcile the medical doctrine of Galen with the biological doctrine of Aristotle. There are many who would consider Avicenna's contribution to philosophy even greater than to medicine. The close link between medicine and philosophy so eloquently initiated by the Italic school of ancient Greece was brought into renewed focus in the pages of Avicenna's Canon. The legacy of Aristotle almost alien and lost to the West after the fall of Rome was rescued by this Islamic scholar. Under the aegis of Arab culture this legacy was renewed in Spain and Sicily and thence re-established in the rest of Europe.

ALBUCASIS

Cordoba was the flourishing centre of Arab culture under the Caliph Abd al-Rahman (912–961) of the Omayyad dynasty in the tenth century. The city was an important medical centre with over fifty-two hospitals and a number of doctors looking after its one million inhabitants. Among these doctors now appeared the greatest surgeon of Islam, Abu'l-Quasim, also called Albucasis, in the Latinised form. He was born at El Zahra near Cordoba and wrote an encyclopedic work called *al-Tasrif*, or the *Method*. Gerard of Cremona translated this treatise into Latin. The most interesting and informative aspect of Albucasis' treatise was on surgery. It presented a great deal of information on surgical practice, and on surgical instruments used by the Arabs. The work contained 200 illustrations of different surgical instruments and their method of use. Albucasis' text dominated the teaching of surgery in European universities till the advent of Ambroise Paré.

Albucasis was humble enough to recognize the limitations of surgery in his era. He correctly attributed these limitations to the ignorance of anatomy resulting from the lack of direct experience in the dissection of human bodies. His treatise described the use of cautery, trephining, amputations, lithotomy, herniotomy and operations for fistula, goitre and arrow wounds. He advised the use of silver catheters instead of the usual bronze catheters for bladder disorders, and in edentulous individuals recommended artificial teeth made of beef bone. In obstetrics and gynaecology, direct examination of females by males was forbidden. Female operators were therefore made to work under his guidance. His treatise described several procedures to correct abnormal foetal presentations and discussed the use of instruments to aid delivery.

During the reign of the Cordovan Caliphates there lived, in the twelfth century Ibn Zuhr, also called Avenzoar (AD 1091–1162), a famous scholar and practitioner of medicine. He was born in Seville in an aristocratic family. He was a staunch opponent of quackery and questioned the validity of many doctrines propounded by the great men of the past. He paid greater emphasis on practical experience and preferred to disregard metaphysical explanations. In this regard he was more in tune with the Hippocratic school of medicine. Avenzoar criticized Avicenna's Canon; he was amongst the very few scholars who also dared to criticize the works of Galen. His major work in medicine was titled *al-Taysir*, which dealt with features and management of specific diseases including heart disease, pericarditis and otitis media.

Averroes

Another great physician of the Arab world was Ibn Rashid, latinized as Averroes. He was born in Cordoba in AD 1126, and came from a long line of lawyers. He studied philosophy, law and medicine. He was as much or more a philosopher than a physician. He became a magistrate in Seville and Cordoba, and finally, governor of the province of Andalusia. Averroes was also the personal physician to the ruling Almohad family. He is best remembered today for his great and detailed commentary on the works of Aristotle which drew great praise from Dante. Averroes was bold enough to express his disbelief in the immortality of the soul. He held Aristotle's view that the soul after death merged into universal nature. To Islam this was an unforgivable heresy. His teachings were banned and he was banished for his impiety. He died in Marrakesh in 1198. His philosophy and teachings, however, influenced scholastic thought in Islam. Averroes' famous work in medicine, an encyclopedic work in the Galenic tradition, was titled *al-Kulliyat* (the *Book of General Principles*). It consisted of seven books dealing with all aspects of medicine including anatomy, dietetics and hygiene. It became a companion to the book *al-Taysir* written by his colleague Avenzoar. The *al-Kulliyat* and the *al-Taysir* were translated into Hebrew and Latin (*Colligei*) and printed in Venice in 1482. The *Colligei* (*Collections*), remained an influential medical text in Western universities for many years.

MAIMONIDES

Averroes' most famous pupil was Musa ibn Maimun (1135–1204) also known as Maimonides; he was not an Arab, but a Jew. Like Avenzoar he was a non-conformist. In his philosophical attempts to reconcile faith with reason he went against some of the traditional Jewish beliefs arousing the ire of the orthodox believers. In 1148, the Almohads, a fanatic sect, replaced the Omayyads in Cordoba and expelled all Jews and Christians who refused to be converted to Islam. Maimonides, who was just thirteen years old fled with his family, lost all his possessions in a shipwreck and finally settled in Cairo, Egypt. The intolerance and bigotry of the Almohads was a major factor in the subsequent decline of Cordoba.

Maimonides in the old Greek tradition, was a scholar well-versed in philosophy, astronomy, theology and medicine. His main theological work written in Hebrew was *Mishneh Torah*. His ten medical texts were chiefly written in Arabic. One of his best known medical texts was titled *Fusul Musa* (Latin, *Aphorisms*), a collection of 1500 aphorisms extracted from Galenic writings, together with about forty of his own pithy observations and remarks. He also wrote a treatise on haemorrhoids and a book on poisons and antidotes. He gave one of the best early descriptions of bronchial asthma.

Maimonides also wrote a renowned treatise on sexual intercourse (Latin: *Ars Coeundi*), comprising nineteen chapters. Maimonides became famous as a physician in Egypt and was appointed as court physician to the Caliph Saladin the Great, the famous opponent of the Crusaders and the strong but chivalrous foe of England's Richard I, also called the Lion-Heart. King Richard sent him an offer to join his court and become his physician, which he politely refused. One of his most famous and influential texts was written for the melancholic eldest son of Saladin. It was titled *Regimen of Health*; it embodied rules on hygiene and dietetics also discussing the influence of climate on health.

Maimonides was perhaps an even greater philosopher than a physician. Many consider his lasting fame to be based on his philosophical thesis—*Guide to the Perplexed*. This work is believed to have influenced Thomas Aquinas and the development of Christian thought and scholasticism. It is of interest to quote one of his thought-provoking tenets: "Employ your reason and you will be able to discern that which is said figuratively, hyperbolically and what is meant literally."

Philosopher, physician, theologian, Maimonides was a shining light in the Arab world whose free-thinking intellect soared above the constraints of all religious beliefs and doctrines. His tomb in Tiberias is a place of pilgrimage for all who value intellectual excellence and integrity, combined with the humanism of a good physician.

Arab culture introduced a large number of drugs into medicine, making a significant original contribution to pharmacology. The Arabs also initiated the first pharmacies where drugs were dispensed and where physicians and pharmacists gathered for discussion and debate. Mention has already been made earlier of the mysterious Jabir who improved on methods of evaporation, filtration and sublimation. He also devised the chemistry to produce mercury, arsenious oxide, vitriols, alum, lead acetate and a combination of sulphuric and nitric acid termed *aqua regia*. The writings of *al-Kindi* (AD 800–870) described many Persian and Oriental drugs unknown to the Greeks. His work was the primary source for future Arab treatises on pharmacy, pharmacology, botany and minerology.

The best known and most complete book on materia medica in the Middle Ages was titled *Corpus of Simples*. It was written by Ibn al-Baitar (1197–1248), a great botanist from Malaga who collected plants and drugs along the whole Mediterranean zone and the Middle East. Dioscorides' materia medica which was valued even more than the Hippocratic *Corpus* in the Arab world included about a thousand items from the plant, mineral and animal kingdoms. Ibn al-Baitar listed over 3000 drugs derived chiefly from plants and minerals. In the eleventh century the *Kitab al-Sayadanah fi al Tibb* (the *Book of Pharmacy in the Healing Art*) written by al-Biruni described more than 1000 drugs. The most authoritative of all medieval texts on the art and science of pharmacy was written by a Jew, Kohen al-Attar in Cairo in 1259. Remarkably enough this book was written with the intent to provide education and instructions to his son; it remained the standard reference in materia medica for over 300 years. Among the numerous new medicines introduced by Arabs to the world of medicine were camphor, nux vomica, rhubarb, senna, ginger, amber, myrrh, musk, cloves, nutmeg, betel nut, sandalwood, laudanum, naphtha and alcohol.

The Arabs were the first to initiate the opening of pharmacies in all major cities. Besides dispensing drugs, they dispensed herbs, honey, essence of flowers (a favourite of physicians for washing hands), poultices and plasters. Several pharmacies displayed beautiful artistically exquisite ceramic drug jars and bottles. Some pharmacies had an elegant Moslem architecture, with courtyards and fountains, and became centres for discussion and debate on drugs and their uses. In the Middle Ages and even beyond, there flourished a rich trade of drugs and simples between the pharmacies of the Arab world and the West. This commerce contributed to the growing wealth of some of the Italian maritime cities, notably of Venice.

The Arab world made one more significant contribution to medicine. It was in the establishment of hospitals both for care of the sick and for the teaching of the art of healing. Perhaps, to an extent, these hospitals might have been inspired by Christian monasteries which offered relief to the sick. Yet the hospitals of the Arab world were large institutions, humane, efficient for that time and age, and well-organized. The first large hospital as mentioned earlier was founded in Baghdad in AD 805 by Harun al-Rashid. By the twelfth century all major towns in the Arab world could boast of a hospital. The major ones were in Baghdad, Damascus, Cairo and Cordoba. The most famous hospital of the Arab world was built in AD 1283 by al-Mansur in Cairo. It had a special ward for mental diseases, and had separate fever wards cooled by fountains. It contained lecture halls, a library, a pharmacy, male and female nurses, and had both a Christian chapel and a mosque. Musicians helped patients to sleep and story-tellers distracted patients from their suffering. The hospital even provided money to the poor and deserving patients to help them during their convalescence. The al-Mansur hospital was still functioning when Napoleon entered Egypt in the late eighteenth century.

Christian pilgrims to the Holy Land were impressed and amazed at the humaneness and organization of hospitals in the Arab world. This probably led to the creation of a hospital in Jerusalem in the eleventh century. The Crusaders expanded this hospital so that it formed the nucleus of the religious order of the hospital of St John of Jerusalem. This famous religious order was called the Knights of the Hospitalers; it played an important role in the Crusades. The *Koran* enjoined humanity and care for the insane and this tenet was followed faithfully. The first hospitals for the mentally unbalanced were created by Islam in the Arab world. Their influence was probably responsible for the establishment of the first European hospitals for the insane in Granada, Spain, in 1365.

The thirteenth century witnessed the decline and fall of the Arab Empire. Ferdinand II of Castille captured Cordoba, the centre of Islamic power and culture at the western end of its dominions in 1236; this was just twenty-eight years after the death of Maimonides. The Moslems were steadily pushed out of Europe. The Mongols invaded the Arab world from the east and sacked Baghdad in

1258. The Empire lay in ruins, and, as with Rome, the basic cause was a cankerous rot within its body politic. The Christians under Ferdinand II and the Mongols under Genghis Khan merely delivered the *coup de grace* to a wounded civilization. The Ottoman Turks who dominated the Levant in the next two centuries, were more concerned with conquest and the physical luxuries and pleasures that accrued from these conquests, than with intellectual pursuits of science, philosophy or medicine. Art flourished; Ottoman architecture was impressive but was still a mere extension of Islamic architecture in the old Arab world. There were, however, no great thoughts, no great discoveries or inventions that added to the intellectual or spiritual glory of man.

The Arab heritage to the world has a rich and important place in the history of man. A recognized fact is that it saved for the West and also for the rest of the world the invaluable treasures amassed by the Greeks not only in medicine but in so many other fields of human endeavour. It must be noted that physicians and other scholars under Islam came from many ethnic sources. They drew their inspiration not only from Greece but also from Rome, Syria, India and even China. Had it not been for this act of salvage (in which the Christian Church also participated), the footprints of the progress of man would have been almost completely effaced in the strife, disorder and gloom of the Dark Ages. The clock of Western civilization would then have stood still for perhaps many centuries, and would have been forced to start all over once again.

The Arab mind was both receptive and creative. It was receptive in that it appreciated, and, at times, was enamoured of the work of pagan civilization. It systematized, analysed and presented these works afresh to the world. It was creative in that it made original contributions to chemistry, mathematics, alchemy, botany, pharmacology, and pharmacy. It conceived of humane patient care in large hospitals expertly administered, and of kindness and compassion in the care of the insane. It may not have contributed significantly to the science of medicine, but enriched its art and enhanced its teaching and practice. Islam evolved its own language which had its basic roots in the desert sands of Arabia but which became increasingly expressive, rich and virile with the growth of its civilization. Latin became the language of Europe; Arabic remained the language of science in a vast territory stretching from Spain in the west to India in the east. The Arab heritage was not only to preserve and contribute to medicine and other human affairs but to make medicine international. It linked the old with the new and bridged the East with the West.

The clash between the Christian and Moslem worlds for two centuries during the crusades was an unmitigated economic disaster. Yet it further enhanced the cultural and medical links between the centres of learning in both worlds. By the time the Arab world lay dying in the thirteenth century, it had succeeded in passing on its message to the world; it had sowed the seeds of learning in many centres. The seeds were to blossom and flower in the sunlit garden of the Renaissance.

24 Medicine in the Medieval West

Think what a precious thing you work upon. It is the temple of God, his own image, the most precious creature that ever God made.

Guy de Chauliac

Historical Background

The Middle Ages constituted an era of repair, a return from chaos to a semblance of order, from barbarism to a degree of civilization. The Western church took upon itself the onerous duty of building a Christian society out of warring pagans. It stressed on the absolute supremacy of one God, the precedence of the spirit over temporal affairs and insisted on the allegiance of both princes and people to the Vicars of God on earth. A conflict between the papacy and the rulers of the kingdom states in Europe inevitably stained the annals of history in this era. The streams of medicine, philosophy, science which had nearly dried in the Dark Ages were slowly brought to life, first in the churches and monasteries that preserved and translated the works of antiquity and of the Arab world, and later in the centres of learning and in the universities that slowly bloomed in an otherwise barren landscape. The end of the Middle Ages saw the West poised for the joyous leap into the Renaissance.

The transition from the Dark to the Middle Ages saw the establishment of barbaric kingdoms of the Goths, Franks, Vandals, and Celts. In these early centuries before Charlemagne founded the new Western Empire (AD 800), the barbarian kingdoms consisted of a society owing allegiance to a leader. Feudal rules and customs were non-existent. The ninth to the eleventh centuries saw the transformation of the barbarian states into feudal kingdoms with an established feudal society. There was now imposed a hierarchy of order in a society headed by the king and followed by princes, nobles, vassals, burghers, peasants and slaves. Strict rules of code and conduct governed the relationship between these various classes. The Norman conquest of England in the eleventh century introduced a further addition to feudal customs—the feudal power of the manor lord. The peasants were the manor lord's serfs; they owed him their unswerving obedience, tilled his soil for a specific number of days every year, and contributed a share of their own produce to the manor house.

The Middle Ages were characterized by two great social forces. The first and most important was the confrontation between Christiandom and the power of Islam in the Arab world. This confrontation took the form of crusades, the purpose of which was to protect the holy places in Palestine from being defiled by the Moslems. Jerusalem, the holiest of holies in Christiandom, was in Islamic hands—the crusades were a war to capture Jerusalem and hold fast to it against the Moslems. There were thirteen crusades between 1095 and 1291. The early ones were fired by religious zeal; many of the later ones were chiefly motivated by the desire for territorial expansion, greed and loot, rather than by religious devotion. The conflicts make fascinating history. Crimes in the name of religion were occasionally balanced by nobility, chivalry and generosity of spirit. The crusades proved infructuous, the Holy Land lay unconquered, yet they exercised an enormous impact on Western civilization. The European continent was introduced to and cross-fertilized by the culture, art and learning of the East. The crusades also indirectly instilled a spirit of adventure that blossomed towards the end of the Middle Ages into the great voyages of discovery to the New World and to India.

The second social force that shaped the Middle Ages arose as a direct result of the crusades. It was the growth of knighthood which upheld courage, chivalry, honesty and fidelity as opposed to cruelty, treachery and dishonesty that often characterized feudal society. Knighthood became linked to medicine in the Knights Hospitalers, a celibate order devoted to the care of the sick in the Holy Land. Circumstances forced this order to also assume a combatant crusading role, yet it preserved its main purpose of a nursing brotherhood. The Knights Hospitalers besides looking after sick pilgrims, provided free clothing and food. Attached to the nursing brotherhood were physicians and surgeons who enjoyed the privilege of eating with the knights.

MONASTERIES

Christianity represented by the catholic church had been a beacon of hope and light in the crumbling decay of the Dark Ages. The monasteries now assumed this role and became centres of civilization and learning in the early Middle Ages around the sixth and seventh centuries. The central figure in the story of the development of monasteries in Europe was Saint Benedict who lived between AD 480 and 544. He was born of noble parents at Spoletto in Italy. The shadow of decadent times fell upon him, and, like Buddha, he took to a religious life, at first subjecting himself to the severest of austerities. With a hair shirt as his sole worldly possession he lived alone in a cave within a cliff overlooking the river Arno. His position was so inaccessible that food had to be lowered to him on a rope by a faithful admirer. He remained thus for three years and his fame spread far and wide in the West as had Buddha's in the East a thousand years before. He then emerged into the world fired with the mission of action rather than of self-torment. He sent the following message to a solitary recluse who had chained himself to a stone in a small cave: "Break thy chain, for the true servant of God is chained not to rock by iron but to righteousness by Christ."

We find him now in control of twelve monasteries—the resort of a great number of people who wished to learn and be educated. Benedict now moved south to Monte Cassino, halfway between Naples and Rome, a beautiful mountain in the midst of other majestic mountain ranges. At the summit of Monte Cassino stood a pagan temple dedicated to Apollo. His missionary zeal persuaded the pagans to break the temple and establish a monastery that became a famous centre in the lifetime of its founder. Ultimately 40,000 such monastic institutions of Benedictine and various other orders were built over Europe. Members of the Benedictine and other orders took vows of poverty, chastity and obedience. They were a civilizing influence in those barbaric times. They served as centres of learning, preserved for posterity Greek and Latin texts, perfected the art of calligraphy and transcribed these texts. In the centuries to come, particularly in the late medieval era, they fertilized the West with the wisdom of the East, by translating several Arabic texts written in the civilized Arab world into Latin and Greek. Schools, libraries and infirmaries were attached to many monasteries, which from the very start, established the combined tradition of learning and medicine. Thus medicine (called physics) was added to the curriculum of all cathedral schools founded by Charlemagne in AD 805.

In Monte Cassino and in thousands of other monasteries, the early medieval physician was the priest, reminding one of the priest-physicians of Sumer and Egypt. In most cases the monks who combined within themselves the role of physicians had no special training. Compassion and the use of simple herbs from the monastery's herbal garden constituted the practice of medicine. Many monasteries became treasured libraries of medical books. Two hundred such volumes were listed in the monastery of Christ Church, Canterbury, and a similar number in the neighbouring monastery of St Augustus in the thirteenth and fourteenth centuries.

Two other great names besides that of Saint Benedict must be mentioned in the development of civilizing monasticism. The first is Pope Gregory the Great (AD 540–604), a follower of Saint Benedict and the first monk to become a pope (AD 590). He was a capable pope, ruled Rome like an emperor, organized armies, made treaties, but, above all, imposed the Benedictine rule over nearly the whole of Latin monasticism.

The other is that of Cassiodorus (AD 490–585), a patrician by birth who took refuge from the Dark Ages by founding a monastery on his estate and joining a monastic life. Disturbed by the universal decay around him and of the possible loss of all learning and ancient literature in the world, he initiated a movement of preservation, transcription and translation of ancient valuable manuscripts. Cassiodorus advised his monks to read Hippocrates, Galen and Dioscorides. He encouraged experimental science introducing the first gleam of scientific light in the gathering darkness and produced a series of school books on liberal arts and grammar. He was probably as influential as St Benedict in helping to restore social order in the Western world.

Monastic medical treatises included the encyclopaedic *Etymologiae* of the Bishop Isidore of Seville and the writings of the Venerable Bede, Anglo-Saxon prior at Wearmouth. The *Etymologiae* served as a medical text in monasteries for several centuries. It also included theology, mathematics, history, law and almost all branches of learning. Isidore gave a neat summary of Greek science, philosophy and medicine. His writing on medicine closely followed Hippocratic and Galenic views. The cosmos or the macrocosm was constituted of fire, earth, air, water; the microcosm of the four humors—phlegm, blood, yellow bile and black bile. A disturbance in the equilibrium of humors caused disease. A return to equilibrium restored health and this could be achieved by diet, exercise and drugs. It is of interest that Isidore of Seville titled his work *Etymolagiae* signifying his primary interest in semantics—the correct use of words.

Monastic medicine, primitive as it was, declined in the twelfth century when the church authorities felt that monks neglected their spiritual duties, spending far too much time in the practice of medicine. Medical activities were ultimately completely banned in all monasteries in the thirteenth century. But by this time their purpose had been amply fulfilled because the learning and medicine preserved and perpetuated for several centuries within these monasteries had been passed on to the growing schools and universities of the Latin West.

THE TOWN

In the first five centuries of the Middle Ages villages grouped themselves around a castle, an abbey, a manor house or a monastery. There could be no comparison between these rather primitive settlements and the resplendent towns of the Arab world or the Byzantine Empire.

The break-up of Charlemagne's Empire led to a turmoil in Western Europe for over two centuries. Trade then revived, particularly in the Italian communities that lay astride the mercantile routes between the East and the West. The twelfth century witnessed the appearance of the first self-governing towns. They were the forerunners of the powerful city-states of Florence, Venice and Naples. Feudalism still flourished, yet throughout the turbulent twelfth century there was a movement to found communal town governments. The feudal princes and lords felt the growing power of their people, particularly of merchants, artisans, and students who often initiated a ferment of unrest in the centres of learning. The kings or the lords and masters though still powerful, devised means to come to terms with their subject people.

By 1200, a typical European town was built around a castle and was contained within stone walls for protection against rival rulers. Town buildings were constructed of wood, and fires were frequent. The fabric of social and cultural life was more ordered, but boisterous luxury co-existed with poverty, profligacy and debauchery with fiery reformers threatening damnation and the fires of hell.

The medieval town's greatest contribution to medicine was the establishment of hospitals in numerous centres; its greatest contribution to culture was the cathedral. Church architecture through the greater part of the Medieval Ages was Romanesque in style, characterized by the squat rounded arch. The first structure in the Gothic style of architecture was the Choir of St Denis' Abbey near Paris, constructed in 1140. Future cathedrals now soared heavenwards in Gothic style as a paean to God, using the new structural inventions of flying buttresses, rib vaults and pointed arches. Chartres, Rheims, Amiens, and Salisbury witnessed marvels of soaring architecture to the glory of God. Perhaps they were an expression of the urge of man to break through the darkness of several centuries and soar heavenwards to light and wisdom with the help of God. Unnamed craftsmen devoted their skills over a lifetime to build and transform the house of God into a beautiful manuscript of stained glass and stone which even the illiterate could admire and read. It depicted on its walls and its beautiful windows the scriptures, legends of saints, the joy of heaven, the suffering in hell and moral allegories with symbolic meanings. The cathedral also became the fount of music in medieval Europe. Notre Dame in Paris was reputed to be the greatest centre of music in Europe; the earliest polyphonic music had its origin within its hallowed walls.

The darkness of the Middle Ages was now being slowly dispelled, the impetus being provided by centres of learning and by universities that slowly grew to brighten the medieval landscape.

The School of Salerno

Lay medicine in the medieval era was dormant but not dead. It came into prominence and flourished in the School of Salerno in Italy in the tenth century. This was the first medical centre in the Medieval West and several students, teachers and a renowned faculty of physicians, professors, nuns, monks, apothecaries and translators converged upon this school. The infirmaries within the town also housed the many sick who travelled miles to seek succour.

Salerno, situated south of Naples, became a colony of Rome in AD 194 and was renowned as a famous health resort. St Thomas Aquinas dubbed Salerno as the town of medicine, perhaps because doctors with exceptional professional skills practised in that area. The genesis of the Salerno school first observed in history in the tenth century is shrouded in mystery. Fact and fiction, truth and legend seem almost impossible to separate. The school undoubtedly bore the stamp of Greek, Latin, Arabic and Jewish cultures. This led to the belief that the school was founded by one physician-teacher of each culture. The rabbi Helinus, the Greek teacher Pontus, the Saracen Adela, and the Latin master Salernus were all believed to have taught medicine in their own language. Perhaps the truth in the legends surrounding the formation of the school is that medicine must have been taught in all the above languages to accurately convey the contents of the available medical texts written in Greek, Latin, Arabic and Hebrew.

Two main sources were probably influential in the formation and establishment of the school—ecclesiastical and lay. Besides the attraction of the healthy, salubrious climate, Salerno possessed the miraculous remains of St Mathew within the cathedral of the town. In the early Christian period, medicine was closely allied to religious faith and this must have been an additional attraction for the sick and the maimed to seek help at Salerno. Then again, where the sick abound doctors are often found! It is very likely that doctors with good professional skills now gathered at this site, attracted pupils, and that together they organized and founded a school.

Factual information on the Salerno school has come to light following the research on the history of Italian medicine by Salvatore de Renzi. The first medical text for the use of students was titled *Passionarius* written about 1050 by Gariopontus who was a famous teacher of his time. The *Passionarius* included the doctrines of Galen, Alexander of Traille and Paul of Aegina, and contained the basis of modern medical terminology, latinizing many Greek terms. Another important compilation for students was the *Practica of Petroncellus.*

Women also taught in Salerno, one of them being Trotula who wrote an elaborate treatise on obstetrics and gynecology. The real identity of Trotula is debatable for there are some who suggest that she was not a physician but a mid-wife. Another view opines that Trotula was a nickname common to all Salernian midwives and that none of the works attributed to her are original but were written at a later period. Yet the treatise on obstetrics and gynaecology attributed to her remained a standard and oft-quoted text up to the sixteenth century. It was printed in Venice in 1547.

An important work from Salerno in the earlier period was *Antidotarium*, a collection of prescriptions which became the basis of a subsequent pharmacopoeias. The *Speculum Hominis* (*Mirror of Man*) was another text which dealt with diseases in the verse form.

The school of Salerno reached its zenith in the late eleventh and the early twelfth centuries. The scholar-teacher who lent the lustre of great learning to the school was Constantinus Africanus. He was profoundly well-versed in the Arab texts which he introduced to the students in Salerno, thus bridging the gap between Islamic and Christian cultures; Constantinus was called Africanus because he was born in Carthage. He studied medicine and became a scholar in several eastern languages during his travels to Syria, Egypt and India. He then taught in Salerno and was able to convey the basic aspects of Arabic medicine to the West, a century before the more accurate translations of Arabic texts into Latin by Gerard of Cremona. He also translated Hippocrates' sayings and Galen's work on the Art of Medicine. When the Norman duke Robert Guiscard occupied Salerno, Constantinus Africanus became his secretary. He later became a monk and joined the Benedictine monastery at Monte Cassino where he died in 1087.

The Salerno school specialized in diagnosis from an examination of the urine; it also specialized in surgery. Pierre Gilles de Corbeil was French and became a pupil of Salerno in the twelfth century. His poem on the art of diagnosis through examination of the urine remained the best known urological text for three centuries. The best known surgical text was by Rogerius Frugardi. His chapters on head injuries and abdominal wounds were of special interest. In the case of depressed fractures he advocated the trephining of a number of perforations so that the fractured bone fragment could be removed without damage to the covering of the brain. He also advocated moistening protruded intestines following abdominal wounds before returning them into the abdominal cavity.

Salerian anatomy, like the anatomy of Galen, was based on the dissection of animals. Copho in the early period of the school wrote a text titled *Anatomia Porci* (*Anatomy of the Pig*). Magister

Maurus also wrote an anatomical treatise around the same time; his work acquired fame through Gilles de Corbeil who versified the treatise in Latin hexameters.

The school of Salerno introduced a unique novelty never practised either before or after. It embodied its main teachings in verse which rhymed well and therefore could be remembered easily. The popularization of medicine, and its easy access and availability was perhaps one of the greatest contributions of the school of Salerno. Had it not been for Salerno, the knowledge of medicine would have remained barely accessible, esoteric, buried in the pages of musty manuscripts or in huge tomes, difficult to read and even more difficult to comprehend.

The happy inspiration of presenting teaching matter in verse form was best illustrated in the greatest and most celebrated work of the Salerno school. This work was *Regimen Sanitatis Salernitanum* (the *Salerno Book of Health*) and it formed the basis of clinical medicine up to the end of the Middle Ages. The first version of these verses was produced by Arnold of Villanova who lived from 1235 to 1315. It was printed in 1480, and had 362 verses. De Renzi later published a version of 3,520 verses. The *Regimen* is believed to have been dedicated to an unknown king of England. In delightfully rhyming Latin hexameters, it discussed diet, sleep, work, exercise and play. It dealt again in verse with anatomy, physiology, pathology, therapeutics, venesection. It recommended moderation in eating, drinking, eating cheese at the end of a meal, chopped onions for growing hair and using prunes as laxatives.

It is amusing and of interest to quote Harrington's version of a stanza on hygiene from the *Regimen*:

> Rise earely in the morne, and straight remember,
> With water cold to wash your hands and eyes,
> In gentle fashion retching every member,
> And to refresh your braine when as you rise.
> In heat, in cold, in July and December.
> Both comb your head, and rub your teeth likewise:
> If bled you have, keep coole, if bath'd keep warme;
> If din'd, to stand or walke will do no harme.

The *Regimen* was the most widely read, widely circulated medical book in medieval history. It went into 1500 editions and was translated several times. There were eleven versions in French, ten in German and many in English, Italian and a few in other European languages. The Salerno school was officially recognised by Frederick II, the patron of science and medicine in 1231. He decreed that the curriculum of the school should include three years of logic, five of medicine and one year of practice ending in the award of a diploma. Frederick II also decreed that physicians practising medicine in the kingdom of Naples had first to seek approval from the school of Salerno.

After the thirteenth century Salerno slowly declined, perhaps because of strong competition from other new universities. Yet it had succeeded in reviving the Hippocratic traditions, had absorbed the wisdom of the East, had published over fifty works from within its own faculty and had the inspiration to present teaching matter in easily remembered Latin verse. It not only rekindled the flame of medicine, it popularised and spread it over an increasingly receptive Europe and paved the way for the universities of the future.

The Universities

The rise and growth of universities was a memorable and salient feature in the history of the late Middle Ages. Universities began to appear on the medieval scene in the twelfth and thirteenth centuries. This became possible for two reasons—a slowly evolving civilized order which prevailed over the earlier anarchy, and the growth and increasing wealth of the medieval cities. A civilized order lent the necessary safety and stability; wealth provided the means for centres of learning to take root and flourish. The cathedral schools founded by Charlemagne awakened from their stupor and organized themselves into self-governing associations on the model set by the rapidly-growing towns. They were first known as *studia generalia,* i.e., schools teaching many subjects, and were frequented from all parts of the continent. They then gradually established customs and rules to evolve into organized centres of learning called *universities.* A number of these universities had formal authorization by special decrees from the ruling authority in that area—be it emperor, pope, a reigning aristocrat or the community. University establishments were not necessarily run on the same lines. In general most universities situated to the south of the Alps were run by students who would elect their teachers and even decide the curriculum, while those north of the Alps were run and managed by teachers.

It is outside the scope of this book to discuss the genesis of the many universities in this era. The main ones included Bologna, Naples, Montpellier, Salamanca, Oxford, Cambridge, Padua and Pisa. The most ancient and most famous university of medieval Europe was Bologna, where a famous law school was already in existence from the eleventh century. At its zenith Bologna had 10,000 students on the campus. It was run by a commune of the students under democratic rules in which students elected a rector and chose their teachers and professors. The rector had precedence over the dignitaries including dukes and cardinals at official functions.

The ministry of Bologna taught many disciplines, but was specially renowned for its school of surgery and the study of anatomy. Medical students also studied astronomy. It is of interest that Copernicus began his calculations in astronomy in Bologna. One of the great early physicians of Bologna was the Florentine Taddeo Alderotti (1223–1303) quoted in the verses of Dante, who may well have attended his lectures. Alderotti was a failure in Florence and was believed to have earned his living by selling candles at church doors. In Bologna he soon acquired fame and riches as a professor of medicine and as physician to several nobles and popes. He wrote two treatises—*Della Conservazione della Salute* (*How to Stay Healthy*) and *Consilia* which gave a description of clinical cases in Italian rather than Latin. The latter text was replete with practical observations.

To Bologna in the early thirteenth century came Theodoric of Lucca (1205–1298), son of Ugo Borgognoui who learnt his surgery during the crusades. Theodoric was a Dominican friar and had been bishop of Bitonto and Cervia before he came to Bologna. He wrote a text termed *Cyrurgia* (*Surgery*) based on his personal experience and that of his father. His major contribution to surgery was to recommend the primary suture of wounds rather than leave them exposed, which often encouraged the formation of pus. He also advocated the use of sponges soaked with a narcotic such as mandragora to the patient's nose so that surgery could commence only when the patient was asleep.

Another famous surgeon of Bologna was Guglielmi Saliceti (1219–1277). He preferred the knife to the Arab cautery, and favoured suturing of wounds.

It was in Bologna that official dissection of dead bodies was sanctioned, initially on the orders of the magistrature. History records the death of a nobleman in 1302 under suspicious circumstances. Doctor Bartolomeo da Varignana was ordered to determine if death was due to foul play. He performed the autopsy with the help of a colleague and three surgeons. His report excluded foul play or poisoning and exhibited a fair degree of practical knowledge of anatomy.

The king of anatomy in this era was Remondino de Luzzi, also known as Mondino. He was born in Bologna in about 1275, studied medicine and philosophy and then taught at Bologna from 1314 for a decade. He was the first European to systematically conduct dissection of the human cadaver in public. His treatise termed *Anatomia* was the first manual on the practice of dissection. Unfortunately Mondino was an ardent follower of Galen; he therefore did not break the chains that bound anatomy to Galenic doctrines.

The university of Montpellier in France was one of the most ancient and renowned universities, dating from the end of the twelfth century. A famous teacher, who was accused by the church of being a heretic was Arnold of Villanova. He lived from about 1235 to 1316, was a prolific scholar well-versed in theology, jurisprudence, philosophy and medicine, and knew Latin, Greek, Arabic and Hebrew. He was greatly impressed by the rules of diet and hygiene advocated by the school of Salerno and edited one of the versions of the famous *Regimen Sanitatis Salernitanum*. He practised alchemy and magic, questioned the doctrines of Hippocrates and Galen and advocated observations and experiments to determine the truth. Though a physician to kings and a friend of popes he was accused of heresy and would have surely died at the stake had it not been for the intervention of Pope Boniface VIII, who had been treated by Arnold for kidney stones. His books were however burnt and the number of heresies of which he was accused have been lost to history.

Other famous physicians of Montpelier were Raimundo Lulio (1235–1315) and Bernard de Gordon (who died in 1320). Raimundo was a monk from Majorca who wrote about 150 books on medicine, religion and poetry and led three missionary expeditions to Africa. Bernard de Gordon was a follower of the rational medicine of the Hippocratic school even though he believed in magic and astrology. He made the first pertinent observations on the use of reading spectacles.

Pietro d'Abano (1250–1315) was a heretic like Arnold of Villanova. He was amongst the first great teachers of the famous medical school of Padua. A disciple of Averroes, he attempted in a treatise to reconcile the differences between Arab medicine and Catholic philosophy. He was accused by the Inquisition, but died during his trial. Convicted posthumously, the judge ordered his dead body to be burnt at the stake. The story goes that a loyal servant hid the dead body and the Inquisition had to be content with burning an effigy. Pietro d'Abano may well have been a teacher of the great poet Dante. There are some who believe that Dante was a doctor for he was elected prior to the guild of apothecaries and doctors in Florence. This is probably not true even though he may have studied medicine in Bologna and Padua. His *Divine Comedy*, however, does exhibit a fair knowledge of a number of diseases.

The faculty of the university of Paris was renowned throughout Europe. One of the most learned teachers of the Middle Ages who taught in Paris was Albertus Magnus (1192–1280) also called Doctor Universalis for his great proficiency in botany, zoology, astronomy, philosophy and geography. He wrote a number of erudite volumes and his renown was so great that students came from far and wide to attend his discourses. These were often held outdoors to accommodate the large crowd of scholars listening to him. Albertus Magnus was the teacher of Thomas Aquinas and Roger Bacon. He also taught the physician Petrus Hispanus who later became Pope John XXI—the only physician who became a Pope.

The head of the surgical faculty in Paris was a Milanese called Guido Lanfranchi, a pupil of William of Saliceto. Lanfranchi fell foul of the authorities in Milan and fled to Lyons where he wrote the *Cyrurgia Parva* (the *Little Book of Surgery*). He then went to Paris where he became famous for his lectures in surgery. When in Paris he completed the *Cyrurgia Magna* (the *Big Book of Surgery*) in 1296. Surgery was chiefly the domain of itinerant barber surgeons in the West. The physicians felt it was below their dignity to soil their hands with blood and abstained from its practice. Lanfranchi was amongst the early surgeons who brought it a modicum of renown. His belief that no good doctor could afford to ignore surgery and that every surgeon should possess a knowledge of medicine is as valid today as it was in his own time and age.

The first treatise on surgery by a French surgeon was written by Henri de Mondeville, a colleague of Lanfranchi. Mondeville studied medicine in Paris, Montpellier and Bologna. He advocated the suturing of wounds to prevent pus, and because of his skill rose to become physician to the two French kings, Philip the Fair and Louis X.

The most famous surgeon of the Middle Ages was Guy de Chauliac (1300–1368), who took his degree at Montpellier. He wrote his treatise called *Chirugia* and stressed the great importance of anatomy in the practice of surgery. This was the influence of Mondino and his pupils at Bologna where Chauliac had studied. He became a monk, but continued with his surgical practice winning great acclaim. His fame took him to Avignon, the seat of the papacy in that era; he was the personal physician to Pope Clement VI and later to Popes Innocent VI and Urban V.

Oxford University started as a school in the ninth century. The conflicts between the English and the French in the thirteenth century forced many English students to abandon the university of Paris and return home. Many joined Oxford, so the university began to flourish in the thirteenth century. The university of Cambridge was founded in 1271, and gained prestige over the next two hundred years.

The most celebrated teacher at Oxford was the Dominican friar Roger Bacon (1214–1292) also called doctor mirabalis. He was one of the first intellectuals who showed the true spirit of scientific inquiry. He ridiculed popular beliefs and maintained that experiment was the way to determine or verify the truth. Roger Bacon also taught in Paris; he is reported to have invented the magnetic compass, gunpowder and spectacles. But this is not quite true as these inventions had already been made earlier. On his return to England, he was imprisoned because of his attack on Franciscans and Dominicans. He was released just before his death.

MEDIEVAL ENGLAND

In the Middle Ages, medicine in England was strongly influenced by the church. The early well-known physicians were thus the products of schools set up by cathedrals and monasteries on the Continent. Subsequently, students desiring to study medicine could only do so under the direction of the church and had to become clerics to be admitted for training. To start with the English and French medical professors were thus officially celibate. It was only in the fourteenth century that university appointments were granted to married men. Surgery and obstetrics were considered unsuitable for clerics; hence barber surgeons and midwives had their own independent practice. The midwives acted as intermediaries when a female had to be treated by a male physician.

The church in a way exerted a stultifying influence on medicine. Medicine became increasingly theoretical and less practical and there was a great shortage of practising doctors. Folklore medicine thus played an important role, particularly in the health care of people in villages and small towns. Medical works began to be translated from Latin into English, and, as at the school of Salerno, the popularization of knowledge was through the versification of medical facts, as was observed in the poems of Chaucer.

The most famous of the English physicians of the Middle Ages was John of Gaddesden (1280–1361). He was a Fellow of Merton College, Oxford, and became physician to Edward II. He authored a medical text termed *Rosa Anglica* (*the English Rose*); this book contained many medical quotes from Arab and Greek sources, enabling medieval England to become acquainted with both Arab medicine and ancient Greek medicine.

Chaucer wrote his *Canterbury Tales* in the style of the *Decameron*. In these tales, pilgrims take it in turn to tell a story as they journey to the saint's shrine in Canterbury. Gaddesen, who knew the writings of Arab physicians, may well have been the model of the learned doctor depicted in the *Canterbury Tales*.

The Practice of Medicine

The Middle Ages saw the establishment of three important institutions which became the foundations of medicine in the centuries to come. These were the guilds, the pharmacies and the hospitals. In the late medieval era medicine increasingly passed from the control of the church into the hands of the laity. The school at Salerno was the first to start this trend. This transfer of control over medicine was ordered by Pope Honorius III, who strictly forbade his clerics to practise medicine. The physicians, freed from ecclesiastical control, soon organized themselves into professional bodies whose rights were protected by the law of the land. Guilds thus came into existence with rules and regulations that prevented an individual from practising a profession unless he had completed a prescribed training course and was equipped with the requisite knowledge. Guilds were the forerunners of modern medical associations.

The history of barber surgeon guilds is of interest. Barbers performed many functions of the doctor, including blood-letting, and tooth-drawing, and were important figures in medicine right up to the eighteenth century. They probably gained importance in around 1100 when monks went to the barbers for their tonsure, and also for bleeding which was required by church law. The barber-surgeons were well established by the end of the Middle Ages. In 1505, the faculty of medicine in Paris instituted a course for barbers, arousing the ire of the surgeons. In England, in 1462, the Guild of Barbers became the Company of Barbers. The surgeons obtained a special charter protecting their rights and privileges in 1492. In 1540, Henry VIII combined the Company of Barbers with the small and exclusive Guild of Surgeons to form the United Barber-Surgeon Company.

The first public pharmacies were introduced in Venice, Italy. As with pharmacies in Arab lands they were first attached to religious places, for example, the monasteries. Later pharmacies were set up as private shops and became the meeting-ground for physicians to buy and discuss drugs and to confer with colleagues. The pharmacist was often erudite and had a special knowledge of alchemy and astrology.

The Middle Ages also saw the growth of hundreds of hospitals all over the West and in the lands visited by the Crusaders. Here, again, the control of hospitals was initially vested with the church, but passed into lay hands by the beginning of the thirteenth century. Great hospitals that now came up were the proud achievements of rich, flourishing cities. Examples were the Hôtel-Dieu in Paris, Santo Spirito in Rome, and St Bartholomews and St Thomas in London. Great thought and attention were given to their construction, particularly in Italy; the best architects were often commissioned to design them and they were decorated by some of the greatest artists of the land. Outstanding examples of beautifully designed and decorated hospitals were the Ospedale del Ceppo at Pistoia and the Ospedale degli Innocenti at Florence which had magnificent bas-reliefs in coloured glazed ceramics by Giovanni and Andrea della Robbia. Though no longer under ecclesiastical control, the strong influence of the Catholic Church on these hospitals was evident in the names of the institutes, in the religious motifs underlying artistic decorations, and the fact that nursing, as it existed, was solely the function of religious orders. One important feature of the Middle Ages was the widespread foundation of leper hospitals. There were over 200 such hospitals in England and Scotland and over 2000 in France.

DIAGNOSIS AND THERAPY

The practice of medicine was primitive. The basic therapy in Christian belief was prayer, penitence and invoking the aid of saints. Lay medicine encouraged diagnosis through the evaluation of symptoms, examination of the pulse, observation at the bedside, density and smell of blood, smell and colour of the sputum, and above all, the examination of the urine. Uroscopy or diagnosis through urine examination was universally practised; conclusions derived from this examination were exaggerated beyond bounds of reason. Thus, not only was the colour and odour useful to make a diagnosis, but also the layers of sediment formed in the collecting flask. Cloudiness of the upper layer suggested that the seat of disease lay in the head; of the lower layers pointed to disease of the bladder or genital organs. The urine flask was indeed an emblem of medieval medicine; the Jerusalem code of 1090 stipulated that failure to examine the urine exposed a physician to public censure.

Blood-letting, purging, starving, and use of enemas were carried over to the medieval age from the age of antiquity. Therapy was often based on the theory of opposites (*contraria contrariis*) as in Galenic times. Diseases thought to be due to fullness or plethora were treated by blood-letting. Great discussion and dispute often arose over the site of venesection, its relation to the site of disease, the correct vein to be tapped and the amount of blood to be removed. Herbs and medicinal plants were used as therapy. Even so, magic concoctions, bezoars, and the use of amulets were also part of the pharmacopoeia. Organs and excreta of various animals were concocted into potions and medicine. Milk, blood and urine of humans were also used; powdered pearls were thought to be effective against plague.

In medieval surgery dressings were soaked in old wine. Surgical practice included tonsillectomy, trepanning, tracheostomy. Midwives supervised and managed childbirth. Special parturition charms were sometimes used; shaking the mother was thought to facilitate delivery. Caesarian section was known, but not practised.

THE PHYSICIAN

The rise of medical guilds, and the spread of medical schools greatly enhanced the physician's status in society. Famous physicians amassed a great deal of wealth. They began to dress in all their finery—fur-trimmed coats, fancy hats, sparkling rings and silver spurs. Surgeons belonged to a lower rank and often combined the duties of a barber with those of a doctor.

Most people looked upon the physician with awe and respect. But there were the discerning few who could see through his pomposity, sneer at his verbosity and correctly gauge the danger he often posed to those he professed to treat and cure. This is proven by a letter written by the great poet Petrarch to a pope after he had been upset by the arrogance of Guy de Chauliac, a famous French surgeon of the Middle Ages. The letter is remarkable in that its remarks are as cogent for the physician of today as they were for the physician of those times. Petrach writes:

> I know that your bedside is besieged by the doctors. This is the very mainspring of my fears. They never agree among themselves, judging it blameworthy to contribute nothing new or merely to follow in another's footsteps. There is no doubt that they all trade in our lives, as Pliny put it, while hoping for fame as a result of new discoveries. It is a singular privilege of their calling to only say he is a doctor, for

people to put blind trust in him. Yet falsehood is more dangerous in this art than in any other. Beware: anyone may be deceived, so great is the power of hope. There is no law punishing homicidal ignorance and no punitive precedent. They learn and it is we who foot the bill. Only a doctor can commit murder and get away with it. Most merciful Father, think of that hand as enemy forces. Let the memory of the Man who chose this for his epitaph bear witness 'I died of a surfeit of doctors.'

Castigating the doctor even further, Petrach in the same letter goes on to add:

Their art is almost forgotten. . . . They crowd the sick beds of the unfortunate, high flown phrases flowing from their lips. A poor sick man dies and all they do is discourse on Hippocratic this and Ciceronian that, trying to turn all occasions however tragic, to their own advantage. In conclusion let me say that from a doctor intent in his eloquence and not on advice, you must guard your life as you would from an assassin or a sly poisoner.

Petrarch's letter was an unquestionably exaggerated depiction of a pompous and ignorant doctor, yet there is a lot of truth in it. Every practising doctor in the modern world needs to read it.

Black Death and Other Epidemics

By a curious coincidence, the Middle Ages began and ended with two of the most catastrophic epidemics of plague that ravaged Europe. The first was in the reign of Justinian in AD 542 and 543; it originated in the East and spread through Europe, decimating the population. It has been touched upon briefly in an earlier chapter. The second, called the Black Death, struck the West in the fourteenth century with devastating effect. In both these pandemics the mortality was dreadfully high. No reliable figures can be offered with regard to the death rate in the first pandemic. It has been however estimated that a quarter of the population of Europe, amounting to over twenty-five million people, succumbed to the Black Death.

Like the first epidemic in the Justinian era, the Black Death of 1347 to 1351 came from the East, probably originating in China. In 1346, it spread to the shores of the Black Sea where Italian merchants traded with both Central Asia and the Byzantine Empire. The Italian merchants fleeing from the savage Tartars sought refuge within Caffa (now Feodosiya)—a Genoese trading port in the Crimea. Caffa was besieged for three years during which time plague broke out among the Tartars. The Tartars catapulted dead, diseased bodies over the city walls causing an outbreak of plague among the Italian merchants. Those who survived returned home by ship; they were the carriers of the deadly pestilence that erupted in Genoa. Merchant ships sailing from Caffa must have also carried plague-infected rats contributing to the epidemic in Genoa and starting epidemics in other ports of call, notably in Constantinople and within the island of Sicily.

From Genoa, the plague spread throughout Italy. Michele di Piazza, the author of *Historia Sicula abanno 1337 ad annum 1361* (*History of Sicily 1337–1361*) gives a graphic clinical description of the early progress of the epidemic:

In the first days of October 1347, the year of the incarnation of the son of God, twelve Genoese galleys fleeing before the wrath of our Lord over their wicked deeds, entered the port of Messina. The sailors brought in their bones a disease so violent that whosoever spoke a word to them was infected and could in no way save himself from death. Those to whom the disease was transmitted by infection of the breath were stricken with panic all over the body and felt a terrible lassitude. Then there appeared on a thigh or on an arm, a pustule like a lentil bean. From this the infection penetrated the body and violent bloody vomiting began. It lasted for a period of three days and there was no way of preventing its ending in death.

From Genoa the plague spread to Florence in 1348 where it wrought the greatest possible havoc. The population of the city fell from 1,00,000 to 35,000. Giovanni Boccaccio described the total collapse of the moral fabric within the town. Realizing that death was near, the populace resorted to total debauchery, drinking, feasting and pleasing their senses all through the day and night, perhaps in an effort to forget that the morrow would bring an encounter with death. The pestilence struck such dread into people that it was customary to abandon those near and dear who were taken ill. Boccaccio wrote:

> The trouble struck such terrible fear into the hearts of men and women that brothers deserted each other, an uncle left his nephew and a sister left her brother; women often abandoned their husbands and worse, incredible though it is, father and mother acted towards their children as if they were not their own, by refusing to see them or look after them.

From Italy, the Black Death spread throughout Europe decimating the population. Thousands of villages lay abandoned, and many towns were hopelessly depopulated producing a demographic crisis. In 1348, the Black Death reached England; within two years it crossed into Germany and Scandinavia, reaching Poland. It was indeed the greatest and the most devastatingly unsurpassed epidemic that the West had ever witnessed to that day.

An eye witness account of Guy de Chauliac, the most famous surgeon of the Medieval Age makes interesting reading:

> The visitation came in two forms. The first lasted two months, manifesting itself as an intermittent fever accompanied by spitting of blood from which people died usually within three days. The second type lasted the remainder of the time, manifesting itself in high fever, abscesses and carbuncles, chiefly in the axillae and groins. People died from this in five days. So contagious was the disease, especially that with blood-spitting (*pneumonia*), that no one could approach or even see a patient without taking the disease. The father did not visit the son nor the son the father. Charity was dead and hope abandoned.

The West was, of course, confused as to the cause of the dreadful tragedy. The Christian belief held that the Black Death was a visitation from God, a punishment to man for his many sins. The astrologers stated that it was due to an evil conjunction of Saturn, Jupiter and Mars. The Franciscan monk Michele de Piazza wrote that plague was spread by 'infection of the breath'. A polluted environment was thought by some to result in a pestilential atmosphere. Pollution could be from decaying corpses, the filth that accumulated in towns and from the breath of those stricken with disease. The bigoted also postulated that the air could be poisoned by the Jews, who were regarded as enemies. The explanation as to why some individuals escaped the Black Death was sensible. It was related to the body constitution; if strong, one resisted it and if weak, one succumbed to it.

The Black Death tore apart the moral and social fabric of Europe. Demoralization resulted in a morbid psyche which dwelt on death and disease conjuring the Biblical vision of the Horsemen of the Apocalypse. It also led to abnormal collective behaviour as was witnessed in a fraternity called the Flagellants. The Flagellant movement was Franciscan in origin, started first in Umbria and then spread across the continent. These fanatics passed in a procession through the towns and villages of Europe flogging and flagellating themselves with lashes in the hope that God would look down on their suffering and penitence and His mercy would stop the plague. This sect drew converts in their grim passage through Europe, and themselves constituted a plague, indulging in vandalism, loot and arson. The Flagellants denounced Jews as the enemies of the people and of God and accused them of poisoning drinking water. This lead to persecution and massacre. A large number of Jews were burnt or massacred in Basel, Mainz and Frankfurt. By the time the Flagellants reached

Avignon they posed a threat to the social order and even to the papal authority. Pope Clement VII was forced to threaten them with excommunication.

There was nothing that medicine could do to help the victims of the Black Death. Let us consider once again the views of the surgeon Guy de Chauliac who continued to remain in Auvergne throughout the epidemic. This famous surgeon's chief recommendation was to flee the region. Failing that he advised purging, blood-letting, purifying the air with fire, comforting the heart with senna and things of good odour, soothing the humors with Armenian bole, and resisting putrefaction with acid things.

In the early years of the epidemic the population was resigned to its desperate fate. Gradually however some degree of public health measures were introduced. Plague-stricken victims were thus isolated from other dwelling places. Those treating plague-stricken victims were isolated for a period of ten days.

Burial regulations were enforced in Venice, and the sick or outsiders were denied entry into the city. Milan sealed the occupants of infected houses leaving them to die. A forty-day quarantine on an isolated island was instituted by Ragusa (Dubrovnik) in 1347. Marseilles and Venice followed suit, as did Pisa and Genoa many years later. Florence declared a war on all dogs and cats, destroying the very animals which could have kept the rat population in check. Doctors for their own protection dressed themselves in bizarre costumes resembling birds of prey, with a beak-like frontpiece that contained a sponge soaked in vinegar and other aromatic substances held before the nose.

The social effect of the Black Death was far-reaching. The depopulation of Europe hastened the collapse of the feudal system. The tremendous shortage of farm labour meant that the surviving peasants and serfs could dictate to the lord of the manor or the castle. Instead of a hunger for land, there now arose a demand for hands to till and plough the soil and these hands now would not easily submit to the whims and fancies of the ruling lord.

Leprosy

Lepers, like the Jews, were believed to be in league with the devil and assumed to be the cause of the plague. In many parts of Europe, particularly in Switzerland and Alsace, lepers who escaped the plague were massacred.

Leprosy now called Hansen's disease after Armauer Hansen who discovered the *Mycobacterium leprae,* can be a mutilating affliction. It causes sores on the skin, nodular deformities of the face and mutilation of the fingers, toes, hands and feet. The evidence for its existence in the Middle Ages lies in the description of Gilbertus Anglicus:

> The eyebrows falling bare and getting knotted with uneven tuberosities; the nose and other features becoming thick, coarse and lumpy, the face losing its mobility or play of expression, the raucous voice, the loss of sensibility in the hands and the ultimate breakup of the leprous growth into foul-running sores.

The disease dates from antiquity. Egyptian sources two-and-a-half millenniums before Christ contain references to this disease. The Ebers papyrus a thousand years later produces further evidence of its existence in skeletal remains. Though leprosy has existed since biblical times, the term almost certainly must have been given to a large number of non-infectious skin diseases including eczema, psoriasis, as well as infectious diseases like syphilis, and, perhaps, even smallpox. It is possible therefore that at least some of the unfortunate who were dubbed as lepers were in reality suffering from non-leprous disorders.

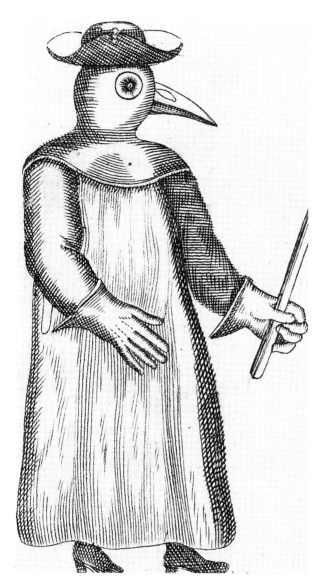

Fig. 24.1   A physician dressed in protective plague costume.

It is indeed a shame that the disease carried a dreadful stigma not only in the Medieval Ages but also well before and after that age. Lepers were subjected to the most shocking and cruel taboos. They were allowed no social contact, could not marry, were refused entry into churches and had to sound a bell warning of their approach. They were segregated in special houses called lazarettos; the sufferers were the dead among the living—or, perhaps, more appropriately, the living dead.

The Middle Ages saw a tremendous increase in the hospitals built to house lepers. By the middle of the thirteenth century there were close to 20,000 leprosaria in Europe serving to shelter and isolate these poor victims. Yet by about 1350, leprosy in Europe was on the decline. The cause of this fall in incidence is not clear. It is possible that the Black Death decimated so many that the reservoirs of infection in the surviving few shrank considerably. It is equally possible that increasing natural and acquired immunity to the disease led to its decline and near extinction. Many *lazarettos* were then converted into houses for the poor or for those suspected of carrying infectious disease; some *lazarettos* were converted into hospitals.

OTHER EPIDEMICS

Other unusual epidemics were observed in the Middle Ages. There was the epidemic of the Dancing Mania also called St Vitus' dance which raged through France and the Low Countries. Another epidemic was dubbed St Anthony's Fire (ergotism) manifesting as gangrene of the hands and feet resulting in death. It was first mentioned in the ninth century and there were many recorded epidemics in the twelfth century. Ergotism was termed St Anthony's Fire when some sufferers praying at the tomb of St Anthony in France were miraculously cured. The disease is now known to be caused by a fungus *Claviceps purpurea* which infects grain and produces a poisonous substance.

THE KING'S TOUCH

When medicine had little to offer, faith often took its place. The 'King's touch' first began to be used to cure scrofula (tuberculous infection of the lymph glands). According to St Thomas of Aquinas the first such 'cure' was by Clovis in AD 496, who on the prompting of an angel, placed his hands on the neck of his sick page pronouncing the words "I touch you, God heals you". This sentence continued to be used with the 'placing of hands' by all subsequent kings of France.

In England the royal touch for healing scrofula was introduced by Edward the Confessor who reigned from 1042 to 1066. The practice continued for over a thousand years. The practice then seems to have died out until the reign of Henry VI who restarted it and also instituted elaborate rituals to accompany the laying of hands. The rituals included the touching of a specially minted gold coin called the Gold Angel. The use of the royal touch and the ceremony associated with it continued through all the reigns up to that of the William of Orange. Queen Anne later restarted this tradition. She 'touched' many—among others also Dr Johnson—but without success.

The royal touch continued to be practised for many more years in France. Louis XVI was said to have touched 2,500 afflicted patients who sought his succour. As late as 1824 Dupuytren, one of the most renowned surgeons of the Napoleonic and post-Napoleonic era presented 121 patients to Charles X for the benefit of the 'royal touch'.

The Medieval Age constituted a trying time for medicine and mankind. It succeeded in stemming the decay and destruction of the Dark Ages consequent to the fall of Rome. It then set out to rebuild the fabric of a broken civilization. The Medieval West rediscovered Greek medicine, accepted the fertilizing influence of the Arab world, rekindled the touch of learning in its universities and built the pillars of modern medicine. The stage was now set for streams that arose from these various sources to merge and form the broad fast-flowing river of the Renaissance. Great must have been the men who though surrounded by a night of darkness and despair strove tirelessly towards the light of dawn. We are eternally indebted to those who conceived the Gothic spires that broke through the darkness to reach out to the sun, to the gifted teachers and students who dispelled the gloom of ignorance, to the music of Dante's verse which soothed a violent world, to the unbroken spirit of man which triumphed through adversity.

Renaissance Medicine

25 Historical Background of the Renaissance Era

The proper study of Mankind is Man.

Alexander Pope

The Renaissance (the Italians called this era *La Rinascita*), or the Rebirth, was a flowering of thought and action, a resurrection of the classic spirit and age after a barbarous interruption of over a thousand years. This splendid period of civilization extended from the 14th century to nearly the end of the 16th century. The Renaissance was an Italian phenomenon born and centred in Italy. Yet like a gentle breeze it spread slowly to exert its influence through the rest of Western and Northern Europe.

In this period of history, man was freed from the shackles of medieval fear, freed from the fear of God and of punishment and hell in his after-life. He believed in God but worshipped beauty in all forms. He loved his immediate existence and ignored his future fate. He became almost hedonistic in his enjoyment of life on earth. The Renaissance age was an age of individualism—its focus centred on the unfettered individual.

The essence of the Renaissance was the concept of *humanism*. The humanists (the Italians called them *unanisti*) were so called because they advocated the study of classic Greek and Roman culture—the humanities (*unanita*). Humanism constituted a total change in the outlook on life when compared to the Middle Ages. It broke dogmas, searched for truth and knowledge, preferred philosophy to religion, studied nature, glorified the individual and believed that—'the proper study of Mankind is Man'. Literature, philosophy, art, and architecture blossomed again as in the classical era of Greece and early Rome. Man was depicted in the image of god in all his strength and beauty of figure and form, in all his joys and sorrows, all his nobility and savagery, his virtue and frailties. The true Renaissance man was steeped in learning that embraced many fields of human endeavour. He was a multifaceted personality who could embrace, with equal aptitude, literature, philosophy, architecture, astronomy and medicine. Yet he had grace, charm, manners, and was often proficient in fencing, hunting, music, dancing and in the courtly arts. Italy led Europe in the development of a genteel society and in the creation of the Renaissance man.

It would however be a gross mistake to consider the Renaissance age as only one of peace and plenty or of happiness and virtue. Unbridled individualism, which was the creed of this period besides liberating the thought of man also bred tyranny, passion and violence. Therefore, this was an era of incredible contrasts—richness and splendour of the human mind contrasted with despicable treachery and meanness; nobility of spirit with a decadent moral code; beneficence with extreme cruelty. Yet for some inexplicable reason when we turn back the pages of history and contemplate on this era, its violence and cruelty fall into the shadows, and the splendour and glory of its achievements rise before our eyes like a breathtaking vision—the vision of being lost forever in a sun-drenched beautiful garden.

Causes of the Renaissance

How did the Renaissance come about? What caused the gloomy, dark, never-ending night in the history of human affairs to be transformed into a sunlit glorious day of beauty and splendour? The Dark Ages did not open into the Renaissance with a sudden clap of thunder or a fitful burst of sunshine. The Renaissance had its gestation, its prelude, which lasted for the greater part of the fourteenth century before ascending to its full glory during the fifteenth and early sixteenth centuries. Most great events in the history of human civilization have been preceded by challenging thoughts or a change in thought. Great thoughts and perhaps great dreams have been the forerunners of great words and great deeds. The Renaissance was no exception; its prelude lay in the thoughts and words of the poet Petrarch and the author Boccacio. Petrarch sang his unrequited love for a woman in beautiful metre and rhyme gathered in manuscript copies as a *Cazoniere* (*Songbook*). His songs were on the lips of the whole of Italy. They were musical, melodious, filled with a subtle and beautiful imagery, songs that sang of the beauty of women, of art, and nature; songs that subtly urged man to break the shackles of past ages and to concern himself with his present life rather than his after-life; songs that spoke of living and loving with a stress on mortal glory than on future immortality. Petrarch was the first humanist of this age—he was indeed the Father of the Renaissance.

Boccaccio began to write his renowned *Century* of seductive tales in 1348. Remarkably enough, this was the year of the Black Death— the plague that decimated the population of Italy and Europe. It was against this desolate backdrop that his tales took shape and form. He named these tales the *Decameron*. Like Petrarch, he wrote in the beautiful native Italian language where prose read like poetry and a poem was like a song. The Decameron was a book that showed a Rabelaisian zest and love for life. Boccaccio portrayed with relish and satire the certainties and uncertainties, fidelities and infidelities, humour and pathos, deceit and honesty that go with the rough and tumble of loving and living. The book was a reflection of the times. In spite of the parodies, caricatures and exaggerations that filled it, the European world identified itself with the book and delighted in it. The book remains a jewel in the literature of the world—a jewel that has lent lustre to the works of many subsequent littérateurs—Molière, Racine, Rabelais, Shakespeare and many others who admiringly partook of its thoughts and style.

There were a number of other causes that contributed to the liberation of thought and the freedom of action, which characterized the Renaissance. Columbus sailed the seas to discover America, Magellan for the first time circumnavigated the world, Vasco da Gama opened the sea-route to India. These were voyages of discovery that shattered forever the small finite limits of the European world. Copernicus showed that the earth was not the centre of the universe and that contrary to belief it was not the sun that moved around the earth but the earth that moved round the sun. The immensity of these discoveries must surely have had a freeing effect on the straitlaced, trammelled minds of the people of Europe. The classical culture of Greece and Rome, the rational philosophy of Plato and the observations and wisdom of Hippocrates were brought into Italy with the scholars who fled Constantinople after its fall to the Turks in 1453. The yearning to recapture the glory and spirit of the classical age increased.

Perhaps the most important single factor in the spread of thought and learning was the invention of printing and of paper. Printing was invented by Laurens Janszoon Coster of Haarlem, Holland, and Johann Gutenberg of Mainz, Germany. Paper made the revival of Europe possible. Paper originated in China probably as far back as the second century BC. The Arabs learnt the art from the

Chinese around AD 750. The manufacture entered Christendom through Greece or through the capture of paper mills during the Christian conquest of Moorish Spain. It was however only in the fourteenth century that the manufacture reached Germany—around the same time as the invention of printing. Printing presses were soon set up in many cities of Europe producing books at a speed unheard of and with a beauty rivalling that of handwritten manuscripts. The printed word spread fast and far and wide; old thoughts and new now gushed forth like a torrent, a flood, and were readily absorbed at first by hundreds, then by thousands, and later by hundreds of thousands of minds.

Medical learning profited a great deal from the printing of ancient medical manuscripts in book form, and from the humanists of the Renaissance who were familiar with all fields of human knowledge and endeavoured reconciling art, philosophy and science with the practice of medicine.

It took, however, more than a revival of antiquity, more than the liberation of thought and the invention of the printing press, for the Renaissance to happen. On a mundane but very important level it took a growing economy with bourgeois money in abundant supply, money that came from a progressive increase in trade, from investments, loans and interests. Yet it required a certain refinement of thought and of the senses for this money to be spent in worthy pursuits, for wealth to be transmuted into beauty. Indeed it required a magnanimity of spirit and a true appreciation of beauty in all forms to be patron to a Leonardo, a Michelangelo, a Donatello, a Titian or a Brunelleschi. The true Renaissance man who had wealth knew how to 'perfume a fortune with the breath of art'.

Renaissance Society

Northern Italy was the centre of the Renaissance and the city of Florence its heart beat. This was partly due to the fact that Venice, Milan and Florence were strategically situated, straddling the natural trade routes between the Orient and Europe. It was also due to the fact that these cities were ruled and dominated by enlightened princes. Thus, for example, Lorenzo de Medici of Florence and Lodovico of Milan encouraged the genteel graces and graciousness of a civilized society, creating the image of the universal Renaissance man—accomplished in humanities and science, courteous, well-mannered, yet bold and brave. The most widely read book of the age was Count Castiglione's *Libro del Cortigiano* (the *Book of Courtiers*) which elaborated on conduct, etiquette and the intellectual accomplishments of a well-bred individual whose guiding principle was *L'onore* and *virtu*. Yet in striking contrast, the Renaissance was also the age of unbridled individual violence never seen before or after. Princes and popes poisoned or assassinated those who came in their way. Wives poisoned husbands, lovers stabbed mistresses. Witches were hired to poison or to cast evil spells. Assassins were available for hire, for any nefarious acts of violence and murder to settle personal scores. It was a society of contrasts.

In Italy, the feudal system of the Middle Ages was replaced by city states independent of the Emperor or Pope. The city states often fought each other for trade routes, commercial gains or for any cause that would add to their wealth or power. Diplomacy was often deceitful and deceit in diplomacy was cultivated to a fine art. Niccolo Machiavelli wrote *Il Principe* (*The Prince*)—the book stressed that the Prince (a head of state) should be guided in his dealings and actions not by honesty or sincerity, not by truth or virtue, not by law or any moral code. His actions should be motivated solely to further his own interests and that of his state. This book was the bible of Renaissance rulers.

Northern Europe and Spain witnessed in this great era a struggle between kings and powerful princely vassals in order to establish a central suzerainty that Italy lacked. England was consumed by the War of the Roses—a bloody contest for power between the Houses of York and Lancaster. Germany saw the establishment and growth of the Hapsburg dynasty. Outside Italy, countries in Europe began to evolve as separate nation states—a feature that has been consolidated in our present era.

There was also constant dispute and sporadic wars between the papacy and kings. Papal taxation alienated the people of many countries. Popular discontent led to the first heresies of John Wycliff in England and John Huss in Bohemia.

Yet through this maelstrom of political discomfort and upheaval, through the rivalry between the city states of Italy, through the chaos that changed the Middle Ages, there prevailed a flowering of thought, a quest for learning, a thirst for beauty and art, a way of life that was unique for this era in the history of civilization. Perhaps the ascent of Man is to an extent conditioned by competition, rivalries, confusion and even some degree of chaos. How else does one explain this phenomenon?

Renaissance Economy

The economic structure of the Middle Ages was totally transformed into the beginning of modern capitalism. Italian merchants developed a banking system, technique of credit and exchange and had widespread trading links with the Orient. A secular, well-educated middle class grew both in numbers and in economic strength. Economic strength lay in the circulation and use of money, replacing the medieval economic system based on the ownership of land. Trade and industry also spread from Italy to Northern Europe as witnessed by the increasing power of the Netherlands, the Hanseatic League merchants of northern Germany and the development of England's trade economy through the wool trade. Money multiplied and circulated all over Europe—it was a key factor in the flowering of the Renaissance.

26 Medicine and Humanism

The great physicians of this era were primarily humanists. The accomplished Renaissance physician was a scholar, a man of letters, as much or more learned in arts, philosophy and literature as in medicine. Doctors belonged to a wealthier class, were often educated in the famous universities of Padua, Bologna and Ferrara in northern Italy. These universities (Padua particularly) attracted a number of foreign students from different countries of Europe. The constitution of almost every university in Italy vested great powers in the student community. It was the students who elected the officials and who debated and decided on the course and curriculum of studies. In the true spirit of the humanist movement, one by one the universities became increasingly secular, freeing themselves from religious dogma and ecclesiastical control. In 1565, Pope Pius IV decreed that the doctorate of medicine could only be conferred on Catholics. The Venetian senate which had earlier granted admission to the university of Padua to Jews and Protestants opposed this decree, insisted on secularism in universities and appointed a procurator to confer degrees on all worthy students regardless of caste, creed or faith.

Humanist physicians abounded in the Renaissance. Niccolo da Longino (1428–1524) was famous for his vitriolic attack on the Galenic doctrine. He is also remembered as an author of one of the earliest medical texts that gave a clinical description of syphilis. He undertook the correction of botanical errors in Pliny's *Natural History* and founded a medical school in Ferrara where he was an outstanding clinician. Geronimo Cardano (1501–1576) was a physician, mathematician, astrologer, musician and author of a great Renaissance autobiography *De Vita Propria Liber*. He wrote scathingly about doctors and healing, winning opprobrium and scorn from his fellow physicians for his treatise *The Bad Practice of Healing Among Modern Doctors*. He was the forerunner by over 400 years of Ivan Illich's *Medical Nemesis*. Thomas Linacre (1461–1524) was a humanist and physician who established chairs of philosophy in Oxford and Cambridge and who founded the Royal College of Physicians of London. He was physician to Henry VIII, and to Cardinal Wolsey, and a close friend of Desidarius Erasmus—one of the great humanist scholars of this age. Another physician to royalty was the great French physician and humanist Jean Francois Fernel who served both Henri II and Catherine de Medici. He was an anti-Gallenist who espoused that the cause of illness was within the body and not by fluids produced by the disease. His masterpiece *Universa Medicina* was read for over a century.

Unfortunately it is true that the spirit of scientific inquiry in both the natural sciences and in medicine lagged far behind the arts and humanities in this era. Medical teaching by and large continued to express the flawed views and dictums of Galen and Avicenna. Though the anatomy of organs of the body had begun to appear in print, the illustrations in books printed in the late fifteenth and early sixteenth centuries were mere copies of old Medieval Age manuscript drawings. These drawings illustrated anatomy under five schematic heads—skeletal, nervous, muscular, arterial and venous, with the body in a half crouched position. The dogmatic Galenic teaching in anatomy of the foetus in utero was a thousand years old and persisted unchanged up to the end of the fifteenth century.

It was Leonardo da Vinci and Andreas Vesalius who finally demolished Galenic dogmas and gave anatomy the long-awaited scientific foundation. Amazingly, the artists and sculptors of fifteenth century Florence seemed to know more anatomy than doctors, as judged from the superb portrayal of human figures. Giotto, Massachio and many others studied perspective and human proportions with assiduous zeal and took an active interest in dissection by joining the Florentine Guild of Physicians and Apothecaries. Artists, apothecaries and physicians now formed a common single fraternity that was eager to unravel the secrets of human anatomy.

The treatment of disease in the Renaissance was no different from Galenic times and from the Dark Ages. Side by side with the humanist Renaissance doctors, quacks flourished, superstition abounded and astrology often reigned supreme. Princes, city-states, popes and even universities all had their coterie of astrologers. A few enlightened men would say *vir sapiens dominabitus astris* ('the wise man is master of the stars'), but the vast majority succumbed to the guile of astrologers.

The year 1543 saw a brief but important triumph for Renaissance science. This remarkable year saw the publication of Andreas Vesalius' *Fabrica* and Nicholas Copernicus' *Di Revolutionibus Orbium Celestium*. Nicholas Copernicus (1473–1540) of Thorn, in Poland, was a mathematician, astronomer, theologian and physician. He studied theology in Bologna and medicine in Padua. He practised medicine at Frauenberg in East Prussia and at the same time discharged his religious duties as canon of the town cathedral. He received on his deathbed the first printed copy of his work which demolished the Ptolemaic theory that the earth was the centre of universe. He substituted the correct theory that it was the earth that moved around the sun. He died a happy and fulfilled man.

27 Art and Anatomy

Pre-renaissance art in painting was flat, lacking in perspective, austere and religious in its theme. Renaissance painting introduced perspective and rejoiced in the strength, shape and beauty of the human form. The artist, the physician and the apothecary (from whom the artist purchased paint) as mentioned earlier, formed a closely knit fraternity that sought to unravel the anatomy of the human body. Perfect anatomy, with special reference to line, form, muscles, ligaments, joints and the superficial veins, was depicted by Andrea de Verrocchio (who had Leonardo as his pupil), Titian, Perugino, and Raphael in painting, and by Signorelli, Donatello and Michelangelo in sculpture. Often physicians would select a vein for blood-letting after studying the veins painted on the canvas of artists such as Giotto or Raphael.

The Renaissance Man

The greatest man of the Renaissance and one of the greatest men of all times was Leonardo da Vinci. He was a genius unsurpassed in his versatility. Perhaps it required a background of Renaissance thought and the Renaissance way of life for the world to have produced a human of such great distinction. He combined within himself the excellence of all the arts and of all the sciences. He studied nature as he would a book, with curiosity, patience and close observation. He had no pre-formed concepts of ancient learning or wisdom; he only believed in what he found or discovered through meticulous study and experiment. As an artist and a painter he had a thirst to unravel the secrets of human anatomy; to learn the laws of proportion and perspective, to study the composition, reflection and absorption of light, to study the chemistry of oils and paints used for his canvases. The artist within him brought out the scientist so that art and science mingled and reinforced each other to forge a splendid unity.

To study anatomy, Leonardo dissected more than thirty dead bodies by candle light in the mortuary of Santo Spirito. He was then in the service of the Borgia family in Rome. He wrote down what he saw during his dissection and of 6,000 closely written pages in his diary, 190 pages are devoted to anatomy. He left 750 illustrative anatomical drawings, of which fifty illustrated the structure of the heart. He described the auricles but did not grasp the place and significance of the septum separating the left from the right ventricle. Had he done so, he might well have discovered circulation. He made beautiful drawings of the coronary arteries and understood the significance of valves within the veins. He analysed the muscular system to perfection—the origin of each muscle, its insertion and its action; he illustrated this through copious notes and superb drawings. He was the first anatomist to attempt to trace the course of the cranial nerves and to dissect the foetal membranes. It appears from his drawings and notes that he planned a major treatise on anatomy in conjunction with Marcantonio della Torre of Verona. This was not to be because of the premature

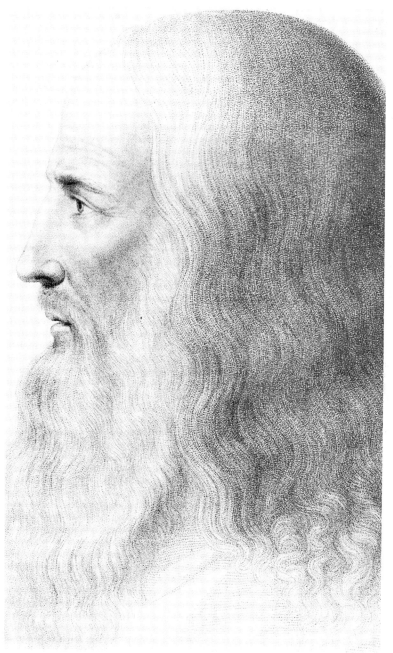

Fig. 27.1   Leonardo da Vinci.

death of della Torre. Leonardo was recognized in his lifetime and forever after as an artist, sculptor, architect, inventor, engineer, scientist, and philosopher. He would have surely been considered the father of modern anatomy if his notebook had not remained undiscovered for two centuries.

How should we rank Leonardo in the history of Man? Which one of us possesses the knowledge and talent in science and art to gauge so rich and multifaceted a personality? Many would say that Titian and Raphael left greater treasures of painting, that Michelangelo was a superior sculptor, or that there were superior engineers and scientists before and after him. Yet Leonardo was the man who was all of these together and rivalled the best in each field. No canvas of Raphael, Titian or Michelangelo could match the beautiful composition, the poignant portrayal of thought and feeling in Leonardo's 'The Last Supper', no drawing could surpass the beautiful lines of 'The Virgin Child and St Anne', no philosophy at least of the Renaissance times could compare with Leonardo's conception of natural law. Leonardo died at the age of sixty-four on 2 May 1519. A friend who witnessed his death wrote "The loss of such a man is mourned by all, for it is not in the power of nature to create another."

We can only marvel at his achievements; he renews our hope and faith in the ascent of man.

When we speak of Leonardo da Vinci, it becomes impossible not to recall Michelangelo Buonarotti. Art and anatomy were closely united in the works of this great painter, sculptor and architect. Michelangelo, like Leonardo, also dissected cadavers (obtained from grave-diggers) in a cell in the monastery of Santo Spirito. By the light of a candle he dissected and studied muscles, tendons and ligaments. His sculptures were endowed with strength and passion, with powerful torsos and muscular limbs, in postures that evoke strong emotion. His sculpture of David in the Academy, of Moses in Rome and of the beautiful Pieta in St Peters Church in Rome, his canvas of *The Virgin and Child* and

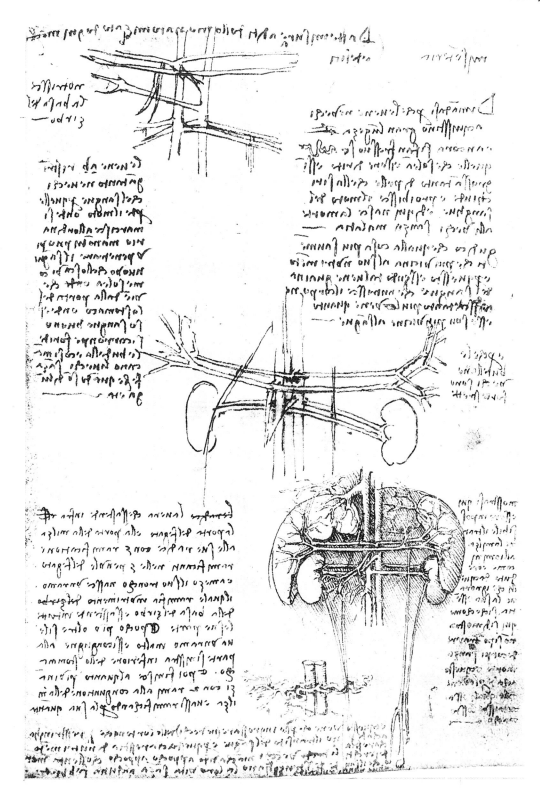

Fig. 27.2   Studies of the abdominal blood vessels and arteriosclerosis.

the monumental painted figures on the roof of the Sistine Chapel beautifully illustrate how his knowledge and appreciation of human anatomy embellished the beauty and the virile vigour of his art.

28 Diseases in the Renaissance

Smallpox, plague, malaria, tuberculosis, typhoid and other water-borne infectious diseases occurred sporadically and in epidemics—a legacy to mankind since civilization began. Outbreaks of relatively new diseases were also noted. Scurvy occurred in epidemic form in sailors voyaging to distant countries. It was not a new disease, for it had also been noted to occur in the Middle Ages, when besieged cities were short of food supply. Rickets was a common affliction of children in the Renaissance. Ambroise Paré described the deformities of *genu valgus* and *genu varus* produced by rickets.

A new devastating scourge often occurring in an epidemic form, and characterized by fever, rash, severe prostration, with circulatory collapse and death was accurately described by Girolamo Fracastoro. This scourge was typhus and this disease occurred when human beings lived in crowded unsanitary conditions in the cold of winter. The Spanish suffered severely from typhus during the siege of Granada, losing over 17,000 soldiers. In 1529, typhus nearly decimated a French army besieging Naples.

A new and mysterious disease broke out in an epidemic form in the summer of 1483. It first appeared in Wales along the Welsh coast and spread to London. John Caius, physician to the English Court, has written a good description of what came to be named the 'sweating sickness' or *sudor anglicus*. The illness was sudden in onset with profuse sweating, neck pain, shivering, severe pros-tration, intense thirst, and miliary skin eruptions. Death frequently occurred within twenty-four hours; if the patient survived the early phase, recovery occurred in over one to two weeks. This mysterious illness erupted in five major epidemics over the next six decades. One of these epidemics decimated the population of Oxford and Cambridge by more than half. It has never occurred since, and though the aetiology is almost certainly an infection, the nature of the infection to this day is obscure.

The Story of Syphilis and of Girolamo Fracastoro

The 'great pox', later named syphilis made a sudden dramatic entry on the Renaissance stage. It was a dreadful, lethal scourge very akin in ferocity and spread to plague and small-pox. The first great epidemic of this 'great pox' or syphilis was observed in the soldiers of Charles VIII of France when his army laid siege to Naples in 1493. It was then termed the Neopolitan disease (*mal napolitain*). Naples surrendered without a fight, and disbanded soldiers, mercenaries and their camp followers returned home to spread the disease all over Europe. The disease, characterized by repulsive rashes and disfiguring ulcers, had various names. The Italians as a taunt to the French, called it *mal francese*. Other terms were *morbus gallicus, mal lusitano, mal spagnole—morbus gallicus* was the term in general use.

In 1530, Girolamo Fracastoro published a poem *Syphilis Sive Morbus Gallicum* (*Syphilis or the French disease*) in which a shepherd Syphilus insults the Greek god Apollo. Apollo seeks revenge by striking the shepherd with a scourge, which causes the flesh from his limbs to decay and fall, revealing his bones, his teeth to break loose, his breath to become foetid and his voice to fail and be reduced to a whisper. The great pox now universally became known as syphilis.

It was and still is a common belief that syphilis was introduced into Europe and the world from America through Columbus' sailors. A Seville physician Ruy Diaz de la Isla, who treated these sailors, was of the opinion that the sailors contracted the disease during their halt in Haiti. Yet there are Renaissance documents that referred to this disease well before Columbus discovered America. A typical syphilitic crural ulcer has been depicted in a 1461 painting, and medieval medical manuscripts describe cases of venereal leprosy which could well have been cutaneous syphilis. Fracastoro noted that the disease appeared simultaneously in many countries and cast doubt on the popular theory that it came from America with Columbus' sailors. This doubt is indeed valid today. It is very likely that the *Treponema pallidum* causing syphilis existed in the Old World prior to the discovery of America. Perhaps it underwent a worldwide mutation in the fifteenth century to become extremely invasive in hosts (both in Europe and the Orient) who were hitherto resistant to infection. There might thus well be a close analogy between the outbreak of syphilis in the fifteenth century and the spread of HIV infection in the late twentieth century. There are a few historians who believe that commercial interests encouraged the belief that syphilis came from America. Guaiac, the holy wood, was being used by the natives of America and was brought by the Spanish sailors to Europe as an effective therapy for syphilis. Even Fracastoro was enthusiastic about the guaiac treatment for syphilis, though it was ultimately proved to be useless. Trading companies in the Baltic controlled the import of this 'cure' from America, and belief in the worth of this 'New World' cure was perpetuated by this trade.

Within a few decades of its description, it was established that syphilis was related to sexual contact. Doctors in Scotland were amongst the first to recognize this fact and the town council of Aberdeen threatened to brand women of ill-fame if they continued to work as prostitutes. The enigma of the horrific spread of this disease was now solved, for conditions in Europe were ideally suited to sexual spread. Rome earned over 30,000 scudos a year from a tax levied on the brothels in the city. Venice had a population of 3,00,000 of which over 12,000 were proclaimed prostitutes. Prostitution and a hedonistic moral code that pervaded the Renaissance period undoubtedly fuelled the spread of syphilis far and wide. Various city states and different countries brought forth legislations for its prevention. In 1497, the authorities in Paris issued an order in which all those infected with syphilis, who were not residents of Paris, were to leave. There was a campaign against brothels and prostitutes. Some countries made the examination of prostitutes compulsory, others sought to quell prostitution and expel prostitutes. Special hospitals sprang up to treat the great pox and at some of these the community provided free treatment. Besides the use of guaiac imported as a cure from America, the only treatment available was the application of mercury as an ointment. The 'greasers of pox' who were mere charlatans and quacks smeared the whole body with the Saracenic ointment promising cure. Blood-letting, purging and hot baths to promote sweating, were the age-old methods to eliminate the syphilitic vapours and poisons from the body.

Girolamo Fracastoro

It would be both worthy and deserving to pause briefly before this humanist *par excellence* who adorned the Renaissance. Fracastoro was a wealthy Veronese gentleman who studied with his

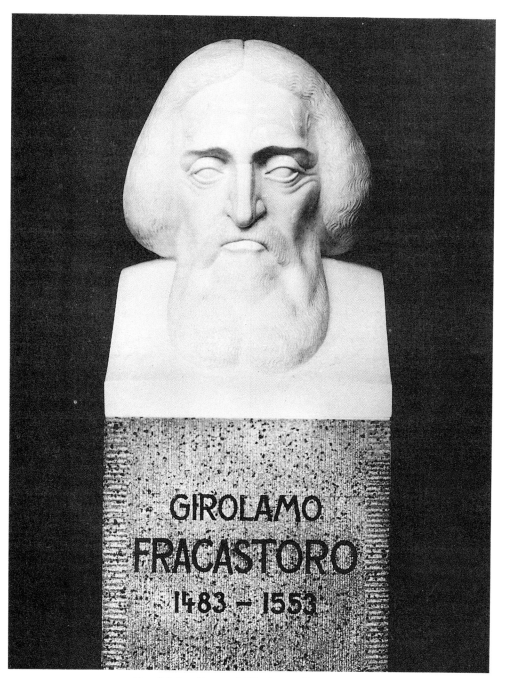

Fig. 28.1   Bust of Girolamo Fracastoro.

fellow student Copernicus in the university of Padua in the early years of the sixteenth century. He then lived as a country squire and a practising physician on his country estate in Verona. He was also a poet and playwright and was known to carry a volume of classics to read as he made his leisurely rounds precariously perched on the back of a mule. After practising medicine for 20 years, he returned to literary pursuits. He wrote poetry, plays and also treatises on literature, geography and astronomy. He also wrote two major medical works. The *love sickness* or rather the *love pestilence* excited his interest as a physician and an epidemiologist. His poem (mentioned earlier) on *Syphilis Sive Morbus Gallicum* ran into three volumes and was published in 1525 and

1530. It was written in Latin and it described the disease, its origin and its treatment; it is perhaps the most widely known poem in medical literature. Fracastoro's second and greater contribution to medicine was his volume *De Contagionibus et Contagiosis Morbis* published in 1546. This book enunciated the early principles underlying contagious diseases. He suggested that invisible germs called *seminaria* caused contagious diseases and he stressed the need to destroy these *seminaria*. He described three forms of contagion—simple direct contact, indirect contact by way of clothing, linen, personal belongings and utensils, and finally contact through distance propagated by germs in the air.

This Renaissance Man was the first to give an excellent description of typhus and to differentiate typhus from plague. He also emphasized the infectious nature of tuberculosis, which was rearing its ugly head once again in Europe. With reference to tuberculosis he wrote:

> Were it possible to destroy seminaria with caustics, there would be no better remedy; but as these substances cannot be used without endangering the lungs, treatment could be tried through neighbouring organs.

Without perhaps being aware of it, Fracastoro was both a brilliant humanist physician as also a pioneering epidemiologist in medicine.

The Great Renaissance Rebels in Medicine

The Renaissance humanists blazed an unrivalled trail of splendour and beauty in painting and sculpture, architecture, literature and philosophy. Medicine unfortunately trailed way behind. There was no brilliant discovery comparable for example to William Harvey's discovery of circulation in the seventeenth century, no breakthrough in diagnosis or treatment, no great drug that helped conquer suffering and disease. Yet there strode on to the Renaissance stage three great rebels in the field of medicine, each of whom in his own way sounded the death-knell of Galenism and who changed the path of medicine from dogma and doctrine to that of true scientific inquiry. They were Andreas Vesalius, the anatomist, Paracelsus the physician, and Ambroise Paré, the surgeon. It behoves us to summarize the achievements of each of these rebels with a passing reference to some of the lesser luminaries in the above respective fields.

Andreas Vesalius

This Flemish scientist born in Brussels in 1514 is celebrated the world over as the Father of Anatomy. His magnum opus *De Humani Corporis Fabrica* published in 1543, is one of the greatest books in medical science. Vesalius was the son of the apothecary of Charles V and came from a family of distinguished physicians. He lived at Wesel on the Rhine and took his surname from this small town. He first studied at Louvain and then successively at Montpellier and Paris. At the university of Paris he was known along with other students, to raid the cemeteries and bring back parts of corpses for dissection and study at home. In 1537, Vesalius went to the university of Padua and received his university degree with distinction in the same year. Remarkably enough, the day after he received his university degree he was appointed professor of anatomy at the same university, and the day after this appointment he commenced his lectures, demonstrations and discourses on human anatomy. His brilliant dissection, his sketches whilst dissecting and his scholarship drew students, physicians, surgeons, clergy, courtiers, and scholars from all over Italy and the European world. In 1538, he published the *Tabulae Anatomicae Sex* (six anatomic plates) for his students' benefit. Strangely enough, at this point of time both the illustrations and text of these plates perpetuated some of the age-old Galenic mistakes. In the following year he described the venous system of the thorax, discovered the azygous vein and noted its entry into the superior vena cava. After five years of brilliant dissection, experimentation and observation, Vesalius ultimately discarded the old Galenic dogmas of anatomy and published his magnum opus *De Humani Corporis Fabrica Libri Septem* (seven books on the structure of the human body). In 1543, Vesalius introduced the concept of 'living' anatomy. With the help of his fellow contemporary Van Calcar and perhaps also with the help of Titian and other artists of the Titian school, Vesalius drew his anatomical sketches of corpses in the living position using the Padua landscape as the background. The sketches were engraved on wood, and 300

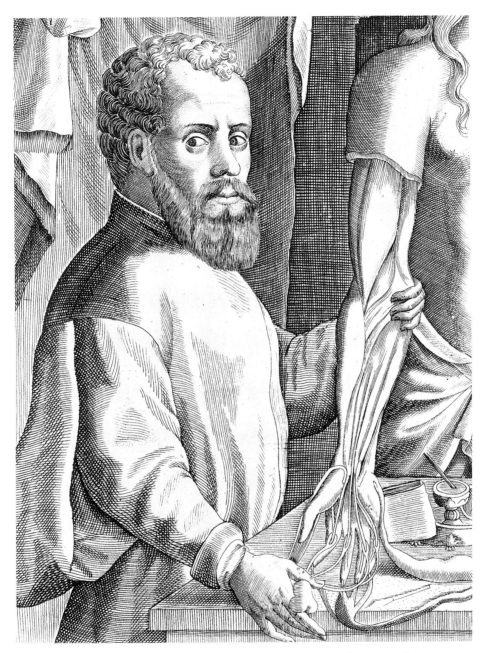

Fig. 29.1   Portrait of Andreas Vesalius dissecting the forearm of a corpse.

printing blocks of these engravings were sent on mule-back across the Alps to the master printer Johannes Operinus. This monumental work in the history of medicine was written by a man who was then just twenty-eight years old. Galenic myths were shattered (he corrected 200 Galenic errors), particularly in relation to the anatomy of the liver, bile ducts, uterus, the upper jaw and in relation to the anatomy of the skeleton with special reference to the sternum, sacrum and the cartilages of the knee. The *Fabrica* was not however without mistakes. To enumerate a few—Vesalius believed that there were only seven cranial nerves, that the vena cava arose from the liver and that the lens was in the centre of the eye. The book nevertheless demolished hallowed concepts in medicine that had been well-nigh incorporated into religious beliefs.

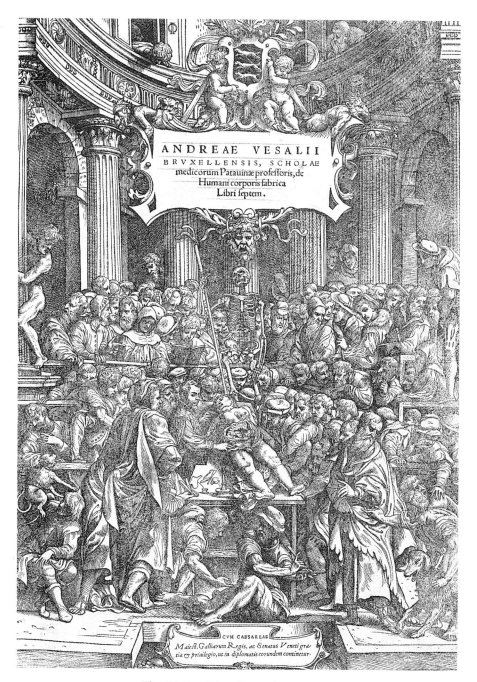

Fig. 29.2   The dissection scene.

The shock in the world of medicine was profound. How could this upstart just twenty-eight years old challenge Galen and his 1,500 year old doctrines on anatomy! The greatest heresy was Vesalius refuting the Galenic theory of blood from the right ventricle reaching the left ventricle through pores in the ventricular septum. No such pores existed. Like many great discoverers he was ridiculed and even hounded by his fellow colleagues, and accused by the church and clergy of heresy for challenging what till then was the gospel truth. He was even accused of practising vivisection in humans, a charge that was levelled by two of his most bitter Galenic enemies in France. These Galenists, Dulaurent and Riolan, accused him of vivisecting a Spanish nobleman in the wrong belief that he was already dead. It seems impossible that a man of Vesalius' stature with his knowledge of anatomy would ever commit a mistake of this kind. Unable to withstand the torments hurled at him from all sides, Andreas Vesalius made a bonfire of all his remaining unpublished works and fled Padua to become physician to Charles V and then to Philip III of Spain. In 1563, he journeyed on a pilgrimage to Jerusalem. On his return his ship was wrecked on the island of Zante in the Ionian sea. He died on this island probably of typhoid in 1564. Thus was destroyed a great man in his prime— destroyed by the bigotry, jealousy and hate of lesser mortals of our world.

Lesser luminaries also contributed to the scientific tempo in anatomy. Gabriel Fallopio (1523– 1562) belonged to the Ferrara school of medicine; he taught at Pisa and ultimately was professor of anatomy at Padua. Fallopio recognized the genius of Vesalius, but proceeded to correct a few of his mistakes. He was the first to describe the semicircular canals in the ear, the chorda tympani, the lacrimal duct, and the inguinal ligament. He gave an authentic account of the muscles of the eye and of the cranial nerves, and described the clitoris and the fallopian tubes which bear his name. His most important work was *Observationes Anatomicae* which was published in Venice in 1561.

Fallopio was succeeded by Gerolamo Farbrizio D' Acquapendente, also called Fabricus. Fabricus was a great surgeon and the first to give a good description of valves in the veins, though he opined that the blood flow in the veins was away from the heart. He also studied reproduction, childbirth and the anatomy of the foetus. William Harvey, the discoverer of circulation, was a student of Fabricus at Padua.

An unusual figure of the Renaissance was the Spanish Michael Servetus (1511–1550). He was a humanist, a theologian and a man of medicine. In a theological treatise, *Christianisimi Restitutio*, produced almost as an aside, he briefly described the pulmonary circulation. His theological treatise was judged to be heretical by the church and this brave man who thought differently from the general herd of humanity was burnt at the stake for his heresy.

Paracelsus

The foremost and most famous rebel physician who declaimed fearlessly against the teaching and practice of the traditional dogmas and doctrines in medicine was Philippus Theophrastus Bombastus von Hohenheim. This peripatetic iconoclast who became the sworn enemy of bigotry and tradition named himself Paracelsus, suggesting that he was even greater than Celsus the renowned aristocratic Roman physician who practised and wrote extensively on medicine in the early years of the Christian era. He was of Teutonic descent and was born in 1493 in the town of Einsiedeln in Switzerland. His father was a doctor who soon left Switzerland for Austria, and the young Theophrastus was introduced into the mysteries of alchemy and astrology by the Abbot of the monastery at Wurzberg. He then briefly studied at Vienna, Paris and Montpellier and finally took his medical degree in Ferrara in 1519. Then he embarked on his travels across the greater part of Europe. Judged from his extensive writings, he must have visited Poland, Russia, Lithuania, Spain and the greater part of Western Europe. He communed with the common people wherever he went—barbers, alchemists, quacks, and bath-keepers. He wrote: "I have not been ashamed to learn from tramps, butchers and barbers things which seemed of use to me." He observed, experimented and wrote medico-religious works that challenged traditional views with truculence and arrogance. Though brilliant, his precise ideas were often couched in obscure language. His writings were a potpourri of medicine, natural science, religion, astrology, magic and alchemy. Perhaps his early years of tuition with the Abbot of Wurzberg and his travels to distant exotic lands were responsible

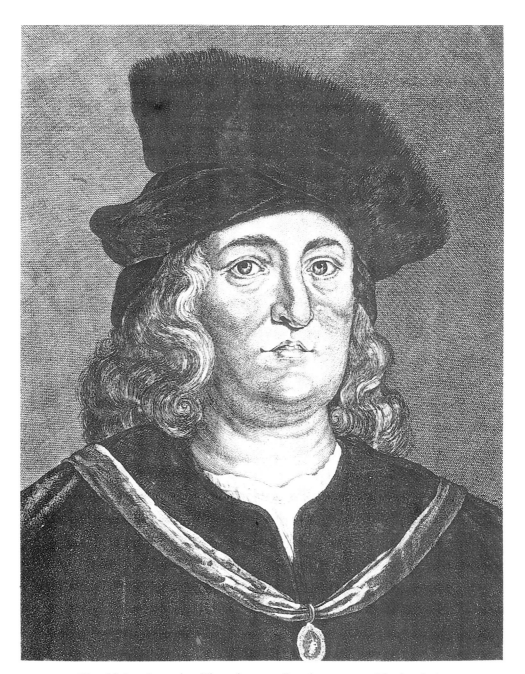

Fig. 29.3   Aureolus Theophrastus Bombastus von Hoohenheim.

for his extravagant concepts. He was a classical example of a strongly opinionated individualist of the Renaissance who combined humanity and knowledge with violence and intolerance. Coarse in his behaviour, often drunken in his habits, he alienated friends and made many enemies. He was violently opposed to Galen, yet erred in postulating that all matter was composed from sulphur, mercury and salt. His alchemical concept maintained that these elements were the outcome of distillation; the condensed vapour in the alembic was sulphur; the dense liquid distillate was mercury; and the dry residue was salt. His travels ceased when he was requested to treat the Basle humanist and master publisher Johnnes Frobenius in 1526. Frobenius had an inflamed leg and had

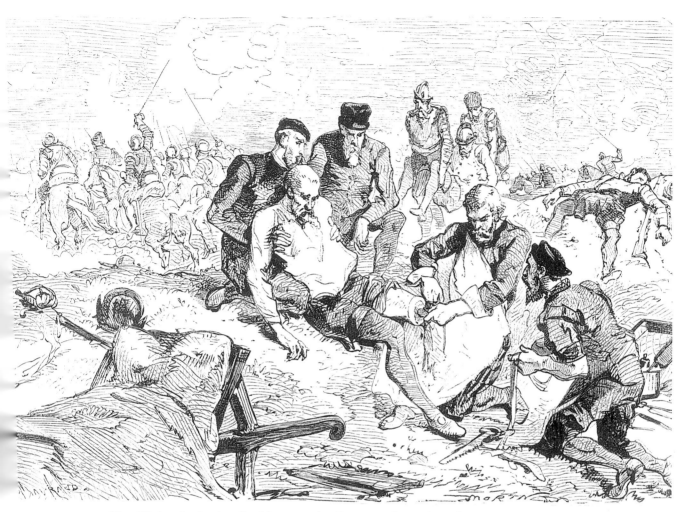

Fig. 29.4   Ambroise Paré invents the ligature of arteries after an amputation.

been advised amputation to save his life by several physicians. Paracelsus treated and cured him. Soon after, the great humanist Erasmus described his own illness in a letter to Paracelsus and requested his advice. Paracelsus again cured him. These were two famous cures that catapulted him to good fortune. He was now offered a university chair in Basle and was appointed municipal doctor to the town council of Basle—a far cry from his earlier wandering existence in the company of the meek and the lowly. Even so, Paracelsus remained true to his iconoclastic self. His first speech as a university professor instead of being in customary Latin was delivered in his native German to a shocked audience. He followed this breach of tradition by a heresy that many never forgave him. He publicly burnt the works of Galen and Avicenna condemning the slavish mentality that had hindered the progress of medicine for nearly 1,500 years. He also publicly denounced and castigated his colleagues for propagating dogma, and falsehood instead of searching for the truth. He kept his post in Basle for two years during which he fostered controversy and dispute and then reverted to his vagabond existence. He died in 1541 at Salzburg when he was just forty-eight years old.

In spite of his eccentricities and his egoistic arrogance he was eternally true to his own self and was a great Renaissance man. He devised no great and enduring system of medicine, but he broke the shackles that bound medicine to the wrong tradition and pointed to the true path. He himself did not take more than a few steps on this new path, yet opened the way for future generations to follow. He must have been a great physician of his time and age, for he looked at medicine with fresh eyes. His concept of disease was that of a living process that often came from without. Disease occurred through a weakening of the vital principle and his therapy was based on the curative powers of nature—an ayurvedic-cum-Hippocratic teaching. He replaced ancient polychemical and dangerous ancient formulations for the treatment of disease with simple medicaments— essences and tinctures such as those of laudanum and turpentine. He was always experimenting and searching for new cures; he introduced preparations of metals in the pharmacopoeia and was indeed the forerunner of medical chemistry. He denounced as useless the use of guaiac in syphilis and pointed to the usefulness of mercury in this disease. Paracelsus also wrote on disease afflicting miners—probably the first treatise on occupational disease. He discussed at length, insanity—under diseases that deprive man of reason. He wrote on epilepsy, on the connection between goitre and cretinism, and of the 'dancing mania' which was widely prevalent in that period. He strongly believed in the ethics of medicine and upheld the Hippocratic tenet that the place of the physician was at the bedside of his patient. He intuitively grasped the role of the physician in medicine when he wrote: "The most famous thing we physicians possess is our art, and next comes our love for our patients, hope being the keystone of both." His legacy to our world was a spirit of flaming rebellion against untruths and half-truths, even if they were sanctified by tradition or religion.

A less known and less recognized rebel in the Renaissance period was the Dutch physician Johannes Weyer. His rebellion was in psychiatry and he voiced his belief in the basic human rights of men and women with deranged minds. Even during the humanist age, belief in witches was universal. People of unsound mind, the manics, schizophrenics and the depressed were often burnt as witches. The time of the infamous Catholic Inquisition was the time of burning, especially after the Inquisitors Sprenger and Krämer published their infamous treatise *Malleus Maleficarum*. The treatise was a penal code that legalized and regulated the unmasking of witches and codified the horrendous punishments for those convicted of witchcraft. Countless mental patients with disorders of the mind were convicted as witches, tortured and burnt to death. The Inquisition also became a ruse to destroy personal enemies or those considered enemies of the state or church. It is believed that over a million people in Europe were tortured and burnt as practitioners of witchcraft. Johannes Weyer regarded witches as individuals with disorders of the mind who often suffered from hallucinations. They were ill patients, only in that the disease was in the mind and not in the body. This brave rebel, at great risk to life and liberty, started an almost solitary crusade against the hunting and burning of witches. He spread his belief through the printed word by writing and publishing his famous book *De Praestigiis Daemonum et Incantationibus ac Venificiis*. His crusade was carried forward by Juan Luis Vives.

Ambroise Paré

In the year 1536, Francis, king of France, cast his covetous eyes on rich Turin and on the duchy of Savoy in northern Italy. He marched his army into Piedmont attacking the forts defending that area. The carnage was great and the battlefields were strewn with the dead and the wounded. The wounds were chiefly gunshot wounds and the surgeons in the French army had a great deal of work on their hands. Ambroise Paré was then a young barber army surgeon who had just joined the service of the king of France. He grew in later years to be the most famous and renowned surgeon of the Renaissance and one of the greatest surgeons of all time. His baptism into surgery was indeed by

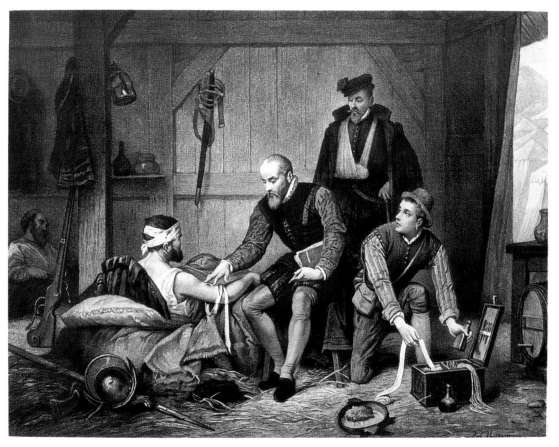

Fig. 29.5 Ambroise Paré.

fire. He had never seen gunshot wounds before, but had been taught that gunshot wounds were poisonous because of the gunpowder in them and that the treatment of such wounds consisted of cauterizing them with burning oil of elder mixed with treacle. Realizing the agony that this would cause to the wounded, he asked his senior surgeons what they used for their first dressing. When told that they poured burning oil into the wounds, Ambroise Paré with great trepidation did likewise. Fortunately, both for him and the wounded he ran out of oil. Perhaps a lesser person in his predicament would have searched for more oil or would have surreptitiously sought the comfort of a campfire to escape the horrors of the battlefield. Ambroise Paré through intuition, perhaps through innovation and invention, or perhaps through sheer chance (we shall never know), began to apply a mixture of egg yolk, oil of roses and turpentine to the wounds. He awakened before daybreak with the fear that those who had not been cauterized would probably have died. To his great relief and happy surprise he noted instead that those on whom he had used his mixture felt little pain and their wounds were not inflamed, whilst those cauterized with burning oil were in great pain and their wounds were markedly inflamed. He vowed never to use burning oil on gunshot wounds. A mere novice of a barber surgeon thus exorcised forever the cruel practice of scorching wounds with burning oil or with a red hot iron.

Barber surgeons were at that period of history the lowest in the medical hierarchy. Besides shaving customers, they also concerned themselves with cauterization, incision of abscesses, blood-letting through the application of leeches, cupping of vessels, and in other operative procedures. Unlike most humanist physicians of the Renaissance, barber surgeons lacked education, were ignorant of Latin and were unable to enter universities. Ambroise Paré was born in 1517 in Mayenne. His father and uncle were both barber surgeons and it was the ardent wish and ambition of young Ambroise to join the fraternity of barber surgeons. Unable to go to a university he learnt his art and craft from experience as an apprentice with a relative barber surgeon, and then as a resident surgeon at the Hôtel Dieu in Paris—an old hospital founded by monks in the Middle Ages. As an army surgeon his young mind had not been prejudiced by the tradition and dogma of earlier centuries. He had no reverence for Galen or Albucasis. In his treatise on gunshot wounds written in French he says: "I do not wish to be able to boast of having read Galen in the Greek or in the Latin; God was not pleased to be so kind to me in my youth so as to provide for instruction in the one or the other of these languages." He learnt from observation, experience and experiment. In fact lack of old knowledge was probably an asset to this young surgeon. But it was not just the excellence in his art and craft that alone characterized him. He was compassionate, considerate, innovative and above all singularly modest for a surgeon of such brilliance. He realized that his hands were the gift of God and that he was merely His instrument. In his first encounter with death and suffering during the French Piedmont campaign, a badly wounded officer named Le Rat was brought to Paré. The young novice barber surgeon saved his life and when asked how, made the historic remark: *"Je le pansay, et Dieu le guérit"*—I dressed him, God healed him. This is the remark that has been aptly engraved on his tombstone. It was indeed a profound remark—an expression of his innate humility and devoutness, of hope, faith and trust in God and in the healing powers of Nature.

Ambroise Paré wrote extensively in his diaries on what he saw and did. The illness of Marquis D'Aurel detailed below illustrates not only his approach to diagnosis and management but also his faith in the healing powers of Nature and his close communion with a very sick man—factors that promoted healing and recovery in what seemed a mortal illness.

Marquis D'Aurel had his femur shattered by a gunshot wound and in spite of being treated for several months by several doctors was at death's door. The king of France requested Paré to treat him. Paré describes beautifully the clinical features of infection: "The young Marquis had a high temperature, his eyes were sunken in their sockets, his face yellow, his tongue dry and spotted, his body wasted and voice feeble as that of a dying man." Paré found a deep filthy suppurating wound with many bone fragments embedded within. The patient had extensive bedsores, got no rest by day or by night, was emaciated, feeble and close to death. His sheets were incredibly dirty, stained and had not been changed for months for fear of causing pain to the patient. Paré writes, "It looked as if there was little hope of avoiding death. However, to give him hope and strength, I told him he would be well with the help of God, his physicians and surgeons." Paré incised and drained the suppurating wound, removed the bone fragments embedded within, ordered a good bath, a clean bed and positioned him skillfully to relieve both pressure and discomfort from his bedsores. Paré devised a device whereby drops of water falling into a basin made a sound like rain, thereby lulling the patient to sleep and allowing him the rest he had been denied so long. He also ensured that the air of gloom in the household was replaced by good cheer, by song and sweet music. Marquis D'Aurel recovered and lived to write his tale.

Ambroise Paré in his later years wrote a great deal of his experiences in surgery. His major text was titled *Oeuvres de M Ambroise Paré, Conseiller, et Premier Chirurgien du Roi*. It was a magnificent volume of a thousand pages published in Paris in 1575. We would be failing in our duty to this great man if we did not briefly list some of his more important achievements in surgery. Besides revolutionizing the treatment of gunshot wounds, he practised vascular ligation of arteries to arrest haemorrhage, devised the haemostatic forceps and other surgical instruments. He popularized the operation for hare-lip, performed a herniotomy without castration, wrote on obstetrics, and was probably the first to put into successful practice podalic version to correct abnormal foetal positions. In fact Paré was a pioneer and founder of modern obstetrics. His *Generation de L'Homme* combined Hippocratic principles with his own observations and was a classic obstetric work of his times. Paré was also interested in cripples and devised a number of aids and prosthesis for cripples including an ingenious artificial hand. Paré lived through the wars of the Reformation initiated by Calvin and Luther. Some historians considered him a Huguenot, but this is unlikely. Whatever may have been his faith, he was a true Christian with Christian motives and Christian charity within his heart. He was brave enough to treat the leader of the Huguenots, Admiral Coligny. This was considered as a well-nigh mortal sin by the Catholics at the time of the massacre of St Bartholomew. His life was spared only through the king's intervention.

Destiny ultimately beckoned this humble barber surgeon to worldly glory. He became councillor in state and surgeon to four kings of France—Henry II, Frances II, Charles IX, and Henry III. He died in 1590, revered as a great surgeon and a great man. Ah would to God that more surgeons were cast in his mould!

The other surgeons of the Renaissance were lesser mortals who pale into insignificance when compared to Ambroise Paré. Yet mention must be made of Gaspare Tagliacozzi (1546–1599), professor at the university of Bologna, who made significant advances in plastic surgery, particularly in the operation of rhinoplasty. His technique (often referred to as the Italian method), consisted of using a strip of skin and subcutaneous tissue from the arm of the patient to restore the nose. The patient's arm was strapped to his head so that the flap remained attached to the face until it was ready to be detached surgically after it had taken. The church charged him with impiety and the operation was banned. It was revived in the early nineteenth century.

30 The Renaissance Ends

Just as the sun rises, it also sets. It set over the Renaissance age in the last sixty years of the sixteenth century. There were many causes for this decline and it is appropriate to touch upon these before concluding this section. The fierce rather unbridled individualism which characterized the Renaissance and which was partly responsible for its intellectual and artistic brilliance was also responsible for a moral decay. Increasing wealth resulting from Italy's strategic position on the trade route between the rich Orient and Europe reinforced this decay. The ascetic ideal advocated in the formative period of the Christian church was shattered. Men and women resented a way of life, born of poverty and fear because it ran counter to their individualistic hedonistic instincts— instincts and urges that could now be easily satisfied by increasing wealth. The charm of the good life—of wine, women and song—increasingly prevailed over the threats, fears and prohibitions of religious teaching. Another important cause of the decline of the Renaissance was the political turmoil and uncertainty of the times. France and Spain, increasingly united under powerful kings, seemed to have rediscovered the riches and political weakness of fragmented Italy. Invasions by foreign armies, ravages of war, strife between the city states of northern Italy, the rule of despots who suppressed legitimacy with autocracy and force, led to social and political chaos. The church and the rulers who ruled the city states were a law unto themselves; neither could they protect the common man, who therefore took the law into his own hands and protected himself through craft, cunning or force of arms. Men found themselves unmoored, struggling in an uncharted sea of disorder and violence.

The moral laxity of the Roman Catholic Church in that era of history certainly contributed to the decline of this glorious era. Even worse than this moral laxity were the murderous activities of the Inquisition which started in Spain and spread to Italy. Men either questioned the prevailing tenets of the Christian religion or turned from religion to pursue an epicurean, bacchanalian existence. The decline of Roman Catholic influence spawned the revolt led by Luther and Calvin—a revolt termed the Reformation, which led to the founding of the rival Protestant Church.

The lights now slowly dimmed over Italy. France, Spain and the papacy carved the greater part of this country among themselves. Ravages of war and the opening up of sea-routes to the Orient and to America slowly but surely adversely affected Italian trade. The final factor in the fading of the Renaissance was the counter-Reformation enforced by a strict catholic church, which shed the laxity that imperilled its own existence, and enforced a rigid orthodox conservatism that laid strong restraints on free thought, speech and inquiry. There was an intellectual retreat and the voice of individualism and humanism was smothered in the clash of militant faiths and warring nations. Yet the echoes of this voice can still be heard reverberating in the passages of time.

And through the veils and mists of past centuries, we can still picture the triumphant smile of Vesalius on the front piece of his Treatise after he had shattered ancient Galenic myths; still gaze with never-ending rapture on the smile of Mona Lisa, wondering how mankind could have produced one such as Leonardo da Vinci, who strove undauntedly for truth and beauty. We can still absorb a fraction of the humility of Ambroise Paré, as he dressed the wounds of the wounded; still picture Michelangelo, who with a million strokes of his hammer and chisel turned stone into everlasting beauty. These were the men who gave meaning to life, nobility to thought and who held forth a light to our world which has remained undimmed through the centuries.

Medicine in the Baroque Period

31 Historical Background of the Baroque Period

The place of medicine is in the stream of life, not on its banks.

René Sand

By the beginning of the seventeenth century the urge of the western world to return to the civilization and culture of classical antiquity seemed to have been satiated. The stage was now set for a ferment of ideas and events that shaped the sociopolitical, scientific and intellectual foundations of our modern world.

The political scenario was characterized by intrigue, turmoil and frequent wars. Powerful nation states crystallized under autocratic monarchs who claimed to rule with absolute power through the divine right of kings. The balance of power in Europe was remoulded again and again through conflicts and wars, which saw a slow decline of the once powerful Spanish Empire with France emerging stronger than ever under the Sun King, Louis XIV.

Perhaps the greatest political tragedy of the century was the thirty years war fought between the Bourbons of France and the Hapsburgs of the Holy Roman Empire. The battlegrounds were in Germany and this tragedy resulted in untold suffering, starvation and disease. The increasing power of France in the latter half of the century was however balanced by the growing power of England, Russia, Holland, and Sweden.

The century witnessed the murderous clash between the Ottoman Empire and Peter the Great of Russia, and the entry of Russia on to the European stage. It also witnessed the last decisive battle between Islam and Christendom— the sea battle of Lepanto where the Venetians and their allies defeated the Ottomans, thwarting forever the expansion of Islam into Western Europe.

Many crimes were committed in the name of religion in this era. Catholics and Protestants spilled blood for the last time in an internecine conflict. Religion did not isolate itself from world events— it spread its tentacles into the political fabric of the western world. Thus the feud between Protestantism born of the Reformation of the previous century and the counter-Reformation of the Catholic Church led by the Jesuit order influenced political decisions, events and conflicts. England, Germany and the Low countries sided with the Reformation, whilst Spain, France, Austria and the Papacy with the counter-Reformation. Wars were thus ignited by the breath of religious fervour.

One of the foremost features of the age was the rise of capitalism. The merchant princes of the Renaissance were now replaced by powerful Dutch and English mercantile companies. The vast increase in the volume of trade could no longer be financed by individual banking families like the Medicis of Italy and the Fugers of Germany, as in the Renaissance. Trade was often financed by the State, so that the politics of a country was wedded to the idea of expanding trade, thereby increasing its wealth and power. Thus the rise of England and Holland was due to increasing commerce, encouraged and protected by powerful navies.

Yet, through all this turmoil, literature, art and architecture evolved its own Baroque style, philosophy prospered, and science, as we understand it today, was born and flourished as never before. The Baroque era was indeed the golden era of science. Its light shone bright and strong all through this century; the arts and humanities evolved within its shadow. The Baroque era also witnessed one great discovery and one great invention in medicine. William Harvey discovered the circulation of blood—a discovery that is one of the most important foundation stones in the edifice of modern medicine. The invention was that of the microscope. Its use led to the visualization of a fascinating, hidden, undiscovered new world that for the first time was laid bare to the inquiring eye and mind.

Society

The Baroque era was characterized by splendid, spectacular and often vulgar display. Society was stratified and acutely class conscious. In descending order, there were the monarchs and princes of royal blood, the nobles, aristocrats and clergy, the landed gentry, the bourgeois class who had, within its fold, both the rich and poor, the working class in the cities, and finally the peasants in the countryside. Climbing up the social ladder was for many the greatest ambition in life.

The upper classes made a great outward show of exaggerated courteous manner and etiquette, of pomp and ceremony. Honour at any cost was the accepted credo. The glance of an eye, a gesture or a word could lead to a challenge to a duel, which was honour bound and had to be accepted. Thousands perished by the sword or the pistol in these senseless duelling encounters. For the rich, the bold and the powerful, the world was a grand stage and they were the actors—actors who strutted across this stage with all the pomp and ostentation they could display. Barring notable exceptions they were shallow lives bereft of true magnanimity, or a sense of vision and beauty that the rich and powerful of the Renaissance Age possessed. On the other hand, for the peasantry the Baroque century was one of unmitigated suffering and disaster. The ravages of frequent wars across the fields of Europe spread untold misery, starvation and death among these poor people. Their sad plight was worsened by the direct and indirect taxes levied upon them to enrich the coffers of the state or to fill the pockets of the upper classes.

Architecture and Art

Architecture was on a grand monumental scale, with a sense of luxury and exaggerated ornamentation. The classic straight line and the proportional elegance of line and space that characterized the architecture of ancient Greece and Renaissance Italy, were replaced by the dynamic flowery curve. It was as if the western world now exulted in movement and motion and it expressed this movement with an exaggerated flourish. Corners of monuments or buildings which in Greek and Roman antiquity were bare and geometrical, now had flowing swirling contours, often embellished and filled with patterns or figures. The spirit of the age expressed itself in the urge to build grand manors, stately chateaux with opulent curves and formal manicured terraced gardens.

The outstanding architects of the age were Lorenzo Bernini and Christopher Wren. Bernini's first revolutionary work was to construct, under Michelangelo's great dome of St Peter's in Rome, a bronze canopy 100 feet high resting on four gigantic beautiful twisted columns.

After the destruction caused by the great fire of London in 1669, Christopher Wren rebuilt St Paul's and many other churches in the Baroque style. Perhaps the grandest, most magnificent, yet the most elegant example of Baroque architecture is the Palace at Versailles, constructed under the direction of Louis XIV by Le Vau. This king whose style and life epitomized the Baroque period, converted and expanded a hunting lodge of his father into this most famous palace in the world at a stupendous cost of 60 million livres.

Baroque painters continued to paint scenes from antiquity, classical history, mythology with sumptuous ornamental backgrounds; portraits painted against lavish backgrounds were also in great demand. They also painted life as it was in that era—rogues, vagabonds, peasants, self portraits, still life, domestic scenes.

One of the greatest artists of the early Baroque period was El Greco (1548–1614), the Greek who made his home in Toledo, Spain. He was strangely modern in his art, which had a strong streak of religious mysticism within it. As his models for saints he used the insane within the mental asylum of Toledo.

Some of other greats of the Baroque era were Rembrandt Von Rijin (1606–1666), whose masterly perception of light and shadow on canvas remains unsurpassed to this day, Peter Paul Reubens (1577–1640), whose nudes captured the lustiness of this epoch, Franz Hals (1584–1666), whose art was rooted in the daily life of ordinary people and simple peasants, and Diego Velasquez who epitomized the heroic style of Spanish Baroque.

Baroque painters for some remarkable reason also portrayed deformed specimens of humanity and those afflicted with disease. Velasquez, in particular painted numerous dwarfs and achondroplasics. A careful study of his achondroplasic in his great painting Las Meninas is more instructive than reading a description of this deformity from a medical textbook. Dutch painters depicted cripples, deformed creatures, dwarves, and blind men and portrayed diseases and illnesses, such as chlorosis, dropsy and melancholy. The Dutch school also indulged in art depicting medical themes—urine inspection, the doctor at the patient's bedside, the costume and attire of the physician of this age and the anatomy lesson as illustrated by the famous painting of Rembrandt titled 'The Anatomy Lesson of Dr Tulp'.

The spirit of the Baroque age also significantly influenced music and the composition of music. Music thus combined a formal well-nigh mathematical tonal balance with an increased expression of emotion and feeling. This age saw the development of the opera, the oratorio, and of the concerto and the overture in solo and orchestral music. The major technical improvement was in the development of the organ and of the violin as we recognize them today. Music was no longer a solely amateur exercise—it grew to be increasingly professional in its scope. The opera was indeed a clear mirror reflection of the Baroque—the stage, the splendour, the spectacle, the display, the lustiness, the concept of honour, and yet the invariably tragic end. The ballet and the masques were the offshoots of the opera and were frequently indulged in by the rich and the powerful.

The pomp, splendour, gravity and the feeling of honour, pathos, and tragedy were expressed by authors and poets in rich, often flowery, ornate language. William Shakespeare bridged the gap between the Renaissance and Baroque in English literature, Miguel de Cervantes did the same in Spanish literature. His great classic Don Quixote is not just for the Baroque period but for eternity. It expounds the romanticism, the idealism, the chivalry of man and contrasts these with grotesque reality. Jean Racine and Pierre Corneille captured the Baroque century in their tragedies. The thin but clear streak of mysticism which originated in the Middle Ages but which was still distinctly visible in the Renaissance and Baroque periods was kept alive in the works of John Milton, John

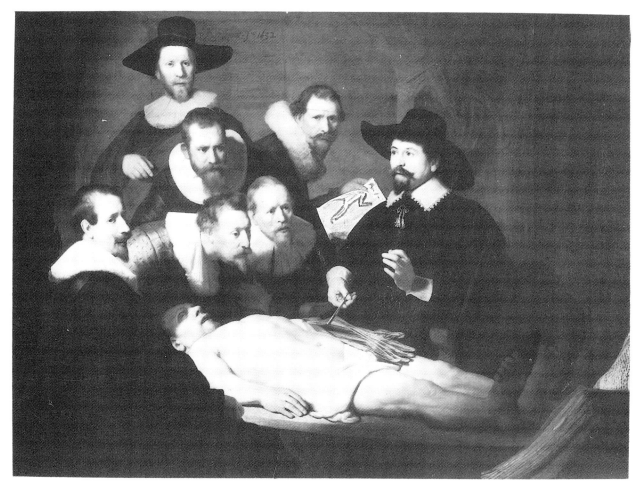

Fig. 31.1   The anatomy lesson of Dr Tulp.

Bunyon and John Donne. An important work on medicine in relation to ethics and religion was the *Religio Medici* by Sir Thomas Browne (1605–1682) a gentle country physician from Norwich, England. There is the rhythm of poetry in his prose and a beautiful philosophy of life and living in relation to medicine that lifts this work into the realm of great medical literature. He ends his treatise on *Religio Medici* with beautiful lines that carry a universal message: "Bless me in this life with but peace of my Conscience, command of my affections, the love of Thy self and my dearest friends, and I shall be happy enough to pity Caesar."

Philosophers and Scientists

Great thoughts penetrated the turmoil of the sixteenth century. The physician philosopher John Locke (1632–1704) believed and wrote that primitive men were equal and happy, and that a state must follow natural law and protect the rights of the individual. His thinking ran counter to the policy of absolute power wielded by monarchs of kingdom states in Europe. The thoughts of this physician philosopher found a responsive chord, not in the Baroque century, but, in the works of Rousseau over a hundred years later. An ardent supporter of the postulate of absolute power of the state was England's Thomas Hobbes (1588–1679). He expounded the view in *Leviathan* that men must

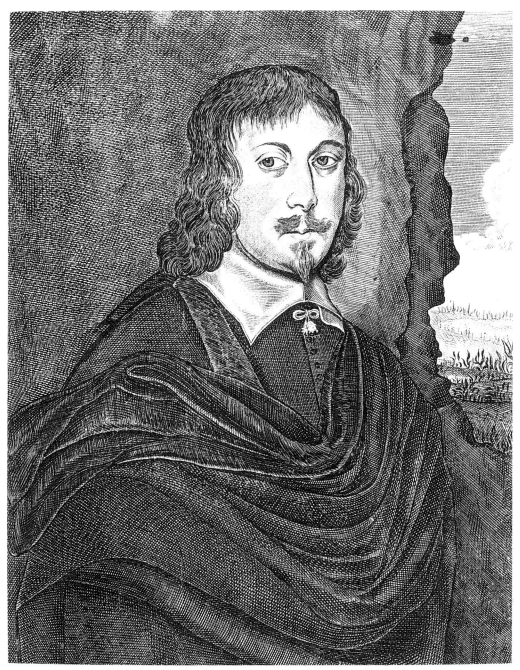

Fig. 31.2   Sir Thomas Browne.

surrender their individual rights to the state and submit to the absolute rule of the sovereign if anarchy
and strife were to be prevented. Descartes (1596–1650) was perhaps the foremost thinker of his age
who not only influenced many aspects of the Baroque era (including the concept of medicine) but
also the succeeding ages. He was born in Normandy, France, and his first loves were mathematics
and physics. As a young man he enlisted as a soldier, but later settled in Amsterdam where he
continued his studies in science, philosophy and medicine. Descartes was a thinker who wedded
philosophy to science. In his *Discours de la methode* (1637), he resolved to doubt all, to pursue truth
and to reconstruct natural philosophy on self-evident principles. He started on the one premise he

could not doubt—his own consciousness. He summed this up in a famous sentence—*"Cogito, ergo sum or Je pense, donc je suis"*—I think, therefore I am (exist). His philosophy was deductive, but he recognized the importance of observation and experimentation in the path towards truth.

The study of medicine was crucial to the study of the natural sciences. Descartes, living near the butcher's quarters in Amsterdam dissected several animals and wrote three medical treatises—*Tractatus de formatione foetus* (1664) (Treatise in the formation of the foetus), *La description du corps humain* (1649) (Description of the human body), *Traité de l'homme* (1662) (Treatise of Man). He postulated the concept of dualism where mind and matter were separate entities, their only link being through God. His scientific method was based on mathematical rationalism and he endeavoured to explain the complexities of nature through algebraic and geometric formulae, forms and equations. He was anti-Galenic, anti-Aristolean and aganist the concepts of the presence of humor within the body. He considered both the physical world and the human body as machines—as matter in motion in accordance with mathematical laws. The human body was however a machine influenced by thoughts. He offered a rather bizzare, purely speculative explanation that the pineal body situated at the base of he brain mediated this influence. Even so, his mechanistic philosophy on the world and on the workings of the human body had a significant impact on medicine and on the natural sciences in the years to come.

A great philosopher and scientist of this age was Francis Bacon, Lord Chancellor of England. He postulated that the way to truth was clear thinking. He postulated the use of inductive logic in scientific research. In the *New Atlantis,* he considered science to be the foundation of all knowledge

More brilliant than all facets of human activity and endeavour was the brilliance of science in the seventeenth century. The great names of this era who blazed a trail of truth and glory were Johannes Kepler (1571–1630), Galileo Gallilei (1564–1642), and Isaac Newton (1643–1727). Their discoveries dealt with basic observations on nature, and on the universe—they were easily understood, expressed lucidly and quantitated by simple mathematical formulae. As always, their beauty lay in their inherent simplicity. Keppler exemplified this when he stated that nature loves simplicity, loves unity and there is nothing superfluous in it. He studied the systems of Copernicus and Tycho Brahe and formulated three fundamental laws to explain planetary motion.

Galileo studied medicine at the university of Pisa, but took to mathematics, and later was professor of mathematics at Padua. He fell foul of the Church which persecuted him for supporting the Copernican theory that the planets revolve round the sun. He was the first to apply mathematics to the study of mechanics. He proposed the law of uniform acceleration for falling bodies, and suggested the use of the pendulum for clocks. He developed the astronomical telescope with which he discovered craters on the moon, sun spots, the satellites of Jupiter, the phase of Mercury. He showed that the Milky Way was composed of stars.

Newton, even today, is considered by many as the greatest scientific genius of all time. He discovered calculus, discovered the components of white light, formulated the three fundamental laws of mechanics, and enunciated the epoch-making laws of universal gravitation. His two great works are *Opticks* and *Principia Mathematica*—the latter being written when he was just twenty-seven years old.

There was a true revolution in science in the Baroque era. Natural science evolved into an independent intellectual entity. Diligent observation without prejudices or dogma was its first requisite. Experimentation to verify a hypothesis was the next requisite. Quantitative measurements replaced qualitative impressions of nature and nature's complexities. Science became both rational and mensural, so that scientific observations were condensed into fundamental mathematical formulae. It was not just the great discoveries made by the geniuses of the era that mattered. The methodology that they introduced, the technique of experimentation, and the scepticism over scientific results, inculcated a mental habit or a scientific temper that was a *sine qua non* in the search for truth—both in the natural sciences and in medicine. It is this invaluable legacy that we have inherited from these great men; a legacy that forms the framework and background of science and medicine in our modern age and in the many ages to come.

32 Medicine in the Baroque Period

The influence of research and discoveries in the natural sciences had a decisive influence on medicine. The methods of investigation, the testing of hypothesis by experiment and the concept of science as measurement postulated by Galileo and the other great figures of science, percolated into the field of medicine and was responsible for important medical discoveries. Yet the gulf between these discoveries in medicine and the practice of medicine as translated into patient care was never so wide before or since.

Schools of Thought

The two principle schools of thought in medicine were Iatrophysics and Iatrochemistry—the study of physics and chemistry in relation to medicine. These schools were offshoots of the advances in the natural sciences, reinforced perhaps by philosophic-cum-scientific views of thinkers such as Descartes. To these could be added the individual approach of the systematists. These schools of thought and the individual systematists were at scornful variance with one another.

The iatrophysicists believed that the human body was a machine and that physiology of living and the state of disease could be explained by the laws of physics. Iatrophysics was encouraged and influenced by the genius of Galileo with his penchant for measurements and by the development of instruments of significant use in the service of medicine. It received a strong impetus in the abstract arguments of Descartes who authored perhaps the first treatise in physiology titled *Traité de l'homme* in 1662.

Descartes was among the first to recognize the truth of Harvey's discovery of circulation. He regarded the human body as a machine, which was activated by the heat extracted from the blood flowing through it. The blood reached the brain carrying with it the vital spirit, which activated the brain permitting it to receive impressions of external objects as also those of the soul.

Circulation, respiration, digestion and locomotion were all machine-like mechanical actions obeying physical laws. A champion of iatrophysics was Sanctorius Santorio (1561–1636), the father of metabolic physiology, who was professor at the university of Padua. He invented a clinical thermometer and a platform with scales that enabled him to measure alterations in body weight during rest, work, digestion, emotion. The platform with scales was large enough to accommodate him, his bed, his work table and all the necessities of daily living. He experimented upon changes in his body weight for endless hours, discovered insensible perspiration as being due to loss of water vapour from the skin. He published his work in *De Statica Medicina* (1614). The measurement and quantification that he used for the first time in experimental physiology was the forerunner of modern metabolic physiology.

Another leading proponent of iatrophysics was Alfonso Borelli (1608–1679), a pupil of Galileo and a teacher of Malphigi. He explained in mechanical terms the principle of muscle action, of respiration and of energy spent in muscle action in his book, *De motu animalium* (1679). He believed that digestion was a mechanical process, the secretion of gastric juice being induced by blood pressure, and that symptoms such as fever, pain and convulsions were related to mechanically defective motion of nerve juices.

It is indeed amazing how individuals endowed with intelligence and the spirit of inquiry should have so abandoned the basic tenets expounded by the great figures of the natural sciences of the Baroque era and allowed themselves to be swayed by flights of fancy. It is equally amazing how strongly they believed in the correctness of their views in the realm of medicine.

Iatrochemistry was under the leadership of a strange individual—the Belgian, Jan-Baptista Van Helmont (1577–1644). He was described as pious, learned and famous; he was the sworn enemy of Galen and Aristotle. The sick never lingered long in his care; within a few days they were dead or they were well again! Van Helmont first thought of studying magic, but then decided to study the stoic philosophers. He later took to medicine and then became an ardent follower and avid reader of Galenic works. Then there occured a rather amusing incident. A lady dropped a glove which he picked up and returned with all courtesy and chivalry. But the lady had scabies and Von Helmont contracted scabies. He followed Galen's treatment of repeated strong purges to rid himself of the disease. His scabies got worse, he was enfeebled with the treatment and he developed a hatred for Galen. He however did not abandon medicine and ultimately cured himself by a prescription of Paracelsus, whose ardent follower he now became.

Van Helmont postulated that all physiological processes were controlled by ferments and were thus purely of chemical origin. Each physiological process had its own special ferment, controlled by a particular archeus or spirit. All the archeus spirits were controlled by the soul located in the solar plexus. His therapy in medicine consisted of diet and chemicals in small doses, contrasting strongly with lethal doses used in that age. In 1624 he was accused of heresy by the Inquisition, imprisoned for two years and then fortunately released. His book *Ortus medicinae* was printed and published in 1648 in Amsterdam—a Protestant town that did not fear the Inquisition.

The iatrochemical school was further consolidated by Francois de la Boe (AD 1614–1672), a professor at the University of Leyden who disregarded and disbelieved a number of notions held by Van Helmont. He explained physiology in chemical terms and had students attending his clinic from all over Europe. He was one of the rare good teachers who believed in the Hippocratic doctrine of teaching medicine at the patient's bedside.

De la Boe's most famous pupil was Thomas Willis, an exponent of iatrochemistry in England. He was professor of natural philosophy at Oxford in 1660, and six years later moved to London where he acquired a large and lucrative practice. His work *Cerebri Anatome* (1664) illustrated by Wren was in that age the most accurate and best study on the anatomy of the nervous system. He described the spinal accessory nerve for the first time as also the circle of communicating arteries at the base of the brain known as the circle of Willis. Willis was undoubtedly a good clinician. He was the first in the Western world to notice the sweetish taste and characteristic odour of diabetic urine (1670); he gave the first description of epidemic typhoid, puerperal fever and was the first to describe the disease now known as myasthenia gravis (1671). He made the original observation that some deaf people can hear in the presence of noise (*paracusis willisii*) and wrote neurological works on general paralysis of the insane, and on hysteria.

Willis was one among about a dozen learned men who met weekly in a tavern to discuss medicine, science and philosophy. This group included Boyle, Hooke and Wren. From these meetings was born the Royal Society.

Systematists

Not a single discovery in the natural sciences or in medicine in the seventeenth century made any significant difference to the practice of medicine. The main objective of medicine is patient care and consists of relief of suffering or healing of disease. Systematists were engaged in the practice of medicine and were unconcerned with the experiment and observation that went into the unravelling of nature's secrets. By and large their concept of the practice of medicine was still Galenic. Barring a few exceptions, they were mediocre characters or outright quacks. Those who had obtained degrees were full of obsolete theories and many had never seen a patient before starting practice. In the large cities of London, Paris, and Leyden they were dressed ostentatiously wearing a square bonnet on the head, a wig, a long robe and high-heeled shoes which showed below the robe. They spoke pompously, often in Latin, a language which the common man could not comprehend. These men often invited scorn and formed perfect subjects for satire by playwrights such as Molière. Molière ridiculed doctors in five of his comedies. In *Le Malade Imaginaire* he indirectly, through the character of the doctor, contrasted the uselessness of medicine as it prevailed in the seventeenth century with the wisdom of the ancients who tended the sick. Perhaps his prejudice against medicine and doctors was due to his belief that the death of his only son was due to antimony prescribed by the physicians.

A professor at Cambridge would earn 40 pounds per annum; a popular but not necessarily wise physician would earn up to 250 pounds yearly. The most coveted post was that of a court physician who would be handsomely rewarded if a king, prince or noble was cured of an illness. More often than not, the cure was not because of the court physician but in spite of him!

The treatment for all patients with any disease remained the same; the patient was either starved, purged or bled through venesection. Blood-letting was used for almost every ailment—it was often done repeatedly, with disastrous consequences particularly when it was combined with purging and starving. Treatment therefore was inadvertently designed to help departure from the world rather than to promote healing and care. The old tenets of Ayurveda and of Hippocrates to help nature and not thwart it were safely buried within the rubbish that passed for truth.

The Pharmacopoeia

The Baroque physician did use drugs for his patients—almost every one was an unmitigated poison. It was popularity and not efficacy judged by reason or science that determined its use. Antimony, for example, was the most popular drug in use in the seventeenth century. This metal was known to Paracelsus as stibium, but its popularity soared after the publication of a book titled *The Triumphant Chariot of Antimony* (1604) by an alchemist Johann Tholde. Tholde observed that pigs fed with antimony flourished and grew fat. He therefore tried antimony on a group of emaciated monks, and all of them died! This stirred a controversy over the use of the drug—a controversy which was unfortunately settled in favour of the drug when Louis XIV of France developed typhus fever. He was given antimony as treatment and he survived. It is indeed amazing that the thought did not occur that he could have survived without antimony; in fact he survived in spite of antimony! But the outcome of the illness of Louis XIV dictated treatment in medicine. The use of antimony flourished in the Western world and was almost certainly responsible for the premature demise of many patients.

One of the few useful drugs in the pharmacopoeia of the age was quinine, but again it suffered from indiscriminate overuse. The discovery and use of quinine in Western civilization is interesting. A Jesuit missionary priest in Peru, South America, had been cured of malaria by a concoction administered by an Inca medicine man. The medicine man would not reveal the ingredients or the source of his medicine. The Jesuit, determined to find this for himself and after a great deal of search, discovered that the medicine came from the cinchona bark. Quinine was introduced in Europe in 1632 under the name of Jesuit bark. The Jesuits held the monopoly for the export and supply of quinine to Europe, thereby earning a great deal of money. Quinine is an example of a useful drug discovered for a disease (malaria) about which nothing was known in that era. The apothecaries thrived on its use for all illnesses and of course both doctors, alchemists and apothecaries were ignorant of its side-effects. The drug was often dispensed in fanciful ways. Robert Talbot (an apothecary's apprentice) became famous and rich by dispensing quinine mixed with rose petals, lemon juice and water. His services were asked for at Versailles in France where he is reported to have cured the king and the dukes of Burgundy and Anjou. Remarkably enough, quinine, besides its excellent efficacy in malaria, served fortuitously and by accident one other purpose. It struck one more nail in the coffin of Galenism. Galenic doctrines dictated that effective treatment of most diseases was purgation, which expelled toxic material. While they argued that the success of mercury in syphilis was related to both salivation and purgation which expelled syphilitic toxins, no such argument could be offered in relation to the use of quinine.

Besides quinine, only two main drugs were of use in medicine. The fox glove plant (*digitalis purpurea*), which was effective in dropsy due to heart failure, and opium which was a sedative and analgesic and which could offer significant relief from pain and suffering. However, there were numerous poisons in use which passed for drugs. Some of these drugs were said to possess magical properties—a throwback to prehistoric times and archaic civilizations. Crushed worms, lozenges from crushed vipers, crabs' eyes, moss from the skull of a victim who had suffered violent death, are some examples of these useless and dangerous remedies. Some of these drugs were priced exorbitantly and those dispensing them made huge fortunes. A good example was the prescription of Scott's pill which was a purgative made of aloes, jalap, gamboge and anise. It was introduced in 1635 and continued to be dispensed and used till the end of the seventeenth century. Another example of an exorbitantly priced concoction was Goddard's drops, prescribed by no less than Sydenham. It was said to be made from raw silk and was bought by Charles II for over 5000 pounds!

Syndenham—the English Hippocrates

Great minds of the era were engaged in the unravelling of the secrets of natural sciences, or were thinkers indulging in abstract philosophy. Physicians influenced by the experimentation and observations in natural science grouped themselves as iatrophysicists and iatrochemists, explaining health and disease either through mechanistic physical laws or through chemistry and chemical processes. The iatrophysicists and iatrochemists had no concern for the care and treatment of patients. Little did they realize that many of their postulates were figments of imagination and fancy with little or no truth in them. Similarly, physician thinkers were busy philosophizing and physician scientists remained engrossed in experimental observations and in the formulation of hypothesis. Clinical medicine, which in essence is the care of the sick thus stood sadly neglected in the hands of mediocrities and quacks. However, there stood out one man in this century, who was a great clinician, who learnt and practised medicine at the patient's bedside and who championed the cause and practice of clinical medicine. He was Thomas Sydenham (1624–1659); he was rightly called the English Hippocrates, because he practised medicine in accordance with the principles laid down by Hippocrates.

Sydenham was born in Dorset in 1624, and belonged to a Puritan family. He studied at Oxford and Montepellier and then joined the parliamentary army as a soldier in the civil war. He later went on to study medicine at Cambridge and received his doctorate in a year's study. He soon became a Fellow at the All Souls College and commanded sufficient authority to espouse the cause and practice of Hippocratic medicine. After some years he went to London where he had a lucrative practice.

Sydenham remained totally aloof from the raging controversies of the age. He believed neither in the iatrophysicists nor in the iatrochemists. He ignored the teachings of Galen yet did not join forces with the anti-Galenists. He did not wax eloquent over Vesalius nor did he show undue interest in Harvey's great discovery of the circulation. In a way, he was strangely nihilistic yet was obviously influenced by both Descartes and Bacon, for he believed in what he observed directly from his patients, and he applied the method of inductive logic propounded by Bacon for the study of natural sciences to the bedside study of medicine. His favourite author was Cervantes and he once remarked to a friend that he could well learn medicine by reading Cervantes' *Don Quixote*. His practical and Hippocratic attitude to medicine is illustrated by the following incident. He was visited by a man sent to him with a letter of introduction from a close friend. The letter of introduction stated that his visitor was a good scholar, a first rate botanist and a fair anatomist. Sydenham remain unimpressed with these attainments and remarked that the women in Covent Garden knew more botany, his butcher more anatomy; he advised his visitor to go to the bedside and learn from his patients.

His views on disease were simple and easily understood. He believed that the cause of disease was extraneous to the organism and resided in nature, and that nature had the inherent propensity to heal. He thus shared the Hippocratic faith in the healing power of nature. He was a keen observer at the bedside and followed meticulously the natural history of disease. He gave lucid descriptions of smallpox, rheumatic fever, scarlet fever, dysentery, pneumonia, malaria and St Vitus' dance (Sydenham's chorea). He left a classic description of gout from which he himself suffered.

His therapy consisted of diet, fresh air, horse riding for tuberculosis, iron for chlorosis, and opiate in the form of Sydenham's drops which were particularly useful for heart failure. He faithfully avoided the poisons that passed as drugs in the prevailing pharmacopoeia, but was among the first to recognize the therapeutic value of quinine.

Sydenham was a good teacher—his teaching was chiefly by example. One of his pupils was Walter Harris (1647–1732), physician to Charles II. Harris authored one of the first books on children's diseases.

Mention must be made of a few other clinicians in other parts of Europe. They were not as great as Sydenham but were cast in the same mould. De Le Boe (the iatrochemist) has been already referred to earlier (pp. 195)—he was a famous teacher of clinical medicine in Leyden and Giorgio Baglive taught medicine in Rome. Giovanna Larcese (1654–1711) was an Italian clinician who was considered a pioneer in public health especially with his suggestion of reclaiming marsh lands. He advised an extended course of study for medical students and advocated that they become familiar with the use of the thermometer and the microscope.

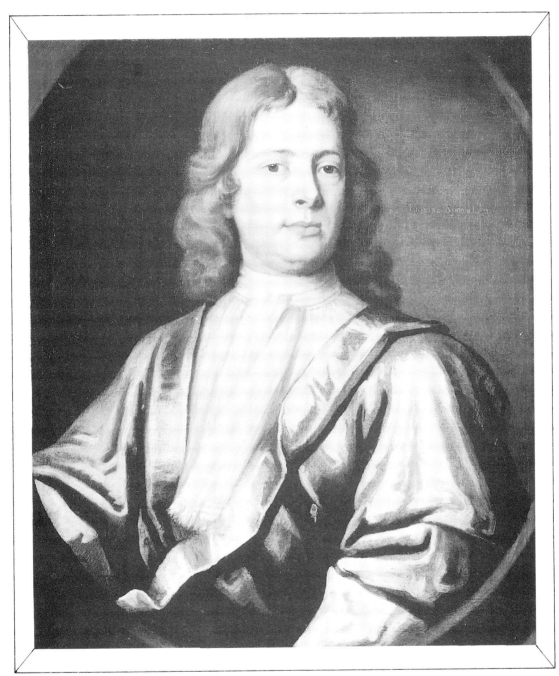

Fig. 32.1   Portrait of Thomas Sydenham.

An entirely new school of legal medicine was pioneered by Italy's Fortunato Fedele, who discussed in his work the jurisprudence of poisoning, of lethal wounds and the attestation of virginity.

Bernardino Ramazzini (1633–1714) pioneered the science of occupational diseases. He described mercury poisoning, lead poisoning in children, antimony poisoning and silicosis in stone masons and in miners working in mines.

The Founding of Scientific Associations

The Baroque period saw the establishment of scientific associations which increased the perception of scientists and physicians through meetings and publications. The first association was the Accademia dei Lincei founded in Rome in 1603. Cardinal Richelieu created the French Academy in 1630. The Accademia del Cimento (Academy of Experiment) was established by Prince Leopold in 1637 for the purpose of promoting natural sciences. The Royal Society of Medicine was founded in 1662 and Leibnitz persuaded Frederick I to found the Berlin Academy of Sciences in 1700.

Medical publications also started in the seventeenth century. They appeared in the *Philosophical Transactions of the Royal Society*, in the *Journal de Sçavans* in France and the *Giornale dei Letterati* in Venice. Interestingly enough, the first political newspaper in the western world was the *Gazette de France*, founded in 1631 by a doctor Theophraste Renaudot. The first medical review titled *Journal des nouvelles decouvertes sur toutes les parties de la medicine* was started in 1679.

33 Surgery

Surgery was even further in the backwoods as compared to medicine. The brilliant new exposition of anatomical facts by Vesalius in the sixteenth century was not made use of by the surgeons in the practice of their craft. Whereas physicians went to universities, were often versatile in natural sciences or in philosophy and had a high social standing, surgeons in this era were an uneducated, underprivileged class akin to the barbers and ranked very low on the social ladder.

In England, the company of Barber Surgeons was inaugurated in 1540. The barber surgeons were permitted dissection in their own hall and nowhere else. In France surgeons had a higher standing and at times assumed the pomposity and attire of the physician but he was still an inferior individual. Guy Paten (1601–1672) the dean of the medical faculty in Paris was scornful of his pompous upstart surgical colleagues: "Mere booted lackeys—a race of extravagant coxcombs who wear moustaches and flourish razors."

An unusual event in Paris in 1686 however served to boost and favour the standing of surgeons in France to a significant extent. This was the surgical cure of the anal fistula of Louis XIV by the surgeon Felix. What the great Ambroise Paré could not achieve in the earlier century with all his brilliance, dedication and work was amazingly enough achieved by the surgical cure of the lower end of a powerful king! Surgeon Felix was rewarded with an estate, a fee of 3,00,000 livres, three times that paid to the royal physician.

Surgical operations generally led to death from agonizing pain, shock, blood loss or infection. The most fashionable operation was lithotomy. Blood transfusion was first described by a Padua professor Giovanni Colle. Jean Baptiste Denis, the French court physician transfused blood from a lamb to a patient exsanguinated by repeated blood-letting in 1666. The patient first improved but then died. The Paris Faculty of Medicine and a Papal Bull subsequently banned transfusion.

An outstanding German surgeon of this era was Wilhelm Fabry, the designer of the stick twisted tourniquet. England produced a famous surgeon—Richard Wiseman (1622–1684). He wrote his *Several Chirurgical Treatises* in 1676; the book dealt with scrofula, ulcers, tumours, anal disorders, fractures, dislocations and gunshot wounds.

Obstetrics

The seventeenth century saw the introduction of the forceps by the Chamberlain family. In 1647 Pierre Chamberlain designed a pair of curved forceps to assist delivery in difficult labour. The invention was kept a great secret within the family and the instrument helped the Chamberlain family to amass a great fortune through a lucrative and highly successful practice. Hugh Chamberlain decided to sell the secret in Paris, but unfortunately its use on a patient resulted in death from a bleeding uterine laceration. He later successfully introduced the forceps in Holland, but it was several years before the forceps was accepted for general use.

Francois Mauriceau (1637–1709) was French, practised in Paris and was the greatest obstetrician of his age. He wrote a treatise on the female pelvis, a standard work translated into several languages well into the eighteenth century.

Public Health and Diseases in the Seventeenth Century

There were two major reasons for the prevalence and spread of disease in this century—poor or absent sewage disposal with no appreciation and awareness of public hygiene and the frequent wars which brought starvation and disease in their wake.

Public sewage disposal services were nonexistent. Sewage was meant to be disposed off by individual communities and often contaminated water supply causing epidemics of water-borne diseases. Wars swept over Europe again and again spreading death, disease and destruction. For the first time in history armies grew to an enormous size consisting of brutal mercenaries who raped and

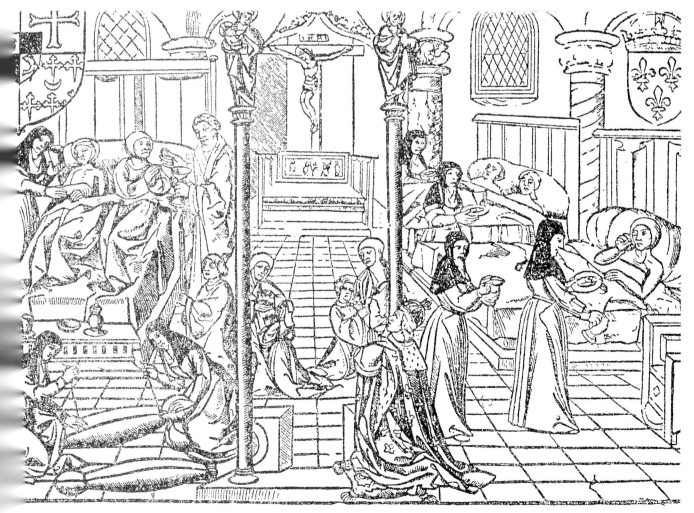

Fig. 34.1   The Hôtel Dieu Paris: Interior showing patients being nursed by monks.

pillaged the countryside with impunity. In between conflicts, groups of disbanded brigands often terrorized parts of Europe. Epidemics of various diseases at some time or the other were an established feature of the Baroque era.

Typhoid, typhus and dysentery were at their peak during the 30 year war in Germany and France and in the Low countries. These diseases surfaced again as epidemics towards the end of the century. Small-pox was all-prevalent—a violent epidemic ravaged Eastern Europe and struck England around 1650. Smallpox crossed the ocean when the colonists settled in America and the disease took root in that continent as well. Laryngeal diphtheria was epidemic in Spain, and, about the middle of the century, spread to Europe. Scurvy was common in Germany, Northern Europe and the Scandinavian countries. Malaria was endemic in Europe particularly in Italy at the start of the century. This was related to the presence of vast tracts of undrained marsh lands. In Italy 40,000 deaths were related to malaria alone. The disease recurred in England in the middle of the seventeenth century. Syphilis however had ceased to exist in an epidemic form in this century, and leprosy too was on the wane, so that lazar houses in France were converted to charity hospitals.

The most devastating epidemics of disease however, were the outbreaks of bubonic plague—the Black Death. They were as horrific as the epidemics of the fourteenth century. Plague decimated more than half of the population of Lyons in France. Over a million deaths occurred in Northern Italy; 5,00,000 died of it in Venice. The decline of Renaissance cities of Northern Italy in this century, particularly of Venice, was significantly related to the ravages of plague. From France and Italy plague spread to Germany and the Low countries, invaded Eastern Europe around the middle of the century and reached a ghastly peak in London, in 1665, killing more than 75,000 people.

Doctors were of no use in these epidemics. The plague doctor was masked, gowned, gloved and wore high heels. His mask was provided with a long beak in which was filled an antiseptic solution for his protection. He carried a long cane and made pretence to feel the pulse by touching the tip of his cane to the radial artery.

Public health was pioneered by Italian physicians—notably by the Roman clinician Giovanni Maria Larcisi (1654–1720). He thought undrained marsh lands in Italy were important causes of epidemic disease and strongly advocated drainage of these lands as an important method in prevention of disease.

35 William Harvey and the Discovery of Circulation

The discovery of circulation by William Harvey (1578–1657) will rank as one of the greatest discoveries in science and medicine. Harvey was the most brilliant star in the Baroque century. His epoch-making work outshone every discovery of the past and formed the foundation on which many subsequent discoveries in medicine were made.

Harvey was the son of an alderman in the English fishing port of Folkestone. He studied humanities at Cambridge and went on to study medicine at Padua—a centre of learning to which flocked the rich and poor from all corners of Europe. In Padua he was the student of Fabrizio D'Acquapendente. He and his fellow students seated within the tiered lecture hall of this university must have heard and seen with breathless admiration Professor D'Acquapendente lecture on anatomy and demonstrate anatomical facts through dissection. Fabrizio D'Acquapendente was the first to describe valves within the venous system and this was of great interest to his pupil William Harvey.

The scientific temper of Harvey must surely have developed in this university, which was famous for its free thinkers, its great teachers and the renowned scholars engaged in unravelling the secrets of nature. The great Galileo was also working and teaching at Padua in this era. Harvey was acquainted with his work—perhaps he peered at the heavenly bodies through the telescope devised by Galileo and acquired an interest in their motion and in the principles underlying motion and movement. Significantly, the study of movement and motion (e.g., of falling bodies, of planets, of the pendulum) was all-consuming in this era. Even though Harvey was a physician, the impact of the above studies in natural sciences may well have had a conscious or subconscious effect on his resolve to study the motion or movement of blood in the human circulation.

On his return to London in 1602, he married the daughter of Lancelot Browne, physician to Queen Elizabeth I and James I and joined the staff of St Bartholomew's hospital as reader in anatomy and surgery. He spent almost all his time in research and investigations on the vascular system and announced his discovery of circulation in 1616. His classic work *Exercitatio anatomica de motu cordis et sanguinis in animalibus* was published 12 years later in Frankfurt in which he described circulation, as we know it today.

The stupendous magnitude and significance of this discovery can only be understood if one contrasts Harvey's concept of the circulation with that prevailing in the early seventeenth century. The old Galenic concept taught that venous and arterial blood were two distinct types of blood with different pathways and different functions relating to three major organ centres within the body—the liver which was responsible for growth and nourishment, the heart controlling vitality, the brain responsible for reason and sensations. The venous blood originated in the liver, and was disributed to all parts of the body through venous channels; it was used up and mediated growth and nourishment. The arterial blood contained blood plus *pneuma* (air) due to an intrinsic 'pulsatile faculty' within the arterial system. Galen explained the composition of arterial blood (venous blood

+ air) in the left ventricle by postulating invisible pores in the interventricular septum through which venous blood reached the left ventricle. He explained the presence of air in this blood by postulating that air was conveyed to the left ventricle from the lungs via the pulmonary vein. The latter also served as a channel through which sooty vapours formed by the mixing of blood with air in the left ventricle travelled back to the lungs and were exhaled. Galen had no concept of the pulmonary circulation and his doctrine was therefore theoretical, lacking both in observation and experimentation. However bizzare his concept may appear to us, it afforded a plausible explanation in that day and age.

Harvey's concept of the circulation was revolutionary when compared to the then prevailing concept. He postulated and proved through experiment and observation that the blood was expelled out by the left ventricle through the aorta and was distributed by the arterial system to all parts of the body; it then became venous and was carried by the veins to the right atrium and from there to the right ventricle. It was now propelled by the right ventricle, through the pulmonary artery and its branches, into the lungs where it was

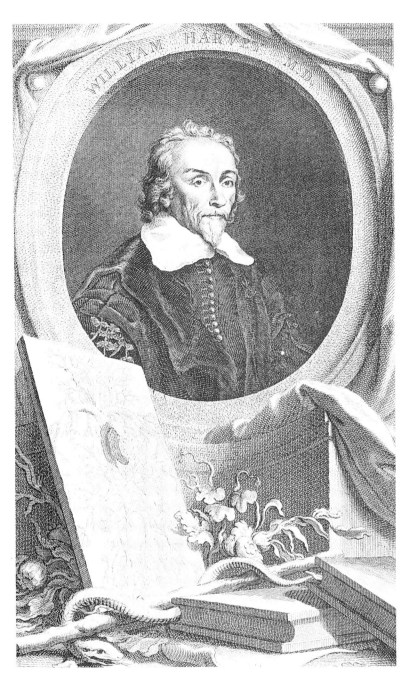

Fig. 35.1   Portrait of William Harvey.

transformed into arterial blood. After passing through the pulmonary veins, it entered the left atrium and then returned to the left ventricle. The blood was therefore in constant motion, in continuous circulation.

Like all great discoverers Harvey had his precursors. The Galenic doctrine that the left ventricle contained air or blood mixed with air, which reached it from the right ventricle through the invisible pores in the septum had been refuted by both Leonardo and Vesalius. Michael Servetus, a Spanish theologian and physician had postulated the existence of the pulmonary circulation and denied the porosity of the septum. Realdo Cremona (1516–1559) of Cremona who succeeded Vesalius to the

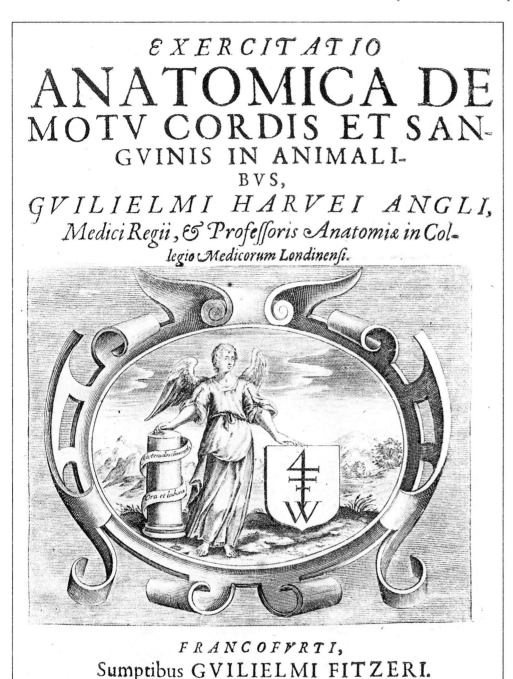

Fig. 35.2   William Harvey: Exercitatio anatomica de motu cordis et sanguinis in animalibus.

chair of anatomy also denied the permeability of the septal wall. Andrea Cesalpino of Arezzo (1524–1603) botanist and physician discovered sex in plants and gave a correct concept of the circulation in the human body. His concepts were embodied in his work *Des Plantes* published in 1583. His house in Arezzo bears a plaque—'here lived Andrea Cesalpino, discoverer of the circulation of the blood and the first author of the classification of plants'.

Harvey crystallized earlier ideas into a definite hypothesis proven by numerous observations and experiments which were lacking in the postulates of earlier workers. The principles of research in natural sciences followed by Galileo, Newton, Keppler were, for the first time, applied with astounding

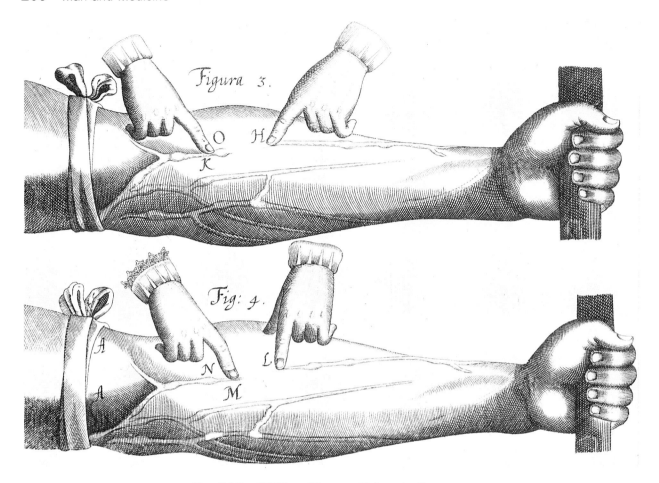

Fig. 35.3   William Harvey: Valves in forearm.

results to medicine. Harvey experimented on over 80 animals to measure the rate of blood flow. He calculated the blood flow to be 8640 oz/hour—a quantum that could not be replenished by food or by tissues hour by hour. He thus deduced that blood flowed continuously in a circle through the heart to the arteries, to the veins and back to the heart. Keppler, Galileo and Newton studied with mathematical precision the movements of falling bodies on earth and of heavenly bodies in space. Harvey studied the movement of blood in the human body, showed that it moved in a circle and used mathematical calculations to deduce this result. Harvey did not rest' his theory of circulation solely on the mensurations stated above. He performed scores of animal experiments using cannulation, ligation and perfusion. He announced his discovery in the Lumelian lecture of 1616 delivered from notes in English and Latin, stating that the heart was a force pump that drove the blood in constant circulation through the vessels. It contracted when it emptied and forced blood into the vessels, and dilated when it filled on receiving blood from the veins. His epoch-making book on circulation *Exercitatio anatomica de motu cordis et sanguinis in animalibus* was published rather shoddily in Frankfurt, years later. It immediately divided the medical world into two hostile camps.

The most violent opposition to Harvey's view on the circulation was from the medical faculty in Paris. Jean Riolan of Paris declared that if dissection had proved Galen wrong, it was because nature had over the centuries changed. Guy Paten, Dean of the Paris faculty of Medicine dubbed Harvey's theory as 'paradoxical, useless, false, impossible, absurd, harmful'. Harvey was stoutly defended by numerous physicians from England, Germany, France and Holland, many of whom proved his experiments correct. One of his great defenders was Descartes who in his treatise in physiology in AD 1662, stated that blood in the body was in a state of perpetual circulation. In fact, he felt that Harvey's concept of circulation of blood supported his mechanistic philosophy. Descartes, however, differed from Harvey in his explanation of the significance of the action of the heart. He believed (and he was of course in error) that the chief activity of the heart was in diastole, when its innate heat rarefied and expanded drops of blood within its chambers forcing these into the arteries. These very small drops of blood became animal spirits, which, on reaching the brain, nerves and muscles induced perception and motion. The heart was thus akin to an engine imparting motion to the body.

Harvey's other great original work was in embryology. His book *Exercitationes de generatione animalium* was published 8 years after his death. Harvey postulated very correctly the theory of epigenesis stating that all living beings develop from an egg: *omne vivum ex ovo*. Thus the organism does not exist as a preformed entity within the ovum but develops gradually with the building up of various tissues and organ systems. Harvey postulated this concept without the use of a microscope and was proved correct by Von Baer who had the advantage of its use.

Harvey rose to be the royal physician to the Stuart kings James I and Charles I. He kept aloof from all political and religious controversies, but sided with the Royalists during the civil wars. His house during the civil war was sacked by a violent mob, with the loss of valuable scientific notes. After the execution of Charles I, Harvey returned to his brother's country house where he died in 1675. His books and possessions were donated to the Royal College of Physicians to fund a library and to establish an annual Harverian oration in his honour.

The only lacuna in Harvey's postulate of the circulation was the link between the arterial and venous systems. Though he could not prove the presence of this link directly through observation, he concluded from simple ligation experiments on the forearm that such a link must exist. He also proved, by similar experiments, that the function of the venous valves was to direct blood always towards the heart. The direct proof of a link between the arterial and venous circulation was provided by the discovery of capillaries by Marcello Malphigi in 1661. The circle postulated by Harvey in the movement or motion of blood was now complete.

Finally a mention should be made of discovery of the lymphatic system. Gaspare Aselli (1581–1626) discovered lymphatic vessels which he called *venae albae et lacteae*. The Frenchman Jean Pecquet (1622–1674) discovered the thoracic duct, and Swede Olav Rudbeck (1630–1702) discovered intestinal lymphatics and their connection to the thoracic duct.

One of the most brilliant of Harvey's pupils was Francis Glisson (1597–1677) who studied the anatomy and physiology of the liver. His name is commemorated in Glisson's capsule, the fibrous capsule of the liver. Glisson also researched on rickets, and published his *De rachitide* in 1650.

36 The Microscope

The study of natural sciences in the seventeenth century through experiment and observation, brought in its wake the invention of instruments. Man had an urge to multiply the power of his vision so that he could unveil the secrets of nature. Galileo developed the astronomical telescope and brought the large far-distant heavenly bodies closer to the eye. The microscope enabled the scientist to magnify objects invisible to the naked eye. In all probability, the microscope was invented in 1590 by Johannes and Zacharius Jansen of Middleburg in Holland. The instrument was significantly modified for the better by Van Leeuwenhock who has been erroneously described as its inventor. The advent of the microscope was an important milestone; it marked a rapid progress in the natural sciences and medicine.

Perhaps the microscopist who contributed the most to medicine in this era was Marcello Malphigi (1628–1694)—a brilliant physician and scientist who contributed not only to the study of man but also to the study of animals and plants. Malphigi took his medical degree in Bologna, taught at the university of Pisa. He learnt mathematics and physics from Giovanni Alfonso Borelli to whom in exchange, he taught anatomy. After these years in Pisa he returned to Bologna where he made extensive observations and studies through the microscope. In 1661, Malphigi solved the only lacuna in Harvey's theory of circulation by the observation through a microscope of blood flowing through capillaries. The capillaries linked the arterial with the venous system.

> I saw the blood flowing in minute streams through the arteries, in the manner of a flood, and I might have believed that the blood itself escaped into an empty space and was collected up again by a gaping vessel; but an objection to the view was afforded by the movement of the blood being tortuous and scattered in different directions and by its being united again in a definite path. My doubt was changed to certainty by the dried lung of a frog, which to a marked degree had preserved the redness of the blood in very tiny tracts, which were afterwards found to be vessels, where by the help of a glass I saw not scattered points but vessels joined together in a ring like fashion. And such is the wandering of these vessels as they passed from the vein on this side and the artery on the other that they do not keep a straight path but appear to form in a network joining two vessels. Thus it was clear that the blood flowed along sinuous vessels and did not empty into spaces but was always contained within vessels the paths of which produced its dispersion.

Malphigi made several other brilliant discoveries. He studied the microscopic anatomy of the skin, spleen, kidney and of the alveoli of the lung. His findings such as the Malphigian bodies in the spleen and Malphigian layers of the skin, commemorate and honour his name. He was the first to observe red blood cells in the capillaries and also discovered the papillae of the tongue and intestinal glands.

Like other pioneers in the medical and scientific fields of this era, Malphigi was ridiculed by his conservative colleagues at the university of Bologna and even assaulted for teaching and propagating outrageous concepts in anatomy. It is fascinating to observe that even in the seventeenth century—the golden age of science—academicians in some universities refused to accept concepts proven by experimental study and observation. Malpighi ultimately prevailed, his findings were accepted outside Italy and he was invited to the Fellowship of the prestigious Royal Society of London.

One of the foremost pupils of Malpighi was Antonio Valsalva (1666–1723), who in turn was the teacher of the great Morgagni. Through numerous brilliant dissections Valsalva laid bare the detailed anatomy of the ear—the middle ear, the ossicles and the semicircular canals.

Another brilliant baroque microscopist was a Jesuit priest Anthanasius Kircher (1602–1680). He was also a mathematician, orientalist and a musician. He was probably the first to use the microscope to investigate the causes of disease. He postulated that contagious disease in an organism was caused by minute living creatures, which could pass into a healthy organism and reproduce the disease. This was the doctrine of *contagium animatum* in infection.

Jan Swammerdam (1637–1682) was a brilliant physiologist and microscopist. He was the first to describe red blood corpuscles and to identify valves in the lymphatic system. He used plethysmographic methods to study the movements of the heart, lungs and muscles.

A great deal of the work of microscopists was only possible because of the contribution to science made by an amateur who had no formal education, but who was brilliant in innovation and invention and who was imbued by an unquenchable curiosity to search for the truth. He was Anton van Leeuwenhoek, a draper born in Delft (1612–1723). He never left his native city, never visited a university and knew no language other than Dutch. He first used the lens in his business to count the threads of fabric. He ground his own lenses and mounted these between metal plates. He personally made over 400 microscopes improving the instrument so that he ultimately achieved a magnification up to 200 times. He spent hours at the microscope looking down at various animate and inanimate material. In 1676, he saw ciliate organisms under the microscope and sowed the seeds of microbiology. He wrote amusingly that he saw under his microscope graceful little animals more numerous than all the inhabitants of the Low Countries, when he examined a bit of food found between his teeth. Thus a humble uneducated draper for the first time showed that the ecological environment of man also included extremely small animate organisms invisible to the naked eye.

Van Leeuwenhoek through his microscope discovered a fantastic world of protozoa, bacteria of various kinds, which for another 150 years were termed infusoria. He was also the first to discover spermatozoa, striped voluntary muscle and the crystalline lens; he also confirmed the presence of capillaries and capillary circulation discovered by Malpighi, by microscopically observing these in the tail of a tadpole. The world indeed owes a great debt to this humble amateur who was blessed with honesty, integrity and a thirst for true scientific inquiry.

Regnier de Graaf (1641–1673) was a contemporary of van Leeuwenhoek. He studied the microscopic anatomy of the female reproductive system in mammals and about the same time as the Dane. Neils Stensen (1638–86), described the Graafian follicle—a vesicle housing the unfertilized egg on the surface of the ovary. He termed the female gonad the ovary, and contended that the ovum played a key role in reproduction. This led to fierce controversy against the 'ovist school' of thought. The 'animalculist school' contended that the spermatozoa discovered by Leeuwenhoek were the key to conception. Some workers claimed to have discovered a miniature organism within the unfertilized ovum, and others claimed a similar discovery within spermatozoan cells in the semen. Thus arose the 'preformation theory' that the new unborn individual was fully developed within this tiny homunculus at the very moment of conception. The preformation theory ran counter to Harvey's more realistic view on the development of the embryo as has been explained earlier.

The Baroque age drew to a close spilling over imperceptibly into the age of Enlightenment (18th century). It had left a rich heritage in science, art, architecture. The work of its thinkers, scientists,

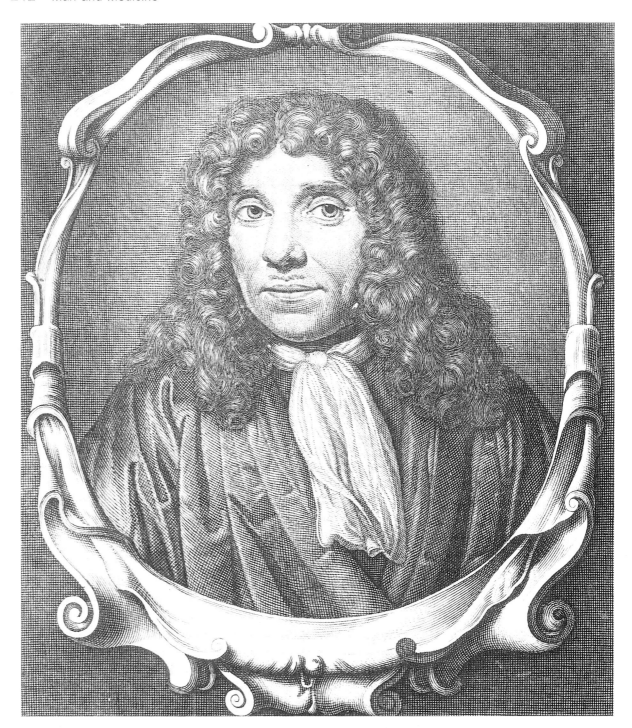

Fig. 36.1   Portrait of Antonius van Leeuwenhoek.

mathematicians, physicians had sown the seeds of great discoveries that were to be made in medicine and the natural sciences in the next two hundred years. The Baroque period also sowed the seeds of medicine in America for it was in this era that the Mayflower pilgrims embarked for the New World. More than half these pilgrims died within a few months of their arrival chiefly because of a hostile environment and the ravages of disease such as typhus and smallpox. The struggle to survive was certainly a factor in establishing medicine in the New World. It must however be conquistadors in South America. The conquistadors conferred in Peru the first degree in the New World of Doctor of Medicine. The first chair in medicine in the New World was founded in Mexico and the first textbook in medicine in the New World was also published in Mexico.

The growth of medicine in America had one great advantage. It was unfettered, unhindered and unconditioned by the doctrines and dogmas of the past. It built anew, ignoring the past but assimilating what was currently known. It was uncluttered and had ample room for fresh thoughts and new discoveries which were pursued with great fervour and vigour. America was rich in natural resources and it grew richer with the years, so that in the centuries to come when science and medicine required to be funded, the country was rich and powerful enough to do so with a lavishness that could not be easily matched by the rest of the world.

Medicine in the Age of Enlightenment and Reason— Eighteenth Century

Historical Canvas of the Age of Reason

Medicine is a science of uncertainty and an art of probability.

Sir William Osler

The eighteenth century witnessed an age of enlightenment, of reason, of intellectual ferment. The western world glowed with the light shed by the new thoughts and new ideas of the great thinkers of this age who were keen to reshape the world to their heart's desire, in the quest for man's happiness. They were supremely optimistic in their utopian search for a perfect society, for perfect governance and a perfect state—alas a search unfulfilled and utopian to this day. Reason reigned supreme, science was deified, and an attempt was made to apply the immutable physical laws of nature to politics, philosophy and economics. Gifted men contributed to physics, chemistry, biology and the natural sciences—contributions which indirectly helped the progress of medicine.

The age of enlightenment and reason was not free from political conflicts and wars. These chiefly revolved around dynastic rivalries and colonial aspirations of powerful kingdom states, such as France, England, Austria and Prussia. The Ottoman Empire was crumbling but the power of Russia was on the rise and under Peter I and Catherine II, this country exerted an increasing influence on the map of Europe. The balance of power between kingdom states was maintained as in the previous century through force of arms, intrigue and a Machiavellian diplomacy that was devoid of even a shred of honesty and integrity.

The political system operating during the greater part of the eighteenth century was that of absolute rule based on the divine right of kings. No regime ruled with greater absolutism than the Bourbons of France. The kings and the aristocracy of France became increasingly divorced from and unconcerned with the degradation and poverty of peasants and the bourgeois working class. Yet France was the centre of the enlightenment; its thinkers and philosophers championed the rights of man, urged a philosophy of politics that hoped to remove the prevailing inequality so that it could be universally acceptable to all states. The ordinary people of France avidly absorbed this message, and resolved to act upon it. Rumblings of discontent, often subterranean and sometimes overt, were ignored by the king and the state. In 1789, the pent-up discontent and anger of the people of France burst forth in a torrent of rage and violence, into a bloody revolution. On 14 July 1789 the people of Paris barricaded the streets, stormed the Bastille—a castle prison that was the symbol of the absolutism of the Bourbons. The streets of Paris ran blood. Louis XVI the reigning monarch, Marie Antoinette the queen, and the young dauphin—heir to the throne were done to death. A number of physicians were involved in the revolution, including Jean-Paul Marat, a rabid revolutionary, and Dr Joseph-Ignace Guillotin, who with Dr Louis, invented the guillotine—a huge razor sharp blade that became the symbol of terror that the revolution had unleashed. Republican France sent a tremor of fear and outrage in the other kingdom states of Europe. The fear was justified. The ideas underlying the revolution spread slowly and surely all over Europe so that in the decades to come the monarchs of the ancient regimes tumbled from their thrones one after the other.

Architecture, Literature and Art

The style in architecture was rococco, which combined classical lines with subdued ornamentation. The Pantheon in Paris and the Royal Palace in Madrid are examples of eighteenth century architecture. In England architecture developed the elegant lines and proportions of the Georgian style which also prevailed in the American colonies. Landscaped gardens were a passion, particularly in France; terraced gardens with clipped yew hedges were ornamented by playing fountains, grottoes and colourful lights.

A subdued elegance in dress and furnishings was observed in this century. Furniture was in the rococco style designed and fashioned by expert craftsmen. Craftsmanship in the designing and making of jewellery and in the making of clocks and watches rose to great heights. Porcelain factories of Dresden, Sèvres and Wedgwood produced the most delicate and beautiful porcelain ware the West had ever seen.

Literature, art and music in the first half of the century were influenced by classicism, and later by romanticism. The reading public had by now increased considerably all over Europe and the power of the pen was being increasingly realized. Romanticism in literature was ushered in the middle of the eighteenth century by Jean Jacques Rousseau with his idealized portrayal of the 'noble savage.' Rousseau stressed the importance of feeling and emotion in life—that it was the heart that mattered even more than the intellect. In 1774, Johann Wolfgang Von Goethe published the *Sorrows of Young Werther,* an autobiographic novel of his unhappy love for Charlotte Buff. Goethe was a many-splendoured personality, a true Renaissance man and a friend of the German poet and dramatist Friedrich Schiller. His drama titled *Faust* was published in the early nineteenth century and ranks as among the greatest in world literature.

Art flourished, particularly under royal patronage. Boucher extolled the beauty of the female form; Fragonard and Watteau depicted the gaiety and elegance of the court. Yet there were others who painted life as it was. William Hogarth and Francisco Goya were amongst these brilliant artists whose palettes depicted vagabonds, crowds and the ugliness of the society they lived in. The end of the century witnessed the return of art to the classicism of David, who was an artist of the Revolution and of the Napoleonic era.

Music rose to celestial heights in the works of Wolfgang Amadeus Mozart, a child prodigy born in Salzburg in 1756. Music was polyphonic, with perfect tonal balance and possessed the fineness, beauty and elegance that could be likened to gossamer silk.

Philosophers and Thinkers

This age of enlightenment or age of reason should also aptly be termed the age of philosophers and thinkers, for it was they who shed the light of new ideas that shaped momentous events in this era. Philosophy was no longer abstruse, intellectual, theoretical to be understood only by the elite, nor did it merely deify reason and promote scientific inquiry. For once it carried a strong social message.

Jean Jacques Rousseau (1712–78), who was a great thinker and a political theorist, in his revolutionary booklet *Social Contract* wrote: "Man is born free but he is everywhere in chains."

Philosophers wrote on the inequities and wrongs perpetrated on man by his fellowmen and the state. They discussed the relation of a ruling state with its subjects, championed the basic human rights of man to liberty and equality. Their writings influenced all aspects of living—art, literature, science and medicine. Above all, the social message conveyed either directly or palpably evident between the lines, fuelled an ideology that heralded the French Revolution, shattering the political framework of France and sending tremors of impending change all through Western civilization. These challenging ideas and thoughts were not confined to Europe; they spread far and wide, lending support to the American people in their war of American Independence (1775–83), which culminated in the founding of the United States of America in 1783.

A monumental literary event of the eighteenth century was the compilation of the *Encyclopaedia* (28 volumes) in France under the editorship of the thinker and philosopher Denis Diderot, whose objective was to bring philosophy to the people. *"Hâtons-nous de rendre notre philosophie populaire,"* said Diderot. The *Encyclopaedia* was epoch-making. It contained, in alphabetical order, and classification the sum and substance of all that the eighteenth century man knew in every sphere of thought, learning, inquiry and activity. Some of the greatest and most fertile minds in France took it upon themselves to steer this work to completion. Baron de Montesquieu whose work *L'Esprit des Lois* influenced the ideology behind the French Revolution; Jean Le Rond D'Alembert who in the preamble expressed his thoughts on the laws of nature; Francois-Marie Aronet (Voltaire), who with his barbed wit spread new ideas all over Europe. The *Encyclopaedia* had an enormous influence. It democratized knowledge and stimulated the growth of a cultured bourgeoisie fostering debate and exchange of ideas not only in formal scientific and academic meetings but also in popular cafés often patronized by learned and literary people of this age.

Scientists

This age did not produce a Newton or a Keppler or a Gallileo but it did produce a number of individuals who contributed to the natural sciences.

The leading astronomers of the age were Sir William Herschel (1738–1822) who discovered the planet Uranus, and Edmond Halley who not only discovered the comet that bears his name but also calculated its orbital motion.

In natural sciences the two great luminaries were the Swedish doctor and botanist Carl Von Linne or Linnaeus (1707–1778) and the French zoologist Compte de Buffon (1707–78). Carl Von Linne for the first time devised a system of classification of plants and animals according to the now universal binomial method. He wrote his *System of Nature,* classifying man, apes, lemurs, bats in the order of primates and named man as *Homo sapiens.*

Compte de Buffon's life long interest in zoology culminated in the writing of his fifteen volume *Natural History,* which was an encyclopedic classification of all known animal life. It was Buffon who wrote the popular aphorism *'The Style is the Man'.*

Physics continued to make progress, the Newtonian trend of measurement, experiment, direct observation continuing into the new century. There were important contributions to the physics of sound, hydrodynamics and optics. The excitement of the century was electricity. Static electricity was known for many centuries, but in 1746, it was discovered at Leiden university that electricity could be stored in a jar and could be used for experiments.

The great chemist of this era was Antoine-Laurent de Lavoisier (1743–1794) of France. He studied the chemistry of combustion and showed that it involved oxidation. He demonstrated that respiration was a form of combustion and that chemical processes were important for life and living.

Charles Cavendish of England analysed the composition of water showing that it consisted of oxygen and 'inflammable air'. Lavoisier showed that the 'inflammable air' was hydrogen.

38 Schools of Thought in Medical Science

As in the previous centuries, medical science lagged far behind when compared to the advances in physics, chemistry, mathematics, astronomy and other natural sciences. Also, the domination and paramountcy of medical centres in Italy were now challenged not only by centres in France but also by other quickly growing centres in the western world—Leiden, Halle, Vienna, London, Edinburgh, and, in the late years of this century, Philadelphia. Why should medical science have consistently lagged behind the natural sciences? Perhaps because in medicine the subject of study was as complex a mechanism as man. After all, the principles of mathematics, physics and chemistry did not necessarily always explain life in health and disease. Perhaps because medicine, particularly when translated to patient care was not all pure science but contained a significant measure of art, which could neither be measured nor expressed as a mathematical formula. There was just no single uniform school of thought in the science of medicine. In fact there were a number of streams of thought in different centres often heading in different directions. These different schools arose from the conflict between new ideas and traditional beliefs. The new ideas of the thinkers and philosophers of the eighteenth century deified science and made reason their *raison d'être*. Science with Reason could explain nature, could unravel the secrets of life—provided science was based on the Newtonian and Galilean principles of mathematics, measurement, experiment and direct observation. These ideas clashed with the traditional belief of the earlier centuries where religious, theological doctrines were used to help explain the working of the human body. The scientific concept triumphed, but the conflict threw up three main schools of thought in medicine—the mechanistic school, the animistic school and the school of vitalism.

The mechanistic school had its origin in the iatrophysicists and iatrochemists of the Baroque period, and was further strengthened in the eighteenth century. This age of reason prompted physicians to propose that man was in essence a machine in motion—that he could be explained according to the laws of mathematics and science. Julien Offray de la Metrie (1709–1751) unabashedly said that man was solely a mechanism. He wrote in his *L'homme machine* (1748) that matter thinks, that there was no need for a soul, and that the body is a machine that winds its own springs. There were indeed very few (Metrie was perhaps the exception) who equated man 'in toto' to a machine, even though they felt that the basic laws of nature working in the human body were mechanistic and explicable on scientific principles.

The mechanistic view of medicine was given support by the great Dutch physician professor Herman Boerhaave (1668–1738) who straddled both the Baroque and the eighteenth century. He viewed health and disease in terms of altered forces, weights and hydrostatic pressures. A balance of internal fluid pressures resulted in hydrostatic equilibrium and good health; an imbalance of these pressures led to disequilibrium and disease. Boerhaave also distinguished between diseases involving solids and those involving 'humors' and 'liquids'. Tuberculosis was a disease due to a weakness of solids, and blood clots were due to an abnormality of the blood and humor with rigid fibres. The treatment for weak fibres was milk and iron, whilst blood-letting was advised for rigid fibres.

Boerhaave, in spite of his mechanistic views on health and disease, like most others holding similar views accepted dualism—i.e., the presence of a soul. However the interaction between the body (the machine) and the soul was left to the realms of imagination and fancy.

The animistic school of thought in medicine was a counter to the mechanistic view. It was championed by a German doctor and philosopher Georg Ernst Stahl (1660–1734). He was a student of G W Wedel of the iatrochemical school. Stahl opposed the dualism of Descartes who had proposed the demarcation of the physical body from the soul. He countered that the soul (*anima*) was God–given, and was responsible for all forms of life. It was the source that regulated and worked the body, so that on death when it left the body, the body putrefied. Stahl fired a strong dissenting salvo against the machine-like, mathematical mechanical view on medical science; there was no activity possible without the guidance of the soul. The soul (*anima*) regulated life processes and disease was an expression of the soul to expel morbid matter and thereby restore bodily functions.

Stahl who taught medicine, botany and pharmacology at the university of Halle was challenged by his friend and colleague Friedrich Hoffman (1670–1742), also a pupil of Wedel with regard to the direction medical science should follow. He believed in the animist school but took a more mechanistic view of man, and published his concepts in a nine-volume work *Medicina Rationalis Systematica*. A follower of the German philosopher Leibnitz, he argued that the ultimate causes were beyond our comprehension, and knowledge was limited to what was directly appreciated by our senses.

Hoffman described the body as consisting of fibres with the ability to contract or dilate under the influence of a nervous fluid distributed throughout the body by nerves. This ether-like vital fluid was perhaps secreted by the brain. Alteration in this ether-like fluid led to disease. Acute disease was spasmodic and needed to be treated by sedatives; chronic disease was atonic and required stimulant medicines. He also opined that the chief cause of disease was a 'fullness', which he termed *plethora* acting indirectly through the stomach and gut to which, therefore, treatment should in the main be directed. Hoffman, however far-fetched his thinking may appear in our time, was a scholar who exchanged scientific notes with colleagues in other centres and who considered medicine to be international rather than regional.

The third major school of thought was vitalism; it was midway between the mechanistic and materialistic school on the one hand and the animistic school which leaned on religion and theology on the other. It postulated the presence a of special vital principle quite distinct from the body and the soul. An important proponent of this school was Theophile de Bordeu (1711–1776). Bordeu felt that each organ contributed a vital substance to the blood and the body; health and integrity were dependent on these secretions. Barthez introduced the term vital principle and its control over body functions.

William Cullen (1710–1790) was a brilliant vitalist of the Edinburgh school, and he held that it was the nervous system which regulated all body functions through a nerve fluid which controlled the tone in the various solid parts of the body. Changes in tone produced either spasm or atony and this determined disease.

Unquestionably the most towering personality of the eighteenth century who indirectly supported the vitalist school was Albrecht Von Haller, a man of great distinction who divided all fibres according to their reactive properties—the irritable and the sensible. There was an aspect of vitality or inherent vitalism in their response. Haller is more fully discussed in the next chapter.

John Hunter was also a vitalist and believed that blood contained a life principle which promoted health and living and which distinguished living organisms from inanimate matter. France also had its vitalists—in particular the students of Jean Astruc (1684–1766), who taught at Montpellier. Theophile de Bordeu, mentioned earlier, was one such brilliant student. Mention must be made of an unusual offbeat school of thought that held considerable sway in some parts of Europe for many years. John Brown (1735–1788) was a Scottish parson turned physician who felt that the chief property of life was excitability and that the degree of excitement controlled disease. Increased excitement produced sthenic disease and decreased excitement caused asthenic disease. Treatment for asthenic disease was a stimulant such as alcohol, and for sthenic disease sedation with laudanum. His school and system of medicine was the rage in Italy and parts of Germany and was adopted by Benjamin Rush in Philadelphia. There were strong proponents and equally strong opponents of John Brown—brawls and duels in Italy and Germany were said to have caused deaths comparable in number to those in the French Revolution!

The Investigators

The trail of scientific inquiry and discovery blazed by Harvey in the Baroque period was eagerly followed by a number of investigators in the eighteenth century. They did not make any epoch-making breakthrough as Harvey did, but they contributed significantly to medicine and medical science.

Albrecht Von Haller was born in Berne in 1708 and is chiefly remembered for his contribution to physiology. He must have been an amazing child prodigy, for at the age of nine he had produced a book on Chaldean grammar, compiled a Greek and Hebrew dictionary, and had written poems and biographies. He grew up to be a man for all seasons, a truly universal man. He began studying medicine at the age of fifteen at Tubergen and then went on to Leiden. When still below twenty years, he qualified with a thesis that disproved the belief of Professor Coschwitz of Halle that the lingual vein was a salivary duct. He then studied in London and, Paris. In Basle he was the student of the famous Jean Bernoulli (1667–1748) a great mathematician of this age. Haller soon became professor at the university of Gottingen, where for seventeen years he taught all branches of medicine and then returned to Berne. His output was incredible. He wrote twelve books on physiology, four books on anatomy, seven on botany. He also wrote on theology, and compiled a vast ten-volume bibliography on botany, the medicinal properties of herbs and the practice of medicine.

Multifaceted as he was, his forte was physiology and his best work was in the physiology of the nervous system. His *Primae Lineae Physiologiae* (1747) (*First Lines in Physiology*) became the standard textbook on physiology and was translated into several languages. His magnum opus was *Elementa Physiologiae Corporis Humani* (1757–1766) (*Elements of the Physiology of the Human Body*), an eight-volume encyclopaedic work which reviewed the past and elaborated upon the current concepts of the subject.

As mentioned earlier, through experimentation, Haller established that irritability was a property inherent in muscle fibres, and sensibility a property inherent in nerve fibres. The pulsatile activity of the heart was thus explained by inherent myogenic irritability, the heart being made up of muscle fibres. These inherent properties of muscle and nerve strengthened the vitalist school of thought in medicine. Haller also made valuable contributions to the study of blood vessels, to microscopic anatomy and established the importance of bile in the digestion of fat.

A man of medicine and of the natural sciences, a linguist, a poet, a writer who carried on a voluminous correspondence with eminent contemporaries of his era (including Voltaire and Giovanni Casanova), he reminds us of some of the great men of the Renaissance. He designed botanical gardens, established churches, founded an orphan asylum, improved public health and finally became head of his native canton of Berne.

There were other physiologists of note in the eighteenth century. Stephen Hales, an English clergyman was the first to experimentally measure blood pressure in the arterial system using a glass tube inserted into a horse's artery. He noted that the arterial pressure was far greater than the venous pressure.

René Antoine de Réaumur, besides inventing the thermometer, studied the physiology of digestion. He trained a pet kite to ingest fine metal tubes filled with food closed at either end by wiremesh. The kite after a while regurgitated these tubes and Réaumur showed that digestion was not a process of trituration and putrefaction of food as was till then believed. He demonstrated it was the gastric juice that dissolved food. Further work on digestion on the same lines was continued by Lorenzo Spallanzani (1729–1799). He experimented on himself by swallowing thin cloth bags containing nutrients. He vomited these and established the solvent power of gastric juice as also the solvent power of saliva. Maria Theresa recognized his talent and he was installed in the chair of natural history at the university of Pavia. Spallanzani was also a pioneer in experimental morphology and demonstrated that tadpoles, earthworms and lizards could spontaneously regenerate parts of their anatomy (the tails) after these were severed.

Luigi Galvani (1737–1798) pioneered electrophysiology. He described experiments in his *De Viribus electricitates in motu musculari* (1791) (*Electrical Power in the Movement of Muscle*), wherein he suspended the legs of skinned dead frogs by a copper wire from an iron balcony. As the feet touched the iron uprights the muscles contracted and the legs twitched. There was thus a strong suggestion that the inherent properties of sensibility and irritability postulated by Haller could be 'fired' by an electrical impulse. Count Alessandro Volta (1745–1827) professor at the university of Pavia expanded on these experiments and showed that a muscle could be sent into continuous tetanic contractions by repeated electrical stimulation. These early experiments were the forerunners of modern electro-physiology. Perhaps they also influenced Mary Shelley's *Frankenstein*—a science fiction book in which life is created by an electrical spark.

The eighteenth century witnessed pioneering work on respiratory physiology. The air we breathe was recognized to be not one single gas but a cocktail of gases. Joseph Black discovered carbon dioxide in 1757; Henry Cavendish discovered hydrogen in 1766 and Daniel Rutherford discovered nitrogen in 1772. Oxygen was isolated by Joseph Priestley in 1772. The issue of oxidation was for sometime confused by Stahl's belief that substances on burning, i.e., on oxidation, were supposed to lose a substance called phlogiston even though an increase in weight was observed. Priestley called oxygen dephlogisticated air. It was finally Antoine Laurent Lavoisier, a great chemist and a distinguished physiologist who discovered the true nature of respiration—Lavoiser compared the physiology of respiration to the process of combustion, with the utilization of oxygen (oxygen being taken up by the blood in the lungs) and the production of carbon dioxide and water. Lavoisier also demonstrated that oxygen was indispensable for life and that the greater the activity of the body the greater the oxygen consumed. Antoine Laurent Lavoisier an aristocrat by birth was guillotined in the blood bath that followed the French Revolution in 1789. His friend Lagrange said in anguish. "It takes a second to sever a head. Perhaps a century will pass before there is another like his."

Giovanni Battista Morgagni (1682–1771) was the student of Anton Maria Valsalva (1660–1723) who was famous for his anatomical dissections and description of the middle and internal ear. Morgagni's expertise in dissection must have been sharpened under the tutelage of his teacher. Morgagni was appointed to the chair of anatomy at Padua in 1773 and at the age of near 80 years, he published his great work *De sedibus et causis morborum* (1761) (*On the Sites and Causes of Disease*). He described in this work his findings on 700 autopsies and together with his seventy letters to a friend (medical information was often exchanged in this age through letters), detailed the anatomy of organs in various diseases. He showed that a disease produces anatomical distortion and change in one or more specific organs and that any anatomical change in an organ system was accompanied by a change in function. His case histories included autopsies on bandits and bishops, prostitutes and princesses—a veritable encyclopaedia of disease and the specific organ systems afflicted by different diseases. He correlated the symptoms in his case histories with his findings at autopsy and noted how different diseases sprang from alteration in the anatomy of specific organs. He was truly the father of modern pathology; a luminous star in the firmament of medical science. He was also a fine archaeologist and the author of the biography of his teacher Anton Valsalva.

Morgagni made a great number of discoveries. He noted that a stroke was caused by disease of the cerebral vessels and that hemiplegia occurred on the side of the body opposite to that of the damaged cerebral hemisphere. He was the first to observe that syphilitic disease could affect the cerebral vessels. It is of interest that pyramidal decussation in the medulla had been earlier described

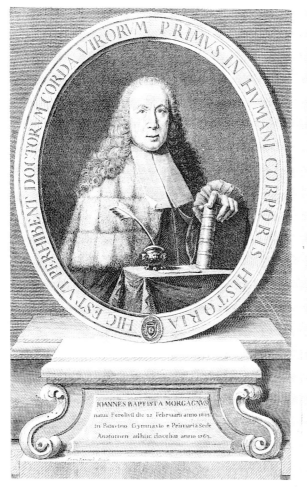
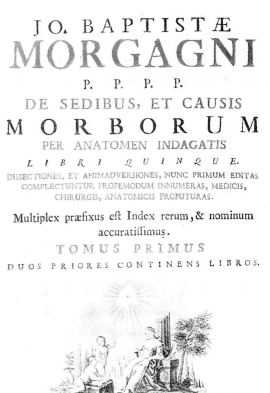

Fig. 39.1   Giovanni Battista Morgagni.

by Mestichelli in Rome in 1710 and that crossed hemiplegia had been also described earlier in the Smith's *Papyrus*, in Hippocrates' *Cranial Fractures* and by Aretaeus of Cappadocia.

Morgagni described the syncope associated with heart block—Morgagni Stokes Adams syndrome. He gave excellent descriptions of angina pectoris, subacute bacterial endocarditis, cirrhosis of the liver and renal insufficiency, and distinguished clots in the heart which were post-mortem from those that were ante-mortem. Morgagni also wrote on tuberculosis of the lungs and described a caseating liquefying tuberculous lesion.

Morgagni had his counterpart in England. Mathew Baillie in 1793 published *Morbid Anatomy of Some of the Most Important Parts of the Human Body*. Baillie was the nephew of the Hunters.

trained at his uncle William's anatomy school of Great Windmill Street and at St Georges hospital. He became the owner of this school on uncle William's death. He also became physician to St Georges hospital and physician to George III. His *Morbid Anatomy* contained excellent descriptions of disease. He described gastric ulcer, noted the relation of alcohol to cirrhosis of the liver, gave an excellent description of ovarian cysts, of emphysema and of grey hepatization of the lung in pneumonia.

Marie François Xavier Bichat (1771–1801) of France studied in Paris at the height of the Terror and had ample surgical practice after joining the army. He is believed to have conducted over 600 autopsies, living and sleeping in the anatomy hall. He however never held any hospital attachment and died at the young age of 31 years. Bichat went a step further than both Morgagni and Baillie and considered the tissue to be the basic unit of a living organism and the basic site of pathology in disease. He believed that life consists of a group of functions that resist death and described 21 tissues with specific properties. He is regarded to be the father of modern histology.

The best known investigator in embryology was Caspar Friedrich Wolff (1733–1794). He restated Harvey's theory of epigenesis—the gradual development of the parts of the body. He wrote his *Theoria Generationis* (1759) (*Theory of Generation*), stating that living beings are compelled to grow by an essential force (*vis essentialis*)—a basic principle of vitalism.

40 Medicine in the Age of Reason

The Physician And The Practice Of Medicine

In this enlightened age the physician was a respected member of society. He was often educated at university, was a man of letters, who could also have studied philosophy, mathematics or natural science. He was well attired and the more successful ones sported a gold cane and were elegantly dressed and wigged. If he was fortunate enough to be appointed as physician to royalty he could amass a great deal of wealth, acquire a title and vast estates. A successful physician in a large city such as London would easily earn £5,000 per annum. His fee for an office consultation averaged a half guinea, for a house call two guineas, but his main income was from prescriptions which he would often prescribe (in cafés or on a promenade), on a mere history even without examining the patient.

Ironically enough, even in an enlightened age, the faith of man on lotions, potions, pills, useless and often poisonous though they may be, was immense. As of today, the reputation of the practicing physician was often dependent on his attire, his demeanour and bedside manner, only occasionally on his learning. The physician was also perfectly capable of promoting himself by subtle or overt means over his colleagues. Some engaged in pamphleteering to draw clientele to their office. This often led to arguments and duels. An argument over 'bilious fever' was settled with swords and pistols leading to the death of two physicians. Richard Mead challenged a colleague to a duel over the treatment of smallpox; to every one's relief the duel was aborted.

Yet the profession was also known for its charity and magnanimity towards the poor, to younger colleagues and to literary men. The profession also gave generously to a worthy cause. The most notable example was Sir Hans Sloane who was a reputed physician, a great natural scientist and a collector *sans pareil* in this age. He was made a baronet (the first physician to be so honoured), became a Fellow of the Royal Society and donated his private museum and library to form the nucleus of the British Museum. William Hunter bequeathed his famous anatomy museum and his vast library valued at £1,00,000 to the university of Glasgow.

The art of diagnosis was still primitive by our present standards. A careful history (an art which the modern physician of today is in the process of losing) and close observation preceded a calculated inference. Careful observation chiefly took note of the traditional 'five senses'—feeling the pulse, observing skin and eye colour, detecting abnormalities in breathing, sniffing for gangrene and tasting the urine. The more experienced the physician, the more accurate the inference. John Floyer (1649–1734) in his *Physician's Pulse Watch* had advised counting the pulse rate by checking the pulse against a special second hand. This quantitative measurement was by and large ignored—it was the nature and feel of the pulse that was emphasized. It is in a way amazing why a physical 'hands on' examination of the patients was not seriously considered or practised; perhaps prevailing etiquette and social mores particularly in relation to the examination of females, were responsible for this lacuna.

The most important new technique in bedside examination in the eighteenth century was the discovery of the importance of percussion of the chest by Leopold Auenbrugger (1722–1809) of Vienna. His father was an innkeeper and since childhood he was familiar with the percussion note over full and incompletely filled barrels of wine. He could thus detect the extent to which a barrel was full or empty from the percussion note over it. He translated this technique to the percussion of the chest and in his *Inventum Novum* (1761) described the difference between the percussive note of healthy chests from that obtained in diseases of the lungs or the pleura. His discovery was unfortunately ignored up to the beginning of the nineteenth century.

The Thermometer

In Hippocratic times the importance of body temperature was realized, but the physician used only his hand to feel the skin temperature. In 1592, Galileo constructed what was probably the first thermometer. It gave only gross temperature changes and was cumbersome. Galileo was not interested in the medical implications of this device. Santorio however was greatly interested in measuring body heat and devised ingenuous but cumbersome instruments for thermometric measurements.

The impetus to thermometry came after the discovery of the Centigrade scale by Christiaan Huygens (1629–95) in 1665 and the Fahrenheit scale by Gabriel Fahrenheit in 1717. It was Herman Boerhaave in Holland and his students van Sweiten and De Haen who routinely used thermometry in clinical practice. They recognized the importance of monitoring temperature in a patient's illness. The Swedish astronomer Anders Celsius (1701–44) reintroduced the Centigrade scale and this was followed by significant improvements in the design of the thermometer. Karl August Wanderlich (1815–77) studied numerous cases and maintained that fever was a symptom and not a disease and that in many patients the measurement of temperature was as important as the pulse.

The early thermometer was long and required contact with the skin for over twenty minutes to register temperature. Aitkin, in 1852, narrowed the glass tubing above the bulb so that the column of mercury did not fall back after the thermometer was withdrawn. In 1870, Thomas Clifford Allbutt gave the thermometer the design in use today.

Specialities of Medicine

The eighteenth century saw the early beginnings of what in the next two centuries blossomed into specialties. The seed of cardiology as a speciality was planted by Antonio Guiseppe Testa (1764–1814). Jean Baptiste Sénac, a French clinician recognized asthma, orthopnea, oedema of the legs, haemoptysis as being related to cardiac insufficiency. Many would consider Jean Nicholas Corvisart (1755–1821) the founding father of cardiology. More is written about him in chapter 44. He was the first individual to call himself a heart specialist and to coin the term 'carditis'.

Obstetrics and gynaecology had already taken root in the Baroque era. A famous teacher and practitioner in the eighteenth century was the Scot William Smellie (1697–1763). He was strongly resented by the midwives who considered obstetrics their sole domain and prerogative. Smellie had a large practice in London. He was innovative and improved the design of Chamberlain's forceps and made forceps delivery easier. He taught obstetrics and wrote his book on *Midwifery* in 1752. To his house came William Hunter who was freshly trained in Paris. Hunter now trained further with

Smellie and moved on to Glasgow as Cullen's pupil. He then returned to London and started his lecture courses in anatomy, surgery and obstetrics. Many a surgeon obstetrician was trained by Hunter and as the eighteenth century progressed the field of obstetrics came to be increasingly dominated by male-midwives also called accoucheurs. Under the influence of accoucheurs mothers were encouraged to deliver in open rooms with fresh air and bright light. Newborns were no longer wrapped in multilayered clothes and mothers were encouraged to do away with wet-nurses and breast-feed their own babies. These points on child-birth and infant care were emphasized by William Cadogan (1711–1797) in his book *An Essay upon Nursing and the Management of Children*. The rise of the male accoucheur along with changes in the management of childbirth and baby care were observed chiefly in Britain. In Germany midwives and wet-nurses were still in charge. In France, Spain, Italy, Austria, the Catholic church was all for female modesty, and accoucheurs made no headway against the traditional midwives.

Ophthalmology was also born in this century. Advances in the anatomy and physiology of the eye, pioneered by Leonardo da Vinci in the Renaissance, were made by a number of this century's physicians. These advances in combination with the study of light and colours by eminent physicists established ophthalmology as a special field in medicine. Jacques Daviel demonstrated and taught the surgical procedure for cataract extraction. In 1773, Maria Theresa the empress of Austria established the first school of ophthalmology on the continent.

In Germany Haller's friend and fellow poet Paul Gottlieb Werlhof (1699–1767) unwittingly started the study of diseases of the blood—haematology. He gave the first original description of *purpura haemorrhagica*—a bleeding disorder now known to be related to a quantitative or qualitative defect of the platelets in the blood.

Boerhaave and his Students

Straddling the Baroque period and the age of enlightenment was a great physician and a gifted teacher. Herman Boerhaave was born near Leiden in 1668. He was the son of a clergyman who desired that Herman followed his footsteps. Herman Boerhaave therefore first studied theology and philosophy but later changed to medicine. He studied at the university of Leiden and in 1701 was appointed to the Chair of theoretical medicine, which also involved teaching physics, chemistry and botany. Over the years he built a great reputation as a physician and a teacher. As a physician he focused attention on patient care in the true tradition of Hippocrates. The eighteenth century was an era of conflicting schools of thought. Boerhaave was not above contributing to these conflicting thoughts on the science of medicine. It was however his clinical approach at the bedside, his meticulous notes on each patient's history, his observations on each patient's illness and above all the care and concern he lavished on all those entrusted to him that marked him out as a giant among the physicians of the western world. He advocated the setting aside of all academic theories and preconditions in the actual practice of clinical medicine and maintained that the aim of medicine was to care for and cure the sick. His practice was legendary; he was respected by his colleagues for his eclectic intellect and his character, loved by his students and adored by the public. It is said that he was so loved by the people of Leiden that when he recovered from a particularly nasty attack of gout, the bells of Leiden tolled long and loud and the city was brightly lit with torches. Boerhaave amassed a fortune through his phenomenal practice, leaving over 10 million florins on his death.

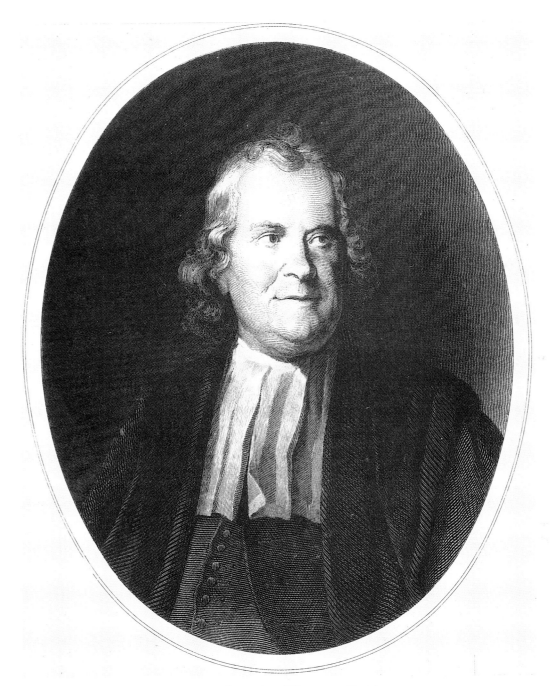

Fig. 40.1   Portrait of Hermann Boerhaave.

As a teacher Boerhaave reigned supreme. Students from Edinburgh, London, Paris, Padua, Vienna and all other centres of learning attended his clinics in his 12-bedded ward at Leiden, spreading his Hippocratic teachings to all corners of Europe. Eminent people waited for his consultations or at the door of his lecture theatre to hear him discourse on clinical medicine. It is said that the Czar Peter the Great was one of them. One of his greatest pupils was Albrecht Von Haller who called Boerhaave 'The Common Teacher of all Europe'. Another student who was to become famous was the Dutchman Gerard Von Sweiten (1700–1772) who as we shall see later founded the school of medicine in Vienna. Boerhaave's two major contributions to medical literature were *Institutiones Medicae* (1708), a textbook of physiology, and *Aphorisms* (1709). Both these slim volumes were read all over Europe, and they went into numerous editions and were translated into several languages including Arabic.

Herman Boerhaave made no great discovery, no great invention, yet he was the greatest physician of the eighteenth century. Like Hippocrates of yore and Sydenham of the seventeenth century he brought back the focus of medicine on the care of the sick, emphasized the importance of the doctor at the bedside, and the healing power of mother Nature. At 61 years of age, due to a crippling attack of gout, he retired from teaching chemistry and botany but continued to teach and practise medicine till his death from cardiac failure in 1738.

Schools of Medicine

In the early eighteenth century Leiden was a famous medical centre, chiefly because of the reputation of Boerhaave, known as the *Communis Europae praeceptor,* the 'medical instructor of Europe'. Leiden was particularly famous for its clinical teaching—two small wards of six beds each in a charity hospital were designated for bedside teaching of patients and for clinical demonstrations. This was an innovation as it was rare for hospitals in that age to set aside wards for teaching.

Boerhaave's pupil, Dutchman Gerhard Van Swieten (1700–1772) founded the old school of Vienna. The Austrian empire of the Hapsburgs in the eighteenth century was a powerful kingdom stretching west to Flanders and including a part of Northern Italy. In 1744, Maria Theresa's (the Empress of Austria) sister fell ill and Van Swieten was consulted. Maria Theresa was so impressed that she invited him to be her personal doctor and to set up a medical school in Vienna. Van Sweiten was the natural successor to Boerhaave in Leiden, but being a Protestant, he felt his chances of succeeding to the chair of medicine slim in a Catholic country. He accepted Maria Theresa's offer and set about organizing the faculty of medicine. The university of Vienna, though founded in 1365 had no medical tradition of any consequence, so Sweiten had to build a sound medical faculty where there was none.

He separated the departments and teaching of anatomy from surgery, created a chemistry laboratory, a botanical or herb garden and organized the clinical teaching of medicine along the style of his mentor Boerhaave in Leiden. As in Leiden two six-bedded wards (one for male patients and the other for female patients) were set aside for clinical teaching. The old Viennese medical school was funded by the state, which appointed the faculty, paid the salaries of the staff and granted diplomas on completion of study. Sweiten was a clinician in the mould of his teacher and he had taken notes on his teacher's comments on different cases during ward rounds in Leiden. He used these notes to publish five volumes titled *Commentarea in Boerhaave aphorismos.*

The old Vienna school further enhanced its reputation through the work of other doctors, notably Leopold Auenbrugger (1722–1809) who discovered the art and science of percussion as a help to physical diagnosis—a discovery which came into use only a year before he died.

The medical school of Edinburgh grew into increasing prominence in the eighteenth century. It was the Leiden of Scotland—the school dating from the appointment of Leiden-trained Alexander Munro to the chair of anatomy in 1726. Both the university (noted for its teaching of human sciences and philosophy) and the faculty of medicine gained increasing renown in the next hundred years. Three generations of Munros (all called Alexander Munro) ruled anatomy from their professorial chair. Munro II succeeded his father in 1758, Munro III succeeded Munro II in 1798, and occupied the chair till 1846. The Munro family held the chair for 120 years! The standard of anatomy teaching is believed to have declined under Munro III who is said to have used his grandfather's (Munro I) notes quoting verbatum remarks such as, "When I was in Leiden in 1719".

There was an abundance of other talent in the Edinburgh school which clearly outshone the medical schools in London, Oxford, Cambridge and in many cities of Europe. It attracted students from Europe; many leading American physicians of the eighteenth century were also trained in the school. Training in Edinburgh was well-organized and was particularly excellent in anatomy, physiology, surgery and in the theory and practice of medicine. Dissection in anatomy was however hampered by a shortage of corpses, leading to illegal acquisition of cadavers through violation of graves and body-snatching, and even through murder. Clinical teaching was pioneered at the Royal Infirmary. Professor John Rutherford initiated clinical lectures in 1740 and a special clinical ward was started at the Infirmary in 1750, the students being encouraged to visit a patient's bedside and study the notes and reports. A three-year course in the medical school enabled a student to step out and practise as a family doctor or a general practitioner—reasonably adept in both medicine and surgery. Students at the university attended and paid for only those courses they desired. There was no obligation to graduate, the courses of study being practical and oriented to student demand. In the late eighteenth century, Edinburgh attracted 200 medical students each year. The Edinburgh Royal College of Surgeons was founded in 1778 and attracted a number of students in surgery from its first year of inception.

Medical teaching in London developed outside the university, in private anatomy schools and in the teaching hospitals. Though the chief private schools were in anatomy, practical private courses in materia medica, chemistry and obstetrics were also taught. The capital's most famous private school was the anatomy and obstetric school set up by William Hunter in 1768. This school trained a number of famous individuals including John (the brother of William Hunter), Willian Cruickshank, Mathew Baillie and William Hewson.

Hunter's school was as brilliant as its founder and teacher. Lectures and demonstrations in anatomy were avant-garde as they dealt with findings not yet in print. Thus descriptions of the placental circulation, the gravid uterus and the surgical anatomy of aneurysms were the topics of lectures in this school, renowned for the anatomical prowess of its teacher.

The Enlightenment had aroused awareness of the sufferings of the poor and the sick. This led to the establishment of many dispensaries and municipal hospitals. A number of large teaching hospitals in London were also founded in the eighteenth century—Westminster (1719), Guys (1725), St Georges (1734), the London (1740) and Middlesex (1745). For the first time hospitals were opened to students for clinical teaching on patients admitted to the wards.

British schools of clinical medicine produced William Heberden (1710–1801) who first described angina pectoris as a 'sense of strangling and anxiety brought on by exercise, relieved by rest and nitroglycerine and associated with a tendency to sudden death'. Heberden published his *Medical Commentaries in the History and Cure of Diseases* (1802) giving excellent accurate clinical descriptions of disease.

William Withering (1741–1799) discovered the use of digitalis in the treatment of dropsy caused by cardiac failure. A brief account of this important discovery is mentioned in the next section.

James Lind, also of the British school, in his *Treatise of the Scurvy* (1753) showed that this deficiency disease could be prevented in sailors on ships if they were provided with lime and lemons. He persuaded the Royal Navy to take this important preventive measure.

Therapy

The studies on physiology by Haller and the studies on the anatomy of disease by Morgagni and Bailly did not open the doors of healing and cure in the eighteenth century. Therapeutics barring a few exceptions, remained archaic. Dieting or starving, purging, blood-letting or cupping and often a combination of these were the mainstays of treatment and obviously more often than not led to death rather than a cure. An ardent supporter of blood-letting was Benjamin Rush of Philadelphia. He believed that disease was caused by a hyperactive state of arteries, which he termed hypertension. Cure therefore lay in bleeding, which reduced hyperactivity. Rush's reputation as a politician unfortunately made this absurdity even more acceptable to physicians in America so that this pernicious therapy caught on in the New World. Authors, playwrights and thinkers were among the first who through satire, poured doubt and even ridicule on the wisdom of blood-letting. Le Sage in France wrote a satirical play in the early eighteenth century termed *Adventures of Gil Blas*. Dr Sangrado, a doctor was consulted by a cleric for his gout. Dr Sangrado, remarked that it was a vulgar error that blood was of any use to the system. He instructed the surgeon to do a massive 'blood-let'—'six porridges of blood, and more three hours hence and to repeat the process the following day!'

Purging was through herbal remedies and through the use of mercury, which was not only used in massive doses for the treatment of venereal disease, but also in the form of pills as a laxative. Again an ardent supporter of mercury as a universal medicine was the Philadelphian Benjamin Rush. Calomel (containing mercury) remained popular right up to the twentieth century as a purgative that 'cleared the system'.

The Hippocratic tradition of helping nature heal was fortunately practised by a few wise physicians. Temperance, exercise, diet, regular evacuations with purges, and baths were advocated as part of the healing process. Hydrotherapy perhaps carried nature's diktat a step too far. Sigmond Hahn and John Floyer were ardent advocates of cold baths in a variety of ailments. James Currie's management of typhoid fever included pouring cold sea water over the patient again and again!

Advising travel was often the prescription for the rich and famous. The increased incidence of tuberculosis prompted doctors to advise the phthisical rich to winter in southern Europe. Horse-riding was the exercise favoured for consumptives. The founder of Methodism, John Wesley (1703–1791) believed that he would keep healthy if he was always on horseback and he followed this belief by delivering his sermons on horseback even when eighty-five years old! Travel was often combined with 'taking the baths', of course to the delight and pleasure of the hotel-owners and doctors who often centred around these places of pilgrimage—a feature which persists to this day. Gambling, dancing, music and other entertainment were also offered in these spas, so that what we today call a consumer industry grew in and around such centres. Fashionable spas in Europe included Baden-Baden and in England the most popular was Bath (founded by the Romans), which provided facilities for bathing in spring water or in the sea.

Primitive electrotherapy followed the discovery of electricity. By the end of the eighteenth century many hospitals had electrostatic machines. Christian Kratzenstein in Copenhagen used electricity in the treatment of paralysis.

The pharmacopoeia barring a few exceptions remained medieval and poisonous; it was essentially the same as in the Baroque era. This was unfortunate, the more so because people were becoming increasingly dependent on potions and lotions and pills, rather than going back to nature to help healing. Newer additions to the pharmacopoeia in the century included Fowler's solution

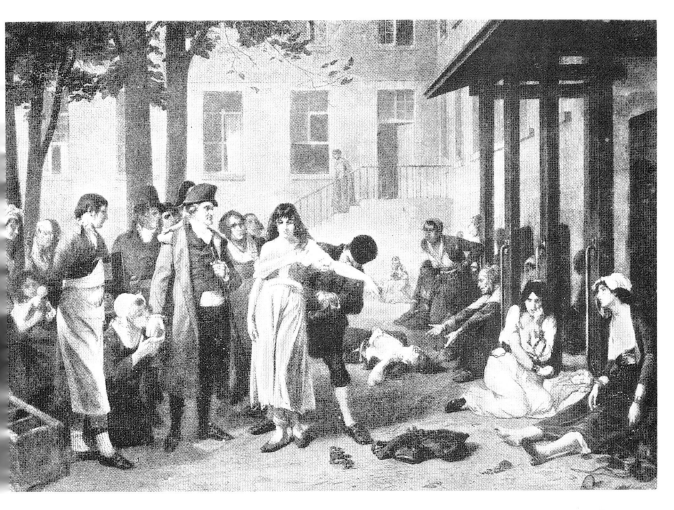

Fig. 40.2   The visit of Dr Pinel to the Salpêtrière, Paris, in 1795, when he ordered the chains
to be taken off insane patients.

containing arsenic, Hoffman's anodyne, Gregory's powder, quassia, balsam, the buccaneer physician's famous Dover's powder containing opium and liquid paregoric which was liquid opium. Antimony still flourished, and mercury used as calomel was the purge of choice. The oral use of mercury and its application as an ointment continued in the treatment of syphilis. Amazingly enough the use of Fowler's solution and Dover's powder continued well into the twentieth century. Opium was indeed an invaluable drug in this era, for it relieved pain and suffering, induced sleep, and was noted to relieve the breathlessness of heart failure. However, the dependency and addiction to opium was now being observed. Samuel Taylor Coleridge and others who to start with used opium as a medicine ended up suffering terribly from hopeless addiction.

The two most useful and important discoveries in therapy in the eighteenth century were digitalis for heart failure and the willow bark (*salix alba*) for fever. Digitalis was discovered by William Withering (1741–1799). A product of the London school. Withering was a medical botanist who had studied the works of Linnaeus. He practiced in Shropshire and heard from a village woman of a 'herbal tea' which was a family secret and which was useful in both dropsy and heart failure. The 'herb' the woman mentioned was the foxglove plant (*digitalis purpurea*). Withering gave a decoction of this foxglove plant containing digitalis to a fifty-year-old man with asthma and with fluid in the abdomen. He noted that his patient passed a great deal of water, that his breathing became easier, his abdomen flatter and that within ten days he was much better and had started to eat well. In 1785 Withering published *An Account of the Foxglove and Some of its Medical Uses etc; with Practical Remarks on Dropsy and Other Diseases*. He noted that digitalis had a stimulant effect on the heart, reducing the dropsy that frequently accompanied heart failure. Digitalis was included in the Edinburgh pharmacopoeia in 1783 and in the London pharmacopoeia twenty years later.

The use of the willow-bark for fever was discovered in 1763 by Revd Edmund Stone. The willow-bark grew in wet damp areas where fevers abounded and Stone's religious faith led him to believe that if God had thought it fit to place the willow-bark in these areas, it would be useful for fevers. His religious view was further strengthened by the bitter taste of the bark resembling the bitter taste of the Peruvian cinchona bark which was successful in the treatment of malaria. He administered the willow-bark to fifty patients with symptoms of rheumatic fever and reported good results. He reported his results to the Royal Society but was ignored. Willow-bark contains salicin and has an effect similar to aspirin—a drug of proven use in rheumatic fever.

The Therapy for Madness

The last decade of the eighteenth century brought dramatic relief to patients suffering from mental disease. Till then insanity was an affliction due to a demonic possession but not a disease, and the mentally ill were chained and treated with utmost cruelty in filthy lazarets. Philippe Pinel (1745–1826) of France was the son of a country physician who first studied theology and then turned to medicine and natural science. He studied and worked at Montpellier, embraced the vitalistic school of thought in medicine and achieved fame by his classification of disease according to botanic methods and principles. He became physician to the Bicêtre Hospital in Paris and believed that the insane behaved like animals because they were treated worse than animals. In 1796, he obtained permission to unchain fifty insane patients, arguing that insanity was a mental disease.

Pinel is famous for his three books *Nosographie* (1798), *La Médicine Clinique* (1804), and *Traité Médicophylosophique sur l' Aliénation Mentale* (1801) (*Medicophylosophical Treatment on Mental Alienation*). He had read the philosophers Locke and Condillac and was truly an enlightened man reflecting an enlightened age. He believed in the role of psychological factors in mental disease but considered that a derangement of understanding was generally the effect of an organic lesion in the brain.

In Italy, Vincenzo Chiarugi, in 1793, presented one of the first works diagnosing and classifying mental disease. Another pioneer in Europe was the German vitalist Johann Christian Reil, who around the same time described the island of Reil (the insula in the brain) and believed in the brain's functional independence. The vital principle or life force, according to Reil, was a chemical interaction between body fluids.

An interesting 'mad patient' in the eighteenth century was George III. It is now certain that His Majesty's madness was due to a metabolic disease porphyria, though this was of course not known in that era. The madness of King George not responding to the ministrations of court physicians was ultimately entrusted with some trepidation to the Revd Dr Francis Willis who ran a madhouse in Lincolnshire. In spite of opposition from his defeated medical colleagues he managed a complete physical and psychological domination over the King, employing fearless methods of using a strait jacket, a gag and a restraining chair during His Majesty's fits of madness. Besides physical intimidation he managed to gain the King's confidence and in due course the madness remitted, with

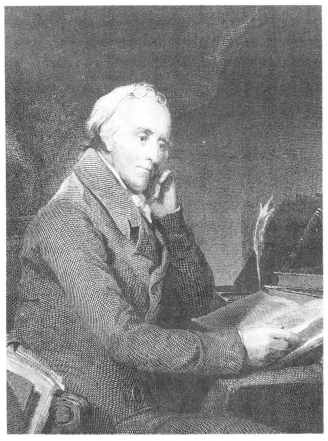

Fig. 40.3   Benjamin Rush.

Willis encouraging the king to recite Shakespeare and to shave and dress himself. This remission, now known to occur in porphyria, was then attributed to Willis and his methods of treatment. Willis thumped his chest with glee to claim credit for His Majesty's cure. William Pitt, the then prime minister rejoiced, as the country was spared regency and had parliament vote £1,000/year for 20 years as the reward to Willis. Willis took the celebrations one step further and ordered medallions to be made with the inscription 'Britons Rejoice, Your King's Restored'.

The effect of King George's cure at least in Britain, started the use of physical treatment in the treatment of insanity—not that these methods restored sanity in the insane! Bloodletting, purging became prevalent as in physical diseases. Shock treatment included the use of ice cold showers. Fast rotating chairs and swings were used in the hope of dispelling fixed ideas and thoughts, and when all else failed, there was always the straitjacket to fall back upon.

The well-run madhouse or lunatic asylum became increasingly popular as the abode of the insane. Of course the badly run ones were ghastly death traps for the unfortunate patients. In some of the better-run madhouses a form of instructive psychotherapy was practised, madness being viewed as a defect in understanding and a disturbance in thought processes rather then an affliction of the soul—a view clearly reflecting the philosophy of John Locke. It was to be corrected by the will, understanding and psychological domination of the keeper of the asylum, who in addition, provided a suitable environmental control. The Revd Dr Francis Willis' asylum in Lincolnshire was a surprise to the unwary traveller—the workers on the surrounding farm, all attired in formal dress of black coats, silk breeches and stockings worked away at ploughing, threshing, gardening. They were the mad inmates of Willis' lunatic asylum!

The Great Illusionists

Franz Anton Mesmer (1743–1815) was an unusual figure in the history of medicine. He was born in a village on Lake Constance in Switzerland and studied medicine as a pupil of Van Swieten in the school of Vienna. He graduated from Vienna with a thesis entitled *De Planetarium Influxu*, according to which planets influenced health and disease in the human body. Mesmer discovered his 'mesmeric' powers almost fortuitously after starting practice. Franzisca Oesterli was Mesmer's patient who suffered from seizures, fainting fits, temporary blindness and attacks of paralysis. When Mesmer placed magnets over certain parts of her body there was a convulsive response followed by a remission. When the procedure elicited the same response again and again Mesmer was convinced that he had made a great discovery.

He postulated a theory that every living being possessed a magnetic fluid that was capable of producing a bond between human beings and was also capable of energizing both the living world and inorganic matter. He called this aetherial fluid 'animal magnetism' and felt he had unravelled one of nature's fundamental secrets. Health was dependent on the free flow of this fluid in the body, disease resulted when the flow was obstructed. He claimed to have devised a therapy that removed the obstruction to the free flow of the fluid in disease, thereby curing it. He called his therapy magnetic therapy; it consisted of laying hands on ill patients, and perhaps through the power of his own magnetic fluid effecting a cure.

In Vienna, Mesmer became a friend of Mozart and of the rich and the famous. In 1763, a girl named Maria Paradies who was said to be blind since the age of three had her sight restored by Mesmer after he had treated her by his methods. The doctors in Vienna became hostile to him after this incident and he thought it best to leave for Paris. In a short while Mesmer became the rage of Paris, particularly among the rich. People came to him in droves waiting for weeks or months to obtain a consultation. He would lay his hands on them, perhaps induce a trance-like state and claim a cure. He amassed a huge fortune, enjoying the patronage of Marie Antoinette, the queen of France and of King Louis XVI. Writers, generals (this included General Lafayette), politicians, aristocrats, dukes, nobles and princes waited on him. Patients were ushered into a luxurious room where they found others around a bath filled with dilute 'magnetized sulphuric acid' or some other innocuous chemicals. Curved iron bars protruded from the rim of the bath. Patients joined hands forming a circle around the bath and in contact with the curved iron bars. Mesmer in a scarlet robe would then touch each patient on different spots (including the erogenous zones in women). Though Mesmer claimed animal magnetism as the basis of his method he probably induced a hypnotic trance during which a cure was suggested. On leaving Mesmer the patients would be convinced they were better.

The medical profession in France was of course anti-Mesmer—almost certainly it was envy rather than their concern for the ethics of medicine that prompted them to press for an inquiry into his system of treatment. A commission was set up with four members of the Academy of Medicine, including Benjamin Franklin of America and Lavoisier the great French chemist. After due consideration the committee came to an unfavourable conclusion: "Nothing proves the existence of magnetic animal fluid; imagination without magnetism may produce convulsions; magnetism without imagination produces nothing." Mesmer almost certainly effected his cures through hypnotism and so far probably acted in good faith.

The adulation of people and his immense clientele had by then probably gone to his head. When he could not personally cope with seeing the numerous patients that demanded to be seen and cured by him, he thought of ways and means which clearly smacked of chicanery. He would thus claim to magnetize a chair or table or any other object and ask his patients to be near and touch this magnetized object so that they could be cured. He went a step further and claimed that he could magnetize trees, and standing beneath these magnetized trees could also effect a cure. The final 'coup' was when he claimed to magnetize the very air patients breathed to effect his cures. This to us seems well beyond the bounds of reason but the gullibility of the people in that tumultuous pre-revolutionary era in Paris was incredible.

At last the clouds burst. Paris reeled under revolutionary fervour and one by one his rich patrons and clients went to the guillotine. He knew his journey to the guillotine would surely come; and so, leaving behind all the wealth he had amassed, he fled to London, then to Vienna and finally returned to Switzerland on the shores of Lake Constance. He continued to practise and died rather forlorn and forgotten in 1815.

A picturesque quack and also one of the great entrepreneurs of the century was James Graham, a Scotsman who was an Edinburgh saddler's son. He studied in Edinburgh under the first Munro, then went to Philadelphia where he became acquainted with Benjamin Franklin's discovery of electricity. He returned to London to build in 1780 under the patronage of the Duchess of Devonshire an edifice termed the Temple of Health. This temple (situated just off the Strand) contained statues, paintings, incense burners and other furnishings and decorations that created a sensuous erotic environment. Its 'tour de force' was an electrified, celestial bed which promised sexual rejuvenation for the impotent and guaranteed conception for the childless. The master or rather mistress of ceremonies in this Temple of Health was a dancer named Emma Lyon who was to later become Lady Hamilton the mistress of Lord Horatio Nelson.

In the wake of Mesmer came a number of quacks who played upon the gullible and earned substantial fortunes. One of the best known of these was Guiseppe Balsano (1743–1793) a native of Palermo, also called Count Alessandro di Cagliostro. He was both a doctor and an occultist, and was a favoured physician in the court of Louis XVI at the same time as Mesmer. He claimed miraculous cures through his occult powers. Cagliostro came to disrepute and disgrace following an involvement in a scandal with the Cardinal de Rohan and Countess de la Motte, a lady in the service of Marie Antoinette. He fled to Rome but was arrested as a heretic, a swindler and freemason. He was incarcerated in the Castle of San Leo where he died.

American Medicine

Doctors in America had been trained chiefly in England or Scotland. Many had studied medicine at the university of Edinburgh. The influence of the Edinburgh school of medicine spread and flourished in the new world and there was no distinct American medicine until after the war of American Independence, when the United States of America came into being. James Morgan (1735–1789) was trained by both William Hunter of London and the first Munro at Edinburgh. On his return from Edinburgh in 1761, he published a *Discussion on the Institution of Medical Schools in America*. In the same year he founded the medical school in the university of Pennsylvania and was appointed to the Chair of Medicine. He gained fame and prestige as the director-general and surgeon-general of the American army. William Shippen Jr. was also trained in Edinburgh. He was Morgan's colleague in Philadelphia, was professor of anatomy and surgery and was appointed the second surgeon-general of the American army. Shippen opened his own private lying-in obstetric hospital—the first in the country.

The first general hospital for the sick poor was started in Philadelphia in 1751. Benjamin Franklin tried hard to raise private subscriptions to build this hospital. When sufficient private funds were not forthcoming, the Assembly gave a matching grant of £2000 to enable the Pennsylvania General Hospital to be built. The New York Hospital was established twenty years later and the Massachusetts General Hospital in 1811. The Harvard Medical School was initiated in 1783. The school gave diplomas on completion of study, and, twenty years later, a Harvard diploma served as a license to practise in the state of Massachusetts.

The most prominent and rather controversial figure in American medicine was Benjamin Rush (1745–1813). He was born in Philadelphia, and, like many Americans, studied in Edinburgh and on his return was appointed professor of chemistry and later of medicine in the Philadelphia school of

Medicine. He went into politics when the American colony rebelled against Britain and was a signatory to the American Declaration of Independence. He was the founder of a number of societies, a good teacher and a fairly astute clinician. Some hailed him as the American Sydenham—a comparison in my opinion rather unfair to the great Sydenham. His passion for blood-letting as a panacea for many diseases and his theory that a hyperactive state of arteries was the underlying factor in disease has been commented upon earlier. Rush considered calomel a universal medicine and strongly advocated the use of calomel (mercurous chloride) purges.

When yellow fever struck the eastern coast of North America, Philadelphia came under the grip of this epidemic. Benjamin Rush first believed that the disease was contagious and could perhaps be spread by mosquitoes. He later changed his mind and attributed the epidemic to an infectious miasma arising from a cargo of coffee on the quayside.

41 Surgery in the Age of Reason

Surgery up to the eighteenth century carried no prestige. Surgeons in contrast to physicians knew nothing of liberal arts, of natural science or philosophy and were often caricatured as barbers with whom they were earlier apprenticed and associated, or even worse were compared to butchers. By the mid-eighteenth century the leading universities of France, Germany and England started professorial chairs in surgery and barbers were at last separated from surgeons. The first country to do so was France.The Royal Academy of Surgery was founded in France in 1731 and, by a royal dictat, barbers were forbidden to practise surgery. The first president of this Royal Academy was Jean-Louis Petit (1674–1760). He invented the screw tourniquet and devised an operation for mastoidectomy.

In London, an outstanding surgeon was William Cheselden (1688–1752). He was also an architect and he designed the Surgeon's Hall in London. He was reputed to work with the speed of lightning and could perform a lithotomy in 54 seconds! Cheselden's greatest pupil was John Hunter (1728–1793). John to start with joined his already famous brother William who had established his school of anatomy at Picadilly in London. He soon became an avid dissector and under his brother's tutelage he grew to be one of the most skilful surgeons, and perhaps the most brilliant surgical investigator, researcher and experimenter of his age. He made invaluable contributions to pathology, surgical anatomy, and comparative physiology; he pioneered studies on inflammation and on diseases of the vascular system. He described phlebitis, shock, gunshot wounds and aneurysms of arteries, and distinguished the hard chancre of syphilis (Hunter's ulcer) from the soft chancroid ulcer. However, like others before him he confused the issue between syphilis and gonorrhoea. This confusion arose from a self-experiment when he injected the discharge from a patient with gonorrhoea into himself and observed that he developed a syphilitic chancre. He concluded from this self-experiment in his book on *Venereal Disease* (1786), that gonorrhoea and syphilis were the same disease. This wrong conclusion was due to his inability to realize that the patient must have been infected with both gonorrhoea and syphilis and the discharge that he inoculated into himself contained the germs of syphilis. Hunter unwittingly perpetuated the confusion between gonorrhoea and syphilis—a confusion which continued for another seventy years.

Hunter found time to operate, to experiment, to investigate and yet still had time enough to write extensively on his work and experience in surgery. His main surgical treatises were on *Observations on Certain Parts of the Animal Oeconomy* (1786), *Treatise on the Blood,* and *Inflammation and Gunshot Wounds* (1794). Perhaps his greatest innovation in surgery was the treatment of aneurysms involving arteries supplying the extremities. He advocated the use of a single proximal ligature rather than amputation, perhaps thereby saving the limbs of a number of individuals.

In his personal life, he was both unconventional and eccentric. He had built himself a large unusual house in Earl's Court which became a menagerie for all kinds of animals, including leopards and lions. Over the years he meticulously amassed an incredibly huge personal collection of anatomical specimens and skeletons not only of humans but of various animals. He guarded these zealously in his private house. Hunter thoroughly enjoyed his reputation for eccentricity, sometimes fostering it, as on the occasion when he is said to have driven a buffalo in harness through the streets of London.

In 1783, Hunter acquired a prize specimen to add to his collection. He had frequently expressed a great and morbid desire to acquire the skeleton of the Irish giant John Byrne and kept a close watch on the whereabouts of this giant. When Byrne did die (all giants generally die young), Hunter with cleverness and a great deal of cunning did finally manage to acquire this skeleton. About 13,000 of the specimens in the Hunterian collection became the core of the Hunterian Museum of the Royal College of Surgeons.

Hunter trained many students who were to gain eminence. His most distinguished pupil was Edward Jenner. Others included Astley Cooper, John Abernethy and Henry Cline. He also trained Philip Syng Physic who took the Hunterian surgical skills he had learned to New York and the New World. His students carried the banner of Hunterian surgery into the next century. Hunter continued with his work in surgery till his death. He was a quick-tempered man and suffered from angina. During one such episode of angina, he looked at himself in the mirror and noticing the

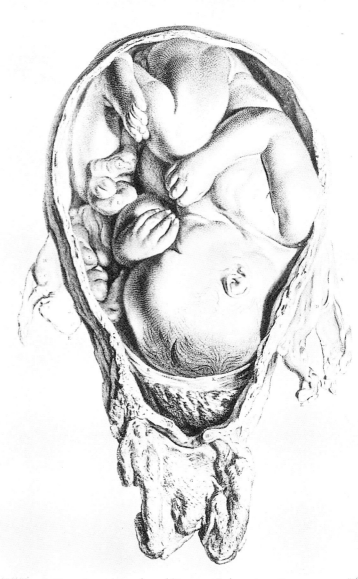

Fig. 41.1   The anatomy of the human gravid uterus exhibited in figures.

pallor on his face remarked, "It was as if a dead man was looking at himself." He had predicted that his life was in the hands of any rascal who chose to annoy him. His prediction proved correct, for he died following a public debate during which he was vastly angered by the contradictions of his colleagues.

John Hunter signalled the arrival of surgery as a science—no longer was it a craft; it was a discipline based on sound scientific principles. Did Hunter not prove that the ideal surgeon could think, investigate and experiment like a physician and could also use his hands and fingers to greater effect? The surgeon could finally look the physician in the eye.

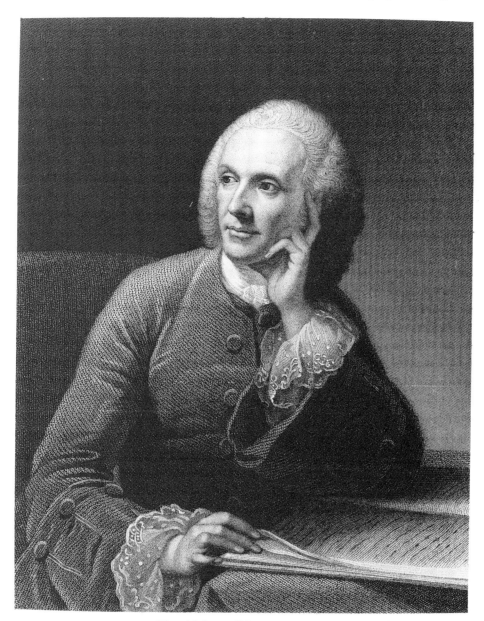

Fig. 41.2   William Hunter.

John Hunter's contemporary in London was Sir Perceival Pott (1714–1788) who wrote a classic account of the occupational hazard of scrotal cancer in chimney-sweepers. He also wrote treatises on hernia, hydrocele, fistula and head injuries. When he was confined to bed by a fall in the street, he wrote his description on fractures of the tibia and fibula above the ankle—Pott's fracture.

The technical skills in surgery were however vastly limited by the pain inflicted on the patient as also by infection. William Cheseldon who lectured in surgery and anatomy at the St Thomas' Hospital, in London made the bladder stone his speciality, publishing his *Treatise on the High Operation for the Stone* in 1723. It is interesting to briefly recapitulate the history of lithotomy first reported in the western world by Celsus in the first century AD. Celsus incised the neck of the bladder through the perineum, and with one finger in the rectum the stone was pushed out through the incision—a technique known as apparatus minor, as no special instruments were necessary.

Mariano Santo of Barletta (1485–1550) dilated and incised the urethra just anterior to the bladder neck and with a special instrument removed the bladder stone—the technique was called apparatus major because special instruments were involved.

Jacques de Beaulieu (1651–1719) was an untrained individual who as an itinerant practitioner sold his expertise from place to place. He was also called Frère Jacques because for reasons of safety he travelled in Franciscan attire with a large broad-brimmed hat of a Franciscan friar. He performed lithotomy with the patient in the lateral posture, cutting through the perineum into both the bladder neck and the bladder to remove the stone. He also operated upon hernias, undoubtedly had great skill and greater speed and is reported to have done over 4,000 lithotomies and 2,000 hernias in a twenty-year span. Cheselden in the eighteenth century substituted the lithotomy technique then prevailing for the technique in the lateral posture which had been followed by Frère Jacques. Cheselden could remove a stone in a minute. He probably reflected the general feeling of many surgeons when he exclaimed that he endured great anxiety and sickness before an operation, but that his uneasiness vanished when he started to operate.

Other new surgical techniques included the extraction of the lens from within the eye—a technique perfected by the French surgeon Jacques Daviel (1696–1762). He performed several hundred such operations with success.

The teaching of surgery now took on as firm a footing as medicine. Surgery, was thus taught with medicine in Paris and by Alexander Munro in Edinburgh. In far-away Madrid, Spain's Antonio de Gimbernat in 1793 founded the Royal College of Surgery. Pedro Virgili, his contemporary, founded the Royal College of Surgeons in Cadiz. The Enlightened Age had to an extent enlightened surgery.

Public Health, Jenner and the Discovery of Vaccination

The devil or the evil spirits controlling disease (the ancients believed in these spirits) must have laughed at the attempts of man to enlighten this age and relieve suffering. Epidemics continued to rage as in previous centuries. Bubonic plague decimated 3,00,000 in Prussia in 1709, and exanthematous typhus killed 3,000 French in 1741. Malaria, diphtheria and pertussis were widespread and took a heavy toll. Yellow fever endemic in Africa made its presence felt for the first time in Europe in 1723. Water and food-borne infections, cholera and typhoid continued as in the previous centuries and tuberculosis, particularly involving the lungs, was alarmingly frequent.

Though eighteenth century cities were an improvement on crowded, medieval towns—public health and hygiene continued to be primitive. There was no sanitation, excrement being thrown into the streets. Sewers were few and when present were open and unpaved; sewage often found its way into sources of drinking water causing repeated epidemics.

The greatest scourge of mankind besides bubonic plague was smallpox. It was an infectious disease and in the case of an epidemic, spread like wild-fire respecting neither prince nor pauper, neither the strong and rich, nor the weak and poor. A severe attack was invariably fatal; survivors were scarred and hideously pock-marked for life. Queen Mary of England (1662–1694) and Louis XV of France (1710–1774) died of smallpox. Periodic epidemics in Europe and in other parts of the world would decimate populations of cities and villages. In bad years smallpox alone was responsible for more than a tenth of all the deaths in Europe.

An attack of smallpox conferred immunity from this dreaded disease for life. In ancient India and in Ottoman Turkey attempts at prevention and protection took the form of variolation, wherein a very small amount of material of a patient's pox was scarified into the skin or inserted into the nose of a healthy individual, or as in Turkey pushed into a vein. The aim was to produce mild disease without inviting a full attack of the hideously deforming pox. In 1713, a Greek physician Emanuel Timoni of Constantinople had submitted a report on variolation to the Royal Society but had been ignored. The idea of variolation gained attention only after Lady Mary Montagu, wife of the British Ambassador in Turkey, wrote a letter in 1713 that she had her three-year-old son innoculated in the above fashion. Three years later during an epidemic in London she had her five-year-old daughter also undergo variolation. She urged this protection on the royal family. Human experiments on condemned felons followed and the Prince of Wales who was later King George II had his daughter undergo variolation. In England the Sutton family, Robert (1707–1788) and his son Daniel (1735–1819), surgeons in the countryside who claimed to have standardized variolation, 'variolated' a large number of people with a small death rate.

In France variolation was supported by the philosophers. Thomas Dimsdale (1712–1800) an English surgeon variolated Catherine the Great and her family and was amply rewarded for his services. But the overall spread of variolation by the method stated above was slow. Perhaps this was partly related to religious and moral objections and partly to the uncertainty of the results. The risk of death from severe smallpox after variolation was always there and though played down by its protagonists could have been quite significant. Variolation as practised above could never possibly be standardized satisfactorily and almost certainly a wider use of this method would have caused severe disease and a number of deaths from smallpox. Smallpox in spite of the above attempts at prevention continued to ravage the world.

Then came Edward Jenner (1749–1823), a man who has probably done more for the benefit of mankind than any human being before or after. Edward Jenner was born in Berkley in Gloucestershire, and from his childhood was keen to become a doctor. He did not enter a university and perhaps was not well acquainted with the liberal arts. At the age of thirteen he apprenticed himself to a surgeon in Bristol learning practical surgery for a period of six years. One fine day a countrywoman came into the surgery and made a profound remark on smallpox: "I cannot get this disease because I have had cowpox." This remark probably made a great impression on young Jenner's mind, and he noted its truth in his practice among the farming families that he looked after. Jenner at the age of 21 years then moved on to London where he became the student and later a friend of the great surgeon John Hunter. Perhaps Jenner learnt the basics of experimentation in medicine from Hunter, perhaps he was inspired by the investigative skill, tenacity and intellect of this great surgeon. Jenner discussed his views with Hunter on innoculating cowpox (so common in

milkmaids milking cows infected with this pox) with the idea of preventing smallpox. The chance remark of his patient on cowpox during his Bristol days must have made an indelible imprint on his mind. Hunter is said to have remarked "I think your solution is just. But why think? Why not try the experiment?" After spending two years (perhaps tired of life) in London, he returned to Berkley in Gloucestershire to practise as a country doctor.

Jenner again confirmed the immunity conferred by cowpox to an attack of smallpox. He studied the problem systematically for 20 years before performing his decisive experiment. On 14 May 1796 he took the contents of a pustule from the hand of a milk-maid infected with cowpox and innoculated it into the arm of a healthy eight year old boy. This had no ill effects. Six weeks later Jenner innoculated the same child with the contents of a pustule from a victim of human smallpox. The eight year old boy remained well and did not contract smallpox. One can imagine the deep anxiety and trepidation and yet the courage of his conviction which made him perform a human

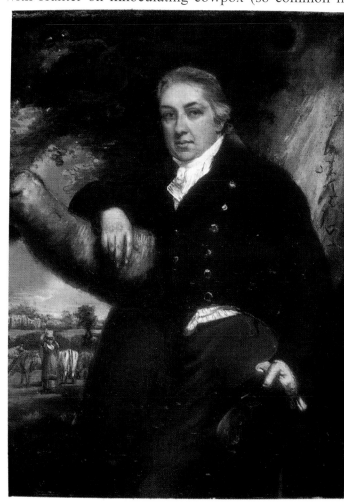

Fig. 42.1   Portrait of Edward Jenner leaning against a tree, with a milkmaid in the background.

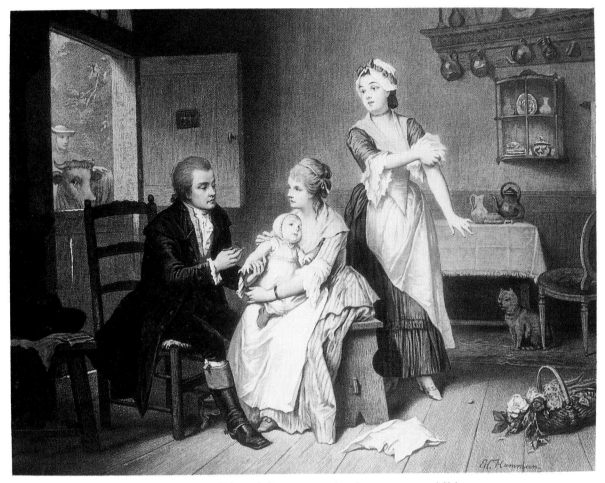

Fig. 42.2   Edward Jenner vaccinating a young child.

experiment, which if repeated under the same circumstances in today's time could bring shame and opprobrium on the experimenter. Jenner repeated his experiment on several others and confirmed his findings. He reported his results to the Royal Society of which he was a member on the strength of his zoological work. The Royal Society advised him to forthwith stop his experiments, warning him that he was endangering the reputation he enjoyed. But this country doctor, perhaps not supremely intelligent, yet humble, and extremely practical ignored this advice, continued his work and finally published in 1798, a small book titled *An Inquiry into the Causes and Effects of Variolae Vaccinae*.

Violent emotions for and against Jenner and his practice of vaccination in the prevention of smallpox raged for a time all over Europe. But the results were there for all to see and vaccination against smallpox spread first all over Europe and then all over the world. Jenner was lionised in his country, was voted a grant of £10,000, and in 1808 was appointed as the director of the Institute of Vaccination. Although he was modest, unpretentious country doctor, he was a good observer and an excellent experimenter. However there were many more gifted men in this age who achieved little by comparison. Is it not strange that the Lord should have chosen a man such as Jenner to confer one of the greatest benefits to mankind? Perhaps because he was aloof from the controversies of the various schools of thought in medicine, perhaps because he was intellectually honest for he refused to theorize as to why vaccination with cowpox should prevent smallpox. Strange again that the greatest triumph ever in preventive medicine should have stemmed as an empirical fact deduced from mere experiment and observation. It would be over a hundred years before the basic features of immunity would explain Jenner's discovery. Jenner in a way was a hundred years before his time. He in my opinion is among the greatest immortals that walked this planet, and he must not have even dreamed that it would be so.

Europe and the United States of America saw a sharp decline in the incidence of small pox after the widespread use of preventive vaccination. Smallpox however had world-wide prevalence. In those days of poor communication and slow travel how did the rest of the world fare? Poorly indeed, in spite of the evangelical spirit of a few doctors. To give just one outstanding example, a Spanish physician, Francisco Javier de Balmis took twenty-two children who had been innoculated on a 'vaccinating journey' around the world innoculating hundreds of thousands of persons in South America, Philippines, Macao and Canton. Smallpox however reared its ugly head again and again in the poor developing Third World countries till just a few years ago. It not only required the genius of Jenner who discovered vaccination in 1796, but the financial clout and vast administrative network of the World Health Organisation together with the will to succeed in Third World countries that has finally rid the world of this scourge.

Public health towards the end of the eighteenth century became a concern for the state. There was a purposeful decline in monastic hospitals in Austria, the money meant for these monasteries being used to improve the hospitals in Vienna. The most famous general hospital on the continent towards the end of the eighteenth century was the Vienna Allgemeines Krankenhaus rebuilt by Joseph II in 1784. The hospital looked after 1,600 patients, reserved 18 beds for clinical teaching, and catered specially to the needs of the poor sick of Vienna. Similar large state-financed hospitals were built by Joseph II in Linz and Prague. The increasing population of the major cities of the world and the increasing awareness of the poor and sick of their rights in this age of enlightenment made it imperative for the state to finance public health. As mentioned earlier, most of London's great general hospitals had already been founded by 1760. Attention was next directed to special hospitals e.g., for venereal disease, for smallpox and for special groups, e.g., seamen. A cancer ward was endowed by the brewer Samuel Whitbread to the Middlesex hospital in 1791. A similar trend was observed in state-sponsored hospitals on the continent. The Berlin Charity Hospital was built in 1768, and Catherine the Great (1762–1796) built the state-owned Obuchow Hospital in St Petersburg.

The eighteenth century also saw reforms in prisons and dungeons which were hell-holes with subhuman conditions. John Howard (1726–1790) was an Englishman who after suffering imprisonment in France, was a man obsessed in improving prison conditions. He travelled thousands of miles all over Europe visiting its prisons and dungeons, and in 1789 wrote an influential indictment titled *Account of the Principle Lazerettoes of Europe,* arousing the pressing urgency for prison reforms.

Public health required data on populations, birth rates, death rates and death rates in known epidemic diseases. The Prussian army chaplain Johann Peter Sussmilch (1707–1777), pioneered vital statistics collecting data in relation to life insurance, epidemics and public hygiene. Peter the Great of Russia organized a census in Russia, but with the selfish motive of ensuring taxation rather than for reasons of public health. Sweden established a centralized system for collecting birth rates, death rates and other vital statistics in 1748, whilst the the United Kingdom did so in 1801. The principles of preventive disease were extended to important groups of societies like the army and the navy. The history of many wars had clearly shown that more men had died from disease than from battle. Sir John Pringle (1707–1782), was a Leiden trained Scotsman who was a doctor in the

British army. His observations on the *Disease of the Army* published in 1752 described basic preventive measures for common illnesses such as dysentery, typhoid, typhus and scabies. Pringle will perhaps be better remembered for securing the neutrality of military hospitals during battle. He proposed to the French commander at the battle of Dettingen, in 1743, that hospital tents on each side be spared from attack. The proposal was accepted and prevailed to some extent in future battles as well.

Sailors at sea often suffered severely from scurvy, a disease which was noted to be widespread even in the Baroque period. Lord Anson (1697–1762), during his world expedition of 1740–1744, lost close to 1,000 of the 1,950 sailors from scurvy by the time the expedition returned. The disease caused swollen gums, bruises, swollen joints, lassitude and death from bleeding or heart failure. James Lind (1716–1791), a Scottish naval surgeon investigated this disease and in his *Treatise on the Scurvy* (1753), concluded that citrus fruits were effective for cure. He supported his thesis by what was probably the first controlled trial in medicine performed on the HMS Salisbury in 1754. Lind chose twelve scurvy patients—two were given vinegar, two sea water, two had a quart of cider a day, two a mixture of garlic, radish, balsam and myrrh, two had oil of vitriol and two had oranges and lemons. Those on oranges and lemons were cured in six days, and Lind put them to work to nurse the other ten who remained ill. Lind did not realize that scurvy was due to a deficiency of vitamin C. He postulated that scurvy was due to moist air clogging the sweat pores and preventing escape of toxins because of blocked perspiration. Lemon juice he felt acted as a detergent which split toxic particles to a very small size allowing them to squeeze through the sweat pores in the skin. Lind's recommendations were not followed to start with, and scurvy remained an occupational hazard in the navy. James Cook (1728–1779) and other naval commanders stressed the importance of an integrated approach with proper diet, exercise, good ventilation, cleanliness, and the use of lemons, lime and oranges. Cook also stressed the antiscorbutic properties of onions, cabbages and malt. The navy finally issued lemon juice as a compulsory item to all sailors and scurvy disappeared from the British fleet. Perhaps the claim made by some historians that lemons were as responsible as Nelson for the defeat of Napoleon may have a modicum of truth!

The Age of Enlightenment came to an end with a clap of thunder. The French Revolution unseated the Bourbons and shook the other monarchies of Europe. The power of the aristocracy was increasingly challenged by a burgeoning middle class all over Europe. The first half of the century had deified reason. The end of the century saw the expression of a fervid romanticism breeding unreasonable dogmas. There were no earth-shaking scientific discoveries in medicine comparable for example to that of Harvey's discovery of circulation in the preceding century. Yet the spirit of scientific inquiry prospered—its flame burnt bright and strong. There came a prodigy such as Haller, as universal a man as almost any produced by the Renaissance, there came Morgagni who fathered modern pathology, Hunter who fathered surgery and surgical anatomy, Boerhaave who brought Hippocrates to life and there came a number of greater and lesser stars keen to ferret out the secrets of life, disease and nature. Yet man's destiny was for ever threatened by disease and early death. Medical science translated to patient care continued to have a dismal record. But yes, there was one broad beam of light that illuminated the practice of medicine. It was the discovery of vaccination in the prevention of smallpox—the first discovery in medicine which sounded, however faintly, the possible death-knell of a dreaded disease, the first hope in medicine that has indeed been fulfilled in our time.

Modern Medicine

43 Historical Background of the Modern Age

A physician is obligated to consider more than a diseased organ, more even than the whole Man—he must view the Man in his world.

Harvey Cushing

Modern medicine as we know and practise it today can be traced to the beginning of the nineteenth century. Medicine from now on did not advance in small, slow, struggling steps as it had done in the past two thousand and more years—it appeared to move forward by leaps and bounds.

Discoveries in medical science multiplied, particularly during the last three decades of the nineteenth century, spilling over into the first quarter or more of the next. Confining the history of medicine solely to the nineteenth century and then proceeding to the twentieth century would interrupt this narrative. Also attempting to trace and describe every aspect of the changing face of medicine during this period would perhaps result in a cataloguing of a mass of details, in which the essence and far-reaching effects of major discoveries could be blurred. This section encompasses the major events and the men and women who shaped these events in the nineteenth century, and in the first twenty to thirty years of the next. The section on Contemporary Medicine covers the remaining years of the twentieth century medicine. Both the nineteenth and twentieth centuries could be termed the centuries of revolution or of revolutionary change that influenced all fields of human thought and endeavour, encompassing politics, economics, philosophy, basic sciences, technology, medicine, art, architecture and literature.

This period of man's history spanned an enormous gap between the world of horse-drawn coaches, mounted couriers and sailing ships, to the world of railways, trans-atlantic liners, aeroplanes and the radio; between imperialism, and a world pulled apart by capitalism, communism and socialism; between the treatment by massive blood-letting in the early part of the century, and the use of anaesthesia and asepsis by the second half of the nineteenth century.

The past 200 years also illustrated the intrinsic and indivisible link between the history of man and the history of medicine. Medicine did not change in an isolated milieu or as an isolated phenomenon. It was merely a part of a change that altered the whole fabric of human society; and each aspect of life and living influenced the other so that a new picture of the world emerged—a picture that even today is changing faster than it ever did, so that if we were to revisit the world even a hundred years from now, we would perhaps find ourselves on an alien planet. To appreciate the history of medicine in this period we must therefore look at all the basic features of the overall history of man and the world he inhabited.

Historical Background

The last decade of the eighteenth century and the first fifteen years of the nineteenth century in Europe were dominated by Napoleon Bonaparte. It was the age of Napoleon, one of the greatest geniuses of all time, superior to all other men of action by virtue of his far-ranging intelligence, his leadership and his sense of reality coupled with an imagination on which great men thrive. Rousseau perhaps fathered the French revolution, Napoleon was its child, its soul force, its incarnation; he first defended it and then became its 'uniformed missionary', spreading its seeds and its ideals far and wide all over the world. As a general, as a consul, and till the early days of the Empire, he was cast in a heroic mould. But then absolute power corrupted him. He made grievous mistakes, aroused the hatred of many conquered people, and unleashed counter-forces that engulfed and overwhelmed him. Like a meteor he flashed brilliantly across the sky and crashed with a thunder that resonated all over the world. A man of vision, it was he who believed in one Europe albeit under France's suzerainty, he who visualized a possible under-sea tunnel connecting France to England—now a reality.

He opened the doors of opportunity in all fields of human endeavour to the ordinary people of France giving the country a new foundation which has stood the test of two centuries. In transforming France he left a continuing, indelible influence on the western world. Medicine flourished under his influence and patronage and the medical school of Paris gained renown, influencing medical schools in all major centres of Europe.

The post-Napoleonic era (after the Treaty of Vienna in 1815) was shaped by important political and economic forces. The important political forces dominating this century were the continuing

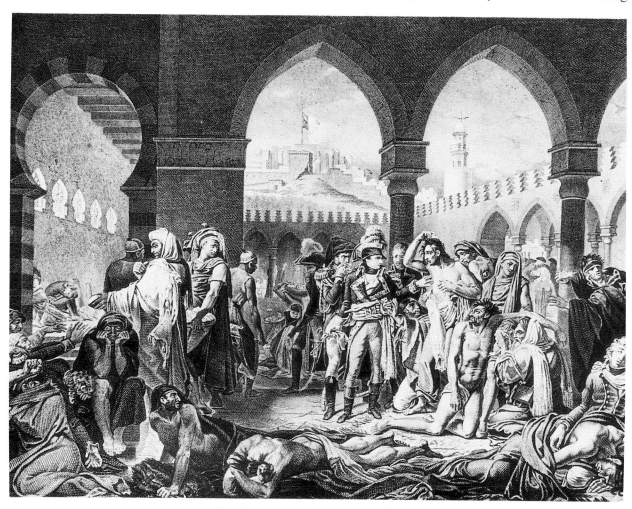

Fig. 43.1   Napoleon Bonaparte visiting plague-stricken soldiers at Jaffa in 1799.

struggle of republican movements against monarchy and feudalism, the growth of nationalism in countries under alien domination, and the continuing growth and establishment of colonial empires by powerful countries such as England and France.

The surge of nationalism reshaped the map of Europe. Between 1815 and 1850, the Greeks overthrew their Turkish rulers, Poland fought for liberty against Russia, Hungary sought to free itself from Austria, Italy was united as one single country for the first time in its history after breaking its shackles from Austria, and the Prussians sowed the seeds of a unified Germany. By the turn of the century the face of Europe had changed—Germany, Italy, Greece, Serbia and Belgium had become independent nations. The nationalist fervour had spread to South America so that most of the former colonies of Portugal and Spain in that continent were now sovereign states.

Remarkably enough the surge of nationalism in Europe and the Americas was associated *pari passu* with the rise and expansion of new empires. The greatest empire was the British Empire, on which, by the turn of the century, literally the sun never set. British colonial rule extended into Africa, the Middle East, India, South-East Asia, Canada, Australia, and the West Indies. India was the jewel in the British Crown. An Indian mutiny, in 1857, attempted to oust the British from the country but failed. British rule over India persisted upto the middle of the twentieth century. France had its share of colonial rule in Africa and South-East Asia. Russia marched eastwards through Central and Eastern Asia to reach the pacific coast. In the second half of the century trade routes to China and Japan were opened up by western nations; the riches of the East were now at the mercy of the West.

The single most important economic force in the nineteenth century was the Industrial Revolution. Its impact on all human affairs was so immense that the two halves of the century were disparate and appeared almost as two separate civilizations. In a short span of time the light from candles was replaced by the light from gas and electricity, railways supplanted stage-coaches, steam ships and ocean liners took the place of sailing boats; the telegraph, telephone, and radio revolutionized communication. The early automobile, towards the end of the nineteenth century, resembled a horseless carriage careening down at thirty miles per hour on open country roads or along the streets of New York, London and Paris.

Man's dream of flying in the air became an incredible reality. Aviation was born as balloons soared high into the air, and by the turn of the century, the Wright brothers flew in an aeroplane for the first time in history. The science of metallurgy made rapid progress. The manufacture of steel was revolutionized by the Bessemer process—steel became one of the symbols of the age. Agriculture was revolutionized by chemistry and machinery and the yield of crops rose manifold. The Industrial Revolution ushered in the Industrial Age, the Age of the machine and of technology. It is an age which has continued to grow and will probably dominate our lives and our living for many centuries to come.

The effects of the Industrial Revolution from the mid-nineteenth century onwards were enormous. People flocked from the countryside and villages to the cities. Cities grew bigger, almost bursting at the seams. Men, women and even children worked with machines in factories. Often living conditions were deplorable. Sanitation and hygiene grew increasingly primitive, as slums housing the poor workmen mushroomed around factories and in large cities. Disease spread, epidemics of various infections were common, public health was at its nadir. The working class (as these factory workers came to be called) was increasingly exploited. It appeared that there was a human price to be paid if wealth were to increase and that capitalism in this age had an ugly face.

The reaction to this machine age took many forms varying from the Luddites who destroyed the new machines, to the evolution of social and economic thinking that gave birth to both socialism and communism. An important reaction to the Industrial Age was the emergence of humanitarianism. Individuals and organizations championed the cause of the workers, of the poor and downtrodden. Slavery was abolished in the British Empire by an act of parliament in 1833, and a Factory Act limited the working hours of children and young persons to ten hours per day. Charitable bodies organised distribution of food, gifts and necessities to the poor. Factories and mines were pressurized to offer better safety measures at work. The workers themselves formed associations for better wages and better working conditions, culminating in this century in the formation of powerful trade unions.

Women played an important role in this increasing surge of humanitarianism. Mary Carpenter founded the first slum school in 1846, Elizabeth Fry worked for prison reform, Mary Wollstonecroft championed the rights of women. Friedrich Froebel, in 1846, founded the first kindergarten school. Numerous such schools were then founded in the West, as were creches for the children of the working class and foundling homes.

By the middle and later years of the nineteenth century, the power of the aristocracy was increasingly balanced by a new *noveau riche* middle class that arose from the industrial and financial worlds. Queen Victoria of England spread the power and influence of her country far and wide through a parliament ably led by an intelligent visionary prime minister, Benjamin Disraeli. Frederick the Great of Prussia laid the foundation of an increasingly powerful and belligerent Germany. The animosity of England towards France, evident from Napoleonic times, persisted through this century. Bismarck in Prussia ruled with an iron hand, waged war against France, defeating Napoleon III (the nephew of Napoleon Bonaparte) in the battle of Sedan in 1875. This humiliating defeat and the treaty that followed was the forerunner of the first World War that erupted in 1914. The British Empire and France were locked in a death struggle with Germany. They were joined in this struggle by other countries of Europe—Turkey and Russia. Turkey was with Germany, Russia sided with England and France. This cataclysmic war which lasted for four agonizing years, which laid waste the fertile fields of Europe and which spilt the blood of the flower of the youth of so many European countries, was indeed made more horrific by the science and technology available to man. Germany capitulated and the Treaty of Versailles imposed a peace which was so humiliating to the vanquished that it undoubtedly led after the lapse of a decade, to a militant nationalism under Hitler's Nazi Germany.

The 1914–1918 war as a side-effect produced a shattering convulsion in Russia—the Russian Revolution, in which the Romanov dynasty was put to death and communism under Lenin seized power. From henceforth communism and capitalism would be the major contending political and economical forces in our world.

Culture

The first half of the century and in particular the Napoleonic age was dominated by a spirit of romanticism and classicism, the second half by realism. Romanticism witnessed the poetry of Byron, Keats, Shelley, Wordsworth, Chateaubriand, and Heine, and the romantic works of Alexander Dumas, Victor Hugo and Sir Walter Scott. Architecture took neo-Gothic forms. Artists painted historical or romantic themes in the genre that prevailed in the latter half of the eighteenth century.

In the second half of the century, the novelists replaced romanticism with realism, describing the problems of everyday life, the foibles, virtues, passions and vices they observed in society. There was Honoré Balzac with his wit and satire that punctured the prudery and hypocrisy of the Victorian society, Emile Zola, who championed the cause of Dreyfus, Gustave Flaubert, who in *Madame Bovary* explored the psychology of female sexuality.

It was painting however, which was a forerunner of the changing times. The Impressionists produced a form of painting related to the psychology of the times. Painting henceforth in the history of man would reflect the relation and response of society to the world he lived in. Manet, Monet, Degas, Renoir, Gaugin, Van Gogh and several others broke away from traditional painting. The interplay of light and shadow was through the use of colours, producing a strong and often disturbing visual impact. Colour often became the central focus of a picture independent of form or theme. Cézanne, towards the end of the nineteenth century, painted landscapes imbued with an elemental force through an analysis of structure into basic shapes and forms. He was indeed the first to hint at the direction modern art would take in the twentieth century. Painting in the early years of the twentieth century was indeed predictive of the discipline of times to come. Picasso, probably the greatest painter of the modern age, painted in 1907 his *'Demoiselles D' Avignon'*, which aroused shock at the disruption and distortion of the human form that characterized this work of art. Picasso and Braque with several others now graduated into Cubism where the geometry of figure and forms was explored by splitting a composition into its small cubist shapes gathered together to form a whole. The analogy of physicists considering matter to be made of small atoms held together was inescapable. Whilst Picasso, Braque and many others concentrated on exploring form, Matisse explored colours, so that his paintings were like a symphony of gorgeous colours, a sensuous feast for the eyes.

The Philosophers

The leading schools of political and economic thought held two opposing views. One school believed in the power of the state in evolving a utopian society of equality, the other school believed that any form of government was unsuitable and unworthy. George William Hegel (1770–1831) belonged to the first school. He philosophized that the evolution of history was related to the interplay of forces, a thesis resulting in its opposite (antithesis), the two together resulting in synthesis. He philosophized that an organized state could conform to the highest human ideas and could benefit mankind. Pierre Prudhon in France and Michael Bakunin in Russia preached an anarchist philosophy maintaining that all forms of government and all property-ownership was evil and deserved to be abolished.

The philosophic school of politicians believed in the inevitable progress of mankind and of civilization. Its main protagonists were August Comte (1798–1857) of France and Herbert Spencer (1830–1903) of England. At the other end of the spectrum was Arthur Schopenhauer's (1788–1860) nihilistic view that social progress was an illusion, and the destiny of the universe and man was blind and lacked purpose or direction.

Friedrich Nietzsche (1844–1900) was not concerned with good and evil, but he propounded the doctrine of the superman who was above and beyond good and evil. He epitomized his views in *Thus Spake Zarathustra,* and perhaps unwittingly encouraged the Nazis of Hilter's Germany in the twentieth century to consider themselves as a super-race.

Undoubtedly, the most revolutionary thinker of the twentieth century was the great English naturalist Charles Darwin (1809–1882), who in his book *Origin of Species* (1859), expounded the law of natural selection, thereby opening up new vistas in medicine. His theory on the evolution of man was based on the gathering of scientific facts from biological data obtained during his prolonged travels to various parts of the world. He expressed these scientific facts within the framework of a single idea that shook the Victorian world to its foundations, stirring up a storm of furious controversy. This controversy raged all through the second half of the nineteenth century between religion and science, between religious fundamentalists who believed in the creation of man as revealed in the Bible and the others who believed that man evolved from the animal kingdom—his immediate forefather being the monkey. Julian Huxley has perhaps correctly dubbed Charles Darwin as the 'Newton of Biology'.

Basic Sciences

The spirit of scientific inquiry grew increasingly strong and a number of nature's secrets lay unravelled by the end of the nineteenth century. The first quarter of the twentieth century saw monumental discoveries in basic physics—discoveries that altered our concept of the world and ushered in a new era full of both promise and uncertainty. Astronomy flourished as never before, and was largely related to improvement in the construction of telescopes and a burning curiosity to study the universe we inhabit. Astronomers in 1800 had listed about 3,000 stars; by the turn of the century, 45,000 astral bodies had been mapped and documented!

The century opened with John Dalton in 1803 reviving the ancient Greek theory that elements were composed of small invisible atoms. Dimitri Mendeleyev, the Russian chemist had published his periodic classification of elements. Modern chemistry and biochemistry were pioneered by Germany in the early twentieth century. In 1828, Friedrich Wohler (1800–1882), in an epoch-making event produced urea from ammonium carbonate. This was a startling discovery, as till then it was believed that organic compounds could only be formed by living tissues and stood distinct from inorganic compounds. Wohler's discovery destroyed this sharp distinction between inorganic and organic compounds. This was the beginning of organic chemistry and biochemistry. Justus Von Liebig (1803–1873) investigated many organic chemical compounds derived from food and waste products and discovered chloral and chloroform. Numerous hypotheses were advanced to explain the chemical structure of organic compounds. In 1865, the German chemist Friedrich Kekulé von Stradunitz worked out the theory and structure of the benzene ring—a discovery of fundamental importance in modern chemistry. By the turn of the century 70,000 chemical compounds had been discovered and analysed.

Pioneering studies on plant physiology were conducted by Jagdish Chandra Bose (1858–1937) from India. Bose devised sensitive instruments that detected minute responses in living organisms enabling him to note the parallelism between plant tissue and animal tissue. His research on plant behaviour showed astounding results. He observed through extremely sensitive automatic recorders capable of recording the slightest movement, that plants had feelings exemplified by their quivering after insult or injury. Bose was also a renowned physicist who contributed to the development of organic state physics. His three major works are *Response to Living and Non-Living* (1902), *Plant Response* (1906), and *Mechanism of Plants* (1926).

The science of physics made phenomenal progress. A vital and fundamental discovery was the discovery in 1845 of the law of conservation of energy by James Prescott Joule and Robert Jules Mayer. This discovery opened the door to the study of thermodynamics and the application of energy released by heat for various practical uses. In 1831, Michael Faraday discovered electricity, electromagnetism and electromagnetic induction, introducing to the world the electrical generator and electric motor. In 1879, Thomas Alva Edison of the United States of America devised the first incandescent electric lamp.

The great advances in this century in optics on the nature of light led to the fundamental discovery of spectrum analysis. This led to the study of the intimate nature of molecules and constituents of stars millions of miles away from the earth. In 1895, William Roentgen discovered X-rays that saw through matter, and in 1898, the Curies discovered radium which was to revolutionize the treatment of cancer.

The early years of the twentieth century saw discoveries being made by some of the greatest geniuses that the world has ever produced. These discoveries changed the concept of the universe. In 1900, Max Planck postulated that the transfer of energy in radiation was not a continuous flow, but through discontinuous small units—*quantums*. In 1905, Albert Einstein (1879–1955), perhaps the greatest genius of our times, published four research papers, each containing a great discovery in physics—the special theory of relativity, the equivalence of mass and energy, the theory of Brownian motion and the photon theory of light. Einstein's theory of relativity was summarized in a simple equation $E = mc^2$. He showed that time and space are not absolute entities as was hitherto believed, but were relative to moving systems. The maximum velocity attainable in the universe was the velocity of light; mass appeared to increase with velocity, and mass and energy are equivalent and interchangeable properties.

Einstein's photon theory postulated light quanta comparable to energy quanta postulated by Max Planck. Neils Bohr, in 1908, extended his theory to the structure of the atom. In 1919, the British physicist Ernest Rutherford, for the first time succeeded in splitting what was till then considered the indivisible atom. He bombarded the atoms of various elements with helium particles forcing them to yield hydrogen. The process of atomic fission, supplemented by the process of atomic fusion, provided a source of power and energy undreamt of in the history of man. That this energy could be used constructively to benefit mankind, and also used for its awesome destructive power which could possibly annihilate mankind, was proved in the years to come.

One of the greatest discoveries of the mid-nineteenth century was the work in genetics by the Austrian monk Gregor Johann Mendel (1822–1884), who experimented on the hybridizing of garden peas in his cloistered garden in a monastery in Bohemia. He published his results in 1868, in an article titled *Experiments in Plant Hybridization,* wherein he enunciated the principles of heredity as observed in his experiments. Mendel was thus the founder of the science of genetics, a science of immeasurable importance to man in the twenty-first century.

44 The Paris School of Medicine

Napoleon exerted a far-reaching influence on medicine in Paris, and, through Paris, to the rest of the world. During the French revolution the anarchy that prevailed in the name of equality also involved medicine so that any individual trained or untrained, for a modest fee, could acquire a legal permit to practise. Napoleon revolutionized the organization, teaching and practice of medicine—more often than not, his views on the subject were dictated from his camp-cot or his travelling-desk on battlefields during lulls between battles. He established two tiers of doctors. The first tier consisted of doctors of medicine or surgery, who after four years of medical education and training, had to pass an examination, following which they were permitted to practise anywhere in France. The second tier consisted of doctors with a lesser level of knowledge and education; these officers *de santé* were restricted to basic elementary patient care and their practice was localized to the region where they had been certified. It was not just organization, nationalization of schools, licensing and training that boosted the standards of medicine in France. Even more important was Napoleon's vision of opening all institutes of learning—schools, colleges, technical institutes, universities to talent. The potential in the populous country of France was immense—he drew on this talent, recognized and promoted it to make France what it was—a leader in almost every field of endeavour. Talented physicians and surgeons at state salary were appointed to the large public hospitals in Paris. These had 20,000 beds (more than all the hospital beds in the whole of England), and stored an immense amount of clinical material, which was taught by brilliant men to the numerous students who thronged the wards.

No longer was teaching restricted to the reading of books. Frequent physical examination of patients gave hands-on experience. Students were taught to arrive at the diagnosis, to determine the root cause of an illness through evaluation of the physical signs obtained at clinical examination. When death occurred, as it often did, a careful autopsy in every case could confirm whether the diagnosis was correct or incorrect. The clinico-pathological correlation was of supreme importance, and pathology became the arbiter and the referee of clinical medicine. It must be stressed that the Parisian outlook on medicine was not an abrupt volte-face from past practices. Sydenham of the seventeenth century, Boerhaave in the eighteenth century and the medical schools of Edinburgh and Vienna had also taught on similar lines, but these were small isolated foci of brilliance. The school of Paris consolidated clinical teaching, clinical examination, clinico-pathological correlation and spread this gospel to all cities of learning in the West. This Parisian influence persists with us to this day.

The school of Paris paid great heed to Francis Xavier Bichat's (1771–1802) basic concept of disease and the underlying pathology in disease. Morgagni had looked at organs as seats of disease, Bichat went a step further, and as explained in the earlier chapter 39, looked at tissues as the basic structure and building blocks of the human body. In his *Anatomie Generale* he wrote that different organs were constituted by a smaller number of tissues which he described in health and disease.

Bichat had a great influence on the most celebrated clinician of the early nineteenth century, Jean Nicolas Corvisart (1755–1821). He was Napoleon's personal physician, and Napoleon loved, trusted and respected him. Napoleon is said to have said of him—"I do not believe in medicine but I believe in Corvisart." Corvisart was the first to describe the symptoms of heart disease and distinguish them from the symptoms related to pulmonary disease. He was adept at the art and science of percussion of both the heart and chest, first advocated by Auenbrugger. In fact, he had translated Auenbrugger's book for the benefit of his colleagues. Corvisart was probably the first cardiologist of the modern age—in fact he called himself so. He was the first to use the term myocarditis and he embodied his clinical studies and experience on heart disease by publishing in 1806, the *Essai sur les maladies et les lesions organiques du coeur et des gros vaisseaux* (*An Essay on the Organic Diseases and Lesions of the Heart and Great Vessels*). Corvisart was an extraordinarily astute clinician. When looking at a particular portrait he is said to have remarked, "If the painter was right the man in this picture died of heart disease." This had indeed proved true; Corvisart had made a correct diagnosis by just looking at a portrait!

Corvisart's greatest pupil was René Theophile Hyacinthe Laennec (1781–1836), a name that will remain immortal in the history of medicine. Laennec was physician to the Salpêtrière hospital in 1814 and became chief at the Necker hospital two years later. It was well known that the heart made sounds when it beat. Corvisart and others would place their ears directly to the chest to hear these sounds. Laennec for many years was obsessed to hear with greater clarity sounds of the opening and closing of the heart valves during systole and diastole. It is said that one day while crossing the Louvre, he saw a boy listening with his ear to one end of a beam to scratches made by another boy with a nail at the other end of the beam. He was struck by the ease with which sound was conducted in this manner. Could he utilize this simple physical principle in medicine? In 1816, a young stout woman consulted him for symptoms suggestive of heart disease. Her young age and obesity did not permit him to put his ear directly to the chest (immediate or direct auscultation). He lightly rolled up a thick sheaf of paper placing one end over the precordium and the other end over his ear. To his delight, he heard heart sounds with greater clarity and distinctness than he had ever heard earlier by placing his ear directly to the chest. Like Archimedes many years before him he must have shouted 'Eureka', for he had instantly grasped the significance of this discovery. He immediately noted that this method of indirect auscultation would 'enable one to hear not only the beating of the heart but likewise all movements capable of producing sound in the thoracic cavity'.

Laennec in his treatise on *Mediate Auscultation* (1819), described his first monoaural stethoscope— a wooden piece 9 inches long 1½ inches in diameter. It was made in two pieces—the detachable earpiece and the chest pieces which could be screwed together. Following minor modifications, by the mid-nineteenth century, rubber tubing was introduced to create a flexible monoaural stethoscope. Finally, the familiar two-ear instrument with rubber tubings was devised by the American physician George P. Cammann in 1852. Laennec made excellent use of his invention, studied both normal and abnormal breath sounds, described them in great detail, and drew conclusions from what he heard as to the nature and extent of the disease in the chest. Above all, he verified his findings with what was revealed at autopsy. He was the first man to create a diagnostic system of auscultatory findings in the diagnosis of both pulmonary and cardiac disease. He described and gave the correct significance to adventitious sounds–rhonchi and râles, and through his system of mediate auscultation diagnosed pulmonary ailments such as bronchitis, pneumonia and tuberculosis.

Laennec's treatise on *Mediate Auscultation* focussed particularly on pulmonary tuberculosis which was rampant all over the world in the nineteenth century. He suggested methods and gave guidance

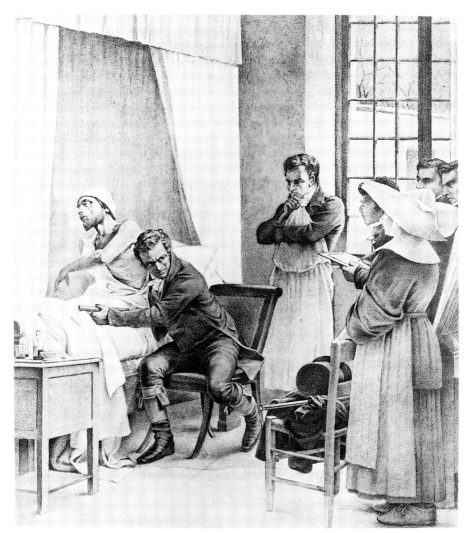

Fig. 44.1   Laennec at Necker Hospital conducting physical examination in
front of his students.

for the early diagnosis of tuberculosis. He noted the presence of the tubercle or the tuberculous nodule which was ubiquitous in every organ affected by the disease. On this basis he postulated that tuberculosis was a single disease which could affect many organ systems. This was indeed a remarkable observation considering that the tubercle bacillus causing the disease had not been discovered in Laennec's time. Laennec unfortunately himself suffered from and ultimately succumbed to tuberculosis—as did many other contemporaries, including the surgical student and poet John Keats. Laennec however did draw a few erroneous conclusions. Thus he denied that tuberculoses was contagious when it was strongly so; he believed that it was often hereditary when it was not so. He felt that psychological factors such as grief, sorrow, and unrequited love played a role in its causation and perpetuation. Laennec's name is also associated in relation to cirrhosis of the liver, which he described in great detail, and which has been known since the time of Hippocrates. He left many superb writings that prompted Thomas Addison, the English physician, to remark that Laennec contributed more to the advancement of medical art than any other single individual.

A great favourite of Napoleon during the Napoleonic wars was Jean Dominique Larrey (1766–1842), the doctor-in-chief of the Grande Armée. He was the first to organize and operate field ambulances (horse-drawn carriages) during the thick of battle, so that the wounded soldiers could be attended to promptly. Besides writing a biography on Ambroise Paré, he also wrote an account of his life as an army surgeon. He was present in all Napoleon's battles; when Napoleon abdicated, Larrey awaited him and joined him on his return to France in 1813. In the battle of Borodinov, fought in 1812 on the plains of Russia, Larrey performed 202 amputations over a continuous period of twenty-four hours, without sleep or rest. The Emperor is said to have said *"C'est l'homme le plus virtueux que j'ai connu."* Napoleon conferred a baronetcy on both his favourites—Larrey and Corvisart—as also on two other surgeons—Pierre Francois Percy (1754–1825) the chief surgeon of the army, who authored the *Manuel de chirurgien d'armee* (the *Army Surgeon's Handbook*), and Guillaume Dupuytren (1777–1835), who was the chief surgeon at the Hôtel Dieu.

Dupuytren was an extraordinary man. He came from humble origins but through hard work and force of personality became the best known and popular surgeon of the age. He started as a demonstrator in the dissection hall; at thirty he was an assistant surgeon, and at thirty-four he rose to be the professor of operative surgery at the Hôtel Dieu. His clinics were extremely popular, he had a phenomenal practice and a large private clientele outside the hospital. Patients came to seek his help from all over Europe, so that he amassed a huge fortune. As an individual he had many drawbacks. He was proud, overbearing, immodest; he intrigued against and persecuted his rivals, so that though respected for his professional skills, he was more feared than loved. Pierre François Percy (1754–1825), the chief surgeon of Napolean's army called him the first of surgeons and the least of men. Dupuytren left classic descriptions of Dupuytren's contracture (a flexion deformity of the fingers of the hand) and of Dupuytren's fracture (a fracture of the lower end of the fibula).

François Broussais (1772–1838), like Laennec, came from Brittany. He exerted significant influence on medicine in the eighteenth century, though in time to come his influence proved to have been more negative rather than positive in its overall effect. Broussais served as a sergeant in the Republican army and then as a mariner before graduating in medicine in 1803. He believed that disease was the result of some irritative process in one or more organs, in particular the stomach and the intestinal tract. He disbelieved the view that poisons or extraneous agents could ever be responsible for illness. Gastroenteritis was thus the initial cause of a large number of diverse ailments. His treatment to counter disease was a regime that purposely debilitated the patient through a starvation diet and through the uninhibited application of leeches—up to fifty at a time—to all parts of the body. Indeed, the demand for leeches soared to a point where there was an acute shortage of these creatures. In 1833, 41,500,000 leeches were imported into France to help meet the medical demand imposed by the belief in Broussais' doctrine. In contrast, in 1822–1823, two to three million leeches sufficed to meet the requirement of doctors who believed in blood-letting. Broussais seemed to have got even more dogmatic and bloodthirsty with age; his extremist views were then abandoned even by his followers, who embraced the more intelligent and moderate teachings of Laennec and others.

Broussais' views on the therapy of disease were scientifically demolished by Pierre Louis (1787–1872). Pierre Louis has however gone down in history as the man who first introduced statistical methods in medicine and who described the significance of the angle between the manubrium and the body of the sternum now known as the angle of Louis. Louis first spent six years in Russia and realizing the futility of medicine in combating epidemic disease returned to Paris, and from then on engaged in teaching and research. He realized that fanciful theories and arguments in medicine could be refuted by careful statistical analysis. Louis was the first to apply mathematical methods to a number of medical problems. He was thus the father of medical statistics—a branch which is

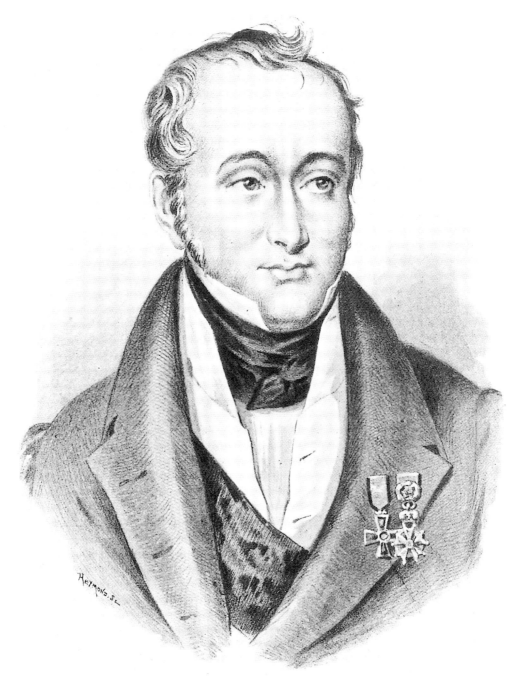

Fig. 44.2   Guillaume Dupuytren.

today of invaluable use in gauging the validity or otherwise of the methodology, results and conclusions in any modern scientific paper. Even in that age, some of his work was of lasting value. An early application of his work by Fournier and Erb proved that both tabes dorsalis and general paralysis of the insane resulted from infection by syphilis.

Louis' statistical methods also came into use to determine if treatment in a particular disease was effective or not. His magnum opus was *Recherches anatomica-physiologiques sur la phthisie* (1825). Based on a study on 2,000 patients with tuberculosis he demonstrated the frequent occurrence of the disease in the apex of the lung. He also wrote a treatise titled *Recherches on typhoid fever* (1829) which gave this disease its present name and finally wrote a blistering attack on Broussais, showing by statistical methods that blood-letting in pneumonia was of no value.

From the physician-statistician Pierre Louis we now move on to Joseph François Magendie (1783–1855), who may perhaps be considered the founder of modern pharmacology. He stressed the importance of conducting animal experiments in the study of medicine. He said: "The aim of science is to substitute facts for appearances and demonstration for impressions." Through animal experiments, Magendie showed the site and mode of action of strychnine and morphine, thus providing a scientific basis for the clinical use of these drugs. Magendie is also remembered for his discovery of the sensory function of the posterior nerve root of the spinal nerves. Interestingly enough, it was Charles Bell the Edinburgh surgeon who confirmed the motor function of the anterior spinal nerve roots.

Magendie's favourite pupil was Claude Bernard (1813–1878). He was one of the greatest figures of medicine in the nineteenth century. A great physiologist, his achievements embraced all aspects of this subject. He made numerous discoveries in various fields, but above all, he had the vision to synthesize many of these discoveries to basic fundamental laws that have stood the test of time.

Claude Bernard was born in 1813 in the village of Saint Julien (known for its lovely vineyards) near Villefranche, Rhone. When eighteen years old, he went to Lyons as a pharmacist's assistant. Pharmacy bored him and he took to literature and playwriting. His amateur works included an amusing play termed *Le Rose du Rhône* and a five-act drama titled *Arthur de Bretagne*. The pharmacist dispensed with his service and Bernard went to Paris. He carried with him the manuscript of his, *Rose*, the first act of his play, and a letter of introduction to a celebrated critic. The critic, a professor at Sorbonne read Bernard's amateur works and is said to have remarked— "My dear you have been working in a pharmacy and your head is full of ideas, it is science you want and not theatre."

Bernard in this fortuitous way now enrolled in the faculty of medicine. After completing his studies he became assistant to Magendie, lecturing and demonstrating at the College de France. These lectures were published in a number of volumes between 1854 and 1878. It would be impossible to describe all the numerous experiments and discoveries in physiology attributed to Bernard. There were some discoveries that were outstanding and these need to be touched upon.

One of his first and most important observations was that the liver had a glycogenic function— could convert glucose reaching it to glycogen and convert glycogen to sugar. He also showed that when an animal was fed a pure protein diet so that no sugar reached the liver (via the portal vein), the blood on circulating through and leaving the liver (via the hepatic vein) contained large quantities of glucose. Evidently, the protein supplied to the liver could be converted within it to sugar—a phenomenon termed neoglucogenesis. Bernard concluded that the body could make its own chemical when it functioned normally. He called this process 'internal secretion'—a term of fundamental importance in the basic concept of endocrinology. Equally important was Bernard's work on vasomotor nerves which constrict and dilate blood vessels under varying conditions to different parts of the body.

Bernard also produced a pancreatic fistula and demonstrated the importance of pancreatic fluid in digestion. Pancreatic enzymes could digest carbohydrates, fats and proteins. He also conducted experiments on the oxygenation of blood, on opium alkaloids and the action of lethal poisons like carbon monoxide (which acted by displacing oxygen from haemoglobin) and curare. He experimented and proved that curare acted on nerve muscle endings, preventing the nervous impulses from reaching the muscles and thereby causing paralysis. He thus postulated that certain drugs could have very specific localized action at well-defined sites.

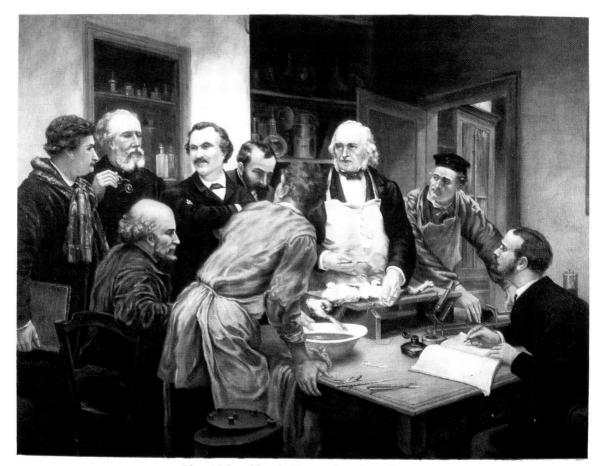

Fig. 44.3   Claude Bernard and pupils.

Unquestionably his great achievement was to synthesize his many discoveries into a fundamental principle or tenet. He formulated this principle in his last and best work entitled *Leçons sur les phenomenones de la vie* (1878), wherein he stated the constancy of the internal environment. Thus the normal physiological processes within the body are so capable of adjustment, that even under extraneous stimuli or stress, the internal milieu changes little or not at all. "The stability of the internal environment is the prime requisite for free independent existence."

Bernard was the great exponent of the use of experimental method in the study of medicine. Physiology, pathology, pharmacalogy were the handmaidens of experimental medicine. Disease was disordered physiology. Both physiology and disordered physiology could be studied to advantage by experimentation in a strictly controlled environment. Bernard's approach to experimentation is contained in his aphorism of taking off one's imagination on entering a laboratory as one would remove an overcoat. His book on the *Introduction à l'Etude de la médecine experimentale* (1865) states that, "One must break the bonds of philosophical and scientific systems as one would break the chains of scientific slavery. Systems tend to enslave the human spirit." Claude Bernard was a great experimentalist and a great thinker. He won renown within his country and from scientists all over the world. He succeeded Magendie as the head of the College of France, and in 1855, gained chairs at the Sorbonne and the Museum of Natural History. He was admitted to the Academy of Medicine in 1861, and became president of the Academie Français in 1868. He was made a senator in 1869.

Bernard's successor at the College de France was Charles Edouard Brown-Séquard (1817–1894), born in Mauritius of an American sea captain father and a French mother. He was truly an international figure for he had studied in Paris, travelled to England and Harvard, taught at Harvard and practised at the National Hospital, Queens Square, London. He returned after Bernard's death to Paris. Brown Séquard, besides describing the effects of the hemisection of the spinal cord, proved that the adrenal glands were essential to life and was thus a pioneer in endocrinology.

The Influence of Paris

Paris in the early years of the nineteenth century reigned supreme in medicine. Students from all over Europe and North America flocked to learn from Parisian professors. Laennec was a great draw teaching over 300 foreign students. An added attraction was the large number of public hospitals in Paris where students had a free hand in examining patients, in performing dissections and autopsies. At the end of their instruction these students returned to their own cities. There were standard-bearers of French medicine in London, Edinburgh, Dublin, Vienna, Madrid, Lisbon and Philadelphia.

In England, an early enthusiast of Parisian medicine was Thomas Hodgkins (1798–1866). He first studied in Edinburgh, then went on to Paris for a year and was so enamoured by Laennec that he returned to Laennec in Paris. In 1825, he settled in London as a lecturer in morbid anatomy at Guy's Hospital, introducing the stethoscope to England and lecturing on the pathology he had seen and learnt in France. His description titled *On Some Morbid Appearances of Absorbent Glands and Spleen* was a classic description of malignant disease affecting the lymphatic tissue which ultimately came to be known as Hodgkin's disease.

There were two other great figures in medicine at Guy's Hospital, London—Thomas Addison (1795–1860) and Richard Bright (1798–1855). Addison will always be remembered for his essay on the "Constitutional and Local Effects of Disease of the Suprarenal Capsules". In this brief essay he gave a brilliant description of adrenocortical insufficiency and also included a short description of pernicious anaemia. His observations gained little recognition during his lifetime.

Richard Bright was a graduate from Edinburgh. He was an artist, a geographer and a naturalist who travelled extensively in Iceland and Hungary. He wrote lucid descriptions of many diseases, but his name will always be associated with his description of glomerulonephritis, which at that time came to be known as Bright's Disease. In 1842 he established what was probably the first research unit at Guy's Hospital, the unit consisting of two wards for patients with kidney disease, an attached clinical laboratory and a consulting room.

In London, the Hunterian tradition was carried forward by Charles Bell, who in 1812 acquired William Hunter's old Windmill Street anatomy school. The accent of the Hunterian school in London was on anatomy, unlike the French school which was on pathology. Charles Bell was against animal experimentation both on moral and medical grounds. It is no wonder that London did not produce a figure of the stature of Claude Bernard of Paris.

It would be of interest at this juncture to relate the problems created by the shortage of dead bodies in the study of anatomy, particularly in London and Edinburgh. Robert Knox (1791–1862) was a famous teacher of anatomy in Edinburgh. Grave-snatching to provide bodies, to which authorities turned a blind eye, was well known. In 1827, an old man died in William Hare's (1792–1870) boarding house. Hare together with his lodger William Burke decided to supply to the anatomists dead bodies, bypassing the grave altogether. Emboldened by success they now turned to murder, suffocating victims so that there was no trace of violence and selling these murdered victims for huge profits. Sixteen murders, with each body sold for £7 went by before they were brought to justice in 1829. Hare turned King's evidence; Burke was convicted, hanged, publicly flayed with his skin tanned and sold by the strip. The first cadaver had been discovered in Knox's dissecting room. The enraged crowd burst into his house. Knox fled to London and died in obscurity.

The Hunterian tradition of superb anatomy remained alive and vital in Britain as exemplified by a splendid work on anatomy produced by Henry Gray (1827–1861), a lecturer in anatomy at Guy's Hospital who died prematurely of smallpox. Amazing as it may sound, his updated version is still in print and is read by students of anatomy all over the world.

Parisian influence in medicine was strong in Vienna. The Viennese school of clinical medicine fairly strong during the time of Van Swieten and De Haen had then gone into a decline. It was the Paris-inspired Carl von Rokitansky who resuscitated its fortunes. Rokitansky was the champion pathologist of this age. He made pathological anatomy a compulsory study. He is supposed to have performed 60,000 autopsies in the course of his career. He wrote, "Pathological anatomy must constitute the groundwork not only of all medical knowledge, but also of all medical treatment; it embraces all that medicine has to offer of positive knowledge." Rokitansky made significant contributions to the pathology of peptic ulcer, pneumonia, and valvular heart disease which he described in his *Handbuch de Pathologische Anatomie* (*Handbook of Pathological Anatomy*). Rokitansky's contemporary in clinical medicine was Joseph Skoda (1805–1881). He was a blacksmith's son who walked from Bilsen in Bohemia to study in Vienna. He was greatly influenced by Laennec, concentrated on the clinical aspects of chest diseases, wrote a major treatise on percussion and auscultation assigning to each of the auscultatory sounds its musical pitch and meaning. He was an excellent bedside clinician and was the first Viennese professor to lecture in his native dialect of German instead of the customary lecture delivered in Latin.

Besides this influence of Paris on the approach to clinical medicine, a more profound influence was exerted on the development of a systematic and scientific education all over the western world and also, to an extent, in America.

45 The German School

The Paris school of medicine was centred in the hospital wards, in bedside observation and in a study of pathology in the autopsy room. The German school was a counter to the school of Paris. The central focus of medicine in Germany was in the laboratory. The stethoscope was not the end-all and be-all of medicine; the microscope was equally important. The laboratory nurtured the science in medicine—the use of the microscope, animal experiments under controlled conditions, chemical investigations in relation to normal and abnormal physiology of the human being. Fortunately, the technical advancement in microscopes enabled the scientist to see with clarity objects, which in earlier years were optically distorted. In 1826, Joseph Jackson Lister (1786–1869), an amateur microscopist and father of the great surgeon Joseph Lister, constructed a microscope with a far higher magnification. This gave an increasing impetus to histology—the microscopic study of tissues and cells.

German universities gave scientific research their first priority. Academic positions were prestigious and eagerly sought. Most big universities had their own attached research institutions or faculties. Encouragement for scientific inquiry was not limited to the academic staff; it was inculcated in all students who became, for example, as familiar with the use of the microscope as their counterparts in France were familiar with the stethoscope. Laboratory research in Germany in the nineteenth century was thus a matter of high priority and was encouraged at all levels. Perhaps clinical medicine was pushed to the background, but in the years to come the fruits of the research projects in Germany came to be applied to the patient at the bedside.

A rather novel approach to medicine in Germany was the research on clinical processes relating to physiology. A pioneer in this field was Justus von Liebig (1803–1873). After studying in Bonn, Liebig spent two years in Paris, and in 1824 was appointed professor of chemistry at the Institute of Chemistry at Giessen University. Like all great men he soon had a number of students and acolytes working with him. Liebig's main study was on the energy produced by various foods through chemical investigations, measurements and analysis. William Prout (1785–1850) of London in his lectures on animal chemistry was probably the first to classify foods into oleaginous material or fats, saccharinous substances or carbohydrates and nitrogenous matter or proteins. Prout was a vitalist who believed that the uniqueness of the chemistry of living beings compared to that of the inorganic non-living world was due to the vital principle which synthesized organic substances from inorganic material.

Liebig related chemistry to physiology by proving that the body temperature or 'heat' was not innate, but was due to the process of oxidation. Oxygen introduced into the blood and tissue through respiration combined with carbohydrates to form energy, carbon dioxide and water; proteins were nitrogenous products that helped to form muscles and other vital body tissues. The waste products after this incorporation of nitrogenous products were excreted via the urine as urea. Food was the fuel for the body resulting in consumption of oxygen, production of carbon dioxide and the release of energy. The ratio between food intake, oxygen consumption and energy produced could be established by experimental work and chemical analysis of animal tissues in the laboratory. Liebig thus laid the foundations of the science of nutrition and biochemistry.

A great embryologist of the German school was Ernst von Baer (1792–1876). He proved that the function of the mammalian ovary was to ovulate and produce an ovum, establishing that ovulation was essential for reproduction. He studied the fertilized egg under the microscope describing the presence of four layers. The organs evolved from these germ layers. From the top layer there developed the external covering and the central nervous system, from the next arose the muscular and skeletal systems; from the third was evolved the vascular system; the fourth evolved into the alimentary tract and associated digestive organ systems. Baer maintained that a study of comparative embryology in different animal species would throw light on morphology and help in unravelling the mechanism of the evolution of the living species from lower to higher levels.

Liebig championed the study of chemistry to fathom the secrets of health and disease, von Baer stressed on the study of embryology to understand morphology and evolution, but perhaps the most influential of German scientists in this era was the physiologist Johannes Müller (1801–1858). He was a versatile investigator in many fields including physiology, anatomy, zoology and pathology. Initially he was professor of physiology and anatomy at Bonn and then at Berlin. He wrote a book titled *Handbuch der Physiologie des Menschen* (Handbook of Physiology). It became the standard text in physiology of the German-speaking world in the nineteenth century. He contributed to the studies of colour vision, of sensation, sensory appreciation and speech. He was an ardent advocate for the use of the microscope, of controlled animal experiments, and of the use of the laboratory for scientific research and inquiry. He was a great teacher and his students were great names in the annals of medicine and science in the nineteenth century. However, like so many of his contemporaries he was a vitalist, believing in the vital principle. Many of his students who followed him abandoned this aspect of his teaching. His protégés included Schwann, Henle, Kolliker, Du Bois-Reymond, Helmholtz, Brache and Ludwig. We must pause to look at a few of these great names.

Jacob Henle (1809–1885) was termed the 'Vesalius of Histology'. He discovered the portion of the renal tubules that bears his name (Henle's loop), described the muscular coat of the arteries, and the microscopic anatomy of the eye. His theories on infection are mentioned in Chapter 48. He was also a great teacher, and stressed the value of experimental physiology in medicine and insisted that students be familiar with the use of the microscope.

Hermann von Helmholtz (1811–1894), professor of physiology at Konigsberg will be remembered for one major discovery and one major invention. His major discovery was in measuring the speed of transmission of nerve impulses. His great major invention in 1851 was the ophthalmoscope which revolutionized ophthalmology. He wrote of the 'great joy of being the first to see a living human retina' through his new invention.

Karl Ludwig (1816–1895) was the most influential teacher after Müller. He disbelieved the vitalistic theory of his mentor. He taught a materialistic science encouraging chemical analysis, quantitative measurements and championed the cause of laboratory science and physiology as being inseparable from the study of medicine. In 1865, he was appointed director of the Physiologic Institute in Leipzig.

In an attempt to study the basic unit of living organisms, he began a microscopic study of cells in association with Theodor Schwann (1810–1882), another of Müller's pupils. The cell theory was first enunciated in botany by the botanist Matthias Schleiden (1804–1881). Plants were aggregates of cells existing as reproducing living units. Schwann maintained that this principle in botany was also applicable to animal and human living beings. Cells were the basic unit of animal and human life.

Debate on the origin of cells and the reproduction of cells in human beings was fiercely controversial. Schwann, for example, believed in the concept of a maturing fluid (the *blastime theory*), out of which cells arose as a result of spontaneous generation.

It was Rudolf Ludwig Karl Virchow (1812–1902) who unearthed the truth on the origin and multiplication of cells and who researched with great effect on the implications of cell theory in relation to disease. Virchow dominated medicine for more than half of the nineteenth century. He was unquestionably one of the greatest pathologists who ever lived, a worthy successor to Morgagni and Rokitansky. He was born in Pomerania, studied medicine at the university of Berlin and began teaching pathological anatomy in 1846. In 1849 he was sent to Silesia to study an epidemic of exanthematous typhus. He was incensed at the deplorable living conditions of the workers and wrote a scathing indictment that displeased the authorities. Perhaps this incident reveals the independence of his mind and the courage he had of expressing his beliefs. He was forced to resign, and spent seven years in Wurzburg. It was in this city that he laid the foundations of his great work. He then returned to Berlin as professor and director of the Institute of Pathological Anatomy of the Charité Hospital. He held this post till his death in 1902.

During his long tenure Virchow personally performed and also directed an enormous amount of work in autopsies, the microscopic study of various organ tissues, the collection of innumerable pathological specimens and the collation and correlation of the clinical features of disease with macroscopic pathology and microscopic histopathology. In 1858, Virchow published his magnum

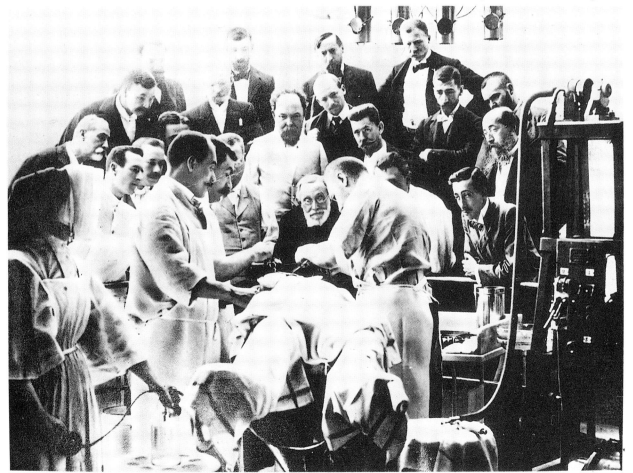

Fig. 45.1   Rudolf Virchow observing an operation on the skull in a Paris clinic.

opus *Di cellular—pathologie*. He stated this famous sentence at the very start '*Omnis cellula e cellula*' ('Each cell from a cell'). Thus all cells came from the first original cell. He thus demolished the theory of an enveloping matrix (or the blastema theory) that supposedly encouraged the spontaneous generation of cells. Virchow further stated that the cell was the basic seat of disease and that it was the abnormality in cells that manifested as disease. The macroscopic and microscopic changes in the human organism in disease were the manifestation of cellular changes governed by the cause of the disease. An analysis and understanding of cellular abnormality was, according to Virchow, basic to the study of cancer and of metastatic lesions.

His unique and brilliant concept not only focused attention on the microscopic study of tissues and of cells constituting these tissues, it also demolished the ancient concept of the humoral theory of disease. Virchow wrote: "The essence of disease according to my idea, is a modified part of the organism or rather a modified cell or an aggregation of cells (whether of tissue or of organs). In fact every diseased part of the body holds a parasitic relation to the rest of the healthy body to which it belongs and it lives at the expense of the organism." It is of interest that though his doctrine negated the ancient humoral theory, he was not aware of the factors that caused disease and the resulting abnormality in cells. It was left to Pasteur and his 'microbe-hunters' to establish the cause of disease.

Besides his studies on cancer, Virchow researched on thrombosis, embolism and elucidated the nature of phlebitis. He proved through experimental work, that emboli within the lungs were due to 'clots' thrown off from venous thrombi generally present within the leg veins. These 'clots' travelled via the venous system and the right heart to plug vessels within the pulmonary circulation.

Virchow like so many great men of medicine before and after him, had other interests besides his professional work. He was a keen anthropologist and in 1879 he accompanied Heinrich Schliemann on an expedition to Asia Minor to excavate the city of Troy. He was liberal in his thinking and was an ardent advocate of good public hygiene and social reform. As an intellectual he displayed a fearlessness in expressing his views. To his credit, he denied the existence of a pure Aryan super race—a concept that had just raised its ugly head towards the end of the nineteenth century. In 1862, he was elected to the Prussian House of Representatives and as founder of the Progressive Party he came into frequent conflict with Bismarck, the conservative.

On his death, he was given a state funeral. He was a great man, great in his profession, great in his achievements, his integrity and his sense of social justice. He belongs with the likes of Vesalius and Pasteur to the Valhalla of medicine.

46 The Control of Pain and the Story of Anaesthesia

The scope of surgery in the earlier years of the nineteenth century was limited. The most limiting factor was pain. Surgeons worked with furious speed and operations had to be completed within five minutes, else the anguish of unbearable pain could result in shock and death. The other difficult problems the surgeons had to face were haemorrhage, post-operative shock and post-operative infection. But the immediate and most pressing problem was the relief of pain.

The latest attempt at pain relief was the use of mesmerism to produce oblivion and a state of unconsciousness free of pain. John Elliotson (1791–1809) was the first to use hypnotism in surgical operations. He published his results in 1843. In 1845 John Esdaile, a Scotsman, used hypnosis to perform 261 painless surgeries on Hindu prisoners in Bengal. He was rather unsuccessful when he attempted to repeat this performance on his own countrymen in Scotland.

The history of attempts at the pharmacological relief of pain stretches into antiquity. Sleep-inducing drugs include Homer's nepenthe, hemp used in the East, Dioscorides' potion and the mandrake used by the thirteenth century surgeon Hugh of Lucca. No single drug was consistently effective, and till the middle of the nineteenth century, a strong dose of opium fortified by a heavy dose of alcohol was all that could be used. Even so, at the first cut of a sharp knife the agony of the surgery became inevitable.

Anaesthesia was one of the great discoveries that brought not only relief from pain but induced a state of muscle relaxation that made the surgeon's task less difficult. Remarkably enough, the first milestone in the discovery of anaesthesia was not by doctors but by a chemist. In 1772, Priestley discovered nitrous oxide. Humphrey Davy in 1800 experimented on himself and on his acquaintances by inhaling this gas. He found that it produced an irresistible desire to laugh, and he and his acquaintances continued to inhale the gas till they would slip into an unconscious state. He noticed that this gas, nitrous oxide, could deaden pain even at the stage where consciousness was not lost. In 1800, Davy wrote a book in which he stated: "As nitrous oxide appears capable of destroying physical pain it may be preferably used with advantage during surgical operations in which no great effusion of blood takes place." Not one physician or surgeon in England or on the Continent or in the United States took any heed of this remark!

In 1818, Michael Faraday the physicist had reported on the pain-relieving properties of an inhaled gas, ether. His observations too went unnoticed by the medical fraternity. In the same year (1800) that Davy wrote his book, there was born in the village of Lady Halton a boy named Henry Hill Hickman. He grew up to be a country surgeon who experimented on the effects of inhalation of carbon dioxide on animals and noted that he could operate on these animals, as they remained free of pain during the period of inhalation. He published his work in 1824 and was convinced that his work would benefit surgery. He concluded in his study that operations could be performed while the patient remained unconscious from the effects of inhaling a gas. Hickman appealed to the Royal Society to recognize the importance of his work. The Royal Society, of which by a remarkable coincidence Sir Humphrey Davy was then the president, ignored his appeal.

All seemed forgotten when nitrous oxide was dragged out of oblivion, once again not by the medical profession, but remarkably enough by show business. Quasi-scientific demonstrations on road-shows were popular in the United States in the 1830s, and a young lad named Samuel Colt who wished to promote the revolver which later made him famous, decided to raise money through these shows. Colt came from Hartford, but advertised himself as 'Doctor Colt of New York, London and Calcutta'. He obtained an apparatus that allowed inhalation of nitrous oxide, and in 1832 began staging demonstrations at street corners and on village greens using as his subject any volunteer prepared to inhale the gas. The entertainment consisted of the strange, hilarious antics that the subjects indulged in after inhaling nitrous oxide. All went well for young Samuel Colt till one fine day in one of his larger shows he administered the gas to six Indians who promptly fell asleep. Sam realized he was in trouble—for his customers (who were many) had not paid him to see Indians take a nap! Resourceful as he must have been, he saved the day by persuading a blacksmith to inhale the gas. The blacksmith fortunately went on the rampage, chased Sam all over the stage and then collapsed in a heap on the sleeping Indians, who awoke to find themselves on the floor. The audience felt that they had their money's worth, but Samuel Colt gave up his nitrous oxide demonstrations altogether.

In 1840, the young people of America had discovered that they could get 'drunk' by inhaling either nitrous oxide or fumes of ether. They would get jolly, laugh, perform hilarious antics, and if they sniffed a bit too much, they would fall into deep insensible sleep. Amazingly, even then, the significance of insensible sleep produced by nitrous oxide or ether went unnoticed by surgeons.

At last came Crawford Williamson Long (1815–1878). He was a young handsome doctor living in the town of Jefferson in Georgia. He was popular with the ladies, went to the ether parties, enjoyed himself immensely and noted that he felt no pain when he bruised himself if under the influence of ether. Long had a patient named James M. Venables, who had two tumors on the nape of his neck. Long offered to remove them, promising absence of pain if surgery was done after inhalation of ether. Venables went through the surgery and had these tumors removed successfully and experienced no pain. The date was 30 March 1842. The doctor's record read thus: "James Venables, 1842, administration of ether and removal of tumour—2 dollars." Unfortunately, Crawford Long made no announcement of any sort either to perpetuate his glory or to offer this method of surgery to the medical fraternity. He made known his results only in 1849, after he had used ether several times in surgery, and after its effectiveness had already been proved by Morton and others.

Two years after Long's surgery on Venables, a young dentist named Horace Wells (1815–1848) attended one of the itinerant science shows. A volunteer named Cooley who had inhaled nitrous oxide went berserk, falling all over the place, bumping into benches, and finally, when the effects of the gas wore off, he collapsed into the seat he had left to get on to the stage. By a strange quirk of coincidence this seat happened to be next to Horace Wells. Wells now requested the owner of the show named Colton to supply him with nitrous oxide, as he felt that a tooth could be extracted painlessly under the effect of the gas. Colton agreed, accompanied Wells to his office, administered gas to Wells, while a colleague pulled out one of Wells' teeth. Wells is said to have exclaimed, "It is the greatest discovery ever made! I did not feel so much as the prick of a pin." Wells felt certain that he was on his way to making a fortune.

Wells was also eager for fame; he was a man in a tearing hurry—and the thought of fame and fortune haunted him. He had an assistant named William Thomas Green Morton who tried to dissuade him from being overhasty. Wells did not listen and arranged to demonstrate the use of nitrous oxide at the Massachusetts General Hospital. One of the students volunteered to be the victim and Wells made him inhale the gas. But there was a fiasco. Either Wells did not give him enough gas or waited too short a time for the gas to take effect—for as he pulled the tooth out, the patient let out a yell of pain. There was pandemonium in the lecture hall and poor Wells dropped his forceps and fled. Wells continued to practise for a time but he was a broken, depressed man and ultimately committed suicide by opening a vein and inhaling ether.

It was left to William Thomas Green Morton (1819–1868) to complete the story of anaesthesia. He started as Wells' assistant and then went on to the Harvard Medical School, where his friend Charles Jackson, a chemist, supplied him with ether and suggested he use it to relieve pain. Morton felt that if ether fumes were inhaled steadily, ether might be the analgesic for which he was searching. He decided to experiment and his experiments literally began at home. He took his wife Elizabeth and their spaniel dog Wig for a holiday. Surreptitiously, he made the unwilling Wig inhale ether and Wig went into senseless slumber from which he could be aroused with difficulty and following which he behaved as if drunk! Next in line were the family goldfish, which he sent into a splendid slumber after they had inhaled ether. His wife Elizabeth saw them prostrate on the ground and burst into tears, but was pacified when Morton threw them back into the water apparently unhurt. All things creepy and crawly from caterpillars to earthworms came under the influence of ether vapour administered by Morton. Finally, Elizabeth found Morton himself stretched on the floor—he had inhaled enough ether to knock himself senseless and even the hysterics of his wife failed to hasten his reawakening. Morton and family returned to Boston and now Morton continued with his experiments on patients. He consulted his chemist friend once again, though by now they were not on friendly terms. He obtained from Jackson a useful piece of information—the vapours of sulphuric ether were more reliable then the chloric ether that Morton was still using. Morton decided now to try sulphuric ether before dental extractions. Eben Frost a musician walked into Morton's clinic for a painful tooth requiring extraction. Morton and his assistant (a dentist named Hayden), got to work. Morton soaked his handkerchief with ether, held it to Frost's nose to render him unconscious, while Hayden focused a lamp very near to Morton to help the procedure, and providentially did not blow up the clinic (neither realized that ether is highly inflammable). The operation was successful and painless. Frost became Morton's ardent disciple, his prize exhibit. Morton now felt that ether could also be used for surgical operations and he dreamt of being the benefactor of all mankind. He therefore first decided to design an inhaler. Next, he decided to meet Dr John Collins Warren—senior surgeon of the Massachusetts General Hospital who agreed to allow Morton to use ether vapour on a patient fixed for surgery. The patient for surgery was Gilbert Abbott who had a tumour in the neck. The day and time of the surgery was notified to Morton. But the inhaler which Morton had designed was not ready and the instrument maker worked frantically to get it functioning on time.

The morning of the appointed day arrived. It was 16 October 1846. The tiers in the theatre of Massachusetts General Hospital were filled by doctors and students right up to the top. The news of a novel approach to surgery had spread through the whole campus. The patient was wheeled in—a pale, consumptive looking young man with a large tumor in the neck behind the temporo-mandibular joint. He was taken to the operation table. Then entered Dr Warren who explained to the audience what was to take place. There was silence after his talk. It was a quarter hour past the time fixed for surgery. Warren looked impatient. There was a titter amongst the spectators which became louder with time. Sarcastic comments on the absence of Morton were heard. Dr Warren then spoke: "Since Dr Morton has not appeared, I presume he is otherwise engaged." He held up his knife and stooped over the patient. At that moment the door burst open and Morton appeared totally out of breath. He was accompanied by Eben Frost. Morton explained that his delay was due to his instrument not being ready but that he had his new inhaler with him and he was ready to begin. Dr Warren after hearing him, replied a trifle sarcastically, "Well sir, your patient is ready."

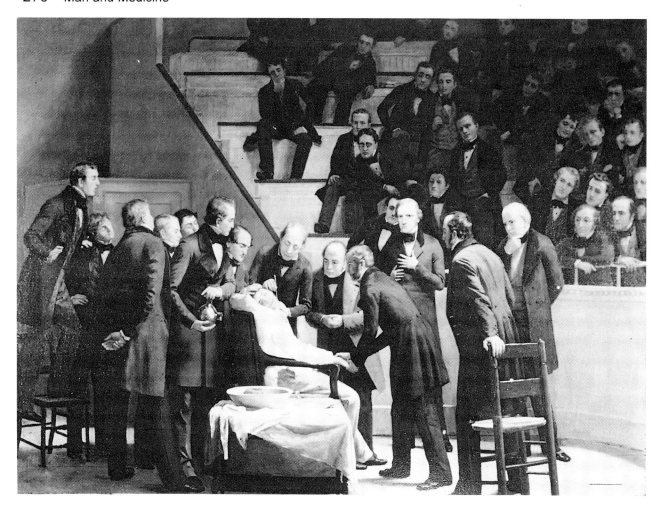

Fig. 46.1   One of the first operations with the use of ether as an anaesthetic agent, performed at the Massachusetts General Hospital, Boston, on 16 October 1846. Morton administering ether.

Morton went to the head of the table and reassured the patient, pointing to Eben Frost who had testified to the successful use of ether vapour on himself. Amidst tense silence the patient followed Morton's instructions. The glass tube of the instrument was inserted into his mouth and he inhaled deeply and evenly. He then began to breathe faster, his face grew flushed, he moved his arms spasmodically and then lay quiet on the operation table. Morton now looked towards Dr Warren and said, "Doctor, your patient is ready."

In the silence of this eventful morning Dr Warren picked up the scalpel and went to work. The tumor was removed and the wound was sutured. Towards the end, Abbott who all this while had laid still, stirred uttering incoherent sounds, but on recovering consciousness admitted that he felt no pain. Warren was deeply moved and turning to the spectators muttered, "Gentlemen this is no humbug." Warren promptly ordered for hospital use the apparatus that allowed ether inhalation from the instrument-maker but was told that this was not possible as Morton had applied for the patent rights on the apparatus. The Massachusetts Medical Society on hearing this felt deeply incensed. They declared that it was unethical to allow an invention that could benefit mankind to be used for private profit and that if some amicable arrangement was not arrived at, the society would ban its use. Warren conveyed this to Morton, who to his eternal glory, wrote the following letter to Warren: "Dear Sir, as it may sometimes be desirable that surgical operations should be performed at

Massachusetts General Hospital under the influence of the preparation employed by me for producing temporary insensibility to pain, you will allow me, through you, to offer to the hospital the free use of it for all hospital operations."

The sequel to the story of anaesthesia now turns sordid. Morton's claim to fame was challenged by Jackson and Wells, each of whom claimed credit for this discovery. A continuing controversy on this issue did not help matters. Morton gave up his practice to study and publicize the use of ether anaesthesia in surgery, impoverishing himself in the bargain. His torment that the recognition due to him continued to be debated both in Europe and America must have added to his agony. Morton sank from poverty to penury, but managed to rescue his house at Wellesley from creditors and supported himself by farming. He died in July 1868 when only forty-eight years old.

The new discovery needed a name. It was Oliver Wendell Holmes who finally gave the acceptable name of 'anaesthesia'. The term in fact was an ancient Greek word used by Plato and Dioscorides and meant insensitivity. Dioscorides' potion, used in antiquity to relieve pain was made thus: "boil roots of mandrake in wine until the liquid is reduced to one third; then administer the decoction in a cup to a patient before operation or cauterization, so that the person is in a state of insensitivity." Mandrake contains alkaloid which like hemp and poppy was used in antiquity for the relief of pain. These drugs were banned in the Dark and Middle Ages because they proved dangerous and could cause death.

The use of ether as an anaesthetic was publicized within a month of Morgan's demonstration at the Massachusetts General Hospital by H.J. Bigelow. Within another month ether was being used in London. The surgeon was Robert Liston, the operation being an amputation. When the patient regained consciousness and realized that he had felt no pain during surgery he dropped back on the operation table weeping with relief. Liston turned to the students and doctors in the theatre and said, "This Yankee dodge, gentlemen, beats Mesmer hollow." Ether thus became popular all over Europe and was in wide use by the end of 1846.

Sir James W Simpson (1811–1820), the Scottish obstetrician, had used ether with great success, but was dissatisfied because of its strong smell and the bronchial irritation it often caused. He therefore experimented with chloroform, a new anaesthetic independently described by Eugene Soubeiran and Justus von Liebig in 1831, and by the American Samuel Guthrie in 1832. Simpson started using chloroform as an anaesthetic agent informing the association of surgeons of Edinburgh about his discovery. This brought the wrath of the Scottish clergy upon him. Labour pains according to the clergy were ordained by God. Did not the *Book of Genesis* state "with pangs shall you give birth to children"? Simpson cleverly responded that the book also stated that God made Adam fall asleep before taking a rib from him to create Eve. God therefore anaesthetized Adam. The medical profession in Philadelphia sided with the clergy, stating that the pain of childbirth was a natural and necessary manifestation and should not be relieved. Simpson, not to be outdone, replied that when they next wished to travel to New York they should walk, as it was the natural thing to do and not take the train! These polemics did not however help the use of anaesthesia in childbirth. It was only when Queen Victoria gave her royal assent to chloroform anaesthesia for the delivery of Prince Leopold her seventh child, that anaesthesia became both fashionable and acceptable. Her obstetrician was John Snow (1813–1858), and his work on chloroform and other anaesthetics gave anaesthesia an increasingly scientific basis.

Technical developments in the administration of anaesthesia and the discovery of new anaesthetic agents kept apace. Ether irritated the respiratory tract. Chloroform was shown to be both hepatotoxic and could occasionally cause cardiac failure. A mixture of nitrous oxide and oxygen was safe but did not always produce deep narcosis and sufficient muscle relaxation. The search for an effective non-inflammable anaesthetic agent that could induce narcosis and relaxation continued. Cyclopropane was introduced in 1929, but was found to be inflammable; trichlorethylene was introduced in 1934. It reduced awareness of pain without rendering the patient unconscious, and was thus found suitable for childbirth.

Improvements in the technique of administering anaesthesia include the first use of endotracheal tubes by Kühn in 1900 and the adoption of the closed circuit system in 1934. Intravenous anaesthesia was first introduced by Ore of Bordeaux in 1874 using chloral. It however came into general use after 1902 when Emil Fischer synthesized veronal. Many other barbiturates followed and of these thiopentone for long has been in general use. The basic use of anaesthesia was completed with the discovery of the muscle relaxant tubocurarine and succinylcholine in 1945, but we have by now unquestionably encroached into the period we have termed 'Contemporary Medicine'. It is interesting that these muscle relaxants originated from the discovery of curare—a poison used by South American Indians. For hundreds of years these Indians dipped their arrows in this poison to shoot down animals which remained paralysed without being killed. The poison prevented nerve impulses from reaching the muscles causing paralysis. The use of the above agents in anaesthesia was a boon to the surgeon as it provided muscle relaxation and easier surgery.

The story of the discovery of local anaesthesia is amusing and interesting. Sigmund Freud, the psychiatrist practising in Vienna, was in 1884 interested in experimenting on the alkaloid of cocoa. He did some experimental work on cocaine. Freud was engaged to a girl who lived in another town and whom he had not met for over two years. He felt it was now time to do so. He interrupted his experiments on cocaine but on leaving recommended to a colleague and friend Karl Koller, who was an ophthalmologist, to experiment with cocaine on the eyes. When Freud returned from his holiday, Koller had researched on the effects of cocaine on the eyes of animals and had demonstrated his results to the Ophthalmological Congress at Heidelberg. Freud thus lost the fame of the discovery to his friend and colleague Koller. The local anaesthetic effect of cocaine was put to use particularly in surgery on the eye and the throat. However, in 1898 August Karl Gustav Bier (1861–1949), of Greifswald, injected cocaine into the spinal canal and obtained analgesia in the lower extremities. Spinal anaesthesia then came to be used widely all over the world.

Another modern invention is the use of hypothermia in major surgical procedures, achieved by lowering the core temperature of the body from 37 degrees Centigrade to 30 or 32 degrees centigrade. Larrey of Napoleonic fame had noted during the Russian campaign, that freezing permitted painless amputation. But the *raison d'etre* of hypothermia in major surgery was to reduce oxygen consumption of the vital organs such as the brain and heart, so that they could be deprived of blood for longer periods of time without suffering damage. The use of hypothermia in heart and brain surgery becomes self-evident. Hypothermia today is not just achieved by physically cooling the patient. It is achieved by the use of drugs such a chlorpromazine and promethazine which inhibit the temperature regulation mechanism within the hypothalamus and allow the body temperature to be reduced to desired levels.

The story of anaesthesia which started in the modern period has spilled into the period of contemporary medicine. The anaesthetist has evolved from a scared individual pouring an unknown quantity of ether on a handkerchief and later into a face mask placed on the patient's nose and mouth, to a highly-trained individual practising a quickly-evolving speciality. He can today maintain the patient at any level of consciousness desired by the surgeon, he can collapse a lung when necessary and reinflate it at the appropriate time. He controls a formidable array of dials and has a number of instruments at his command to monitor the effects of the one or more anaesthetics he administers. He intervenes with appropriate drugs when vital signs change, and he works in tandem with the surgeon for the greater glory of surgery.

47 Antisepsis and Asepsis

The discovery of anaesthesia was a blessing for both the patient and the surgeon. At long last the agony of excruciating pain during a surgical procedure was completely relieved. But the chief cause of morbidity and mortality after surgery was infection. Gangrene was a frequent dreaded complication following amputation and other surgical procedures. It often raged like an epidemic in surgical wards whose air was foul and foetid with the stink of festering wounds and rotting limbs. Secondary haemorrhage, post-operative tetanus, erysipelas, septicaemia and pyaemia contributed even further to mortality. The soldier in the battlefield had almost certainly a better chance to survive in battle, than a patient in his ordeal consequent to surgery.

The cause of festering wounds and of gangrene was unknown in the middle of the nineteenth century. It was attributed to a *miasma,* to something in the air, poisonous humors, poisonous vapours, or even to the oxygen in the air to which wounds were exposed. Though the cause of infection and inflammation was obscure, the mechanism behind these processes was being slowly experimented upon and understood. Thomas Addison in 1849 and the experimental pathologist Julius Cohnheim (1839–1884), had both suggested that the formation of pus in wounds was related to the diapedesis of white blood cells through the capillary walls of the damaged tissue. Cohnheim, using special experimental and histological techniques with the aid of a microscope, saw white blood cells escaping through capillary walls in the damaged mesentery of a frog together with dilatation of this capillary bed and stasis of circulation within it.

Infection and sepsis were equally frequent in mothers after childbirth. This infection called 'childbirth fever' (now termed *puerperal sepsis*), also carried a tragic formidable mortality. Oliver Wendell Holmes (1809–1894) in Boston regarded childbirth fever as an infection and considered it a contagious disease that could be transmitted by birth-attendants. He was disbelieved by his colleagues in Philadephia, who maintained that childbirth fever was neither infectious nor contagious.

The man who disproved the theory of poisonous vapours by careful prolonged observation and study was the Hungarian obstetrician Ignaz Philipp Semmelweis (1818–1865), who qualified in medicine from the University of Vienna in 1844. Two years later, he joined the first maternity ward of the Vienna Krankenhaus as assistant to Professor Klein, a famous obstetrician. In 1840, the mortality of childbirth fever in this famous and largest maternity clinic in the world was forbiddingly high. Semmelweis was increasingly distressed at the many deaths among the mothers in his maternity ward. The mortality rate in his first year of work was about 30 per cent. He searched for clues for this high mortality and discovered that the mortality rate in the second maternity ward was four to five times less. It was highly improbable that poisonous vapours could selectively kill mothers in the first maternity ward. He had also noted that in the first maternity ward where the mortality was high, the mothers after delivery were subsequently attended to by the doctors, whereas the second maternity ward with a low mortality rate was in charge of midwives. He then made the shrewd observation that connected the autopsy room to the high maternal mortality in his ward. It was customary for obstetricians to start the day by first carrying out autopsies on their patients and then proceeding with their ward work. The midwives running the second maternity ward never attended autopsies. He was convinced that early morning visits to the autopsy room by the doctors of his ward were responsible for the high maternal mortality. He felt that the low mortality in the ward managed by midwives was because the midwives never entered the autopsy room.

Semmelweis went for a short holiday to Venice in 1847 and on his return, was saddened to learn of the death of his colleague Kolletschka who was assistant to the great pathologist Rokitansky. Kolletschka had died after a scalpel wound sustained while performing an autopsy on a mother who had died of childbirth fever. Semmelweis attended the autopsy of his friend and was shocked to observe that the lesions in various organ systems were very similar to those observed in mothers dying of puerperal sepsis or childbirth fever. The scalpel had unquestionably transferred infection from the corpse to his poor friend. He was convinced that infections in the maternity ward were conveyed to mothers by doctors who performed autopsies and then immediately visited the maternity ward to examine mothers and aid in childbirth. Semmelweis now gave strict instructions that the wards were to be cleaned with calcium chloride and that before touching a patient everyone was to wash his hands thoroughly. This elementary precaution was followed and resulted in a sharp decline in the mortality rate down to almost zero within two years. He then communicated these findings to the medical society in Vienna, claiming that *puerperal sepsis* or childbirth fever was a form of blood poisoning or *septicaemia*. His observations and his views were fiercely attacked by all obstetricians and also by almost the whole medical faculty. There were however three professors who agreed with him and staunchly supported him. They were the great pathologist Karl Rokitansky (1804–1878), the great physician Josef Skoda (1805–1881), famed for his diagnostic ability and for pioneering the use of percussion and auscultation in Austria, and the dermatologist Ferdinand von Hebra (1816–1880).

The tide however was strongly against him; the obstetricians, in particular almost hounded him and he was forced to resign. A saddened, frustrated Semmelweis returned to his native Budapest. Doctors and students at the Vienna Krankenaus stopped washing and disinfecting their hands and the mortality rate in delivered mothers soared to its original high level. In Budapest, Semmelweis became head of obstetrics at St Rochus Hospital and continued to practise antisepsis in his maternity wards. Not only did he insist on handwashing, but he also insisted that all instruments and dressings be disinfected, that fresh linen be provided for each patient and that the wards be periodically disinfected. Maternal mortality dropped very sharply and puerperal sepsis seemed a nightmare of the past. The rest of this great man's tragic life was spent in his trying to convince the world that the simple act of handwashing could save thousands of lives. He published his beliefs and his work in *Die Aetiologie, der Begriff and die Prophylaxis des Kindbettfiebers* (*The Cause, Concept and Prophylaxis of Childbirth Fever*) in 1881. It was an epoch-making landmark in medicine. It lacked elegance and style, was perhaps rendered a trifle dull by a mass of statistical data, yet its message was direct, simple and had far-reaching consequences. The reaction to the book was extremely hostile. Europe rejected his views; the medical profession scorned his work. Virchow, the greatest name in pathology in the mid-nineteenth century, refuted the observations and conclusions of this great physician. Semmelweis was further embittered, and when he visited one of his few friends, Hebra in Vienna in 1864, he showed signs of mental instability. He was finally kept in a mental asylum, where he died within a few months. A sadder twist to his tragic life was provided at autopsy which revealed that his mental symptoms were related to organic disease.

Castiglioni has described Ignaz Philipp Semmelweis as one of the greatest medical benefactors to humanity. His life was a dark, tragic struggle, during which he made a great contribution to medicine, a contribution whose beauty lay in its elementary simplicity. His views, ridiculed during his lifetime, gained acceptance twenty years after his death. There now stands a monument in Budapest to mark the memory of this great man. It was constructed 29 years after his death in 1894, perhaps to atone for the way the world treated him when he was alive. His everlasting tribute, posthumous though this may be, stems from the benefits he conferred on humanity. What greater tribute could a man of medicine ever wish for?

At about the same time when Semmelweis was unsuccessfully attempting to establish the practice of antisepsis in the obstetric ward in Vienna, Lister was successfully introducing disinfection in the practice of surgery and in the treatment of surgical wounds. Joseph Lister (1827–1912) was a titan in surgery; his imprint in the annals of surgery is probably as great as that of William Harvey in the history of medicine. In an age where the ultimate in surgery was

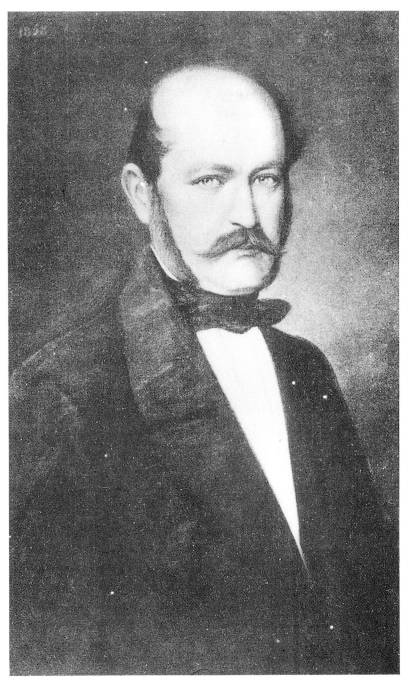

Fig. 47.1   Portrait of Ignaz Philipp Semmelweis.

the cultivation of manual dexterity, speed and daring, Lister followed a different path. He was a man of science, a thinking surgeon, perhaps not over-dexterous with his hands, but experimenting, observing, questioning and enquiring till he established a fundamental tenet that changed forever the practice of surgery.

Joseph Lister was fortunate to be born in an ideal environment that must have helped to nurture his scientific genius. His father, Joseph Jackson Lister was a scientist who had made significant contributions to the improvement of the microscope. He was thus in close contact from his early days with the spirit of scientific enquiry in this age. Both parents were from a Quaker background and imparted the principles of plain living and high thinking to their son. Young Joseph worked hard at his studies but had to be taken away from school for a short period for what was probably a nervous breakdown. We know little about this boyhood crisis, but it may well harbour the secret of some of the personality traits of this great man. Lister was often painfully shy, afflicted by a stammer, could never lecture without notes, and even after days of preparation would continue to work on these notes even as his carriage drove him to the lecture hall. He found it difficult to face an audience and often kept his audience waiting by not arriving at the appointed hour.

Lister graduated from University College, London, and continued his medical studies at the same college. As a first year student he had the fortune to witness the first major operation performed in England by the surgeon Liston using ether. While working at the university hospital, a dreadful epidemic of hospital gangrene broke out in the wards. The surgical wounds instead of healing would turn grey at the edges, fester, spread and eat away into the surrounding tissues. Cauterization was the only known treatment of such gangrenous wounds; some patients recovered, but in many the gangrene would return and kill the patient. It was then the customary belief among many surgeons that contact with oxygen in the air was responsible for gangrene. Lister reasoned that if some patients recovered and some died, even though all had been exposed to oxygen in the air, then oxygen could not be the cause of the gangrene. He looked at some of the grey gangrenous matter under the microscope, made sketches of what he saw but was unable to arrive at a solution to the problem.

Lister finished his studies in 1852 and was made a Fellow of the Royal College of Surgeons of London in the same year. He then went to study under the famous surgeon Syme in Edinburgh, who was one of the best surgeons of his time. He soon became assistant surgeon to Syme at the Edinburgh Infirmary, fell in love with Agnes the daughter of Syme, and married her in 1856. His family belonged to the Society of Friends and he had to break with this Society to marry Agnes, who was brought up in the Church of England.

The Listers set out on a honeymoon, but it was not the sort of honeymoon that would interest most couples. It consisted of visits to all the medical centres of Europe. Strangely, when in Vienna, he did not get to know the attempts of Semmelweis to establish antisepsis in his maternity ward. It is highly probable that had Semmelweis' views been mentioned to Lister, he would have grasped their significance and applied them promptly in the practice of surgery.

After six years of work in Edinburgh, Lister was appointed to the Regius Chair of Surgery in Glasgow. He was appalled at the incidence of sepsis and of gangrene in the surgical wards. He had been busy with research on infected wounds at Edinburgh and continued his studies in Glasgow. He was convinced that the agent which caused suppuration and rotting of living flesh was something which worked from within the wound. He noticed the frequency with which infection first started within a blood clot in a wound, then spreading to the adjacent areas. He also observed that sepsis, putrefaction and gangrene began with inflammation of the wound. This prompted him to study the stages of inflammation, using for his experiments the foot of a frog. He planned his research meticulously, step by step. By now he had laid the foundations which made his later discovery possible.

One day in 1865, Thomas Anderson, a professor of chemistry at the University of Glasgow, placed a scientific paper written by Louis Pasteur in his hands. It was titled *Recherches sur la Putrefaction* (Research on Putrefaction). It was a fateful event, almost destined to happen, for it triggered the genius in Lister to a great discovery. Pasteur in his paper gave proof that micro-organisms invisibly suspended in air caused putrefaction. Lister caught on to the fact that it was these micro-organisms present in abundance in the air of the operating rooms and surgical wards that caused infection, sepsis and putrefaction, and even gangrene in surgical wounds. He realized that microbes could also be carried on surgical instruments, on sponges used to clean wounds and by the surgeon's hands. The secret of success in combating infection was to get rid of microbes, and to seal the wound with a suitable chemical antiseptic dressing till such time as the edges of the wound had healed. This concept did not strike him in one mighty flash. It took a little time, a product of reason, observation and experience. Experience taught him that microbes could enter and cause infection in the smallest wound and that no wound was safe till it was completely healed.

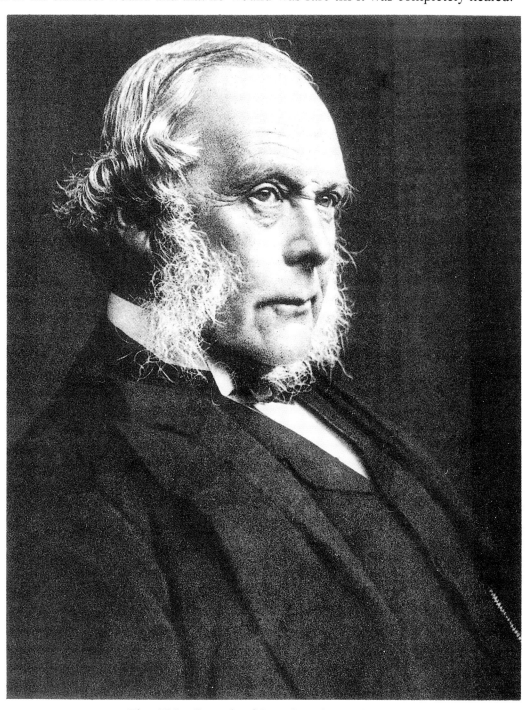

Fig. 47.2   Portrait of Joseph Jackson Lister.

Lister now introduced meticulous cleanliness in his ward and tried out a variety of antiseptic solutions. It was a war against those tiny microbes which he could not even see—an endless war which medicine continues to fight even today and will probably fight forever. He had heard of the town of Carlisle, which had faced disaster because the seepage of sewage into adjacent pastures had poisoned many cattle. The problem had been solved by the treatment of sewage with German creosote, which was an impure form of carbolic acid (phenol). Lister concluded that carbolic acid could destroy bacteria. He requested his chemist friend Thomas Anderson, who had given him Pasteur's paper, to supply him with carbolic acid. His experience in the surgical wards had taught him that whereas a simple fracture healed without infection, a compound fracture with laceration of the skin invariably got infected, and ended in suppurative gangrene. In fact the treatment of compound fracture in that age was amputation, for fear of gangrene setting in. Even so, the stump often became infected and gangrenous. It was obvious to Lister that unbroken skin prevented infection and a lacerated one permitted infection. A chemical barrier to infection was needed when the natural cutaneous one was impaired. A compound fracture was therefore the ideal case to test his theory. In March 1865, a factory worker had a severe compound fracture of the leg. Lister smeared carbolic acid over the lacerated wound; the patient could not stand the shock of injury and died just before the carbolic acid treatment could show conclusive results. Lister bided his time for two more months, when on 12 August 1865, an eleven year old boy James Greenless was run over by an empty cart and was brought to hospital with a compound fracture of both bones of the leg. There was a small open wound which Lister dressed with a piece of lint soaked in carbolic acid. The bones were then set. This dressing was kept in place for four days and the wound remained free of infection. The boy made an uneventful recovery. Nine months later he took up another case and his carbolic acid treatment was again successful. Lister now developed a specific routine for the treatment of wounds. After removing clotted blood, a piece of lint soaked in carbolic acid was introduced by a forceps into the wound. A second piece also soaked in carbolic acid, was placed on top of the wound. Tinfoil was placed on top to prevent evaporation of the antiseptic, and absorbent wool was packed around the wound. Before starting an operation Lister sprayed the operation theatre with carbolic acid, spraying the instruments and also the patient's skin. During the operation the air continued to be sprayed with carbolic acid, soaking all those present with it. The technique involved *antisepsis,* i.e., killing all micro-organisms in the wound, and *asepsis,* i.e., preventing bacteria from entering the wound. He published his successful results of the treatment of compound fractures in the Lancet in 1867. None of his eleven compound fracture patients had died of infection. He claimed in this paper, 'the element of incurability has been eliminated,' a modest statement—its correct interpretation being that his discoveries had saved many, many lives.

The reaction to his theory of antisepsis was mixed. Some ridiculed him but many applauded him. From England, Europe and America, people came to Glasgow in a steady stream—a pilgrimage to see, learn and practise this revolution in surgery. Like Harvey before him, Lister avoided disputes. His results spoke for themselves; his antiseptic technique gave him a new freedom to successfully attempt surgical procedures deemed too dangerous by his contemporaries. Lister had a laboratory at home and continued his research on microbes and on wound infections. He researched on different kinds of ligatures and concluded that catgut was the best material for suturing a wound. Catgut ligatures which are in reality made from the intestine of sheep, were not Lister's invention. They had been tried and discarded earlier because no method had been devised to uniformly ensure their strength and pliability. Lister in addition to giving catgut these qualities, used melted wax containing carbolic acid to ensure sterility, and by trial observed that ageing increased the strength of the catgut. In 1868, Lister with his nephew Richard Godlee, experimented on a chloroformed calf, using sterile seasoned catgut ligature. He noted that the catgut ligature not only served its purpose, but was completely absorbable.

In 1869, Lister succeeded Syme to the Chair of Surgery in Edinburgh and in 1877 he was appointed professor of Surgery at King's College, London. He wrote, lectured and with his wife Agnes, travelled extensively both in Europe and in the United States. When sixty-five years old, he retired from King's College. A year later his wife Agnes died when on vacation in Italy. It was a devastating blow from which he never quite recovered.

Revered and honoured, he was knighted in 1883, elected president of the Royal Society in 1895 and raised to a peerage in 1897—becoming the first doctor to sit in the House of Lords. His eightieth birthday was celebrated all over the western world; he remained at home listening to the stream of people who paid him their respects. At the end of the day he wrote to his brother, "What a change of opinion has taken place in these years in which I have been doing nothing."

He died on 10 February 1912; London witnessed a great funeral at Westminster Abbey, but he was buried according to his wish at West Hampstead beside his wife Agnes. The poet Henley, who had once been his patient, wrote of him:

> A modern Hercules.
> Wrestling with Custom, Patience, Disease
> As his great prototype with Hell and Death.

The surgical revolution initiated by Lister spread to England, Europe and the United States slowly but surely. In the Franco-Prussian war of 1870, of the 13,200 amputations performed by the French, 10,000 died of sepsis and gangrene—a mortality rate of over 70 per cent. Similarly, the post-operative mortality rate in a Munich clinic in the early 1870s was 80 per cent. These dreadful mortality rates fell sharply when Lister's antiseptic and aseptic techniques were introduced. Lucas Championnière in France (1843–1913), Bassini (1844–1913) in Italy, and Billroth in Vienna championed Listerism in Europe.

Newer techniques in asepsis also began to be introduced. Instead of destroying micro-organisms, surgeons aimed at excluding bacteria from operation theatres. In 1886, the German Ernst von Bergmann (1836–1907), developed new methods to sterilize the operation theatre, the surgeon and the patient; he introduced steam sterilization of dressings and surgical instruments.

In the United States, Marion Sims and William Halsted (1852–1922) were convinced of the value of antisepsis and asepsis in the operation room, and in the treatment of wounds. However, it took them a long time to convince their colleagues about this. In 1890, Halstead encouraged the use of rubber gloves during surgery. Berkeley Moynihan (1865–1936) was the first to use rubber gloves in Britain. Interestingly enough. Lister never scrubbed his hands, he merely rinsed them in carbolic acid. He operated in his street clothes—surgical gowns and masks came later. The Polish surgeon Johann von Mikulicz Radecki (1850–1905), first recognized the danger of droplet infection and was the first to use a face mask. Anaesthesia, antiseptic and aseptic techniques, the use of gloves, masks and gowns, and the abandonment of huge amphitheatres crowded by spectators, revolutionized surgery. Surgery was now poised for a quantum leap.

48

The Fight Against Infection—The Microbe Hunters

The middle of the nineteenth century witnessed a great landmark in the history of Man and Medicine—the coming into age of the science of bacteriology and microbiology. This science and those who pioneered it, brought about a true revolution in medicine. It was a revolution that finally resolved age-old controversies on the aetiology and pathogenesis of infections and infectious disease—a group of diseases which at frequent intervals decimated human-kind all over the world, almost since the beginning of the history of man. It began to be shown after 1860 that infections were caused by microscopic organisms—living organisms that invaded the human body with devastating results. It is tempting to compare this nineteenth century revolution in medicine in its far-reaching effects with the French revolution of 1789. The first drastically altered the face of medicine, the second shattered the sociopolitical framework of France and was a prelude to similar changes in other countries of the West.

The cause of infections till that period of man's history was a hot-bed of controversy and dispute. The generally accepted view was that disease (and this included infections as the major cause of disease) was due to 'miasmas', 'humors', or 'vapours', or even the presence of oxygen in the air. This miasmatic theory of the cause of disease was challenged by a few visionaries as early as the Renaissance. The contagiousness of infectious diseases such as plague, smallpox, diphtheria, cholera, typhoid and syphilis, which could spread like wildfire through countries, was long felt to be due to passing of infection from infected individuals to others. As early as 1546, Girolamo Fracastoro had postulated that *seminaria contagiosa* (seeds of disease) from infected patients could produce disease in uninfected individuals through direct contact. He also postulated that these 'seeds of disease' could be carried by the wind and infect individuals not in direct contact with sick patients This was indeed a great vision but a vision that remained veiled and shrouded in mystery for over another 300 years.

The invention of the microscope in the seventeenth century and the discovery by Leeuwenhoek of animals ('wriggling creatures') invisible to the naked eye did not help to solve the problem. The relation between man, his ecology and disease evaded the thrust of scientific inquiry.

Agostino Bassi of Lodi (1773–1857), in the early nineteenth century was amongst the first to suggest the relation between microscopic organisms and disease. He studied silkworm disease *mal del segno* (muscardine) and observed that it was caused by a living organism *Botrytis paradoxa*. He observed white marks on the bodies of the affected worms and concluded that silkworm disease was caused by a living vegetable parasite. On the basis of many other experiments, Bassi asserted in 1846, that disease was not caused by humors but by a living substance—an animal or vegetable parasite. He thus anticipated the great truth on the cause of infectious disease so ably discovered and enunciated by Pasteur ten years later.

The controversies on the theories of infection also involved theories of putrefaction of organic matter, of the decomposition and putrescence of food, vegetable matter and meat. The presence of insects and mites in decaying matter was a recognized feature of putrefaction and putrescence. The origin of these living creatures was however in dispute. There were some who believed in the theory that the putrefaction of matter produced these organisms by 'spontaneous generation'; there were others who maintained that it was living organisms that were responsible for the decay and putrescence. Lazzaro Spallanzani of whom mention has been made earlier, was one who disbelieved the theory of spontaneous generation. He maintained that broth, if boiled and then hermetically sealed, would keep indefinitely without generating any living organisms. There were metaphysical and philosophical overtones in the arguments for and against the theory of spontaneous generation. Religion taught that God created all creatures—if so, how could creatures spontaneously generate? Philosophers like Diderot on the other hand, espoused spontaneous generation. They opposed the all-pervading dogmatism of religion and considered this phenomenon as nature's expression of creating living forms under special circumstances.

Germany was the centre of laboratory research in the West, and two Germans made significant contributions to microbiology before the advent of Pasteur and his discoveries. Theodore Schwann (1810–1882) demonstrated that putrefaction was caused by living bodies and heat could destroy these living bodies. Jacob Henle (1809–1883), who discovered the 'loop' within the renal tubules that bears his name, was amongst the first to declare that infectious disease was not caused by humors or miasmas, but by living micro-organisms which acted as parasites on entering the body. He debunked the theory of miasmas in infections and of spontaneous generation in putrefaction. He also postulated that once the causative organisms of disease were discovered, cure should follow. Henle's views were still speculative and the debate in relation to the causes and mechanisms of infection or of putrefaction continued unabated. Then strode on the stage of history a great man— Louis Pasteur. He was not a doctor but a chemist, yet he unravelled the mystery of infection with a surety that stopped all debate, and that opened up a glorious vista for science, medicine and for the benefit of man.

Before discussing Pasteur, his discoveries and of those who followed him, it is relevant to briefly touch upon the instrument that made their work possible. This instrument was the microscope, invented in the seventeenth century, but which underwent considerable improvement in the early part of the nineteenth century. Compound microscopes which had two lenses suffered from chromatic aberration produced by the prismatic properties of these lenses. Chromatic aberration resulted in fringes of colour around the image. In 1825, Grambattista Amici (1786–1863), the Italian naturalist, astronomer and mathematician, reduced this aberration by improving the achromatic lens. Joseph Jackson Lister, the father of the great Lord Lister, was a London wine-merchant and an amateur microscopist who made considerable further improvements on the microscope around 1830. Further work on the microscope was done by Charles Chevalier (1804–1859), who invented the compound objective lower lens. Amici advocated the immersion of the objective in water which allowed greater magnification, yet reduced the distortion of the image. The technique of oil immersion was later introduced by Ernst Abbé. The refined microscope indeed contributed a great deal to the advances in bacteriology. It was the sword used by Pasteur and many who followed him in the fight against infection.

Louis Pasteur was born in Dôle, in the French district of Jura, on 27 December 1822. He was the son of a tanner who had served as a sergeant in Napoleon's Grande Armée. Pasteur first went to college at Besançon and then went on to Paris to study chemistry at the Ecole Normale, graduating in 1848. His first love was chemistry. He exhibited, from the start, a clarity and brilliance in thought and ideas, a flair for laboratory work, a meticulousness in experimentation and observation, and a refined logic to his many discoveries, that would rank him as perhaps the greatest man of the nineteenth century. His first major research was in chemistry, involving the study of polarization of light in tartaric acid crystals. Tartaric acid crystals were asymmetrical and their solutions could rotate polarized light both to the right and to the left. Molecular asymmetry in the crystals governed this behaviour of light and he concluded that this molecular asymmetry distinguished inanimate forms from animate or living beings. This work led to the development of stereochemistry and secured for him a teaching post at Dijon. In 1852, he became professor of chemistry at Strasbourg and two years later he moved to Lille. His interest now moved from chemistry to biology, from the study of crystals to the unravelling of the mystery of living micro-organisms, and their relation to man and disease. In his inaugural lecture at the university of Lille, he made a profound statement that was indeed so apt in relation to his many discoveries: "In the field of observation, events favour only those who are prepared." His time had come; he was by now prepared to embark on his voyage of discovery. In 1857, he was appointed director of scientific studies at the Paris Ecole Normale and from that point in time his destiny was to be fulfilled.

At the univeristy of Lille, Pasteur began his first studies on fermentation—the souring of milk and the fermentation of wine and beer. The researchist Liebig had maintained that fermentation was a chemical process due to unstable chemical products or ferments. Pasteur postulated that fermentation was a biological process caused by specific living micro-organisms. He continued these studies at the Ecole Normale in Paris. He convincingly demolished the widely held belief that fermentation was caused by the chemical breakdown of dead yeast. He demonstrated that yeast in sugar solutions exposed to air multiplied rapidly, producing little alcohol. When however yeast was introduced into the same solution but not exposed to air, it utilized the oxygen in the sugar, producing a large quantity of alcohol. In his further research Pasteur showed that the decomposition of wine was brought about by living organisms with the production of vinegar, and that milk would decompose into lactic acid under the influence of lactic acid bacilli. He called the process 'fermentation' when the end product was useful, and 'putrefaction' when it was harmful. Pasteur then went on to discover bacilli responsible for butyric acid fermentation. He noted that these bacilli could live without oxygen and flourished in an atmosphere of carbon dioxide. He named these 'anaerobic organisms', in contrast to aerobic organisms which required oxygen to live and multiply.

His research on micro-organisms in relation to fermentation of alcohol and milk also led him to demonstrate through an elegant series of experiments, that the theory of spontaneous generation of organisms as the cause of putrefaction was untenable. An ardent supporter of spontaneous generation in France was Felix Pouchet who based his theory on his own experiments. Pasteur contended that Pouchet's experiments suffered from faulty technique and thus led to wrong conclusions. His counter-experiments proved the immediate and essential role of micro-organisms in putrefaction.

It was widely accepted that broth in a flask would decompose with time and would contain micro-organisms. Where did these micro-organisms come from? Pasteur set out to prove that they came from the air. He passed air through a plug of cotton inserted into a glass tube, the open end of which was exposed to the air outside his laboratory. He demonstrated that on dissolving this cotton, the sediment contained the same micro-organisms as present in fermented broth. Pasteur contended that the organisms in the broth came from the outside air. He then showed that if a stream of air was first heated and then introduced into a sterile solution, the latter remained free of organisms. He thus proved that live organisms contained in the air caused putrefaction, but heat killed these organisms. Finally, he proved with ingenuity that micro-organisms were not present in the same number and density uniformly in air. He took sterile solutions in sealed flasks to different altitudes. He broke the seals, exposed them to air at a range of different altitudes and resealed the flasks. He demonstrated that flasks containing sterile broth exposed to air at high mountain altitudes and then resealed, rarely showed a growth of micro-organisms. Those flasks exposed to air in Paris had a luxuriant growth of organisms. He concluded that mountain air was pure and had very few micro-organisms—city air was rich in micro-organisms.

France followed the usual custom of setting up a court of inquiry into debatable scientific issues. The Académie de France decided to adjudicate between Pasteur and Pouchet in the theory of putrefaction. After listening to arguments on both sides, they pronounced the verdict in Pasteur's favour. The theory of spontaneous generation was thus buried by Louis Pasteur for eternity.

Wine production from grapes was one of the chief industries of France. In 1864, wine producers were disturbed by the frequent souring of wine which led to a great loss of revenue. They approached Pasteur for help and requested him to suggest a remedy. Pasteur researched on this subject and found that the organism *mycetum aceti* was responsible for the fermentation of wine into sour vinegar. He then discovered that bacteria free fluids would remain sterile and free of organisms if properly protected. One way of protection was heat. He then showed that heating wine for a short while to 60° C (108° F) killed the *mycetum aceti* responsible for the fermentation to vinegar without spoiling the quality of wine. Protection of sterility through heat was applied to other liquids, as for example milk, and came to be known as 'pasteurization' in honour of the man who first discovered this process.

In 1865, the silk industry, another important industry in France was nearly crippled and ruined by a disease called pébrine which was destroying silkworms. Pasteur determined that the cause of silkworm disease was a living protozoan present in moths, their ova, as well as in worms. He worked out the life cycle of this protozoan and showed that removing the infected ova prevented the spread of disease.

In February 1878, Pasteur presented his germ theory to the French Academy of Medicine. In a joint paper with Jules Joubert (1834–1910) and Charles Chamberland (1851–1908), he contended that micro-organisms were responsible for infectious disease, putrefaction and fermentation, that specific micro-organisms produced their specific diseases. He concluded that if these micro-organisms could be identified, then specific vaccines could be prepared and could well prevent specific diseases.

In 1879, he had the chance to put his ideas to a practical test. Chicken cholera was raging in several areas of France. He identified the organisms and isolated them in pure culture. He then noted that old cultures lost their virulence and poultry infected with these old cultures were protected when subsequently live virulent cultures were injected into them. He thus showed that poultry infected by old avirulent cultures were immunized and remained protected from contracting chicken cholera. His idea of protection from disease through vaccination was a brilliant thought and he was proved right.

Pasteur now turned his attention to anthrax, a highly contagious disease affecting horses, cattle and other ruminants and spreading to man through contact with infected hides or meat. The death of livestock from anthrax was tremendous and the disease was particularly ruinous to this industry because it persisted and recurred in the fields from which infected animals had been removed. In man the disease produced necrotizing skin lesions or a fulminant fatal pneumonia. The anthrax bacillus had been found in the blood of cattle dying of anthrax by Franz Aloys Pollender (1800–1879) and Casimir Joseph Davaine (1812–1882). Robert Koch, a great bacteriologist, was also studying anthrax around this time and had noted that under certain conditions the bacillus assumed the form of heat-resistant spores. These heat-resistant spores could contaminate the soil of fields and when they reverted to the bacillary form could produce disease. The persistence of anthrax in previously infected fields was thus proven by Koch to be related to the persistent presence of these spores.

Pasteur experimented with ways and means of reducing the virulence of the anthrax bacillus. He finally observed that the virulence was markedly decreased by heating the bacillus to 42° C (75° F). When these bacilli with attenuated virulence were injected into normal sheep, the vaccinated sheep did not develop the disease when subsequently, virulent bacilli were injected into them. Pasteur must have been a remarkable showman, indeed a rare trait for a scientist of such great genius. He resolved to give a public demonstration of the efficacy of the anthrax vaccine on 5 May 1881, near Melun, at Pouilly-le-Fort. He took forty-eight sheep as the subjects of his study. Before a large crowd of farmers, journalists, veterinary surgeons and onlookers, he injected virulent anthrax bacilli into twenty-four sheep previously immunized by his anthrax vaccine, and into twenty-four healthy sheep not immunized by his vaccine. After forty-eight hours all the vaccinated sheep remained unaffected and well; twenty-two of the twenty-four unvaccinated sheep had died of anthrax.

Although crippled by a stroke which paralysed his right side, Pasteur now moved into his last great field of research—the prevention of rabies. This was and remains a dreadful disease, characterized by hydrophobia, with certain death in a few days. It remains as fatal today as it was since antiquity. Pasteur first attempted to identify the organism causing rabies; he failed, not surprisingly, since the disease is caused by a virus only visible through an electron microscope. He noted, however, that in dogs with rabies the infecting organism was present not only in saliva but also in the spinal cord. He now began by injecting spinal cord tissue containing the infective organism into rabbits' brains. When one rabbit after another had been injected with this virus a fixed incubation period of six days was observed. He called the virus acting in this manner a virus fixé. He injected this virus into the spinal cord of rabbits, and after their death, dried the spinal cord. On drying the cord for two weeks, he observed that the virus was well-nigh non-virulent. In 1884, he made fourteen graduated vaccines of increasing potency. On daily injecting one of these graduated vaccines (starting with the weakest and ending with the strongest) into a number of dogs everyday for fourteen days, he conferred immunity to rabies on these dogs. When these immunized dogs were challenged with the live rabies virus after two weeks they remained healthy and did not contract rabies. When non-immunized dogs were challenged with the live rabies virus they all died. He demonstrated to a government commission the efficacy of his anti-rabies vaccine in protecting dogs from rabies. His regret at this stage was that he did not have the opportunity to try the vaccine on human beings.

The day of judgement was however soon to come. In the summer of 1885, Joseph Meister a nine year old boy from Alsace had been bitten several times by a rabid dog. His doctor advised the boy's mother to take him to Pasteur. Ten days after coming to him and twelve days after the rabid dog's bite, Pasteur took the risk of vaccinating the boy with his anti-rabies vaccine. He gave a fourteen-day course (one injection per day) of increasingly virulent and painful injections. Pasteur must have waited with baited breath. Taking a risk of such magnitude must have stemmed from an invincible courage based on strong conviction. Yet what opprobrium, what tragedy, what misery and what a disastrous end to a glorious career of science if Joseph Meister had died of rabies following Pasteur's experiment. But Pasteur was a man born to a great destiny. The boy mercifully stayed well and healthy. What is more, three months after Joseph Meister sought his help, there came another victim to Pasteur's door. He was a fourteen year old shepherd lad from Pasteur's home district of the Jura. He had been badly bitten when trying to save others from the attack of a rabid dog. Pasteur treated him in the same manner with his vaccine and this boy also survived. On 26 October 1885, Pasteur wrote to the Académie des Sciences that Joseph Meister was safe and well.

The story of this human drama between Pasteur, Joseph Meister and the prevention of rabies took the world by storm. Anti-rabies vaccination as discovered by Pasteur became the standard procedure all over the world in the prevention of rabies following a dog bite and other animal bites. His last achievement was the crowning glory of an incredibly great career. He was acclaimed all over the world as a great hero; he symbolized the successful spirit, the essence of science and scientific inquiry. Every discovery he made had led to the benefit of mankind. Perhaps no man of science has been so greatly and so universally honoured in his lifetime as Louis Pasteur. The Institut

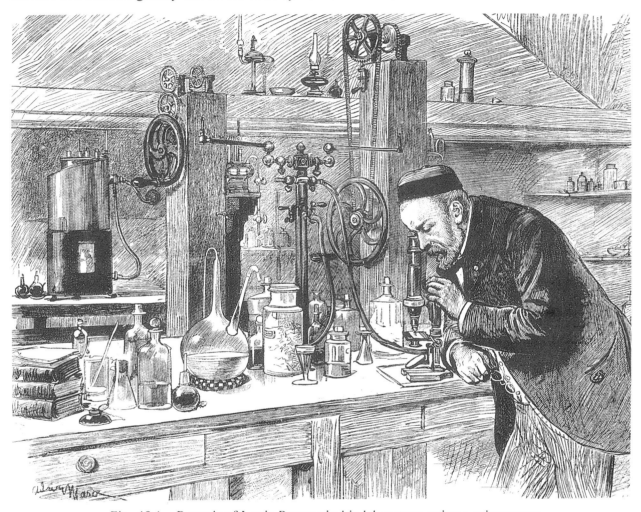

Fig. 48.1   Portrait of Louis Pasteur in his laboratory, using a microscope.

Pasteur was set up in 1888 to enable him to continue his research on micro-organisms and on the development of specific vaccines against disease. There he worked tirelessly to the end of his life, a living legend, gathering around him some of the most famous names in science. He left his immortal legacy to those who worked with him and who shared his travails and joys. Yet it behoves the world to remember that it was a chemist and not a man famous in medicine who became one of the great benefactors of mankind. It is said that a French newspaper put out a questionnaire to its readers as to who they considered the greatest Frenchman of all time. Pasteur, not surprisingly, received even more votes than Napoleon and Charlemagne. Pasteur died at the age of seventy-three in September 1893. The Institut Pasteur remains to this day a living memorial to his name—great scientists have followed his footsteps in the sands of time.

Robert Koch (1843–1910) was a contemporary of Louis Pasteur and made great contributions to the science of bacteriology, conclusively establishing the germ theory of disease. He was born at

Klaustal, Hanover and qualified in medicine in 1866 at the University of Göttingen. His teacher was Jacob Henle. His technical expertise and dexterity were superb, enabling him to pursue his bacteriological research with finesse and exactitude. His initiation into medicine was as a surgeon in the Franco-Prussian war. He then became a district officer in Wollstein, a small town in Prussia. Anthrax was rife in the district and in an almost make-shift laboratory Koch studied its bacteriology. He succeeded in isolating the anthrax bacillus from the blood and spleen of a dead animal, isolated the bacillus in pure culture and worked out its full life history. Pasteur, as stated earlier, confirmed and continued research on anthrax, culminating in the discovery of an effective vaccine against the disease.

In 1878, Koch published a book on the *Aetiology of Infection in Trauma* proving that specific bacteria were responsible for the infection in surgical wounds. In 1880, he was appointed in Berlin at the Kaiserliches Gesundheitsamt (Imperial Health Department). He now contributed a great deal to the technical advances in the laboratory studies on bacteriology. These technical advances have stood the test of time and are in use even today. He used special staining and microscopic techniques for the identification and study of bacteria, making use of the oil immersion lens. He devised and perfected the use of various media (including the solid gelatin and agar media) for the culture of specific organisms.

Koch's greatest triumph was in discovering that tuberculosis was caused by a specific organism Mycobacterium tuberculosis. In 1868, the French pathologist Jean Antoine Villemin had described the pathology of tuberculous lesions and had demonstrated that the disease could be transmitted to animals by the injection of tuberculous material. In 1882, Koch cultured the tubercle bacillus, presenting his results in 1884 to the Berlin Physiological Society. He also presented in this paper his famous 'Koch's Postulates', enunciating a scientific discipline which needs be fulfilled if a specific organism is to be responsible for a specific disease. His postulates were:

- that the organism had to be always found in a given disease;
- that it was to be never found in other diseases or in health;
- that the organism must be grown on culture and that an injection of a pure culture in a susceptible animal must reproduce the disease; and
- that the organism must be present in the animal so inoculated.

Koch through animal experiments convincingly proved that the tubercle bacillus which he had discovered caused tuberculosis. All his postulates were fulfilled in his experimental studies in relation to the specificity of Mycobacterium tuberculosis.

In the following year there was a cholera pandemic and Koch was sent to Egypt to investigate the disease. Also investigating the same problem was a French team headed by Pasteur's colleague, Roux. Roux followed Pasteur's tried method, which was to reproduce the disease in an animal and then look for the organism. Little did Roux realize that cholera only occurred in humans and not in animals. Understandably, he failed. Koch searched for the organism in the excreta of cholera victims, and in 1883 identified the Vibro cholera as the cause of cholera. Koch then went on to Calcutta in India and showed that the organism lived in the intestine and that the disease spread through the contamination of water. He reported his discoveries to the German government. There was unprecedented jubilation, for the Germans felt that in Robert Koch they had the equal of Louis Pasteur of France. The miasmatic theory of infection was now buried and dead, but an occasional die-hard still remained unconvinced. As an amusing aside, the Munich Herr Doctor Pettenkofer refused to believe that the Vibrio cholera caused cholera. He requested Herr Doctor Professor Koch to send him a flask containing a pure culture of Vibrio cholera. Koch obliged, whereupon Herr Doctor Pettenkofer swallowed the contents of the flask. He wrote to Koch in triumph that he was in perfect health and that there was no sign of cholera! Perhaps Herr Doctor Pettenkofer had a high acid content which destroyed the organisms, or perhaps the pure culture he swallowed had lost its virulence!!

The political and economic rivalry between France and Germany in that age crept surreptitiously into science—particularly the science of bacteriology. Robert Koch probably felt impelled to make a climactic discovery that would put even Pasteur in the shade. What better or more difficult subject of research could he choose other than the disease tuberculosis? In that day and age, tuberculosis (also called pthisis or consumption) was the single most important and common cause of death in adults in the West. The disease could be diagnosed clinically ever since the brilliant clinical description of Laennec and Bayle. The morbid anatomy had been determined by Morgagni, Rokitansky and Virchow, the basic pathology being the tubercle. The possibility that tuberculosis was a communicable disease was entertained by a few prominent clinicians and pathologists. The cause of the disease, however, remained a mystery till the advent of Koch, who as stated earlier discovered and proved that Mycobacterium tuberculosis caused the disease.

After his numerous travels to distant countries, Koch went to work in his laboratory to determine the cure for this disease. In August 1890 he announced at the International Congress in Berlin that he had discovered a substance which arrested the growth of the tubercle bacillus both in a test tube and in living human beings. He called his remedy 'tuberculin'. The whole world smiled; for a short euphoric span of twelve months it appeared that there was at last a cure for the dreaded disease.

Instantly after his announcement, Robert Koch was hailed as a hero in Germany, just as Pasteur was hailed as a hero in France. He received the freedom of the city of Berlin and Kaiser Wilhelm personally presented the Grand Cross of the Red Eagle to him. Koch did not reveal the source or nature of his remedy—a rather unethical attitude of a scientist towards his discovery. Tuberculin was administered to thousands of individuals over the next year. The treatment unfortunately, both for Koch and the world, was a fiasco. This was no cure; in many patients the cure worsened the disease. Koch was now denounced for making baseless claims and for not revealing the source of his 'remedy'. It was even rumoured that he had sold his remedy to a drug company at a huge profit. Well after his cure had been proven useless, Koch in a paper published in January 1891 stated that his 'cure' was the glycerine extract of the tubercle bacilli. A few scorned him for a revelation made too late. Yet in years to come, the preparation of tuberculin did have a diagnostic use. An intradermal injection would often produce a strong reaction if the patient in the past or present had been infected by tuberculosis. Koch had tested tuberculin on himself and had noticed a strong reaction. A positive reaction of this nature was determined in a few more years to come to be due to a delayed type IV hypersensitivity reaction to the tuberculous antigen. The tuberculin test even today, is an important diagnostic aid to infection caused by the tubercle bacillus.

In 1891, Koch was appointed director of the Institute of Infectious Diseases and studied methods of the control of water-borne infections by the filtration of water. Notwithstanding his debacle on the use of 'tuberculin', the glory of his early discoveries remained undimmed and in 1905, he was awarded the Nobel Prize. He was revered, though not as universally admired as Pasteur. Like Pasteur, he gathered around him a school of brilliant scientists who in years to come would contribute significantly to the science he had so ably pioneered.

We must now add a postscript to the story of tuberculosis, for the search for a vaccine or other means of immunization against this disease continued and continues to this day. Albert Calmette (1863–1933) of the Pasteur Institute and Jean Marie Guérin (1872–1961) developed a new method of preparing a vaccine. They used a live bovine strain of the tubercle bacillus and on repeated subcultures of this strain noted that the bacillus lost its virulence but retained its protective action.

The vaccine was named BCG (*Bacillus Calmette Guerin*), and from 1924, was tried out on humans. There was a mixed reaction to the vaccine and though thousands of children were vaccinated, its efficacy was controversial. Recent work bears out its usefulness particularly in the prevention of tuberculous meningitis, one of the worst forms of tuberculosis that invariably caused death before the discovery of antituberculous drugs.

Pasteur in France and Koch in Germany had given a great impetus to the continuous progress of bacteriology—an impulse which has persisted to this day. The last twenty years of the nineteenth century saw the discovery of a number of specific organisms responsible for specific major diseases. Identification of a specific infecting organism did not however always result in an effective cure or prevention of the disease. It did however help in the prevention of some of the major infections afflicting mankind—typhoid, plague, diphtheria and tetanus.

The typhoid bacillus was discovered by Georg Gaffky (1850–1898), a pupil of Robert Koch. Immunization by a vaccine, through the use of killed typhoid bacilli was introduced by Almroth Wright (1861–1947). First used on soldiers at war, it strongly reduced the incidence of typhoid in the inoculated soldiers. Paratyphoid A and B were germs allied to the typhoid bacillus, causing a similar but less severe illness. Killed cultures of these paratyphoid organisms were added to the typhoid vaccine and this became known as the TAB vaccine, now widely in use all over the world.

Alexandre Yersin (1863–1943) and Shibasaburo Kitasato (1852–1931) independently discovered the plague bacillus during the Hong Kong epidemic of 1894. Yersin was Swiss, an assistant to Koch, and had worked on diphtheria before commencing his investigations on plague. Kitasato was a Japanese working in the Koch Institute in Germany. Yersin called the plague bacillus Yersinia pestis, recognized that the disease was highly contagious, and demonstrated that it could be experimentally reproduced in healthy rats and then transferred from rat to rat. The rat was the main vector, and extermination of rats would prevent the disease. It was long recognized that plague in man was generally preceded by an epizootic among rodents. The epizootics were now recognized to be due to the plague bacillus which was transferred from rat to rat by the flea *Xenopslla cheopsis*. The flea, after the death of a rat from plague would jump on to a man and transmit the plague bacillus to him, resulting in the disease. An epizootic of plague in a densely populated area was a prelude to an epidemic of plague and epidemics often turned into pandemics that for centuries had decimated mankind. It was the Russian Waldemar Haffkine (1860–1930), who working on plague in Bombay, India, discovered the first effective plague vaccine. His success story is described in chapter 61.

One of the greatest triumphs of bacteriology against disease was in diphtheria, a disease spread by droplet infection. The bacillus causing diphtheria was discovered in 1883 by Albrecht Klebs (1834–1913), a pupil of Virchow, and it was isolated in pure culture by Friedrich Loeffler, an assistant to Koch. Diphtheria was a killer disease among children. It caused a leathery greyish-white exudate on the tonsils, which could spread to the pharynx and larynx and thereby choke the child to death. The disease also produced a systemic illness, chiefly involving the cranial nerves, the heart and the circulation. Pierre Paul Emile Roux (1853–1933), a friend of Pasteur and his successor as the director of the Institut Pasteur, working with Alexandre Yersin, showed that the diphtheria bacillus produced a powerful toxin. The toxin thus produced by the organism within the exudate in the throat was absorbed into the bloodstream, inducing the dangerous systemic effects that killed the patient. In 1890, Karl Fraenkel (1861–1902) injected an attenuated culture of diphtheria bacilli into guinea pigs conferring immunity against the disease. Emil Behring (1854–1917) and Shibasaburo Kitasato, his Japanese colleague showed in 1890 that the serum of an animal immunized against diphtheria could be used to effectively treat another animal that was exposed to this infection and had contracted the disease. Immunity in animals could be conferred by challenging them with gradually increasing doses of the diphtheria toxin. Serum production began in both Germany and France. Roux and Yersin in Paris discovered that large-scale production of diphtheria immune serum was possible by immunizing horses against diphtheria and using the serum so obtained to treat diphtheria in humans. Epidemics of diphtheria were no longer the scourge they used to be.

The Hungarian Béla Schick (1877–1967) showed that when a standard strength of the diphtheria toxin was injected into the skin of the forearm, it could determine whether a child was immune or susceptible to the disease. If the toxin produced a redness or an induration as a reaction, the child was immune; if there was no reaction the child was susceptible. Large-scale immunization programmes in children were now started, so that the incidence of diphtheria was significantly reduced.

The success story of conferring immunity against disease through immunized serum was repeated in the treatment of tetanus and snake bite. Tetanus was and continues to be a dreadful disease caused by the Clostridium tetani whose natural habitat is the soil. The organisms enter the body through cuts or wounds; the toxin produced by Clostridium tetani travels along the axons of nerves, reaching the motor nuclei of the cranial nerves and the motor horn cells of the spinal cord. Rigidity of the skeletal muscles, severe convulsive seizures and death result. It is a killer disease, with a mortality of over 40 per cent. Severe tetanus and tetanus neonatorum (tetanus in the newborn) if not expertly treated even today carry a mortality close to 100 per cent. This disease is still an important cause of death in the developing countries of the world. The tetanus bacillus was discovered in 1880. It can exist in the spore form like the anthrax bacillus, and can grow in the absence of oxygen. Arthur Nicolaier (1862–1942) produced the disease in mice by injecting garden soil. Kitasato isolated the organism in pure culture and obtained a powerful tetanus toxin. This led to the production of an effective antitoxin. Till this point in time, death from tetanus was frequent in soldiers wounded in battle. The organism would enter the body through battle wounds producing disease and death. The compulsory use of tetanus antitoxin for all wounds in battles and wars sharply reduced the incidence of the disease. Tetanus antitoxin as a preventive was first introduced in 1915 during the 1914–1918 First World War; it dramatically reduced the incidence of the disease.

The use of vaccines initiated by Pasteur and the use of immune sera for the prevention and treatment of disease aroused increasing interest in the immune response of the body to infection. The immunity conferred by the above means was termed humoral immunity. Emil Behring and the Japanese Baron Shibasaburo Kitasato published two papers in 1890, proclaiming the discovery of antitoxins and their efficacy in the treatment of tetanus and diphtheria. They laid the basic foundations for all future studies on passive immunity.

Now came on to the scene a great Russian, Elie Metchnikoff (1845–1916). He showed the importance of the cell in the defence of the body to infection, enunciating his theory of phagocytosis. For his outstanding work he was awarded the Nobel Prize in 1905. Metchnikoff researched on comparative physiology and published in 1883, a classic description of defence mechanisms in the lower invertebrates. He carried out his research in Messina, Sicily, which had a rich marine life. Metchnikoff made a special study of the sandhopper (daphnia) a crustacean which was both small and transparent under the microscope. The sandhopper was fed with the spores of a simple type of fungus. After ingestion the spores were noticed to perforate the digestive tract and enter the body cavity. When this happened, the cells in the fluid of the coelomic cavity of the crustacean attacked the spore and ingested it by phagocytosis. They thus removed this foreign invader from the system and the crustacean survived. Metchnikoff proposed that animals and humans had phagocytes which formed an important defence against invading micro-organisms. This was the first step in the study of cellular immunity and of cell-mediated immunity. Phagocytosis was shown to be a function of the white blood cells (leucocytes) and in particular of the polymorphonuclear leucocytes in man and animals. Metchnikoff's theory of phagocytosis opened a new vista in the future study of immunology by other workers.

Perhaps the first great pioneer in the study of immunology, as we know it today, was Paul Ehrlich (1854–1914). He was a scientific genius who laid the foundations of both immunology and chemotherapy. Ehrlich was the son of a Jewish merchant in Silesia. His early years gave no promise of his genius. In fact he was a poor scholar, passed his examinations with difficulty, and was even considered to be a trifle backward by the professors of the faculty of Medicine at Breslau university. He wandered from one university to the other studying first at Strasbourg, Frieburg and then going on to Leipzig where he qualified in 1878. From his very early days, even as a medical student, he was fond of staining techniques, experimenting with dyes and tissue-staining. His doctoral thesis was on the staining of histological specimens for microscopic examination. He demonstrated the use of special dyes to relatively stain and study white blood cells and made the important discovery that the tubercle bacilli stained with carbol fuchsin retained this colour after treatment with acid. Thus there came into medicine the concept of acid-fast bacilli. Ehrlich postulated from his studies on dyes that certain tissues as also certain micro-organisms had an elective affinity for certain dyes and could thus be identified.

Ehrlich was the father of modern immunology. He demonstrated that the anti-toxic effect of immune serum against specific bacteria or their toxins was present not only in animals but also in the test-tube. He showed with his co-worker Julius Morgenroth (1871–1924) that this was due to a heat-stable immune body and a heat-labile substance called complement. Other colleagues added significantly to Ehrlich's work on immune response. Richard Pfeiffer (1858–1945) studied the phenomena of bacteriolysis. He noted that if a guinea pig was immunized against cholera by inoculating it with the Vibrio cholera and if subsequently a live virulent culture of this organism was injected intraperitonealy into the animal, the Vibrios were dissolved. This 'dissolution', called bacteriolysis, was due to antibodies destroying the antigen in the presence of a substance termed 'complement' which was normally present in the serum. The complement was used up in this reaction. The above reaction of antigen, antibody, complement observed in bacteriolysis was also noted in agglutination and haemolysis seen after the transfusion of incompatible blood. Complement fixation was studied by Jean Bordet (1870–1961) and Octave Gengou (1875–1959), who worked out the complement fixation test which is the basis of the Wassermann reaction in syphilis, and the basis of similar reactions used in the diagnosis of other diseases.

Ehrlich was the first to introduce a chemical concept into immunology. The six-carbon benzene ring formula had already been devised by August Kekulé (1829–1896). Ehrlich in his side-chain theory postulated that the protein molecule was analogous of the six-carbon benzene ring. In the case of proteins, unstable side-chains could act as chemoreceptors, so that they combined with bacterial toxins and neutralized them. The immune body was a protein and could be produced in the body and the blood by the stimulus of the antigen (a bacterial toxin in any infecting agent); it would persist in the blood as long as the antigenic stimulus remained. This was a brilliant theory and though it has now been significantly modified by the work of Linus Pauling and Haurowitz it remains an important landmark in immunology.

The science of bacteriology had brought in the beginnings of immunology. It was by now obvious that the mechanism behind the pioneering work of Jenner in the prevention of smallpox was related to the production of specific antibodies through active immunity. The same explanation

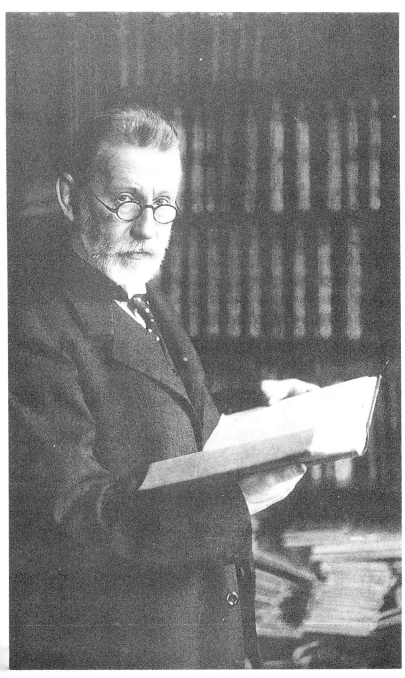

Fig. 48.2   Paul Ehrlich.

underlay the work of Pasteur in the prevention of rabies and anthrax. On the other hand, the prevention of tetanus and diphtheria produced by the injection of immune serum was due to passive immunities. Both active and passive immunity were due to presence of specific antibodies in the blood to specific disease. Advances in biochemistry showed that antibodies were proteins of the gamma globulin group with a molecular weight of 1,00,000 to 10,00,000 daltons. They are disease-specific and were shown to be produced by the lymph glands and the bone marrow. The immunity conferred by antibodies came to be known as 'humoral immunity'. The importance of 'cellular immunity' had already been stressed by Metchnikoff and the property of phagocytosis chiefly exhibited by the polymorphonuclear cell was soon recognized to be the front-line defence against infection by the invading micro-organisms. In time to come, the importance of the mononuclear cell, the macrophage and the lymphocyte in immune response was established. The counterpart of 'humoral immunity' was cellular immunity and cell-mediated immunity. Still later, the link or interconnection between cell-mediated immune response to infection and humoral immunity was established.

Sir Frank Mcfarlane was the first to point out the paradox that cells which destroy worn out cells (like the red blood cells) within the body without production of antibodies, destroy invading foreign organisms or their toxins (antigen) with production of antibodies. This is because cells within the body 'recognise' their own proteins in the blood and in different tissues and do not react against them. This reaction is 'learned' and 'memorised' during the foetal stage of development. If for some reason or the other, the cells active in immune response lose or unlearn their tolerance to one or more proteins in one or more organ systems of the body, they mount an immune offensive against these proteins. This is the mechanism underlying 'autoimmune disease' and there are several such diseases described today. An early description was Hashimoto's thyroiditis, an autoimmune disease of the thyroid gland reported by Hashimoto in 1912.

Immunology has had an increasing role in the history of contemporary medicine. Could infections be countered by means other than passive and active immunization? The attempt to treat disease through herbs and other substances (often noxious and dangerous) date from antiquity. Paracelsus had advocated specific drugs for specific diseases. Many a physician anticipated a future when each specific disease would be countered by a specific drug. Till the early years of the twentieth century, the only effective drugs against infection were the empirical use of quinine (obtained from the Peruvian bark) against malaria and the use of the willow bark (which contained salicylates) against fever, particularly rheumatic fever.

Ehrlich, armed with the new knowledge on bacteriology and the early beginnings of immunology, now used his scientific genius to pioneer chemotherapy. As explained earlier, his studies with dyes had convinced him of the affinity of specific dyes to specific micro-organisms and to specific tissues. He was convinced that biologically active substances must first be attached to a cell before they could act on it. He reasoned that this attachment was through a 'receptor'. If a dye could be attached to a cell because of a special receptor so that the cell was stained by it, a drug could also be similarly attached. His side-chain theory advocated that the reaction between the bacterial toxin (antigen) and antibody was chemical in nature, the antibody 'homing' on and forming a chemical attachment solely to the toxin and destroying or inactivating it. The objective therefore, was to find chemical 'bullets' specific for a particular organism that would latch on through receptors to the organism, destroying the organism without affecting the host.

He first tried methylene blue on malaria with what he considered promising results. He then studied trypanosomiasis (sleeping sickness) caused by the trypanosome, a parasite transmitted by the tsetse fly. He found that the dye trypan-red had some action on the disease. He also used a drug called atoxyl, and other arsenical compounds. These had to be abandoned as they caused neurological complications including blindness as side-effects.

Ehrlich next turned his attention to researching on a chemical that could act on syphilis, a venereal disease caused by sexual contact. Syphilis was distinguished from gonorrhoea, another venereal disease, as late as about the middle of the nineteenth century by Philippe Ricord (1800–1889). Ricord also described the primary, secondary and tertiary stages of syphilis.

In 1905, Fritz Schaudinn (1871–1906) and Eric Hoffmann (1868–1959), two German bacteriologists, discovered the single cell, spiral-shaped motile organism causing this disease, from the chancres of syphilitic patients. They named the organism Spirochaeta pallida, though the current name widely used is Treponema pallidum. Diagnosis of syphilis was made possible by August von Wasserman (1866–1912) by using the complement fixation test. In 1910, Ehrlich reported the discovery of salvarsan also known as preparation 606. This is because it was the 606th arsenical product to be sythesized by his chemotherapeutic institute in an attempt to find a cure for syphilis. Its claim to efficacy was proven after its systemic use on thousands of syphilitic patients. In 1914, Ehrlich claimed that a new arsenical compound neoarsphenamine (preparation 914) was even more effective against syphilis than salvarsan. The arsenical preparations discovered by Ehrlich were a significant advance over the earlier treatment of mercury given orally and applied to the skin as an ointment. Even so, with increasing experience it had to be admitted that repeated courses of painful injections of neoarsphenamine were often required, and in a number of instances, the disease remained unconquered. The world had to wait for penicillin for the conquest of syphilis.

If organical arsenicals had proved to be effective against syphilis, surely there had to be other chemicals active against other diseases. Numerous chemicals were tried for diseases caused by specific cocci and bacilli, but the vision of Pasteur, Koch, Ehrlich, and many other microbe-hunters remained unfulfilled. Up to the middle of the 1930s the only drugs effective against infections were quinine against malaria, arsenicals (and to a lesser extent mercury) against syphilis, and antimony against schistosomiasis. Then came a major breakthrough—Gerhard Domagk (1895–1964) in 1935 reported the discovery of prontosil.

Domagk, like Ehrlich, was searching for chemicals effective against micro-organisms or their toxins causing disease. His research first concentrated on metal-based compounds. He found them both ineffective and toxic. In 1927, he was appointed research director of a large chemical company which chiefly manufactured azo dyes for colouring textiles. He researched on these azo dyes in relation to their effect on microbes and disease. In 1932, he discovered that a particular red dye called prontosil was effective against experimentally-induced streptococcal infection in rats. Domagk then successfully tried out prontosil on his own daughter who took ill with an acute streptococcal infection. Scientists at the Pasteur Institute further researched on prontosil and discovered that the active component of prontosil within the body was a chemical termed sulphonamide. They also determined that sulphonamide did not kill micro-organisms but stopped them from multiplying, the organisms being then killed by the immune response of the body. The action of prontosil, or rather sulphonamide, was termed a bacteriostatic action.

Prontosil was the first drug or chemical to be mass-produced and it was made readily available in the West and later all over the world. The drug acted well against streptococcal, pneumococcal and gonococcal infections. Thus streptococcal tonsillitis, erysipelas, mastoiditis, sinusitis, puerperal fever, as also pneumonia due to the streptococcus or to the pneumococcus now came under control. Gonorrhoea could be cured within a week. Scientists began to look for comparable but better drugs. In 1938, A. J. Ewins (1882–1938), the head of a research team of May and Baker developed M&B 693 (sulphadiazine 693, later called sulphapyridine). It was even more effective than prontosil against streptococcal and pneumococcal infections. It received wide publicity on its successful use on Winston Churchill who took ill with pneumonia during World War II.

Medicine had taken an important step towards the therapeutic control of disease. Yet even as the use of sulphonamides and sulpha drugs spread far and wide, the writing was on the wall. The drug could cause dangerous side-effects and the micro-organisms could become resistant to the drug. The never-ending, never-to-be-won war between man and microbes had just begun.

Man's fight against infections in the nineteenth and early twentieth century must necessarily take note of the close association between industry, science, technology and medicine. Industries (mainly companies) manufacturing drugs opened in the mid-nineteenth century, their performance helped by technology and science. Companies related to drug manufacture were Squibb, Eli Lilly, Merck and Parke Davis. The latter set up one of the first research institutes in 1902. The pharmacological industry flourished best in Germany, there being a close cooperation between science, technology and industry. Thus the Frankfurt Institute Research Laboratories, where Ehrlich worked, had close links with the Hoechst and Farbwerke Casella companies. Even so, the interests of the industry were not necessarily parallel with the interests of science. The former was chiefly interested in profit. The latter solely into getting to know the unknown. Ethical problems and clashes were bound to arise and have continued up to the present time.

The next great step in the fight against infection was the discovery of penicillin by Sir Alexander Fleming, a Scottish bacteriologist at St Mary's Hospital in London. The antibiotic era had arrived and since then there has been a flood of antibiotics introduced into medicine.

49 Military Medicine—The Red Cross and Nursing

From ancient times to the present day wars have brought in their wake pestilence and famine. Armies in the past have been at times defeated by disease rather than in battle. The breakdown of basic hygiene, the crowding of humans in hostile environments and inclement weather, the frequent scarcity of food and water, physical fatigue and mental stress made a formidable combination encouraging violent epidemics of infectious disease that could decimate an army. Soldiers lay wounded on the battlefield, medical and surgical attention was disorganized and primitive, and the mortality in battle wounds from haemorrhage and sepsis was incredibly high. It was only towards the end of the eighteenth century that medical corps were organized and incorporated into the army, and military field stations and army hospitals were established. The Napoleonic wars in the late eighteenth and early nineteenth century witnessed the death of six million French and allied troops. Jean Dominique Larrey (1766–1842), the chief of the medical corps of Napoleon's Grande Armée, was the first to organize field ambulances (horse-drawn carriages) that went into battle with the soldiers, ministering first aid and immediate surgery to the wounded. Though many died in battle, a large number also died of other causes. The necessity for better medical care in wartime was brought home to both the victor and the vanquished. The Crimean War was an outstanding example, where horrendous losses occurred amongst the wounded allied soldiers at base hospitals, till such time as Florence Nightingale arrived on the scene. In the American Civil War twice as many died of disease than from battle wounds sustained in battle.

In 1864, there occurred a rather fortuitous event that significantly altered for the better the miserable plight of the soldiers at war. Henri Dunant (1828–1910), a philanthropist and a Swiss banker was present at the battle of Solferino, fought between the Austrian army and the Franco-Italian army of Napoleon III on 14 June 1859 in Northern Italy. He was shocked and moved by the plight of thousands of wounded soldiers lying unattended on the battlefield. He successfully persuaded the generals of the victorious Franco-Italian army to release the captured Austrian military surgeons to help attend to the wounded of all three countries. He himself went around the battlefield tending the wounded. He repeated *'Tutti fratelli'* (all brothers) to local civilians who resisted giving help to the Austrians. Shattered by his personal experience of war and its sufferings, he wrote his *Souvenir de Solferino* which galvanized European leaders into action. Victor Hugo, the Goncort brothers and Joseph Ernest Renan championed the cause of international humanitarianism. An International Congress of Red Cross Societies was held in Geneva in 1863, each society being a national organization formed to aid the wounded of a country. In the second international conference in 1864, the Geneva Convention was signed by sixteen nations. The convention established the International Red Cross, specifying the regulations that were to apply to the treatment of wounded soldiers. All military and civilian hospitals were to be recognized as neutral territory, and all military personnel and their equipment were to be free from attack, molestation or harm. The protective insignia was a red cross on a white background. The International Red Cross was first successfully baptized under fire when a group of volunteer civilian Red Cross workers went on to the battlefield to care for the Austrians wounded after the battle of Koniggratz in 1866. Austria, who was a non-signatory at the Geneva Convention now joined it.

Not always are good deeds rewarded in this world. In 1867, Dunant became bankrupt, according to some because of lavish spending in founding the Red Cross. He was lost to the world for over fifteen years and was then discovered in Switzerland in a home for the aged, unstable in mind. He was awarded the first Nobel Peace Prize in 1901 and though poor in resources, donated the entire sum to charity.

If care for the soldier at war, right up to the middle of the nineteenth century was poor, care for the ill in large urban hospitals was perhaps just a trifle better and left much to be desired. Hospital mortality was often horrendous, particularly after surgery. Hospital gangrene (the French called it *Pourriture d'hôpital*), often broke out in epidemic form, so that a wound, clean to start with, quickly grew infected, then turned into spreading gangrene with increasing sepsis and death. A foul, putrid odour of pus and decaying flesh often pervaded the wards of many hospitals. John Howard in the eighteenth century had shocked the conscience of the literate with his book *Hospitals and Lazarettos*. It is amazing that even in that era the discerning proclaimed that infections and contagions were directly related to the hospital. Erichsen believed it was the hospital building, or its atmosphere which was responsible for erysipelas and other infectious diseases. The concept of what we today call nosocomial infection had been grasped over two centuries earlier. It was also noted that the mortality of surgery performed on a patient at his home was three or four times less than when in hospital.

An important reason for the sorry state of hospitals in that era was poor nursing. And then there walked into history Florence Nightingale (1820–1910), 'the lady with the lamp', who lit her way into the hearts of the very many she nursed, and who established the profession of nursing as we know it today. Nursing, of course, did not begin with Florence Nightingale. The urge to care for or nurse existed from earliest times. Though nursing was rudimentary and disorganized in the early centuries, the great Charaka by about the second century AD had a perfect concept of the qualifications for a nurse: "Knowledge of the manner in which drugs should be prepared or compounded for administration, cleverness, devotion to the patient waited upon, and purity both of mind and body."

Nursing promptly conjures a vision of gentle caring women. This is indeed true; women have always formed the core of this profession. Yet, in the Middle Ages, men tended to the sick in the hospital. During the Crusades, the Hospitaliers of St John, the Teutonic Knights and the Knights of St Lazarus nursed the wounded and sick, and the mendicant orders of St Francis and St Dominic also acted as nurses in the Middle Ages.

Organized nursing among women was first noticed in nuns of religious orders. Perhaps the oldest religious order devoted exclusively to nursing was that of the Augustinian Nuns in the Hôtel Dieu of Paris. From the Middle Ages onwards, nursing the sick became closely associated with the Church, so that even in hospitals totally unconnected with religion or perhaps even irreligious, the nurses were called 'sisters'. The Reformation, an anti-Catholic movement that swept through many countries in Europe, severed the connection between hospitals and religious orders. The dedicated free services of secular religious groups was now replaced by the paid service of hired workers who lacked both motivation and care. Hospitals as mentioned earlier became increasingly filthy, the hothouses of infection, disease and death. The Enlightenment of the eighteenth century brought back to an extent a humanitarian approach to the care of the sick. But then came the Industrial Revolution, with industry offering tempting wages to men, women and children. The clock turned back once again. The income from nursing was poor. To the uncaring and undedicated, nursing activities were demanding, repulsive and demeaning, so that the inducement to take up nursing as a wage-earning profession ceased altogether. There was now a dire need to improve the quality and training of nurses. In 1840, Elizabeth Fry (1780–1845), an English Quaker founded the Society of Protestant Sisters of Charity, attempting to send nurses to the homes of the sick whether rich or poor, as also to prisons to tend to the sick. Theodor Fliedner (1800–1864), a Protestant minister in Germany and his wife Frederike, were influenced and impressed by the work of Elizabeth Fry. Back in Germany they first organized care for female prison convicts, then for the sick poor. Finally, they acquired a 200-bed hospital in Kaiserwerth, staffed without pay by the deaconesses of the Church. The deaconesses were trained by physicians over a three year period to become proficient in all aspects of nursing. By the time of Fliedner's death, the Kaiserwerth school had trained over 1,500 deaconesses ready to shoulder the onerous responsibility of nursing care. Elizabeth Fry had visited Kaiserwerth and had been inspired by Fliedner's work. She founded the Institute of Nursing in London in 1840. Those who joined were called the Society of Protestant Sisters of Charity. There were protests that this description had the religious overtones of Catholicism and the term was changed to 'nursing sisters'. Nursing sisters, unlike their counterparts in Kaiserwerth, did not receive formal classroom instruction and were only trained in home nursing. There were others who initiated attempts to train nurses and organize the profession but none so brilliant, so gifted and so dedicated as Florence Nightingale.

Florence Nightingale was from a wealthy middle-class family, born during the family's holiday in Florence. She was a shy but intense and stubborn girl who had set her heart as a young girl to serve mankind through nursing the sick. This became an obsession, a magnificent obsession. The parents forbade her to become a nurse. 'We are ducks,' cried her despairing mother, 'who have hatched a wild swan.' At the age of 32 years, her parents relented and allowed her to visit and train at Kaiserwerth. She left Kaiserwerth after three months and went on to spend some time with the Daughters of Charity in Paris. She then returned to London and was appointed Superintendent of the Establishment for Gentlewomen during Illness. She then became the Superintendent of Nursing at King's College Hospital. In March 1854, Britain, France and Turkey went to war against Russia in Crimea—the Crimean War. Amazingly, it was the death and destruction of war that gave Florence Nightingale the opportunity and the occasion to fulfil her childhood dream and compulsion to serve mankind. There was public indignation in Britain that while French wounded soldiers were being nursed by Catholic Sisters of Charity, the British wounded were attended to by untrained male orderlies and were dying by the hundreds. Sidney Herbert requested Florence Nightingale to lead a batch of thirty-eight nurses to Crimea. Hospital conditions were indeed awful at the British base of Scutori across the Bosphorus. One thousand eight hundred men were housed in rat-infested, poorly-ventilated wards with dreadful sanitation. Dirty beds, filthy clothes, poor nutrition and food, no equipment for proper care, and a callous neglect towards the wounded and sick made a mockery of the word 'hospital'. With singular dedication, devotion and against an almost chauvinistic opposition from the officer staff, Nightingale transformed this hell-hole into a clean well-ventilated hospital. The soldiers were now well cared for with regard to diet, cleanliness, medication and the careful dressing of wounds. The death rate among the wounded and sick fell from 40 per cent to 2 per cent. The soldiers loved her for they promptly recognized (as all very sick people invariably do) that here at last was one who truly cared. "We lay there by the hundreds; but we could kiss her shadow as it fell and lay our heads on the pillow again content."

She returned to London in 1856 hailed as a heroine. After the Crimean War, she was largely responsible for setting up the first military medical school in London. She was also the guiding spirit

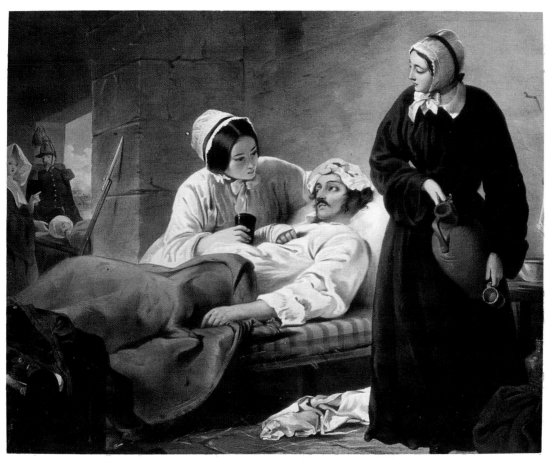

Fig. 49.1   Florence Nightingale.

in the reconstruction of St Thomas Hospital. Her architectural views on the medical aspects governing the construction of hospitals were put into effect during this project. A public appeal to start a nursing school under Florence Nightingale brought in £44,000 and her first batch of students graduated from her school at St Thomas in 1861. Her aim was to train 'matrons'–graduates who in turn, would train raw recruits joining hospitals. She managed thereby, to prise the management of nursing and nurses from the supervision of men, placing them under the control of matrons. Her nursing matrons spread far and wide, both in the West and East, spreading her gospel to several countries of the world. Her extensive notes on nursing, published in 1859, became compulsory reading for all those who joined the profession she founded. The stress in her teachings was on basic hygiene. "Nursing has been limited to signify little more than the administration of poultices. It ought to signify the proper use of fresh air, light, warmth, cleanliness, quiet and the proper selection and administration of diet."

The strain of organizing, travelling, working and writing told on her health. Inevitably there were people who bickered and resented her. She suffered a number of illnesses, perhaps a series of nervous breakdowns. Her health was particularly fragile after she suffered a serious febrile illness (perhaps typhoid or typhus) in the Crimea, but she continued to write extensively and work tirelessly till the end. Amazingly enough, she never believed in bacteria causing disease. She continued to believe in the miasmatic theory of infection, and her focus on bedside care, with scant attention to didactic teaching or scientific discoveries, excited a fair degree of animosity. By all counts, Florence

Nightingale was a great woman. She owed her success to her obsessive motivation, a vision to which she steadfastly adhered, to professional ability and competence, and to a profound devotion to her cause. She transformed nursing from lowly beginnings to a noble and highly respected profession that embodies within itself the very essence of the art of healing. She ensured that the nurse and doctor were equal partners in the fight against disease. She exemplified the care of the sick in her personal odyssey through life, and amazingly also successfully institutionalized care in the nursing profession for posterity. We quote her basic tenets that are equally applicable to the art and science of medicine as they are to the art and science of nursing—tenets that are as compellingly relevant today as they were in her day.

> The art is of nursing the sick. Please mark, not nursing sickness. This is the reason why nursing proper can only be taught at the patient's bedside and in the sick room or ward. Lectures and books are but valuable accessories.

> 'The Lady with the Lamp' had cast an eternal glow on an uncaring world.

50 Physics and Medicine

The close link between basic science and medicine is supremely illustrated by the discovery of X-rays in physics and the application of this discovery to medicine. The use of X-rays to image the body is now termed radiology—a field of investigation which was the forerunner to numerous subsequent imaging techniques, all based on laws of physics.

William Konrad Roentgen (1845–1923) was professor of physics at the University of Würsburg and was engaged in the study of the electrical phenomena described by Crookes and Hertz. His experiments entailed the study of cathode rays induced by the passage of a high-voltage current through a wire, vacuum-sealed in a Crookes tube. Roentgen made his momentous discovery on the evening of 8 November 1895. He noted that while passing a current through such a tube (which had been wrapped in black cardboard to screen out the light it emitted), a sheet of cardboard coated with barium platinocyanide was shining brightly in his darkened laboratory. Roentgen noted that this fluorescence was due to radiation or 'rays' emanating from the tube. He called the radiation X-rays because of the unknown nature of the phenomenon. He then discovered that these X-rays could penetrate dense objects opaque to light waves, giving an image of these objects on a photographic plate as well as on a fluorescent screen. Roentgen experimented with different solid objects which he placed between the Crookes tube and a wooden box which contained a photographic plate. He discovered that the form of each object cast an 'image' or impression on the photographic plate. He also tested the penetration of these newly discovered X-rays against different metal sheets and noted that only lead barred these X-rays completely. He now experimented on his own hands, exposing them to the X-rays and noted that the bones of his hand were clearly outlined on a screen. He repeated this study on his wife's hand catching the 'image' on a photographic plate. The bones of the hands were perfectly visible, together with the ring on her fourth finger, all sharply highlighted against the background of the barely discernible soft tissue of the hand. On 28 December 1895, Roentgen reported his sensational discovery in his preliminary communication to the President of the Physical–Medical Society of Wursburg. He was fully aware of its diagnostic importance in medicine. Within a few weeks, his discovery was greeted all over the West as one of the most important landmarks in medical history. Roentgen received the Nobel Prize for physics in 1902 for this great discovery.

X-rays were used for diagnostic purposes from January 1896 in an increasing number of hospitals. Fractures and bone diseases were now imaged before the eye and the use of these rays soon extended to the imaging of stones in the gall bladder, kidney and detection of foreign bodies like bullets or metal fragments. In December 1896, W. B. Cannon (1871–1945) while still a student at Harvard Medical School, noted that if bismuth salts were fed to animals, they allowed a visualization of the gut on a fluorescent screen. This technique was applied to humans from 1904, barium sulphate being used to opacify the gut so that structural abnormalities in the stomach, duodenum and the rest of the intestine could now be diagnosed.

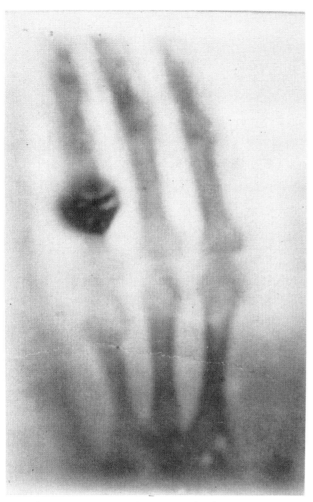

Fig. 50.1   Probably the hand of Frau Roentgen
with a ring.

The early X-ray apparatus emitted poor radiation, requiring over thirty-minutes exposure time to obtain a satisfactory radiograph or picture. The need to reduce this exposure time was evident and was achieved in 1913 by the introduction of the heated cathode, which emitted a far greater number of high-energy electrons when compared to the cold cathode. The use of the X-ray machine with exposure times of less than a few seconds was of immense help during the First World War in the diagnosis of fractures and of bullet and shell fragments within the human body. Technical advances have today cut the exposure time to less than two-hundredth of a second.

Roentgen had noted that prolonged exposure to X-rays caused skin burns, ulcerations, hair loss, dermatitis and skin atrophy. Many radiologists, who pioneered the study of radiology, suffered from X-ray burns involving exposed areas of skin. In fact many of them after a lapse of years suffered and died from cancer and leukaemia, having been ignorant of the late biological effects on the human system caused by prolonged exposure. Soon after their discovery, X-rays were also used to treat skin lesions and skin cancers. In later years when their powerful action on rapidly proliferating and dividing mitotic cells became known, X-rays were focused on areas of malignant disease to arrest the growth of tumour cells. The use of lead shields and accurate dosimetry allowed radiotherapy to become a practical proposition. Earlier problems included lack of penetration to deep-seated lesions, skin burns and inability to accurately focus lesions, so that the surrounding healthy tissue was significantly damaged. All these problems in contemporary medicine have been mitigated to a very great extent.

Within a few weeks of Roentgen's discovery, the great French physicist Henri Becquerel (1852–1908) discovered natural radioactivity whilst researching on the X-ray potential of uranium salts. Becquerel observed that when uranium salts were placed over a photographic plate, the plate was blackened beneath the uranium even if the plate was protected by wrapping it in blackened paper and silver. He concluded that uranium emitted invisible rays that possessed penetrative power akin to Roentgen's X-rays. He was awarded the Nobel Prize in physics for this discovery in 1903.

Further work on natural radioactivity was carried on by Marie Sklodowska, a Polish scientist studying at the Sorbonne. She took as her doctorate thesis a study on the radioactivity of uranium, working as the assistant of a French scientist Pierre Curie (1859–1906), whom she married in 1895. In her research she noticed that pitch blende (uranium oxide ore in tar) was far more radioactive that uranium. She and Pierre, on this finding, postulated the probable existence of a new radioactive element. There now commmenced a frenetic search for this element. They proceeded to refine pitch blende and in 1898, announced the discovery of polonium, named after Marie's beloved country Poland. The research now became even more exciting because the Curies noted within a few more months that even after polonium had been extracted from the pitch blende, the residue still had a higher radio-activity than uranium and therefore, had to contain yet another undiscovered element. In December 1898, they announced the discovery of radium, which when purified, was over 900 times more radioactive than uranium. The Curies received the Nobel Prize in 1904. Marie had accidentally burnt herself when carry-ing a radium phial in her pocket. Pierre purposely studied the effect of radium on skin and body tissue by strapping radium to his arm, thereby caus-ing a severe burn. The

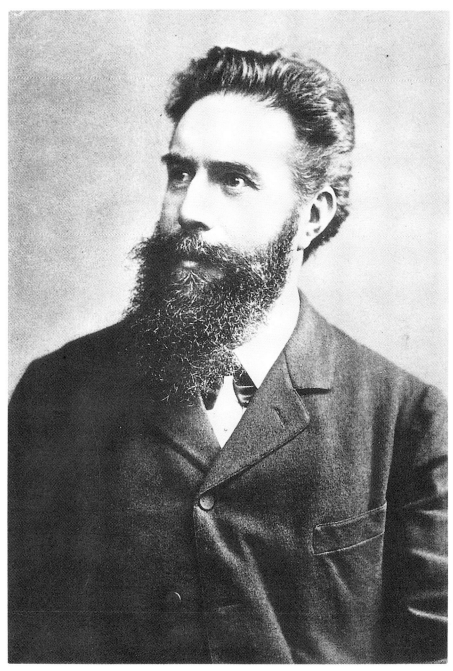

Fig. 50.2   Wilhelm Conrad Roentgen.

destructive effect of radium on malignant and diseased cells was proven in 1904, and this led to the radium treatment in cancer and other diseases. Radium was implanted into areas of malignant disease through radioactive needles, and even today, this modality of treatment is of considerable use, particularly in the management of cancer of the cervix.

In 1906 Pierre Curie was knocked down and killed by a cart whilst crossing a road. Marie was given his chair in Physics and became the first woman professor in the history of the university of the Sorbonne. She was awarded a second Nobel Prize in 1911, being the first and only woman to date who has been so honoured. Her final achievement was the founding of the Radium Institute in Paris, with the help of the Sorbonne and the Pasteur Institute.

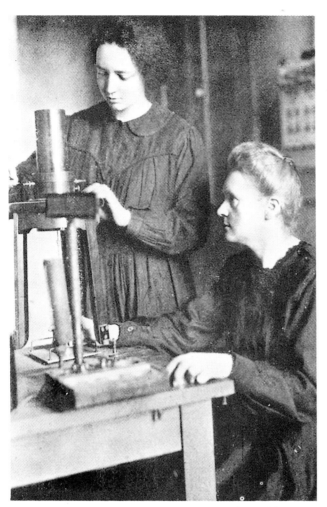

Fig. 50.3   Portrait of Marie Curie and her
daughter, Irene.

The role of physics was not confined to the discovery of X-rays and natural radioactivity. In 1917, Albert Einstein (1879–1955),described the principle of the LASER (Light Amplification by Stimulated Emission of Radiation) and the use of lasers·in surgery has since been assuming increasing importance in contemporary medicine.

Advances in the field of optics have also been responsible for introducing instruments and techniques in the service of medicine. Hermann von Helmholtz developed the ophthalmoscope in 1851 so that the fundus (optic nerve head and the retina) could be viewed with the naked eye. It was the first time that the internal structure of an organ could be so viewed. The oesophagoscope was introduced in 1868, and helped view the inside of the gullet and remove foreign bodies obstructing it. The origin of the gastroscope in the same year was in the form of a half-metre long pipe fitted with a light and lenses. The first gastroscopy was performed by an assistant of Adolf Kussmaul (1822–1910), who engaged a professional sword-swallower to swallow the half-metre long pipe described above! The earlier rigid gastroscopes were replaced in the 1930s by flexible instruments making use of glass-fibre optics which reflected light through a tube by total internal reflection. The inclusion of biopsy forceps for taking pieces of tissue for microscopic examination and of cameras to photograph and permanently record what the naked eye saw, were inevitable advances incorporated into all modern endoscopes. The rectoscope was devised in 1895 by H Kelly (1858–1945); it was soon adapted by the gynaecologists to look into the abdomen and pelvis in the procedure termed laparoscopy.

Advances in the microscope, invented as early as the seventeenth century, continued right upto the present day. The cornea was the first structure to be viewed in the human body through a stereomicroscope in 1899. Twenty-two years later the microscope began to be used in microsurgery—now a standard practice in many forms of surgical procedures. Till the 1920s, in spite of significant advances in the optical system of light microscopes, very small particles like viruses could not be visualized. In 1925, Joseph Bernard, a London microscopist devised the ultraviolet microscope achieving 2,500 times magnification, so that for the first time larger viruses could be seen by the naked eye. The Belgian, L L Morton (1901–1979), used the physical principles of electrons to devise the electron microscope. Electrons have a wave motion similar to that of light, but have a wavelength which is 10,000 times shorter. Objects could now be magnified many times over. By the end of the 1930s a magnification of close to 40,000 times was achieved, so that the innermost secrets of the human cells and of small particles called viruses were laid bare to the scientific eye.

The contribution of physics and other basic sciences to medicine cannot be overestimated. This contribution has gathered pace with the march of centuries, so that in the latter part of the age of what we have termed 'modern medicine', and all through our contemporary era, the science of medicine is inseparable from the science of physics and some of the other natural sciences.

51 Mental and Nervous Diseases

It is of interest to trace very briefly the history of mental and nervous diseases since the beginning of man, before dealing with their historical evolution and advance in the nineteenth and early parts of the twentieth century.

For primitive man mental diseases and physical illnesses were one—inexplicable other than through supernatural explanations. Both were supposedly due to possession of the victims by demons and evil spirits, and a feeling of well-being could return only if these were exorcised. Primitive psychiatry thus involved the use of charms and amulets which incorporated the strengths and virtues of sacred animals or good spirits and also afforded preventive protection against them. Amulets protected not only individuals but as the occasion demanded, afforded protection to communities from disease, famine and death caused by the wrath of gods, demons and malevolent spirits. It is indeed amazing that even today if we scratch the thin veneer of civilization from modern man, we uncover the gullibility and superstitions of the primitive. Charms of various kinds prevail not only in parts of the world where civilization has stood still, but are also noticeably used by the "liberated" civilized man of the twenty-first century.

With the passage of centuries, magic ritual and the compulsions of primitive religion joined forces with the use of magical charms in the treatment of mental illnesses. Magic rituals involved the use of secret formulae, incantations and mystical numbers. The earliest and the most primitive religions in ancient civilizations were given therapeutic power to heal so that the priest combined his religious duties with those of a healer.

The rise of Christianity advocated a different kind of 'magic' for all diseases—physical and mental. It was the 'magic' of implicit faith in Christianity and Christian beliefs that was enough to result in a cure. The attempt to substitute faith for magic formulae and herbal preparations of folklore medicine was never completely successful. Spiritual abstraction and faith coexisted with magic formulae and protective charms. This situation still prevails in many parts of the world. A psychiatric prescription from folklore medicine in Britain around the time of the Norman conquest reads thus "When a devil possesses the man or controls him from within with disease; a spew drink or emetic, lupin, bishopwort, henbane corpleek: pound these together, add ale for a liquid, let it stand for a night, add fifty bibcorns of cathartic grains and holy water—to be drunk out of a church bell." We thus came to a phase in the history of mankind where magic, ritual, faith, prayer, religion, folklore remedies, astrology and other mumbo-jumbo all formed a pot-pourri of cures for mental illnesses. As the Church in the West grew increasingly powerful, it frowned on all cures other than its own. It abrogated upon itself the sole right and power to effect miraculous cures through the exorcism of demons. Nevertheless, the new religion could not quite break the shackles of old learning. Not uncommonly it used charms or talismans, as for example cramp-rings for epilepsy made from coins offered on Good Friday, blessed by prayers and holy inscriptions.

The rational study of mental illness as with so many physical illnesses began with Hippocrates, who asserted that mental and physical disease both resulted from natural causes. Epilepsy till then dubbed a 'sacred' disease was in no way divine and to regard it as different from any other disease was a display of ignorance. The writings of Celsus in *De re medica* included a chapter on the clinical observations and therapy of mental disease. The management of many diseases was remarkable for its practicality. However for the violent patient, Celsus advocated starvation, physical violence and the use of restraints by chains—a practice that continued as an expression of frustration shown by all psychiatrists over the next eighteen centuries.

The scientific study of mental illnesses received an unfortunate setback in the Middle Ages. As the Church grew increasingly authoritarian, any deviation from its beliefs was ruthlessly suppressed. Epidemics of plague and other dreadful diseases decimated the West at frequent intervals producing not only panic but mass hysteria amongst whole communities and populations. The inability of the Church to control these situations led to the persecution of all non-conformist elements in society. Thus there was in the Middle Ages the practice of witchcraft, a discipline which explained non-conformist behaviour and mental illnesses including psychosis, dementia, psychopathic behaviour and criminality as manifestations of being possessed by the devil. Not only were manifestations of psychiatric illnesses stigmatized as witchcraft, but all folklore remedies not compatible with the practice of the Church were suppressed under the same stigma. It was only in the Renaissance that rationality was again restored. A great and to start with a lone voice of reason was that of Johan Weyer (1515–1576), who denounced and condemned witch-hunting and pleaded as Hippocrates had done that the mentally sick should be regarded and treated as any other patient.

Attitude towards the mentally sick changed only towards the second half of the eighteenth century. Physicians began to classify psychiatric illnesses leading to a nosology which could allow a more precise diagnosis. Violent methods of restraint in mental illnesses gave way to more humane attitudes and less cruel therapy. Mad-houses which till then were filthy prisons that housed the wretched and abandoned mentally ill till death delivered them from misery, were replaced in many instances by 'asylums' and hospitals with improved facilities and better care. Vincenzo Chiarugi in 1784, initiated this humanist movement in psychiatric illnesses in Italy, and William Tuke a Quaker merchant founded a retreat for the mentally ill in York, England, in 1794. In France there was the visionary Philippe Pinel, who extended the humanitarian principles of the French philosophers and of the French revolution to the mentally ill. As has been mentioned in chapter 40, Pinel after appointment as physician to the Bicêtre in 1793, released the insane inmates from their chains and restored their human dignity, advocating the use of moral persuasion in place of intimidation and force. Pinel then moved on to the Salpêtrière, where he carefully studied mental illnesses, laying the foundation of clinical psychiatry.

In the early nineteenth century mesmerism was revived and formed an important therapeutic tool in the treatment of psychiatric illnesses. Franz Joseph Gall (1758–1828) introduced Europe to phrenology, a discipline whereby moral and intellectual characteristics could be ascertained from a study of the external configuration of the skull. Absurd as this discipline was ultimately proved, it however focused attention for the first time on the fact that different regions of the brain could serve specific functions. This led to the concept of cerebral localization. The great French physiologist Marie Jean Pierre Flourens (1794–1867), was a strong opponent of Gall. He showed with brilliance that sensation and will were localized to the cerebrum, co-ordination in the cerebellum, and the centre for respiration was within the medulla.

Advances in psychiatry and diseases of the nervous system now occurred briskly and simultaneously. We shall interrupt the history of psychiatry at this point by briefly recapitulating the history of the study of nervous diseases till the early years of the twentieth century. Neurology deals with the functions and disturbances of the nervous system constituted by the brain, spinal cord, autonomic nerves and peripheral nerves. The scientific and rational study of this branch of medicine began with the Renaissance. It however took a great deal of time and research for the fallacious ideas of the previous millennium to be replaced by scientific fact. Galen had correctly noticed that movement or motion and sensation were related to the brain. He also distinguished motor from sensory nerves and attributed control over their functions to the brain. But his great error, unfortunately perpetuated till the seventeenth century, was his unsubstantiated concept of the transformation of the vital spirit in man into animal spirit in the *rete mirabilis*. Even the great Vesalius believed this to be true.

In the seventeenth and eighteenth centuries, Willis as explained in chapter 32, added a great deal of knowledge to the workings of the brain, particularly with regard to the cerebral circulation. Though Willis established the brain as the seat of the will and the mind, he was remarkably enough a demonologist and believed in forcible and often cruel restraint in the treatment of the mentally ill. A great name in the newly developing branch of neuropathology in the eighteenth century was that of William Cullen (1710–1790). He asserted that "life so far as it is corporeal, consists of the excitement of the nervous system and especially of the brain, which unites the different parts and forms them into a whole." He was the forerunner of modern neurophysiology and of the work of Pavlov and Sherrington.

Clinical neurology made rapid advances in the nineteenth century and several disease entities were now described. A classic description was embodied in the essay of a general practitioner and great thinker–James Parkinson (1735–1824), on the 'shaking palsy', soon to be termed Parkinson's disease. Advances in neurophysiology kept pace with clinical neurology. Charles Bell (1774–1842) and François Magendie (1783–1845) showed that the anterior nerve root from the spinal cord mediated motor function and was distinct from the posterior nerve root which mediated sensation. The idea of the reflex arc was expounded by Marshall Hall (1790–1859). The work of Claude Bernard on the sympathetic nerves and the role of sympathetic activity has been dealt with in chapter 44. Brown-Séquard shuttling between France and England taught neurology at the National Hospital in London, and elucidated the sensory and motor function of the cord, illustrating his concept with the clinical features observed in hemi-section of the cord (Brown-Séquard syndrome). Paul Broca (1824–1880) established the association between motor aphasia (a motor disturbance of speech) and damage to a selective portion of the temporal lobe of the left cerebral hemisphere.

Neuropathology did not lag far behind neurophysiology and clinical neurology. Johann Wepfer (1620–1695) of Basel, in 1658, showed that apoplexy was caused by haemorrhage from a cerebral vessel into the brain, and in 1686 Sydenham described the involuntary movements of rheumatic chorea, distinguishing it from St Vitus' dance.

The greatest neuropathologist in the first half of the nineteenth century was Moritz Romberg (1795–1873). He was the director of the Berlin Clinic and chiefly studied diseases of the peripheral nerves, in addition to other long-known diseases such as chorea and epilepsy. He established the Romberg's sign (unsteadiness when standing with eyes shut) in tabes dorsalis, a disease characterized by wasting of the posterior columns of the spinal cord. The syphilitic aetiology of tabes dorsalis was not known then and was only determined later. Tabes was also the subject of the study of Guillaume Duchenne (1806–1875). He wrote and published a masterly treatise on this disease, which came to be known as Duchenne's disease. He localized the neuropathology to the dorsal columns of the spinal cord and established its syphilitic aetiology. Duchenne was the first to describe bulbar paralysis and progressive muscular atrophy.

The second half of the nineteenth century saw significant advances in neuroanatomy and microscopy in Germany and even further discoveries in neurophysiology. Louis Ranvier (1835–1922) studied and reported on the microscopic anatomy of peripheral nerves. Wladimir Betz (1834–1894) described the giant 'Betz cells' in the motor cortex of the cerebral hemispheres, and Willy Kuhne (1837–1900) made an excellent study of the end-plates of the motor nerves in muscles.

Gustav Fritsch (1838–1897) and Eduard Hitzig (1838–1907) were the first to pioneer the knowledge of cerebral localization. They proved that the stimulation of specific areas of the cerebral cortex resulted in the contraction of specific localized muscles. Cerebral localization was the subject of intense investigation by numerous researchers and this proved of vital importance in both diagnosis and treatment. Richard Caton of Liverpool discovered the intrinsic electrical activity of the brain—a discovery which was the forerunner of the electroencephalogram.

One of the greatest neurophysiologists of the nineteenth century was England's Charles Sherrington (1861–1952). His research was embodied in a masterpiece *The Integrative Action of the Nervous System*. Sherrington made a comprehensive study of reflex action, evolving a number of new concepts. His study involved isolation of the brainstem and spinal cord from the higher centres in animals, achieved through removal of the cerebral hemispheres. He proved that reflex contraction of any muscle was not only due to contraction of the agonists, but an active relaxation of the antagonist muscles produced by reciprocal inhibition. Thus he introduced the concept of inhibition and inhibitory impulses as a feature of the central nervous system function.

Sherrington also proved that the conduction of a nerve impulse from one nerve cell to another was delayed by a physiological barrier, which he termed 'the synapse'. He also conceptualized the view of a final common path for efferent impulses to a muscle. Thus impulses from different sensory points on the skin have their own afferent pathways reaching the cord, but if they connect by a reflex arc with a particular muscle they do so only through a common motor nerve to that muscle. Sherrington postulated that reflex action was merely an expression of the integrative action of the nervous system that permitted the body to perform the expected purposeful action. Sherrington's holistic perspective of integrated function of the nervous system was an effective counter to the continuing research on localizing specific functions to specific anatomical areas within the brain and spinal cord.

Ivan Pavlov (1849–1936) was a contemporary of Sherrington. He worked in Russia on a different form of reflex activity—the 'conditioned reflex'. His original experiments were on the secretion of gastric juice in dogs. Nervous mechanisms formed an important stimulus for the secretion of gastric juice. If food was placed into a dog's mouth, gastric juice was secreted. Pavlov termed this reflex as simple and unconditioned. Gastric juice could also be secreted if the dog merely sniffed the food. The reflex involved in secretion was not innate but acquired through experience. Pavlov termed this a conditioned reflex. He then demonstrated that the animal could be conditioned in such a manner to obtain a conditional response or reflex. Thus if for several days a bell was rung just before giving the dog food, the animal was so conditioned that the sound of the bell alone produced gastric acid secretion, even though the food was withheld from the dog. He thus postulated two kinds of reflexes—the inborn or innate, and the conditioned or learned. The former was the subject of Sherrington's study and its centre involved the spinal cord and the brainstem. The latter was learned or conditioned through constant experience; it was unstable, would cease if for a length of time the conditioning ceased, and its centre involved the cerebral cortex.

From the study of reflexes, Pavlov now turned to psychiatry. He induced an artificial neurosis in dogs by presenting two similar conditioning stimuli. He postulated that hysteria and neurosis in patients would result from repetitive stimuli that could upset the balanced and integrated system of the brain. Pavlov in a refreshingly holistic view of central nervous system function theorized that the millions of brain cells in the cerebrum received numerous and often frequently repeated stimuli from the external environment. Over the years these could result in conditioned responses. An integration of these stimuli with their conditioned response could thus determine man's behaviour. Man in other words was a creature of his environment. Pavlov gave neurophysiological evidence to support this concept.

The synthesis between neurophysiology and neuropathology and clinical neurology was achieved by the great French neurologist Jean-Martin Charcot (1825–1893). Under his influence, the Salpêtriére in Paris where he taught, became the centre of neurology and remained so almost till the end of the nineteenth century. He correlated the various clinical nosological entities with disturbances in function of specific localized areas within the central nervous system, as also with the pathological changes observed in these localized areas. He described multiple sclerosis, peroneal muscular atrophy, tabes dorsalis and made a special study of hysteria, and of hypnosis in relation to hysteria. Charcot had a magnificent perspective and vision of neurology. He brought system and order to a rapidly advancing science and was a gifted teacher, whose clinical demonstrations at the Salpêtriére attracted students from far and wide. His *leçons sur les maladies du system nerveux faites a la Salpêtriére* (Lessons on Nervous Diseases Delivered at the Salpêtriére) formed a brilliant exposition of clinical neurology in relation to altered neuro-physiology and neuropathology. Charcot wrote a masterful description of hysteria and hypnotic states, distinguishing hysteria from organic disease of the nervous system by a careful evaluation of the symptoms and physical signs. He studied hypnosis and distinguished between hypnosis and hysteria. Charcot coined the term Parkinson's disease for the 'shaking palsy' described by John Parkinson. He followed up Parkinson's work with a study on tremors, gave an impressive description of paralysis agitans, describing the tremor in this disease with the thumb rhythmically moving over the fingers, 'as when a pencil or paper ball is rolled between them'. He distinguished intentional tremor (tremor observed only on intentional movement) from tremors at rest which disappeared only during sleep.

Jules Dejerine (1849–1917), a younger contemporary of Charcot, worked in Paris for many years describing peripheral neuritis in 1883 and muscular dystrophy in 1888. Muscular dystrophy was a slowly progressive hereditary disorder of muscles characterized by weakness and wasting, starting in the shoulder girdle muscles, followed by weakness and wasting in the proximal muscles of the hips.

It is outside the scope of this book to elaborate upon the historical discovery and description of numerous other clinical and clinicopathological disorders of the nervous system. Mention needs to be made of Jean Cruveilhier (1791–1874), who described the pathology of multiple sclerosis, relating the clinical symptoms to degenerative foci within the spinal cord, brainstem and cerebellum. Friedrich Theodor von Frerichs (1819–1885), made an extended detailed clinical study of multiple sclerosis in 1849. Charcot's triad of ataxia, tremor, and nystagmus aptly summarized the main clinical features of this disease.

Alois Alzheimer (1864–1915) received his medical training in Berlin, Wurzberg and Tuningen. Dementia was till then regarded as a sequel to degenerative changes in the brain from ageing. Alzheimer disagreed and in 1906 described what is now known as Alzheimer's disease, in which progressive dementia is related to structural organic changes in the brain, characterized by senile plaques and neurofibrillary tangles. Alzheimer also gave classical neuropathological descriptions of other diseases, including general paralysis of the insane and Huntington's chorea.

One of the great pioneers of modern neurology was the Yorkshireman, John Hughlings Jackson (1835–1911). He was influenced by Brown-Séquard and joined the National Hospital for the Blind and Epileptic in London soon after its foundation in 1860. Jackson enunciated basic principles in neurology. He considered the brain as an organ system, constituted, arranged and functioning at different levels of evolution. He distinguished between 'irritative' or discharging lesions which cause epileptic fits and the 'destroying' lesions which cause loss of function and paralysis. A lesion could begin as an irritative focus and then proceed to end with a destruction of the concerned area of the brain. The clinical manifestation would to start with, be a convulsive disorder and proceed to paralysis of the affected area. Another of Jackson's principles was that loss of nervous function progressed from that which was the most specialized and therefore the most highly evolved, to that which was the most automatic, least specialized and lowly evolved. Jackson defined epilepsy, a disease of antiquity, 'as the name for occasional, sudden, excessive, rapid and focal discharge of the grey matter of the brain'. A focal fit localized to one half of the face or arm or leg, or to one half of the body is termed a 'Jacksonian fit' after Jackson's eloquent description of this disorder. Jackson was the English counterpart of the French Jean-Martin Charcot. He and his colleagues established excellent standards of neurology at the National Hospital for Nervous Diseases in London. Sir William Gowers (1845–1915) was a colleague of Hughlings Jackson and like him, was interested in epilepsy—publishing a brilliant book on the subject. The journal *Brain*, was co-founded by Crichton-Browne, Hughlings Jackson and Ferrier. It incorporates research publications in neurology and psychiatry and has retained its pre-eminence amongst scientific medical journals to this day.

By the 1930s clinical neurology, neurophysiology and neuropathology were strong advancing sciences. Contemporary medicine (to be described in the chapter 66) saw an even more productive period in each of these disciplines.

We must now complete the history of mental diseases and psychiatry in the nineteenth and early twentieth century, and to do so we must return to the great Jean-Martin Charcot. Charcot besides his studies on organic nervous diseases, made a special study of hysteria and neurosis. He relied greatly on hypnosis to uncover hysteria as also to treat it. He made an elaborate study on numerous manifestations of hysterical reactions. These included hysteria presenting with fits, visual abnormalities, word-blindness, alexia, aphasia, mutism, sensory loss, hyperaesthesia, loss of muscle power and many other disturbances in nervous function. It is likely that the efficacy of hypnosis to uncover hysteria in a number of his patients, as also the hysterical behaviour of some of his star patients, demonstrated to an excited gallery of onlookers at the Salpêtrière, might not be genuine scientific facts and observations. These reactions might have been related to the power of suggestion and the desire to perform and please a personality as strong and overbearing as that of Charcot. Even so, the credit of distinguishing hysteria and diverse hysterical reactions from organic disease of the brain rests with him.

Hippolyte Bernheim (1840–1919), working in Nancy maintained that hypnotism was the intensification of normal suggestion. This view became widely accepted and towards the end of the nineteenth century, hypnotism was frequently used for the treatment of neurosis. The emphasis on neurosis was of considerable importance as it led to the discipline of psychoanalysis. Mention must be made of Pierre Janet (1859–1947), who in his studies on hysteria recognized hysterical dissociation, the existence and role of unconscious factors in hysterical reaction, and the concept of mental automatism in hysteria.

The German school of psychiatry took a different course from that of the French. It searched for organic brain disease as the cause of mental illness. Theodor Meynart (1833–1892) categorized all mental illnesses on an organic basis. Emil Kraepelin (1856–1926) was the exception in the rather dogmatic Germanic school. His clinical studies of numerous patients with mental illnesses enabled him to classify psychosis into dementia precox (later renamed schizophrenia) and manic-depressive states.

Sigmund Freud (1856–1939) discovered and started the discipline of psychoanalysis, throwing light on the unconscious factors governing mental attitude and behaviour in psychiatrically disturbed patients. He first studied neuroanatomy and neuropathology in Vienna, and then went on to the Salpêtrière to work with Charcot on hypnosis as a treatment for hysteria. On his return to Vienna, he was unhappy with the results of hypnosis in his patients. Not all could be hypnotized and the results in those who could be hypnotized were unsatisfactory. He then evolved together with his colleague Joseph Brener (1842–1923) the practice of psychoanalysis, wherein the patient discussed

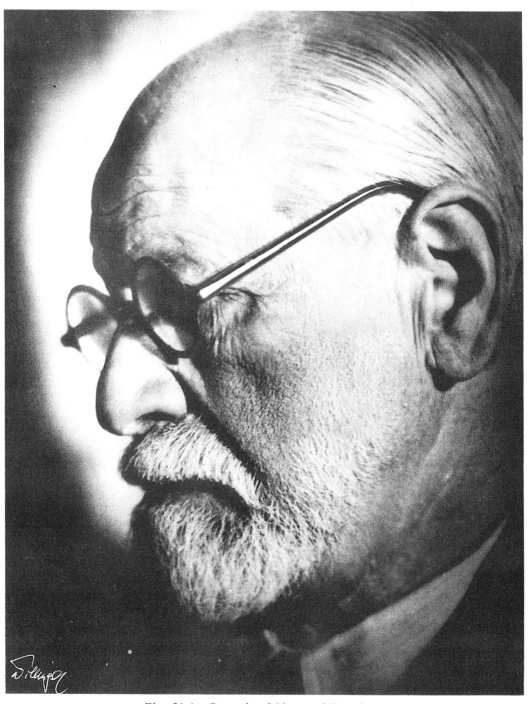

Fig. 51.1   Portrait of Sigmund Freud.

his emotional problems not through hypnosis, but through the process of free association of thoughts that enabled him to bring into open discussion his deep-seated psychic conflicts.

His early experience with psychoanalysis led him to believe, in 1893, that neurosis frequently stemmed from sexual trauma in childhood. He unearthed painful, suppressed memories related to childhood seduction by a parent or another adult, so that the guilt associated with participation in this seduction led to persistent neurosis in later years. He postulated his theory of unconscious motivation, repression and resistance, whereby an experience becomes embedded within the 'unconscious' and its constant repression leads to a disordered mental state, manifesting as neurosis. Freud elaborated and lectured on this novel and shocking hypothesis at a lecture in Vienna in April 1896. However his strong belief in this hypothesis was significantly diluted by 1897. He felt with further experience that many of his patients' stories of seduction were not true but fantasies. This led him to his theory of infantile sexuality and the Oedipus complex to explain the fantasized seduction by the opposite sex. He postulated that the growing up infant passes through three phases—the oral, anal and genital. These phases gratify its main desires. The pre-genital phase ceases at three years, but conflicts in the growing-up phase may cause fixation or regression to an earlier phase. At three, boys became increasingly attached to their mothers and increasingly resentful of their fathers. He termed this the Oedipus complex. The girls in contrast became attached to their fathers and resented their mothers—the Electra complex. The repressed Oedipus complex, according to Freud, was the source of anxiety and mental illness, for it distorted and suppressed adult sexuality and hindered mental balance and reasoned behaviour. Freud further postulated that the mind and its mental function could fall into three categories—the unconscious, the pre-conscious and conscious. He then went on to formulate his theories of the ego (the conscious state of a being), the superego (parental and social conscience), and the id (the source of libido and mental energies). The infant only possessed the id; ego and superego developed with the growing years, either burying or overshadowing the id. Excessive suppression or inhibition of this hidden but ever persistent id led to neurosis or sexual deviation. Sublimation of the id, Freud maintained, could lead to artistic creativity. Freud and Brener now went separate ways. Brener favoured hypnosis; Freud abandoned hypnosis and developed psychoanalysis, investigating free associations of thoughts, as also the symbolic interpretation of dreams, so that the repressed or unconscious mind could be brought out into the open. He considered hysterical reactions as manifestations of unconscious conflicts. An understanding and appreciation of these conflicts through psychoanalysis formed the crux of management. It is indeed a remarkable twist in the history of medicine that Freud's theory on the Oedipus complex, the unconscious function of the mind, the id, ego, superego were only possible because by and large he rejected his original theory of sexual seduction in childhood. The discipline of psychoanalysis thus owes its existence to these changes in Freud's early views.

There was in his lifetime and there exists even to this day, a debate on the validity of many of his views. Yet there is no doubt that Freudian theories for the first time gave a novel interpretation of the workings of the human mind. He delved into its complexities and came forth with startling and challenging thoughts and theories that shook the complacency of the balanced as much as it attempted to restore the stability of the unbalanced.

Psychoanalysis had a fairly ardent following in the United States after Freud's visit to the New World in 1909. Alfred Adler (1870–1937) and Helene Deutsch (1884–1982), emigrants from Europe were its two leading pioneers.

Carl Jung (1875–1961) of Switzerland studied medicine in Basle and then specialized in psychiatry. He joined Freud in 1907 and was, for five years his favourite protégé. He however parted ways from his mentor and developed analytical psychology. He laid much less stress on sexuality as the cause of neurosis. He offered a more balanced view of the psyche, introduced the concept of archetypes, of the extrovert and the introvert. He also postulated the presence of a collective unconsciousness, a repository of centuries of experiences and impressions belonging to a race. It was this collective unconsciousness that could determine attitudes, actions and responses to different situations. Jung's views on analytic psychology are appealing, as they delve into and explore the philosophy of integrated life and living.

52 Endocrinology

It was Claude Bernard who in 1878, in his *Leçons sur les phenomenes de la vie,* introduced the concept of the *milieu intérieur* (internal environment) which is kept constant by several interacting, self-regulating mechanisms. The nervous system he demonstrated was one such regulatory mechanism. The other was provided by chemical messengers (later called hormones), whose study was pioneered by Bernard's work on glycogen metabolism and continued by his successor Brown-Séquard at the College de France.

In 1835, Bernard showed that while the external secretion of the liver was constituted as bile, the internal secretion made blood sugar. In 1856, Brown-Séquard removed the adrenal glands (placed on top of the kidneys) in experimental animals. The animals died, proving that the glands were essential for life. He concluded that these glands must be secreting an essential life-sustaining substance into the bloodstream. Further work on chemical messengers or gland secretions came from the English physiologists, William Bayliss (1860–1924) and Ernest Starling (1866–1927). In 1902, they introduced hydrochloric acid into the duodenum of a dog and noted that the dog started secreting pancreatic juice. They inferred that the duodenum must have secreted a substance which reached the pancreas via the bloodstream, stimulating it to secrete its digestive ferments. They called the unknown substance 'secretin'. It was Starling who coined the word 'hormone' in 1905, for chemical messengers secreted by a ductless or endocrine gland; these 'messengers' reached distant organs within the body via the bloodstream and thus influenced their function.

The thyroid gland had aroused attention since ancient times. Paracelsus associated goitre with cretinism and noted its frequency in those living in mountainous areas. Experimental extirpation of the thyroid gland in dogs and guinea pigs, performed by Moritz Schiff (1823–96) of Switzerland, led to the death of these animals. This therefore was one more gland that possessed a secretory life-sustaining function. In 1860, Bilroth introduced thyroidectomy as the treatment for goitre. His pupil Theodor Kocher (1841–1917) in Bern, improved on Bilroth's technique. The mountainous districts of Switzerland provided him with a large number of patients with goitre. By the time of his death in 1917, Kocher had successfully operated upon 7,000 patients with thyroid disorders, with an astonishingly low mortality of 1 per cent. He had won great fame in Europe as an innovative experimental surgeon and was acclaimed for his superlative surgical skill. He was awarded the Nobel Prize in 1909 for his original contributions to thyroid surgery. Kocher besides influencing surgery in Europe, exerted a seminal influence on two great figures in American surgery—William Halsted and Harvey Cushing.

The first good clinical description of myxoedema was by William Gull (1816–1890) in 1873. He described five adult women presenting with a cretinoid condition. They were slow, sluggish, obese and puffy in the face. They felt inordinately cold, had a slow pulse rate, were hard of hearing and constipated. The condition later came to be recognized as being due to thyroid deficiency and was termed myxoedema. Kocher in a follow-up of his patients subjected to thyroidectomy, noted that a third of his operated patients developed the features described above by Gull. The inference was that myxoedema was caused by thyroid deficiency.

It was not long before the administration of thyroid extract of a dessicated thyroid gland was shown to cure myxoedema. The demonstration of an iodine-containing compound within the thyroid gland suggested that iodine deficiency was responsible for a proliferation of cells within the thyroid gland, causing a goitre to form. The addition of iodine to table salt as a preventive measure reduced the incidence of goitres so frequently observed in mountainous districts.

The role of the adrenal medulla within the human body was elucidated by George Oliver (1841–1915) and Sharpey-Shafer (1850–1935). An injection of an extract of the adrenal gland into a dog sharply raised the blood pressure. The active ingredient responsible for this effect was isolated by Jkichi Takamine (1854–1922) in 1901, and was called adrenaline or epinephrine. Adrenaline on injection was shown to produce the same effect as stimulation of the sympathetic nervous system—constriction of vessels in the skin and digestive system, pallor of the skin, dilatation of vessels in the muscles, sweating, tachycardia, hypertension and dilatation of the pupils.

Walter Cannon (1871–1945) at Harvard studied the effect of strong emotions on the autonomic nervous system. Pain, fright and anger appeared to stimulate the sympathetic nervous system causing exactly the same effects described above. The body was thus prepared or conditioned, through the autonomic nervous system, to 'fright', 'fight' or 'flight'. He further showed that traumatic shock also caused stimulation of the sympathetic nervous system which led to the release of a hormone subsequently called noradrenaline. Cannon coined the term 'homeostasis', a concept akin to that of the constancy of the internal environment proposed earlier by Claude Bernard. He elaborated upon this concept in his book *The Wisdom of the Body (1932)*, discussing the importance of the autonomic nervous system and of the regulation of hormones in maintaining homeostasis within the body.

The pituitary gland had also been known from early times, though its exact function was an enigma till the last quarter of the nineteenth century. In 1886, Pierre Marie (1853–1940) described a disease characterized by prognathism, overgrowth of the hands and feet and kyphosis of the spine. The condition was termed acromegaly and it was noted that patients who died with acromegaly had an enlarged pituitary gland. It was inferred that the pituitary may be the centre responsible for growth within the body.

Henry Dale (1875–1968), in 1909 isolated oxytocin from the posterior lobe of the pituitary. This hormone stimulated uterine contractions during childbirth. In the meantime, experimental work on anterior pituitary extracts suggested that the gland could influence the function of many other endocrine glands. It was Walter Longdon Brown (1870–1946) who called the pituitary "the leader of the endocrine orchestra".

Harvey Cushing at John Hopkins, not only pioneered neurosurgery but also contributed to the understanding of the function of the pituitary gland. He described the effects of over-secretion and under-secretion of hormones from the anterior lobe of the pituitary. Over-secretion produced Cushing's syndrome, characterized by hypertension, obesity, softening of bones, purple striae over the skin, diabetes and hirsuitism in females. Surgical removal of the pituitary gland (which Cushing pioneered) produced a cure. The influence of the hypothalamus on pituitary function came to be proven later in the twentieth century. The hypothalamic–pituitary axis, thus both controlled and fine-tuned the hormonal balance of the body, preserving this balance as far as possible in disease and in periods of physical and emotional stress.

The importance of the pancreas in digestion through the secretion of pancreatic juice was well established by the seventeenth century. Its recognition as an important endocrine gland and its relation to diabetes mellitus were however recognized much later. Diabetes is a disease of antiquity, its clinical features being excessive thirst, excessive urination, weakness and loss of weight. Aretarus first gave the Greek term *diabetes* (Greek for siphon) to these clinical features. The ancient ayurvedic physicians noted that the urine in diabetes tasted sweet. Avicenna made a similar observation on his diabetic patients. It was Thomas Willis who added the word 'mellitus' (Latin for honey-sweet) noting also the excessive thirst and urination that characterized this disorder.

In 1869, Paul Langerhans (1847–88) researching on the microscopic study of the pancreas, observed that besides the acinar cells there were scattered within the organ, clusters of special cells. These cells are now called the islets of Langerhans. The function of these cells eluded him. The relation between the pancreas and diabetes was first recognized in 1889, when Oskar Minkowski and Joseph von Mering removed a dog's pancreas. The dog besides being unable to digest fat and protein developed diabetes. It was Sharpey-Shafer who determined that the substance responsible for regulating carbohydrate metabolism was produced by the islets of Langerhans. He called this hormone 'insuline' (Latin *insula,* meaning an island); it was now apparent that diabetes resulted from a deficiency of insulin.

The isolation of this active principle secreted by the islets of Langerhans was achieved in 1921 by Fred Banting (1891–1941) and Charles Best (1899–1978), in the laboratory of John MacLeod (1876–1935), professor of physiology at Toronto. They injected an extract of the islets of Langerhans from the pancreas of a specially-prepared dog into a diabetic dog close to death. The dog survived. They now enlisted the help of a biochemist J. B. Collip (1892–1965), to obtain purified extracts of the islets of Langerhans. When injected into diabetic dogs, their blood sugar levels fell and the dogs improved. They were now emboldened to use an injection of this extract on their first human patient—a fourteen-year-old boy, Leonard Thompson, critically ill with juvenile diabetes. To their intense jubilation the blood sugar fell, the patient improved from day to day and was well within a few weeks, though needing daily insulin injections. Banting and MacLeod won the Nobel Prize in 1923, though Prof. MacLeod was out on a fishing holiday in Scotland during the earlier phase of this work. Best and Collip went unrewarded. The pharmaceutical company El Lilly in the United States soon went into large-scale production of insulin. This was indeed, a landmark in the history of medicine because though insulin is no cure for diabetes, it has helped to save thousands of lives that would have surely been lost, but for its use.

The hormones secreted by the testes and ovary became known only in the twentieth century. The effects of castration as in eunuchs, were known for centuries. Animal experiments had shown that castrating a cock caused its comb to atrophy. If however the testes were then transplanted into another part of its body, this did not occur. Rejuvenation was, and still remains, the dream of many ageing men. The researcher Brown-Séquard reported to the world in 1889 that he had rejuvenated himself through the injection of extracts of testicles of dogs and guinea pigs. The urge to recapture youth was now given a scientific backing! The first quarter of the twentieth century saw the frequent use of testicular implants, in particular monkey-gland implants in middle-aged and older men.

The male sex hormone was isolated in the 1930s. Androsterone was isolated in 1931 and synthesized three years later. Soon after, a Dutch team led by Ernst Laqueur (1880–1947) succeeded in isolating the pure male hormone from the ground-up testicles of bulls. The hormone was called testosterone.

The ovarian hormones were not so easily isolated. These hormones were from two sources—from the ovary proper and from the corpus luteum. The female hormone secreted by the ovary was isolated in 1931; oestriol and oestradiol were discovered in 1933. A year later, the hormone

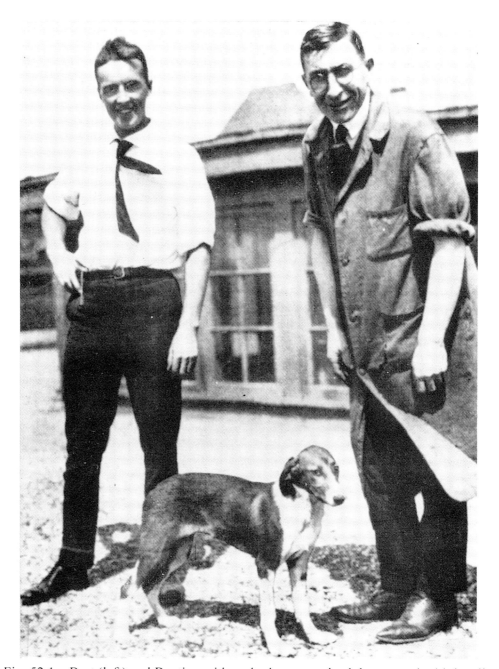

Fig. 52.1   Best (left) and Banting with early depancreatized dog treated with insulin.

progesterone was isolated from the corpus luteum. The function of progesterone secreted by the corpus luteum at the onset of ovulation was to prepare the uterine lining to receive the ovum in the event of fertilization.

Further research on ovarian hormones continued, culminating in the discovery of the contraceptive pill (described in chapter 69).

53 Deficiency Diseases and Nutrition

By the last quarter of the nineteenth century, the humoral theory of disease had been discredited and dispelled. Disease was now most often thought to be due to a number of newly discovered organisms causing infection. It could also be caused by cancer, by physical and chemical agents, poisons and other positive factors. The twentieth century saw the birth of a new concept of disease. It began to be understood that disease could also result from lack or deficiency of essential elements in the diet. A 'lack' or a 'deficiency' causing disease was an unusual concept, as hitherto, it was always a 'positive' factor that was responsible for various pathological conditions within the body.

William Prout (1785–1850) had classified foodstuffs into saccharinous substances (carbohydrates), oleaginous materials (fats) and albuminous or nitrogenous matter (protein). Justus von Leibig had pioneered experimental studies quantitating through careful measurements the energy produced by different foods. The practical corollary to Leibig's work was that it would be possible to formulate an artificial diet of carbohydrates, fats, proteins and mineral salts that would maintain good nutrition and health. This proved to be untrue. When Paris was under siege during the 1871 Commune, a shortage of food for infants prompted the trial of a formula comprising emulsified fat in a sweetened albuminous solution. Though the formula contained enough carbohydrates, fat and protein, it failed to maintain nutrition. Experimental work on animals fed with similar artificial formulae led to similar results. It was against this background that the concept of deficiency diseases took root in the twentieth century.

Amongst the deficiency diseases to be described were marasmus, related to the effects of food deprivation or starvation, and kwashiorkor, which was chiefly due to protein malnutrition. Both occurred chiefly in impoverished Third World countries like India and Africa. Kwashiorkor affected growth and was characterized by muscle wasting, oedema, enlarged liver, diarrhoea, brownish discolouration of the hair and an increased susceptibility to infection.

Pellagra, beri-beri, scurvy and rickets were some other important diseases whose clinical descriptions were well established before their relation to a specific deficiency in the diet was unravelled. In 1755, the French physician Gaspar Casal (1680–1759) gave an excellent description of pellagra in Spain. It was characterized by dermatitis, diarrhoea, dementia, difficulty in walking and early death. The victims were poor and chiefly subsisted on a maize-meal diet. Maize was a plant brought from the New World by the conquistadors and was widely planted in Mediterranean Europe. Pellagra again associated with a maize-meal diet also spread to the poor in Italy, other areas of southern Europe and in the southern states of America. It was also observed in the Middle East, India, south-east Asia and Africa, always amongst the poor and among those consuming maize as their staple diet.

Beri-beri was another disease commonly described in the rice-eating people of Asia. It led to an inflammation of the peripheral nerves causing sensory loss in the hands and feet, weakness of the muscles of the limbs, oedema, an enlargement of the heart, with death (often sudden) from heart failure. People who ate milled rice were more prone to the disease than those eating unpolished rice.

Christiaan Eijkman (1858–1930), who worked in a research laboratory in Jakarta in the 1890s, discovered that chicken developed a neuritis when fed the white rice given to patients, instead of the normal unpolished brown rice chicken-feed. They recovered when they were put back on their unpolished rice feeds. He deduced that the polished rice contained a toxin that caused neuritis and that the husk of the rice contained an antidote to the toxin. His colleague Gerrit Grijns (1865–1944) guessed correctly when he suggested that both beri-beri and fowl polyneuritis were due to an absence from the diet of some essential factor present in rice polishings. He also postulated that this essential substance in rice was destroyed by excessive heat. These views were substantiated when an inquiry into the incidence of beri-beri among the inmates of prisons and asylums in Java showed that there was a strong association between the consumption of polished rice and the occurrence of beri-beri.

Further experimental work pointed to dietary deficiency as the cause of certain diseases. Frederick Hopkins (1861–1947) in Cambridge fed rats with casein, lard, starch, sugar and salt. The diet contained enough carbohydrate, fat and protein for nutrition. Yet they failed to thrive and died, except when small additional quantities of milk were added to the diet. He believed that 'accessory food factors' present in very small quantities were necessary for nutrition and growth. It was Casimir Funk (1884–1967) a Polish biochemist working at the Lister Institute in London, who in 1912 isolated the active substances in rice husk or polishings which could prevent beri-beri. He believed that they were amines (derived form ammonia), and he called these missing but essential elements 'vitamines'.

Vitamines came to be written as 'vitamins' (with the 'e' dropped) when it was realized in the following decade that these missing essentials were not necessarily amines. Funk related not only pellagra and beri-beri but also the diseases scurvy and rickets to vitamin deficiencies. Foodstuffs began to be evaluated and analysed not just for their carbohydrate, fat and protein content, but also in relation to their vitamin content.

Scurvy had been known and described in the eighteenth century and the work of Lind had established the anti-scorbutic properties of many foods, in particular, of fresh lemon or lemon juice. Arthur Harden (1865–1940) of the Lister Institute in London separated citric and other acids from lemon juice, leaving a residue which was highly antiscorbutic. The acids within the lemon juice lacked this anti-scorbutic property. The essential nutrient or vitamin in lemon juice was isolated in 1932 by W A Waugh and Charles King. Albert Szent–Gyorgyi (1893–1986) synthesized this vitamin in the laboratory and named it vitamin C. It was the first vitamin to be synthesized. Vitamin C in 1933, was termed ascorbic acid. In the meanwhile essential elements or vitamins came to be studied. Animal experiments conducted at Yale proved that butter contained a growth promoting factor which was fat-soluble. It was termed vitamin A. Vitamin A was synthesized in 1947. A similar growth factor was shown to be present in egg-yolk and cod-liver oil. Deficiency of vitamin A was increasingly recognized among poor children in Third World countries. This deficiency caused dryness and ulceration of the cornea and was one of the most important cause of blindness in children. Even to this day it remains so.

A growth promoting essential water-soluble factor was also shown to be present in rice polishings, yeast, wheat-germ and cow's milk. This was termed vitamin B; it was isolated in 1926 and synthesized in 1936.

The disease rickets, was known since ancient times. It became widespread when the Industrial Revolution changed the socio-economic face of Europe. The disease became increasingly common in Europe and America in the first third of the twentieth century, being most common among young children living in industrial cities. The cause of rickets was disputed. Some attributed it to infection but there were others who shrewdly observed that diet deficiencies and lack of fresh air and sunlight may perhaps cause the disease. The answer to this came through the work of Edward Mellanby (1884–1955). He induced rickets in puppies by giving them diets lacking a factor found in animal fats. Feeding these puppies with cod-liver oil cured rickets. Mellanby thus established that rickets was a deficiency disease, attributing it to a lack of vitamin A. Human rickets now began to be effectively treated and cured by cod-liver oil or exposure to sunlight. From 1922, vitamin A was believed to contain two factors—the old term vitamin A was retained for one factor and the other factor was termed vitamin D. Vitamin D became the antirachitic factor; its administration cured rickets and its addition to milk prevented its occurrence in children.

Vitamin E was discovered when experiments on rats fed with whole milk showed that though they grew well, they were sterile. An essential dietary factor for reproduction was lacking in whole milk. In 1922, Herbert Evans (1905–1983) of California and Katherine Bishop (1889–1928) showed that this essential factor was present in wheat-germ and green leafy vegetables. It was fat-soluble and was termed vitamin E.

Further research on vitamin B showed that it consisted of several factors. The two factors initially discovered in 1926 by Morris Smith and E.G. Hendrick were the antineuritic factor called vitamin B1, and the growth-promoting factor called vitamin B_2. Vitamin B_1 isolated from rice husks in 1926 and from yeast in 1932, was termed thiamine.

One of the important discoveries in the twentieth century was the relation established between the occurrence of a form of anaemia termed pernicious anaemia and one of the factors present in vitamin B. Pernicious anaemia was first described by Thomas Addison in 1849. It was a progressively severe anaemia, associated with degeneration in the peripheral nerves and the spinal cord, always ending in death. It had no known cause and there was no available cure.

George Whipple (1878–1976), experimenting on dogs reported that the anaemia caused by blood-letting was corrected by feeding them liver, beef or spinach, rich in iron. In 1925, George Minot (1885–1950) and William Murphy (1892–1936), aware of Whipple's work, fed their patients of pernicious anaemia large quantities of raw or lightly-cooked liver. The results were excellent; there was a rapid increase in the red blood cells with a disappearance of anaemia. A cure for a lethal condition had been found; its scientific basis now needed to be discovered. This was achieved through simple yet an elegant series of experiments by William Castle (1897–1990), a young resident physician at the Boston City Hospital. He was intrigued by the work of Minot and Murphy and was aware of the fact that the gastric lining of patients with pernicious anaemia secreted no hydrochloric acid. This was in striking contrast to normal individuals, whose stomach contents were rendered acidic due to the secretion of hydrochloric acid. He presumed that the stomach of normal persons utilized a factor within food and this was equivalent in effect to feeding large quantities of liver to patients with pernicious anaemia. He set about to prove his hypothesis. He fed his patients with steak and lean beef muscle, with no effect on the anaemia. He fed the same meal to normal individuals and recovered their gastric contents through a nasogastric tube. These contents were liquefied and fed through a nasogastric tube to patients with pernicious anaemia. Within a week the anaemia showed clear improvement with an increase in the red blood cells and the haemoglobin. He then went one step further to determine whether it was the gastric secretion of normal individuals or the effect of gastric secretion on the beef muscle diet in normal individuals that improved the anaemia in his patients. He observed that merely giving the gastric secretion was ineffective; it was the combination of the stomach juices of a normal individual with the beef diet that improved the anaemia. He postulated that the stomach lining normally secreted an 'intrinsic factor' in the gastric juice and this interacted with an 'extrinsic factor' within the beef diet. The extrinsic factor was later identified as vitamin B_{12} and the intrinsic factor was shown to be secreted by the normal gastric mucous membrane. The intrinsic factor permitted the absorption of B_{12} across the wall of the small gut (ileum) into the bloodstream. B_{12} was an essential factor in the normal production of blood in the bone marrow. The stomach of patients with pernicious anaemia failed to secrete this intrinsic factor. This could be compensated, as shown in the work of Minot and Murphy, by feeding huge quantities of raw liver. When B_{12} came to be synthesized, pernicious anaemia could be treated by an injection of vitamin B_{12} given just once in two or even four weeks. Work in the second half of the twentieth century went on to prove that pernicious anaemia is caused by auto-antibodies that destroy the cells within the stomach lining which normally secrete intrinsic factor.

The unravelling of important deficiency diseases and the importance of vitamins in diet led to the study of nutrition and of balanced diets. There was now a growing awareness of the poor nutrition in the teeming millions of so many Third World countries. Poverty and malnutrition, together with lack of education and governmental apathy towards public health, led to increasing disease and disability that retarded progress within these poor countries. There were many who realized the inequality and inequities that existed in the world with reference to a need as basic as food. One such idealist was Boyd Orr (1880–1971), who worked desperately through organizations like the United Nations to improve public health through better nutrition. The salvation of the starving and underfed millions in Africa and some Asian countries will ultimately depend on their own efforts to increase food production and ensure its equitable distribution. The debility and illnesses caused by nutritional deficiencies in India were emphasized by the research on nutrition carried out at the National Institute of Nutrition, by Prof. V. Ramalingaswamy at Hyderabad in India. The growing awareness to produce more food has borne fruit in the researches of several individuals in Third World countries. These include M.S. Swaminathan, who through genetic studies, has discovered a form of rice and wheat that allowed a manifold increase in the annual yield of these essential foodstuffs.

It was at the same time realized that nutritional diseases could not be just related to deficiency of basic food and essential vitamins. It could also be due to the over-consumption of food that leads to obesity and the many ills associated with it. The underfed and the grossly overfed, both suffer from nutritional disorders. Excessive consumption of salt is now shown to predispose to hypertension. The present century has seen an almost tripling of sugar consumption aided and abetted by the increased use of processed foods. This has been a major factor in the rising incidence of diabetes. Increased consumption of sugar is now associated with a poor fibre content in the diet, causing colonic disorders and perhaps contributing to an increased incidence of colonic cancer. A rise in the fat content of the diet in the affluent countries of the West is responsible for abnormalities of the lipid profile within the blood and has contributed to the sharp increase in arterial diseases, notably coronary atherosclerosis. Synthetic foods and the use of preservatives and dyes may well pose an additional hazard in the years to come. The frenetic pace of the western world has given birth to junk food, destroying the aesthetics of one of the greatest pleasures of life. Finally, it should haunt and stir the conscience of the world that while the rich countries of the West suffer from a surplus of food, too abundant to consume, the evil sceptre of want stalks millions of people in the poor countries of Asia, Africa and South America.

54 Tropical Medicine

The greater mass of humanity did not live in the West but lived and continues to live in what we now consider to be the poor Third World countries. Many of these countries fall within the tropical belt. 'Tropical diseases' consist of a large variety of diseases. Some of these are common to the West some are more prevalent in the tropics and some appear confined to tropical countries. The discoveries in bacteriology and the triumph over 'tropical disease' constitute according to many, a great and glorious chapter in the history of Man and Medicine. The white man was akin to a knight in shining armour who travelled to distant and dangerous lands and battled diseases that did not concern him, in order to lighten the burden of the poor native. This is indeed far from the truth. The triumphs of tropical medicine were an off-shoot of the colonial conquest of the poor countries by the powerful nation states of the West. The standard bearers of colonial rule in India, South-East Asia, Africa, South America and Oceania had to survive if their imperial missions were to succeed, and if colonial rule over foreign people in a hostile environment had to be sustained. The discoveries in tropical medicine were thus imperative necessities for expanding empires; the conquest of disease that followed soothed their conscience and even became a justification for further colonization.

Many of the diseases that came within the ambit of tropical medicine were also present in the West. These included malaria, plague, smallpox, cholera and typhoid. Malaria, which was endemic in Africa, India and other South-East Asian countries, was also frequent in the low-lying swamps in the Mediterranean region of Europe. Plague had decimated the West several times from the beginning of history. The last devastating outbreak of plague in Europe was as late as 1720 and the last great outbreak of this disease in the Ottoman empire was in Egypt as late as 1850. After this time it disappeared from the West but reared its ugly head again in Asia and Africa. Great epidemics of plague arose in the middle of the nineteenth century in China, spreading to East Asia, Hong Kong, Manchuria and to western India, up to Bombay, killing over a million Indians in 1903. This pandemic also spread to Asia Minor, South Africa and even to the western shores of America. Asia, including India, witnessed epidemics even in the twentieth century. Cholera threatened the West as it raged in epidemic form in the East. Smallpox, cholera and typhoid ravaged both the West and the East in the nineteenth century. Improving economics, education and above all effective measures in public health saw a sharp fall and finally the disappearance of these diseases in Europe, but they persisted well into the middle of the twentieth century in the poor countries of the world.

Tropical medicine came into its own in the last third of the nineteenth century. Patrick Manson (1884–1922) was the first to discover that the transmission and production of disease could occur through parasites transmitted by insect vectors. Incidentally, the possible role of insect vectors in disease had been suggested many centuries ago in Susruta's writings. Patrick Manson studied medicine in Aberdeen and then proceeded to China, spending twelve years in the service of the Chinese Imperial Maritime Customs. In China, he discovered that a disease termed elephantiasis which caused disfiguring enlargement of the lower limbs and genitalia was caused by a nematode worm, the filaria, which blocked the lymphatic vessels. The resulting obstruction to lymph flow led to swelling of the limbs and genitalia, hypertrophy of the soft tissues in this region, causing elephantiasis. In 1877, he made the important discovery that the parasite causing elephantiasis was transmitted to man by the mosquito Culex fatigans. The parasites developed within the stomach of this vector; they then burst through the stomach wall to migrate into the thoracic muscles of the mosquito. They developed further in this region and when the mosquito bit man the parasites were injected into the bloodstream causing disease. He announced his discovery to the medical world in 1877 in a paper titled 'Medical Report of the Imperial Maritime Customs, China'. It was in many ways a monumental discovery—from the epidemiological point of view as well as from the point of studying a completely new breed of living microorganisms in the causation of disease. Manson returned to London in 1899, became physician to the Seaman's Hospital and founded the London School of Tropical Medicine in the same year. He fathered the study of parasitology and tropical medicine. Man was at the threshold of new discoveries in medicine.

The next great discovery was in relation to malaria, the most serious endemic disease afflicting millions in Asia and Africa and a large population group in Europe and America. Charles Louis Alphonse Laveran (1845–1922), a French army surgeon working in Algeria, was the first to observe a protozoal plasmodium as the causative agent in malaria. Ronald Ross (1857–1932) proved that it was the mosquito that transmitted the malarial parasite acting both as host and vector for this disease. In his early years Ross was more fond of poetry than of medicine. He took to medicine due to parental pressure. History proved that this parental choice was to benefit medicine and man. He studied at St Bartholomew's Hospital, joined the Indian Medical Service and served in the third Burma campaign. On leave, he studied bacteriology in London and then returned to India. From 1892 he became involved in research on malaria. On a visit to London in 1894, Ross had met Patrick Manson who felt that the mosquito may well be responsible for the transmission of malaria. He advised Ross to investigate the role of the mosquito. Ross returned to India inspired by his discussion with Manson and continued his research. He soon found the parasite causing malaria in the stomach of the Anopheles mosquito after it had fed on the blood of patients with malaria. He thus proved that the Anopheles mosquito was responsible for the transmission of the disease and succeeded in working out the life-cycle of the malarial parasite. He was awarded the Nobel Prize in 1902 for this discovery. Laveran received the Nobel Prize in 1907 for his discovery of the Plasmodium parasite. This now opened up the exciting prospect of control of malaria by eradication of mosquitoes. The anti-mosquito campaign through the use of chemicals that destroyed their breeding places was promptly successful, first in America and later on in Italy—where the incidence of malaria was still high. Similar campaigns were instituted in South America, Africa and Asia. The advent of dichloro-diphenyl-trichlorothane (DDT), which had high insecticidal powers persisting for several weeks after its use, held out hope that the world would perhaps be rid of malaria. But these hopes were hopelessly dashed, for soon the mosquito became resistant to the effects of DDT, and the plasmodium falciparum resistant to the drug chloroquine, that was introduced both as prophylaxis and as treatment for the disease. The world today witnesses a resurgence of malaria with a horrendous morbidity and mortality.

The role of the mosquito in the transmission and spread of yet another tropical disease, yellow fever, was under study in the 1880s. Yellow fever was originally endemic along the west coast of Africa. It caused fever, severe jaundice due to liver-cell dysfunction, widespread haemorrhages in the skin, mucous membranes, coma and death. The disease spread to the Americas through European traders visiting America for trade, and through African slaves sent by ship to America. By the eighteenth century, yellow fever had made its presence felt in the West Indies, Latin America and along the Atlantic coast of America. The nineteenth century witnessed a spate of epidemics in the southern states of America, particularly New Orleans. The morbidity and mortality in some epidemics was extremely high. In 1882 Carlos Juan Finlay (1833–1915) on the basis of his experimental studies incriminated the mosquito Aedes aegypti in the transmission of the disease. The 1898 Spanish-American war was witness to a severe epidemic of yellow fever in American troops in Cuba. In 1900, the US army appointed a commission to investigate the disease, under the leadership of Walter Reed (1851–1902), from the John Hopkins Hospital. The role of the Anopheles mosquito in malaria had already been proven by now. Walter Reed and his colleagues decided to test Finlay's hypothesis incriminating the Aedes aegypti mosquito. Rather heroically three researchers experimented upon their own selves as no animals were known to suffer from yellow fever. Aedes aegypti mosquitoes after biting patients with yellow fever, were then allowed to bite first Jesse Lazear (1866–1900), then James Carroll (1854–1907), and finally a volunteer soldier who had no contact with yellow fever. Lazear remained healthy and well, James Carroll came down with yellow fever but as he had earlier been in Cuba, the result was inconclusive. The volunteer soldier bitten by the same mosquito came down with yellow fever, proving that the disease could be spread by mosquitoes. An unfortunate sequel to this experiment was the death of Lazear, who contracted the disease through an accidental mosquito bite while working in a yellow fever ward.

Walter Reed and his researchers now conducted a controlled experiment, using soldier volunteers divided into two groups. The first group was allowed to come into close contact with the clothing and beddings of yellow fever victims for several days. The other group was kept in isolation and allowed to be bitten by mosquitoes infected by yellow fever patients. Not one of the first group developed yellow fever, but 80 per cent of those bitten by infected mosquitoes developed the disease. It was fortunate that all survived. Transmission through a mosquito was now clearly established. The commission concluded that the causative agent was an ultra-small, unknown microscopic organism which could pass through a filter that retained all other known micro-organisms. It was the first time in medicine that a very small, invisible, filterable organism (a virus) was implicated as the cause of a disease.

As in malaria, this discovery led to prevention through eradication of the mosquitoes. The breeding grounds as in malaria were stagnant pools of water, ponds, wells and tanks. Kerosene was spread on the surface of water suspected of infection and mosquitoes were destroyed. In addition, the yellow fever patients were isolated, so that the incidence of this disease fell sharply within a short time.

In the early 1900s, an attempt by the French to build the Panama Canal had to be abandoned because of a number of deaths from yellow fever. Malaria too was rampant in this area. The incidence of both these diseases fell sharply proving the great importance of preventive medicine in the control of infectious diseases.

Trypanosomiasis (sleeping sickness) is a killer disease caused by the subspecies of the protozoan haemoflagellate, *Trypanosoma Brucie* and transmitted by the tsetse flies. The disease was and continues to be widely prevalent in animals and man in Sub-Saharan Africa. *Trypanosoma Rhodisiense* produces an acute infection in man while *Trypanosoma Gambiense* causes a more chronic infection. The disease then called 'African Lethargy' was first noted by Arabs and European traders along the western coast of Africa in the fourteenth century. By the nineteenth century vast areas of Western and Central Africa were afflicted with the disease, which in its chronic form caused fever, excessive drowsiness, mental obtundation with progressive blunting of mental faculties (sleeping sickness). Colonial expansion in Africa may well have been responsible for spreading the disease along trade routes into previously uninfected areas. The early 1900s witnessed a horrendous epidemic of sleeping sickness in Zaire and around Lake Victoria causing over three quarters of a million deaths. Sleeping sickness was a great impediment to the progress of colonial expansion in the impoverished continent of Africa prompting an urgent need to unravel its cause and find a cure.

In 1894, Major David Bruce investigating the cattle disease nagana in Zululand, found the protozoan long-tailed trypanosome in cattle blood. He opined that the tsetse fly was responsible for its transmission, and that the disease had a high fatality in animals. In 1901, following a human epidemic of sleeping sickness in Uganda, a sleeping sickness commission was sent out by the London School of Tropical Medicine to investigate the disease. The commission included an Italian, Count Aldo Castellani (1875–1971), and although the investigations on this disease were infructuous, Castellani stayed on in Africa to continue his research in Entebbe in Uganda. He noted the presence of trypanosomes in the cerebrospinal fluid of dying patients.

In 1903, Bruce headed another sleeping sickness commission and both he and Castellani found trypanosomes in the spinal fluid of patients with sleeping sickness. Bruce who has researched earlier on the cattle disease nagana, concluded rightly that the causal agent of sleeping sickness was the trypanosome, and as in the cattle disease nagana, transmission was through the bite of the tsetse fly. Both really deserve equal credit for this discovery. Castellani was the first to note the presence of the trypanosome in the disease. Bruce was the first to attribute the cause of the sleeping sickness to this protozoan parasite.

Preventive measures took the form of the forcible eviction of natives from hyperendemic zones like the shores of Lake Victoria. It is more than probable that this strategy could have further spread infection into uninfected areas. Unfortunately, efforts at treatment were as unrewarding as the efforts at prevention. Ehrlich experimenting with arsenicals advocated the use of atoxyl. The drug had serious side-effects but proved useful in the early course of the natural history of the disease. Suramin is a later drug, now in use for early disease. The treatment of the late stage of the disease is extremely satisfactory and rests on a trivalent arsenical compound, melarsoprol (melaisa oxide with British Anti Lewisite).

Many other exotic tropical illnesses stalked and continued to ravage the poor continent of Africa. Dengue perhaps is of special importance as both Africa, South-East Asia and India are afflicted even today by repeated epidemics. This is a disease characterized by an abrupt onset of high fever with chills, severe headache, muscle pain, pains in the bones ("break-bone fever") and skin rash. In the more fulminant forms the fever is associated with haemorrhage in the skin, mucosa and other organ systems, causing death. It was long felt that the disease was caused and transmitted by the bite of an insect vector, in all probability the mosquito. Even so, its epidemiology and aetiology remained unravelled till the beginning of the twentieth century. In 1905, T. L. Bancroft (1860–1933) and his research team infected volunteers through the bites of the Aedes mosquito. They then injected filtered blood from a patient who had contracted the disease to a healthy volunteer who became ill with the disease. This human experiment proved the role of the mosquito as the vector of the disease. The infectious agent was undetectable by the ordinary microscope because it was a virus. It was as late as in the 1940s that the dengue virus was finally isolated by Albert Sabin (1906–1993). Related arboviruses producing haemorrhagic fever have also now been identified.

There are almost certainly a number of diseases within Africa yet to be researched upon or for that matter yet to be described. Now that colonial expansion and colonial rule are a spent force in the world (including Africa), the *raison d'être* for the rich western countries to research with determination and vigour on these diseases is lost. The victims after all are poor Africans in Africa, who generally speaking do not relate to the whites living many thousand of miles away in the West. Yet the realization that the world is rapidly shrinking, that travel will continue to increase, and that more and more Africans in years to come will leave their shores to visit the West for various reasons, is bound to spur research on disease and death in the Dark Continent.

55 Surgery

In the first half of the nineteenth century, surgery and surgical techniques were about the same as in the time of Ambroise Paré in the sixteenth century. The one difference was that the nineteenth century surgeons were better versed in anatomy and pathology than their colleagues of the Renaissance or the Baroque era. Pain, haemorrhage and infection restricted most surgical procedures to drainage of abscesses, and amputations necessitated by accidents or by tuberculous disease of bones. Skill, speed and daring remained the prime requisites of surgeons. Brilliance was often equated with speed and literally timed by the stopwatch. Sir William Ferguson one of the outstanding surgeons in London, was reported to have said to students, when at work, 'look out sharp, for if you even wink, you may miss the operation altogether.'

The hospitals of large cities like London, Paris, Vienna, and Padua provided huge amphitheatres for the surgeon to display his virtuosity. He was a performer, akin to the *prima donna* of an opera. He walked into this theatre, approaching the operating table (with its leather straps and the sawdust to soak up the blood), to the applause of students, colleagues and numerous spectators who flocked to see the show. Top surgeons even in that era commanded astronomical professional fees. There must have been exceptions, but by and large, they were egoistic, proud, arrogant and ill-tempered. They had a reputation for arrogance. The great William Hunter gave a rather wistful and gentle explanation for some of these traits when he suggested: 'the passive submission of dead bodies, their common objects, may render them less amenable to contradictions."

The Paris School in the early nineteenth century, produced some brilliant surgeons. One of the most illustrious was Guillaume Dupuytren (1777–1835), who is said to have worn a cloth cap and carpet slippers when operating. He has already been commented upon in chaper 44.

The British School of Surgery was also adorned by illustrious men. Perhaps the most famous was Astley Cooper (1768–1841), one of the four great men of Guy's Hospital (the other three being Addison, Bright and Hodgkins). He was hardworking—operating, dissecting, teaching and writing with exemplary brilliance. Even in those pre-anaesthesia days he took pains to demonstrate to his students, as far as possible, every step of a surgical procedure. Cooper's fascia, and Cooper's hernia are two of the designations that have perpetuated his name. He was the first surgeon to perform an amputation of the lower limb at the hip joint, and he did so in twenty minutes. Astley Cooper was a great admirer of Hunter, and dissection was his great passion. His book on *Anatomy and Surgical Treatise of Inguinal and Congenital Hernia* was the product of many years of experience in anatomical dissections and surgery. To pursue his anatomical studies he had out of necessity, dealings with the 'resurrectionists'—people who obtained corpses surreptitiously. He helped to defend them, supported their families and in spite of the sharp antagonism of the general public to body-snatching, his popularity and esteem remained undiminished to the end. Debonair, wealthy and famous, he hobnobbed with high society and was surgeon to the rich and famous. He removed a cyst from the head of George IV and was knighted for this rather simple service.

A different fate was in store for Robert Knox (1791–1862) in Edinburgh. He was a contemporary of Cooper, and also a famous anatomist, who like Cooper had dealings with the 'resurrectionists' or body-snatchers. When the dreadful activities of Burke and Hare who murdered to obtain bodies and sold them for dissection were discovered, Knox was accused of complicity. Although exonerated, he was hounded out of Edinburgh and professionally ruined forever.

Robert Liston (1794–1847) was one of the most skilful surgeons of his time. Daring and speedy, he devised techniques to remove tumors thought to be inoperable by others. A lithotomy would take two to three minutes at most. It is said that during surgery he would at times hold his knife between his teeth so as to allow his hands to work freely. From 1813 onwards, he taught anatomy in Edinburgh. Liston as has been written earlier, was the first to use ether anaesthesia in Britain. James Syme (1799–1870) was Liston's assistant in Edinburgh, then quarrelled with him and became his bitter antagonist. Syme was even more speedy than Liston performing an amputation of the leg through the hip in ninety seconds. Syme developed techniques that permitted the excision of joints, thus preserving the limbs from amputation.

Benjamin Brodie (1783–1862), William Ferguson (1808–1877) and James Paget (1814–1899) were other illustrious surgeons in London. Brodie was versatile—a surgeon, physiologist, writer and a medical statesman. Ferguson however outshone him both in surgery and versatility. He wrote a text on surgery, as also a book on the history of anatomy and surgery. He devised a number of surgical instruments, was an expert at carpentry and metalwork. He played the violin well and was fond of fishing and dancing. James Paget was however the one whose name is best known to future generations. He described Paget's disease of the nipple (a cancerous condition resembling eczema) and Paget's disease of the bones. He was a brilliant writer, and an elegant speaker, and gained the reputation of being the best diagnostician in surgery and of making the most mature decisions on what operation to perform in a given situation. It was often said, "Go to Paget to find out what is the matter and to Ferguson to have it cut out."

Perhaps the greatest surgeon of the pre-anaesthetic, pre-Listerian era was Ephraim McDowell, a country doctor in the wilds of America who pioneered abdominal surgery by successfully performing an ovariotomy on a woman with a huge ovarian tumour. More about him and of his famous co-American, Marion Sims, is written in a chapter 56.

Johann Dieffenbach (1794–1847), professor at Berlin Charité devised a technique for correction of the cleft palate and then turned his attention to the surgical correction of stammering. His operative technique consisted of the excision of a triangular wedge of tissue at the root of the tongue. He tried it first on a stuttering, stammering thirteen-year-old boy. The shock of this surgery must have temporarily stopped the stutter and the stammer! The poor patient is reported to have uttered as soon as the surgery was over (without his stutter): "There is some blood running down my shirt." Dieffenbach's operation for correction of a stammer became a rage all over the West—a classic and unfortunate example of the harm that medicine or surgery has inflicted on man from time to time and through the ages.

The introduction of anaesthesia by William Morton and of antisepsis and asepsis by Lister and those who followed him, brought about a dramatic change in surgery. Pain was conquered; no longer need the surgeon limit his craft to the surface of the body and the skeletal bones. The risks of post-operative infection and gangrene were also significantly reduced. Surgery entered a new exciting era, a brilliant period of exploration and innovation. Its advance in the last fifty years of the nineteenth century and the first quarter of the twentieth century surpassed what had been achieved in the preceeding two thousand years and more.

As late as 1876, the illustrious surgeon Sir John Erichsen declared: "The abdomen, the chest and the brain could be forever shut from the intrusion of the wise and humane surgeon." How wrong he was! Before the turn of the century, all these regions had been explored by bold and innovative surgeons. Operative procedures on the stomach, bowel, gall bladder, biliary tract, liver, kidney, pancreas, and prostate—all forbidden territories just some years ago—now came to be practised successfully with increasing frequency. Surgery on cancers afflicting different organs also came into its own. Surgery had made a quantum leap.

We can write briefly on just a few of the many who blazed this trail. Perhaps the foremost pioneer of his time was Theodore Bilroth (1829–1899), of Germany. Bilroth trained in Gottingen and in 1856, was appointed assistant to Berhard von Langenbeck (1810–1887) at the Berlin Charité Hospital. After four years with the famous German surgeon, Bilroth became professor of surgery at Zurich, and then in 1867 went to work at the German hospital in Vienna, one of the best organized and best equipped hospitals in Europe. Bilroth blossomed into a good researcher, a great innovator and an excellent surgeon. With true German thoroughness he became as familiar with his laboratory and his microscope as with his operation theatre, his surgical instruments and his surgery. He wrote a classic treatise, titled *Die allgemeine chirurgische pathologie und chirurgie* (*General Surgical Pathology and Surgery*), in 1863. The book ensured international fame, ran into sixteen editions and was translated into ten languages. Bilroth pioneered surgery of the gastrointestinal tract. He successfully resected the oesophagus, pioneered partial gastrectomy and successfully bypassed small bowel obstruction—both acute and chronic. Technically he was excellent and was blessed with a temperament ideally suited for a surgeon—cool, bold and innovative. As was to be expected in the earlier years, morbidity and mortality following surgery were high, but with experience and better intra-operative and post-operative care, he produced good results. Bilroth was a versatile surgeon. He loved music, and was a good friend of Brahms, who dedicated two string quartets to him. He gathered around himself an ardent, enthusiastic group of surgeons. One of his trainees was the American William Halsted, who made a name for himself on his return to America.

As always, success with the knife led to its overuse and as always, with the good the knife could do came the harm that it could perpetrate. William Arbuthnot Lane (1856–1943) was an Irish surgeon who performed colectomies as a treatment for constipation. Many a colon was sacrificed at the altar of his unwonted zeal. He saw a sluggish colon as an enemy of the human organism liberating noxious poisons into the system. This flight of foolish fancy was considered sound theory at that time, prompting the surgeon into meddlesome harm. There were other instances when surgical procedures offered as cures were both unnecessary and harmful. It was a fashion at the turn of the century to consider the tonsil as a functionless structure best removed from the human anatomy, even if slightly enlarged. Many children died in the 1930s because of post-operative complications (chiefly haemorrhage) following tonsillectomy. In the same vein hysterectomies were performed not only for diseases of the uterus, but also for emotional and psychological problems. Again when the diagnosis of an illness was not forthcoming it was attributed to a source of hidden sepsis. Out came the tonsils (if they had not already been removed) and out came all the teeth—these were the 'hidden' sources that ignorance blamed.

An important intra-abdominal inflammatory condition was acute appendicitis. The clinical entity had been described by Wilhelm Ballonius in 1734. James Parkinson (1775–1824) described peritonitis as an important complication of acute perforative appendicitis. In the pre-anaesthetic, pre-Listerian era, the treatment was to bleed, use enemas and sometimes to purge (which meant certain death). In the post-Listerian era the treatment of acute appendicitis was appendicectomy. We are not certain as to who should take credit for the first appendicectomy. Robert Lawson Tait (1845–1899) was a pioneer in London and Ulrich Rudolf Kronlein (1847–1940) was a pioneer in Germany. Shortly before Edward VII was crowned king (when he was yet the Prince of Wales), he suffered an attack of acute appendicitis. Frederic Treves (1853–1923) drained the appendicular abscess and was rewarded with a baronetcy for his surgical skill.

Almost all the intra-abdominal organs were being attacked successfully by the scalpel before the end of the century. Cholecystectomy was first attempted by Carl Langenbuch (1846–1901) in Berlin, in 1882. J Knowsley Thornton (1845–1904) performed the first choledocholithotomy (removal of a stone from the bile duct) in 1884. Nephrectomy (removal of the kidney) was infrequently performed. The first successful nephrectomy has been credited to the German surgeon, Gustav Simon (1824–1876), in 1870.

Bilroth pioneered surgery for peptic ulcer. The Bilroth I surgical procedure involved partial removal of the stomach (partial gastrectomy) to remove the major acid-bearing area and then anastomosing the stomach remnant to the duodenum. The Bilroth II operation involved partial gastrectomy, closing the duodenum with sutures and anastomosing the remnant of the stomach with the jejunum. The Bilroth II operation was used for treating both peptic ulcer and gastric cancer. Suturing of a perforated peptic ulcer with successful outcome was first performed by Ludwig Heusner (1846–1916) in 1892.

Radical mastectomy for cancer of the breast was advocated by Sir Astley Cooper in his lecture on the 'Principles and Practice of Surgery'. Bilroth reported a poor survival rate for those who underwent radical mastectomy for cancer.

William Stewart Halsted (1852–1922) was one of the pioneers of modern surgery in America. He was a student of Bilroth in Germany, and after returning to New York became one of the leading surgeons of the country. In the year 1884, Halsted and two of his colleagues started to experiment on the local anaesthetic effect of cocaine. Unwittingly he became addicted to cocaine and try as he would, he was unable to break the addiction. Urged by his friends, he and his two colleagues spent a year in a mental hospital in Providence. He came out a changed man—from being outgoing, social, and gregarious, he was withdrawn, frail, and punctilious with a preoccupation for detail and minutiae. His addiction returned and his work suffered. His friend William Welch realized the tragedy and sent Halsted on a cruise to South America so that he could break his addiction. The withdrawal syndrome on the cruise was unbearable and Halsted is said to have broken into the medical stores of the ship to obtain cocaine. On his return he spent six months in a psychiatric hospital. He appeared cured and now Welch offered him a research post in Baltimore where as professor of pathology he was involved in the planning of the John Hopkins Hospital. He suffered another breakdown and did another stint at the mental hospital in Providence. It is probable that around this time he switched from cocaine to morphine to control his addiction. On his return in 1889, Welch wrongly believed that Halsted was free of his addiction. He was appointed on his recommendation as Associate Professor of Surgery and then rose to become Professor of Surgery and Surgeon Chief of the John Hopkins Hospital. He now embarked on a distinguished surgical career, spanning thirty-three years. His handling of tissues was clean, meticulous and gentle, so that tissue injury during surgery was minimized. He ensured perfect haemostasis so that the operative field was well-nigh bloodless. From being flashy and fast he was now slow but safe. He innovated new surgical techniques in thyroid gland surgery, in surgery of the bile ducts and intestines, and in the Halsted II procedure for repair of inguinal hernias. He is best known for the technique of radical mastectomy (which involved removal of the breast, the muscles of the front of the chest and the lymphatic drainage system of the breast) in the treatment of cancer of the breast. This surgical procedure withstood the test of time for over fifty years after it was first performed.

Halsted trained some of the best surgeons of the succeeding generations. Training started as interns for one year, above them were residents who taught the interns, and at the top was the house surgeon or senior resident who was trained by Halsted himself. His most famous house surgeon was Harvey Cushing who was to pioneer neurosurgery in America.

Posterity will forever remember Halsted for introducing rubber gloves in surgical practice. Caroline Hampton, one of his theatre nurses, complained of dermatitis of her hands following the use of mercury choride as an antiseptic solution. Halsted requested the Goodyear Tyre Company to make thin rubber gloves as a protection. These proved very successful and came into standard use, first in Halsted's theatre and then in all operating theatres. Caroline Hampton married Halsted in 1890. They made an odd, eccentric, but happy couple. In 1912 Halsted died of post-operative pneumonia, following a cholecystectomy performed for gall stones by two of his own house surgeons, using a technique that he

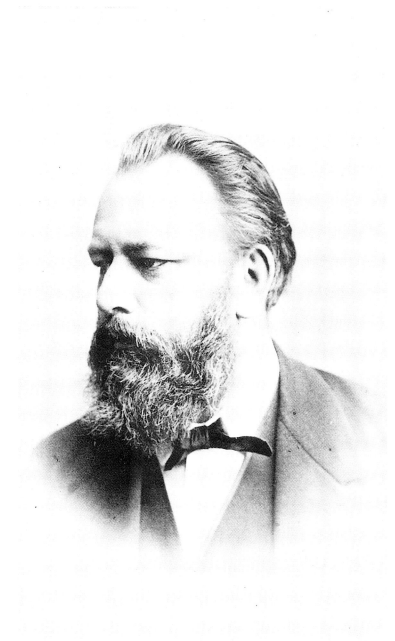

Fig. 55.1   Christian Albert Theodore Bilroth.

himself had devised. It was later revealed that he had never got rid of his addiction and that he had continued to take morphine all through his life. This probably explained his taciturn, withdrawn nature, his sudden disappearance from work, and his sudden long unannounced trips across the sea to Europe. Did his addiction to cocaine and morphine alter to an extent the history of man and medicine? Perhaps the very traits of character related to his addiction strangely enough made him the outstanding surgeon of his country. This clever addict, who became preoccupied with the minutest detail in his work and his life, to the extent that he is said to have selected the beans for his coffee one by one, founded a new school in surgery, where safety was given preference over speed.

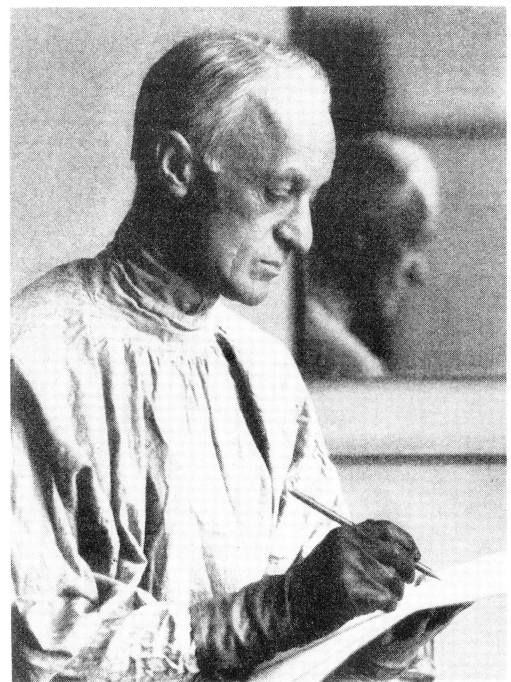

Fig. 55.2   Portrait of Harvey Cushing, in theatre gown and gloves.

Neurosurgery was introduced towards the end of the nineteenth century. The first surgery on a brain tumor was performed at the Queen's Square Hospital in London by Lister's nephew John Rickman Godlee (1849–1925). A walnut-sized tumor was found between the frontal and parietal lobes exactly as clinically predicted. The patient however died of post-operative complications. The first surgeon who selectively specialized in neurosurgery was Sir Victor Horsley (1857–1916), at the Queen's Square. He pioneered brain surgery, writing extensively on diseases and injuries of the spinal cord and brain. His counterpart in the United States was Harvey Cushing (1869–1939), who had his surgical training with Halsted. He had imbibed his teacher's meticulousness, concern for detail and the need for perfect haemostasis to ensure a blood-free neurosurgical field. He invented silver clips to stop bleeding from vessels which could not be easily ligatured. Cushing after studying with Sherrington in England, returned to John Hopkins Hospital in 1901, was associate professor of surgery in 1903 and then went on to Harvard, where he spent the greater part of his professional life. He pioneered the surgery of brain tumor, removing more than 2,000 brain tumors. He also devised the technique for sectioning the sensory root of the trigeminal nerve in trigeminal neuralgia. Cushing studied the results of overactivity of the pituitary gland, which caused truncal obesity, hypertension, diabetes and osteoporosis. He recognized this syndrome, now called Cushing's syndrome, to be due to a tumor in the pituitary gland. He was the first to devise the surgical technique to successfully remove pituitary tumors. He recognized that the pituitary was the master endocrine gland—'a conductor of the endocrine orchestra'. He retired at the age of sixty-seven, the recipient of several honours. His seventieth birthday was celebrated with great éclat and he received the homage of his professional colleagues all over the world. He wrote extensively, fifteen books in all, including the life of his dear good friend, Willian Osler. He was working on the bibliography of Vesalius when he died. Attempting to lift a heavy volume of Vesalius, he was seized with precordial pain. He died the next day on 7 October 1939. Strange are the workings of providence—at autopsy he was found to have a small tumor in his brain.

We are now poised to describe the feats of surgery in contemporary medicine. Surgery was ready for this take-off. Like the explorer making his way through virgin terrain, like the sailor sailing uncharted seas, the surgeon had by now explored the human body, treading into areas where no one had ever set foot before.

56 American Medicine

Medicine in America had taken root in the eighteenth century. The influence of Edinburgh, London and the leading medical centres of Europe, such as Paris, Leiden and Vienna, prevailed in the early part of the nineteenth century. Very soon the impetus to the growth of medicine came from within the country itself. Philadelphia, New York and Boston established themselves as centres of excellence. In keeping with the pioneering spirit of the country, medicine acquired a freshness of thought, a boldness in action and a renewed thirst for scientific inquiry. Great contributions from America included the discovery of anaesthesia, and pioneering work on gastric physiology and in the field of obstetrics and gynaecology.

The most internationally celebrated American doctor was William Beaumont (1785–1853). He was a frontier surgeon in the army, with no medical background and little training. Because of a fortuitous accident he became a physiologist, contributing immensely to the physiology of digestion. Beaumont was a camp surgeon at Fort Mackinae on Mackinae Island, situated at the confluence of Lake Huron and Lake Michigan. French-Canadian trappers and Indians gathered on this island to trade and to sell their pelts. One day in June 1822, an inebriated group of trappers were standing around when a shotgun went off accidentally. Alexis St-Martin, a young nineteen-year-old trapper bore the whole brunt of the blast as he was just a few feet away from the gun. Beaumont the surgeon, was sent for from the nearby fort and attended to the patient within a few minutes. He found the wound to be horrific. It was below the left breast; the left side of the chest had been partly blown off, the lung injured, the diaphragm torn, and the stomach lacerated, with its cavity laid bare, through which food escaped. Beaumont extracted part of the shot, together with pieces of clothing, carefully dressed the wound and pronounced that the man would surely die within a few hours. But Alexis miraculously survived and Beaumont continued to attend to his patient. Alexis recovered, but was left with a large permanent gastric fistula open to the outside. The fistulous opening had to be plugged at each meal to prevent the food from oozing out. It took two years for Alexis St-Martin to regain enough strength to be able to walk around. In May 1825 Beaumont began his experiments on the physiology of digestion. Alexis' stomach became Beaumont's physiological laboratory. He could look straight through the fistula into the cavity of the stomach. Though without academic training, he conducted with impeccable skill and method a successful study on gastric physiology. He observed the peristaltic contractions of the stomach and the changes in the lining mucosa during different phases of digestion. He tested the digestibility of different foods, noting the secretion of gastric juice during the digestive process. He described the appearance and properties of gastric juice and determined the presence of hydrochloric acid and other digestive enzymes within it. Peristalsis within the stomach served two functions—to mix the food with gastric juice secreted by the stomach mucosa and to propel the food through a valve-like opening called the pylorus into the duodenum. The stomach thus emptied itself of the digested food contents. Beaumont continued his experiments on Alexis' stomach at various periods—the last recorded experiment being in

November 1833. Beaumont's studies on digestion won him international recognition and fame. Claude Bernard and Pavlov both acknowledged his influence on their own work.

The pioneering spirit of medicine in America in the early nineteenth century is perhaps best illustrated by Ephraim McDowell (1771–1830), who was the first to successfully remove an ovarian tumor from within the abdomen before the days of anaesthesia and of Lister. McDowell, a Virginian by birth, had studied in Edinburgh but had not stayed long enough to take a degree. He returned to practise in his home of Danville, Kentucky. One day in December 1809, he was called to visit a woman by the name of Jane Todd Crawford, who lived some distance from Danville. She was reported to be in continuous labour pain for two days, but the two doctors attending on her could not deliver her child. McDowell examined her and found that her supposed pregnancy was really an ovarian tumor. He knew that as yet no one had removed such a tumor. The operation in his opinion had a very small chance of success but he was prepared to do it if the patient would accept the great risk involved. McDowell could however attempt such surgery only at his own home. Jane Todd Crawford made her preparations and set out for Danville on horseback with her large tumor propped on the horn of her sidesaddle. She arrived in Danville bruised but prepared for the ordeal. McDowell waited some days for Jane to recover from her journey and decided to perform the most critical and dangerous operation of his life on Christmas day. By this time the community of Danville was aware of what was about to happen and many felt that what their town doctor set out to do was little short of murder. The story goes that a crowd gathered around his house prepared to lynch him if Jane died at surgery.

McDowell was not to be deterred by a mob. He called for his nephew to assist him. Jane was laid on the kitchen table and McDowell opened her abdomen through a nine-inch incision. Jane started singing psalms. As soon as the abdomen was opened, the tumor was visible and the intestines spilled out on to the table. Jane continued singing psalms. McDowell mobilized the tumor and tied a ligature around the stalk. He then wrote: "We cut into the tumor and took out fifteen pounds of a dirty gelatinous substance. After that we extracted the sack, which weighed seven-and-a-half pounds." Midway through the operation, he took time to bathe the intestines in tepid water and keep them moist. After the tumor was removed, he tucked the intestines into the abdomen, turned Jane on the side to drain the fluid and blood and stitched her back. The whole operation took twenty-five minutes and Jane was still singing when the last stitch was in place. She recovered slowly but completely, returning home in less than thirty days, and lived for thirty-two more years, dying at the ripe old age of seventy-nine!

We have described this surgery perhaps in greater detail than was necessary, but it is men such as McDowell who truly adorn the history of Man and Medicine. A country doctor practising in the wilderness of the New World had pushed back and breached the frontiers of surgery, striking a path for others to follow. What must have urged him to undertake a task no one else had ever attempted? Courage, skill, faith, mutual trust between the doctor and his patient and good fortune all blended together to provide a happy and successful outcome.

McDowell waited till he had successfully operated upon other patients before reporting his work. By 1830, he had performed this operation thirteen times, with eight survivors, four deaths and one failure because of inability to remove the tumor due to adhesions. It was indeed a superb achievement. Like most great pioneers he was censured or ignored. Liston called the surgeons who followed in McDowell's footsteps 'belly-rippers'. Dr Philip Physick was one of the best-known surgeons of America. A favourable comment on McDowell's work could have done much for both McDowell and the craft of surgery. Physick chose to ignore McDowell's work altogether. But the tide could not be stemmed. Slowly but surely the abdomen was no longer an unexplored area in surgery. Ovariotomy was now being performed by several surgeons. A famous exponent was Spencer Wells of London, who had performed 1,000 such operations by 1880.

McDowell did not live to taste glory or fame. He went on with his practice of doling pills rather sparingly (for he had little faith in them), and of operating when the occasion arose. In June 1830, he returned from picking and eating berries from his garden. He took ill, with severe abdominal pain and vomiting and was diagnosed by a colleague as suffering from an 'inflammation of the stomach'. He himself felt that he had been poisoned by one of the berries he ate. There is little doubt that the real cause of his illness and death was acute perforated or gangrenous appendicitis, an irony of fate for a man who pioneered abdominal surgery.

James Marion Sims was another great American gynaecologist who pioneered the surgery of vesicovaginal fistula. Sims, a southerner, trained at Jefferson Medical College in Philadelphia and started surgical practice in Alabama. He was called to help delivery in a young slave girl who had been in labour for seventy-two hours. Using the forceps he delivered the child, but the severe trauma of a prolonged difficult labour had left a tear and an opening between the bladder and the vagina. This was a disabling condition for which there was no treatment. He gathered all the cases that he could of similar vesicovaginal fistulae and for four years experimented to achieve a surgical cure. His efforts seemed futile, until one day he made an unexpected discovery. While treating a patient for correction of a retroverted uterus, he placed the patient in the knee-elbow position. The conventional way of correction was by placing a finger in the vagina and another in the rectum. Sims sought to correct the retroversion by placing two fingers in the vagina. In the process of turning his hand to correct the retroverted uterus, the womb seemed to disappear and the patient was relieved. On turning to her side the patient and the doctor both noted an explosive sound of air. He realized that on turning his hand, he had allowed the external air pressure to push the vagina back into the normal position. Sims hurried back to his hospital, put one of his patients in the knee-elbow position, opened the vagina and again heard the air rush in. He wrote: "Introducing the bent handle of a spoon, I saw everything as no man had ever seen before. The fistula was as plain as the nose on one's face." After discovery of the knee-elbow position, later modified to a lateral or side position (Sim's position), he devised a special speculum for vaginal examination, and went on to devise a surgical technique that successfully closed vesicovaginal fistulae. John Marion Sims had laid the basic foundation of the specialist branch of gynaecology.

There were a number of other American physicians and surgeons deserving mention. They were Dr Joseph and John Warren of the Revolutionary War fame, and their descendants, who were leaders in medicine in New England for several generations; Dr Phillip Syng Physick (1768–1837) is credited for the establishment of surgery in America; Oliver Wendell Holmes (1809–1894), a famous practitioner who was also a poet, essayist and teacher. Holmes was the first to suggest that childbed or puerperal fever was contagious. It was however Ignatz Semmelweis who four years later proved this fact beyond doubt.

Medical education in the early nineteenth century left much to be desired. Along with the frontier which crept westwards, medical schools of varying quality mushroomed all over the country. Most of them had inadequate teaching standards, granting proprietary degrees in just a year's study. The school year would ordinarily last for eight to fourteen weeks and the course consisted exclusively of listening to didactic lectures. These schools were dependant on students' fees for income so that very few applicants were refused, and almost all who joined were permitted to graduate. The American Medical Association was founded in 1847. This Association sought to improve teaching standards, establish a code of ethics, suggest measures for public health, and improve the standards and status of the medical profession. It was however only towards the end of the nineteenth century that standards of medical education in America clearly improved. This was partly because of the great strides medicine had made towards the end of this century and partly because of the increasing economic prosperity in America at this time.

A landmark in the history of medicine, medical education and research was the establishment of the John Hopkins University in 1876. The university was endowed with a hospital and a research laboratory, and became a centre for teaching and research in the United States. The medical school boasted of a brilliant faculty—William Henry Welch, William Stewart Halsted, William Osler, Howard Atwood Kelly—the 'Great Four' of John Hopkins. Welch was a renowned pathologist (affectionately called 'Popsy'), and among the first to introduce microscopy and bacteriology into the United States; Halsted (called 'Professor') was a renowned surgeon and Osler was perhaps the best bedside clinician and teacher of his age.

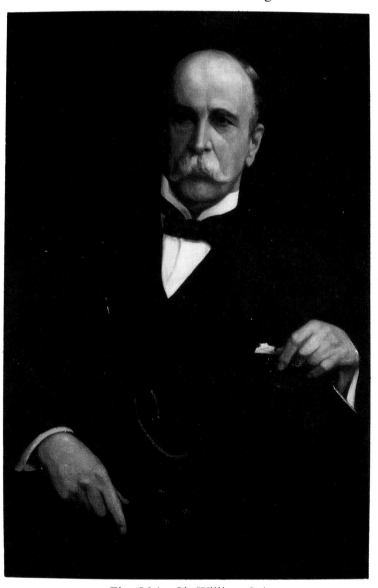

Fig. 56.1   Sir William Osler.

A colourful and peripatetic figure in American medicine was Daniel Drake (1785–1852). He eloquently stressed the need for improved medical education. His brilliant literary masterpiece was *Diseases of the Interior Valley of North America*. The book constituted a masterly study of the climate, geography, flora, fauna, diet, habitat and disease involving the occupants of the Mississippi valley. Seilas Weir Mitchell (1829–1914) was a famous neurologist of Philadelphia, who described erythromelalgia, causalgia and post-paralytic chorea.

Perhaps the greatest teacher of modern medicine was the Canadian, Sir William Osler (1849–1914). In 1875 he was appointed professor of medicine at McGill Medical school in Canada and in 1878, physician to the Montreal General Hospital. He then went on to join the faculty at John Hopkins Hospital in 1888. He raised the standards of clinical medicine to unsurpassed heights. A humanist at heart, he spent time at the bedside, learnt from his patients and taught a devoted band of students the essence of medicine. He was a true physician, caring towards his patients, learned in his own subject, and well-versed in literature and philosophy. He was a teacher cast in the mould of Hippocrates, inspiring generations of students with his intellectual honesty, wisdom and radiant personality. His *Aequanimitas* is a treasure to be cherished by all who have crossed the threshold to embrace the study and practice of medicine. He advocated 'aequanimitas', or imperturbability, as the first quality that needs to be cultivated in a physician or surgeon. "Imperturbability means coolness and presence of mind under all circumstances, calmness amid storm, clearness of judgement in moments of grave peril, immobility, impassiveness, or to use an old and expressive word, 'phlegm'."

Osler's greatness did not just rest on his renown as a teacher or on his clinical acumen in medicine. There have been others in the past who have been his equal in that respect. His greatness lies in his wisdom, humility, humanity and in his practice of the essential spirit and philosophy that is at the heart of medicine. He combined within himself all the ennobling attributes that make a great physician. Besides numerous literary essays, Osler wrote his *Principles and Practice of Medicine* embodying the wisdom of the past with the knowledge of the present. His contributions to medicine include studies on bacterial endocarditis, on platelets, abdominal tumors, cerebral palsies of children, chorea and choreiform movements. In 1904 he was appointed Regius Professor of Medicine at Oxford University and respected by all, he worked tirelessly to the end.

The history of American medicine in the nineteenth and early twentieth century would be incomplete without mention of the brothers William and Charles Mayo, who founded the Mayo Clinic in Rochester, Minnesota. William Mayo (1861–1939) specialized in abdominal surgery whilst Charles (1865–1939) was an expert in thyroid surgery. Their father was a country surgeon known for his flair in ovarian surgery. William and Charles converted the local Minnesota Hospital at St Mary's into the Mayo Clinic, which grew from strength to strength, so that by the first quarter of the twentieth century, the Mayo brothers, through sheer hardwork and professional brilliance had transformed their private clinic into a renowned centre of excellence. The thrust in this clinic to start with was on surgery, but in the years to come it encompassed all branches of medicine providing excellent laboratories and research facilities. Surgery, thanks to the Mayo Clinic and to other surgical centres in the medical schools of Boston, Philadelphia, New York and Chicago, acquired an increasingly high profile by the first quarter of the twentieth century.

The end of the nineteenth century produced two great American surgeons—William Halsted and Harvey Cushing. The story of their romance with surgery has been recounted in the previous chapter. It is of interest at this juncture to briefly mention the Swiss influence on American surgery. Both Harvey Cushing and William Halsted benefited greatly from their interaction with Theodor Kocher, professor of surgery at the university of Bern. Halsted visited Kocher frequently and their relationship was one of mutual admiration, with an exchange of scientific ideas in surgery. He also prompted his student Cushing to work with Kocher in Bern on a neurosurgical research project. This exposure to research and to the skill of Kocher's surgery in 1901 was a great influence on Cushing's subsequent neurosurgical career in the United States. There were other Swiss–American surgeons who contributed to surgery in America. These included Henri Banga in Chicago, who pioneered antisepsis in the Midwest, Nicholas Senn who became professor of surgery at Rush College, Chicago, introducing important educational reforms and Albert J. Oschner, who was professor at the university of Illinois and one of the founder members of the American College of Surgeons.

57 Specialization

The two major groups of practitioners in the early nineteenth century were the physicians practising medicine and the surgeons practising surgery. The compartmentalization of medicine and surgery into different specialities initially caused vehement opposition. For centuries there had been itinerants who specialized in stone-cutting, tooth-pulling or in the treatment of any one particular disease—in particular venereal disease. Some of these even though they lacked training had honed their skills to perfection. Many however were quacks and charlatans who cashed in on the misery of the unfortunate sick. Therefore, specialization at least to start with smacked of quackery and was viewed with suspicion not only by the lay public but also by medical practitioners. It ran counter to the holistic view of medicine that had prevailed since the times of Charaka and Susruta in India, and of Hippocrates in Greece.

Scientific, social and economic factors all played a role in the development of various specialities in the nineteenth century. Voluminous accumulation of medical information and the increasing complexities of surgical techniques made it difficult for one practitioner to encompass all. The school of Paris had highlighted disease afflicting certain organ systems. Morgagni, Rokitansky and Virchow had clearly established pathology as a special field, just as the 'microbe-hunters' established the independence of microbiology and bacteriology in the latter half of the nineteenth century. There were also groups of diseases which came to the fore because they aroused lay and medical sympathy or induced fear and alarm. The large number of blind was thus the spur to ophthalmology; the deaf to the speciality of the ear, nose and throat; the crippled and the victims of trauma to orthopaedics; the sufferers of venereal disease to the speciality of skin and venereal disease; the sufferers in childbirth to obstetrics; and of the female genital tract to gynaecology. The economic principle then in operation was the division of labour. When applied to medicine it encouraged compartmentalization and the growth of specialities. Specialization meant specially lucrative professional fees. The opportunity to earn more, work less onerous hours, and perhaps win greater renown all became incentives for doctors to specialize.

Among the specialities, obstetrics and gynaecology became increasingly important. A historic landmark was the fight against puerperal fever by Oliver Wendell Holmes of America and by the Hungarian Ignaz Phillipp Semmelweis working in Vienna. Their contribution to medicine is detailed in chapters 46 and 47, respectively. Those of the Americans, Ephraim McDowell and John Marion Sims in gynaecology are discussed in chapter 56.

The nineteenth century witnessed a concerted attack on diseases afflicting children, establishing the branch of paediatrics. The German obstetrician Carl Sigmund Crede (1819–1892) introduced the use of silver nitrate drops in the eyes to counter gonococcal conjunctivitis and ophthalmitis of the newborn. John Bunnell Davis (1780–1824) in 1820 opened a children's dispensary and published a book titled *Cursory Inquiry into Some of the Principle Causes of Mortality Among Children* (1817). Infant mortality was attributed to maternal ignorance—a concept also enunciated in the eighteenth century. In 1850, Davis' dispensary had matured into the Royal Waterloo Hospital for Children and Women.

The discovery of the head mirror by the country practitioner Adam Politzer in Vienna in 1841 started the speciality of ear diseases. William Yearsley founded by the mid-century a hospital solely for the ear. William Wilde (1815–1876), the father of Oscar Wilde, established in Dublin the St Marks Hospital for the Ear and Eye. He recommended that the surgical approach to purulent mastoiditis was through an incision directly over the mastoid process. Wilde published his *Practical Observations on Aural Surgery* and the *Nature and Treatment of Diseases of the Ear* in 1853. Mastoidectomy for mastoiditis, as we know it today, was pioneered by James Hinton (1822–1875), a London surgeon, and Hermann Schwartze (1837–1910) of Halle. Joseph Toynbee (1815–1866) was another pioneer in aural surgery, who in 1860 described his experiences in a book titled *Pathological and Surgical Observations on Disease of the Ear.* Manuel Garcia (1805–1906), a singing teacher in Paris, invented the laryngoscope in 1855. The combined speciality of the ear, nose and throat was well established by the turn of the century.

Orthopaedics was an important speciality with its roots in the nineteenth century. Percivall Pott at St Bartholomew's Hospital described spinal caries (now known as Pott's disease). Jacques Delpech (1777–1832) of Montpellier observed that spinal caries was due to tuberculosis. Delpech was among the first to correct a club-foot deformity by tenotomy. The sectioning of tendons with a view to correct muscle contractures and orthopaedic deformities was introduced by George L Stromeyer (1804–1876) of Hanover, and William John Little (1810–1894). Hugh Owen Thomas (1834–1891) devised the Thomas' orthopaedic splint, which helped to immobilize a fractured limb. He was the pioneer of orthopaedic surgery in the English-speaking world, devising a wide range of splints, appliances to ensure that a fractured limb was efficiently immobilized. His nephew Robert Jones (1858–1933), followed in Thomas' footsteps and pioneered in Liverpool the orthopaedic management of crippled children. The use of bone grafts in treating Pott's disease, fractures and deformities was introduced by Fred Albee (1876–1945) in New York. The growth of orthopaedics into an increasingly strong and independent speciality was encouraged following the influx of soldiers with traumatic injuries during the Franco-Prussian war and even more so after the First World War, 1914–1918.

The beginning of ophthalmology had already been formulated in the eighteenth century. The latter half of the nineteenth century saw this branch of medicine firmly established. Of the many pioneers in this era, three deserve special mention. Frans Cornelis Danders (1818–1889), professor at Utrecht elucidated *The Physiology of Optics in Relation to Physics*. The discovery of the ophthalmoscope by Hermann von Helmholtz in 1870 and of the ophthalmometer, revolutionized the study of eye diseases and the use of these instruments enabled one to view the interior of the eye, in particular the optic nerve head and the retina. With time the importance of the ophthalmoscope was increasingly realized not only for eye diseases but also for the diagnosis of certain diseases of the brain and the diagnosis of other systemic illnesses. Albrecht von Graefe (1828–1870), working in Berlin, was another pioneer in ophthalmology. He initiated the treatment of glaucoma by performing an iridectomy and devised surgery for correction of squint or strabismus. By the first quarter of the twentieth century, retinal tears were being repaired by the use of thermocautery, and transplant surgery of the cornea had been performed.

The peripatetic itinerant stone-cutters of ancient and medieval times styled themselves as specialists and in a way they indeed were so. The speciality of urology developed in the latter half of the nineteenth century. Nitz and Luter in Germany, constructed the first cystoscope. The early light source was an exposed platinum wire lit by an electric current. This was later replaced by the electric bulb. Cystoscopy, catheterization of the ureters and advances in prostatic surgery continued apace. A number of these advances were pioneered by French clinicians, trained in the famous urological service of the Necker Hospital.

Dermatology advanced with the histological approach of Ferdinand von Hebra (1816–1880) and his son Hans, of the New Vienna School. In venereology Phillippe Ricord (1799–1889) established the difference between syphilis and gonorrhoea.

Specialities in the years to come began to be identified by the institutions practising them. There was no stopping them. Some of the important specialist hospitals in London were the Royal Hospital for Diseases of the Chest (1814), the Brompton (1841), the Royal Marsden Hospital for Cancer (1851), the Hospital for Sick Children, Great Ormond Street (1852), and the National Hospital for Nervous Disease, Queen's Square (1860). The development of neurology and psychiatry was a milestone in the history of medicine and has been considered at length in chapter 51.

Specialities in the twentieth century bred subspecialities; the opposition to specialization remained and continues even today. Holistic medicine has been replaced in many centres of the West by increasingly compartmentalized medicine. The focus is narrow, the view restricted and technical; the overall perspective of suffering and disease is diminished, and in time to come may well be lost. It all began two hundred years ago.

58 Alternative Medicine

The mainstream of Western medicine is termed allopathic medicine. Alternative systems of medicine came into existence in the West because it was evident to many that allopathy was in the main palliative and could not offer a cure for several diseases. Many regarded the polypharmacy and superspecialization of Western medicine as objectionable and realized that modern medicine with its use of potent drugs and interventional procedures could at times do more harm than good. This was apparent to a few discerning minds over the years, but became increasingly evident in the nineteenth and twentieth centuries.

The earliest important alternative system of medicine which gathered a wide and sympathetic following was homeopathy. Homeopathy was founded, developed and propagated with missionary zeal by Samuel Hahnemann (1755–1833). He was a doctor who received his medical education in Leipzig and Vienna. He graduated in 1779 and was aghast at the dangerous side-effects of drugs indiscriminately prescribed in allopathy. Hahnemann to start with stressed the importance of clean living, diet and exercise for good health. He then enunciated a new alternative form of treatment in *Organon den rationellen Heilkunde* (*Handbook of Rational Healing*). The first principle of homeopathy stated in his work was the 'law of similars'. The drug used to counter a specific disease was likely to be efficacious only if it produced the symptoms of this disease in a healthy individual. The second principle of homeopathy was the use of very small (infinitesimal) doses of a specific drug against an illness. Hahnemann's concern was with drug toxicity and drug purity. He opined that very small quantities of pure drugs were far more efficacious and far less harmful than the large doses of impure drugs used in allopathy. Medicine as practised on homeopathic principles helped the body to heal itself.

Hahnemann now developed his branch of medicine attracting many followers to its study and practice. He found different new medicines for different diseases and published the efficacy of his drugs when used according to homeopathic principles. He was banned from practice in Leipzig. He moved from one city to the other and eventually settled in Paris, where he won a large influential clientele. The system of homeopathy now saw many converts in the West and north America; it then became a world-wide movement. The International Congress of Homeopathic Physicians was founded at the end of the nineteenth century. Homeopathy continues to flourish and remains even today the most widely practised form of alternative medicine. It is a system which is now recognized by licensing authorities in most parts of the world.

Numerous other forms of alternative medicine have sprung up over the last two centuries. Hydrotherapy extolled the healing powers of water. It was originated by Vincent Priessnitz, who founded a spa at Grafenberg in Austrian Silesia. It won many distinguished supporters in England. In the present century hydrotherapy has been modified to a form of 'Nature Therapy'. Besides milder versions of the nineteenth century 'water therapy', nature therapy includes a puritanical vegetarian diet, fresh air, exercise and a regime of clean healthy living. 'Nature farms' of this kind have become increasingly popular in India. The clientele generally consists of wealthy obese individuals who retire to these farms to lose weight, only to put it on in double quick time when they resume their worldly lives.

The osteopathy movement originated in the late nineteenth century and is still in vogue in many cities of the world. Osteopaths healed by manipulation of skeletal parts, particularly the spine. Chiropractic was allied to osteopathy. It was founded in 1895 by David Palmer, who hypothesized that the flow of energy from the brain was a vital force, which, if obstructed, could impair nerve function. Manipulating the spine could restore this flow and restore nerve function.

Mention must be made of Christian science, founded in the nineteenth century by Mary Baker Eddy (1821–1910). She was ill and bed-ridden from a very young age and found no relief with conventional medicine. She entered upon a self-healing process after reading the *Bible,* which revealed to her that all bodily illness was fantasy and that all illness lay within the mind. 'Mind-healing' is the basis of Christian science; if this transpired the illusion of somatic illness would be dispelled. It is amazing that even in this day and age Christian science has its devout followers who refuse to be treated medically even when suffering from a grave illness.

Healing through the laying of hands probably originating in prehistory has been revived time and again in the history of man. The present version termed *reiki* originated in Japan, and today 'reiki experts' abound in most cities of India.

Some alternative forms of medicine have a scientific basis, such as acupuncture and acupressure. Acupuncture for example has been shown to induce the release of endorphins within the body producing an analgesic effect. These form part of the mainstream of medicine in China and many countries of South-East Asia, but are increasingly being used as alternative modes of therapy or as complements to allopathy. Ayurveda which was the system of medicine in ancient India and which is still in use by millions chiefly in the villages of the country is now gaining increasing popularity in the West. Herbal medicine is widely used all over the world and a number of herbal and ayurvedic compounds are now of scientifically proven use.

Unfortunately many systems of alternative medicine have made exaggerated claims with regard to their efficacy. All alternative systems of medicine for example would be disastrous if practised (to cite just a few examples) on a patient with a perforated appendix, a ruptured bowel, acute meningitis, fulminant cholera or other fulminant infections. Yet many illnesses afflicting man are transient and self-healing; they do not require the potent and often dangerous drugs frequently used by practitioners of allopathy. Alternative medicine when used in such illnesses generally does no harm and may even help nature to heal. Clinical practice is also bedevilled with patients suffering from odd ailments or vague but disabling symptoms which defy a semantic label. Sufferers from such problems have tried alternative medicine through desperation or choice and have occasionally found relief. Modern medicine generally scoffs at these claims as they usually do not withstand scientific scrutiny. But then, medicine is both an art and a science and contrary to the currently prevailing cliché medicine need not always be "evidence-based".

Western Medicine in India

59 Historical Backdrop of India

> I know this little thing
> A million men will slay.
> O Death, where is thy sting?
> Thy Victory O Grave.
>
> *Sir Ronald Ross*

The practice of medicine in India before the intrusion of western nations into this sub-continent in the sixteenth century, was confined to the practice of ayurveda by the *vaids* and of yunani medicine by *hakeems*. There is nothing to suggest that western medicine translated to patient care at this point in history was in any way superior to ayurvedic medicine established by Charaka and Susruta and later handed down by the *gurus* to their pupils and protégés over several centuries.

Except for compassion and a trust in the healing powers of nature, there was little or nothing special in the art of healing in that era either in the west or east, that could influence the natural history of disease for the better. There must have been as much quackery in the west as in the east and medicine must have done as much harm as good to man in either half of the world.

There was however one big difference between western medicine and ayurvedic or yunani medicine. Ayurveda remained comparatively static; it was glorious in the time of Charaka and Susruta, but by AD 1400 it became fossilized and uninfluenced by the spirit of scientific inquiry. Western medicine was changing, and strongly influenced by the advances in philosophy and the natural sciences. Though this did not produce an immediate impact on the care of the patient or influence the natural history of disease, it ultimately in the course of the next few centuries did do so.

The introduction of western medicine with the ever-increasing impact of the West, particularly of Britain, in the seventeenth, eighteenth and nineteenth centuries exposed India and its countrymen to an increasingly strong scientific discipline that reinforced the humanist aspect of the art of healing. Sadly, at least to start with, western medicine practised in India was reserved only for the benefit of the colonialists. For the West to have ventured into a tropical climate and into an alien environment without provisions for the care of the sick and measures for prevention of disease, would have surely led to a catastrophe. Research into tropical disease as mentioned in chapter 54, was a compulsion to help combat illnesses alien or uncommon in the west—problems that could have annihilated the westerners in their quest for fortune or conquest.

Many who engaged in research were however noble human beings who almost certainly were as concerned with bringing benefit to mankind at large, as to their own western brethren. In a way there was thus a beneficial fall-out that arose from the impact of the West on the East. This benefit was not confined to medicine; it also involved science, law, economics, the spirit of research and the quest for truth in many fields of human endeavour. The impact of the West on India also brought in its train a set of misfortunes that befell the people of this country. It is a moot point whether the good the West did, offset the harm they inflicted on this vast subcontinent.

Historical and Political Background

The earliest link in history between the West and the East was first established when Alexander the Great invaded Punjab in 326 BC. It was about seventeen centuries later that the Portuguese navigator Vasco da Gama restored the link when he landed in Calicut on the western coast of India in 1498. The Dutch, English and French followed suit in the seventeenth century. The purpose of their adventure, to start with, was trade. The Mughal Empire in India was at its zenith in this period of history and the European merchants carried on their trade after meekly seeking the permission of the Mughal Emperor. It was the English who ultimately ousted the other western trading nations and who exerted a tremendous impact on India.

The English venture into India was through the East India Company, which received its monopoly rights in 1600. Between 1615–1618, the embassy of Sir Thomas Roe to the Mughal court received an accord which gave it the rights to trade and to establish trading factories in the country. The major trading ports and factories were in Surat, Calcutta, Madras, Bombay and the surrounding settlements. There now followed a period of peaceful trading during the seventeenth century.

The Mughal Empire began to decline and disintegrate in the eighteenth century after the death of the Emperor Aurangzeb. Mughal governors began to administer the provinces as independent rulers. There was instability and even chaos in many parts of the country, a situation that was exploited fully by the European merchants. The first stronghold and seat of power established by the British East India Company was in the province of Bengal.

It was the genius, audacity and machiavellian cunning of Robert Clive (1725–74) that opened the vast riches of Bengal to the British. Defeating the Nawab of Bengal at the battle of Plassey in 1757, and the combined forces of the Emperor of Delhi and the Nawabs of Bengal and Oudh at Buxar in 1764, Clive enforced a humiliating treaty on the unfortunate Nawab. The British gained the right to collect all the revenues of this rich province; they exploited this shamelessly. Each member of the East India Company was in addition permitted trading privileges in a private capacity. Intimidation, corruption and nepotism all contributed to the wealth of the British and to the poverty of the Indians. The Nawab became a nominal head and the English became the *ipso facto* rulers of Bengal. An English trading company thus usurped political power in India and laid the foundations of British rule in this country. Even as it was making a fantastic amount of money, Adam Smith wrote about it in the *Wealth of Nations* in 1776: "The government of an exclusive company of merchants is perhaps the worst of all governments for any country whatever." The covetous eyes of the East India Company were now turned to the rest of the country.

With great ingenuity the British played one power within the country against the other, so that they could demolish and subjugate one province at a time. They ensured through concessions the neutrality of the Nizam of Hyderabad and then won control over Mysore after defeating Tippu Sultan at Srirangapatnam. After a protracted struggle, through cunning and feat of arms, the Marathas succumbed and capitulated to them. They next secured their western flank by conquering Sind and bringing Afghanistan under their hegemony. Finally, in the nineteeenth century they prevailed over the brave Sikhs of the Punjab, now exercising suzerainty over the whole country.

It is of interest that the British government realized the stakes involved in India by the middle of the eighteenth century. Therefore through various acts of parliament, it exerted increasing control over the affairs of the East India Company, so that by the nineteenth century it was the British Government which controlled affairs in India through a trading merchant company.

Indian Mutiny of 1857

This was a landmark in the history of India. The old order had been changed by the English largely to suit their colonial designs. The new order did breed a great deal of discontent in the economic and sociopolitical fields. There was also a great deal of discontent among Indian soldiers who were paid poorly and treated indifferently if not contemptuously by British officers. The immediate cause of the mutiny was the greasing of cartridges with the fat of cows and pigs. While loading the new long-range Enfield rifles, the greased covering of cartridges had to be bitten off. This enraged both Hindus and Muslims within the army. The revolt started on 29 March 1857 and spread to the whole of the north; the Indian soldiers who mutinied, together with lakhs of common people who joined them, took Delhi as also the greater part of north India. Bahadur Shah, the aged Mughal Emperor was declared the Emperor of India and the leader of the revolt.

The British crushed the revolt with ruthless precision. Delhi, Kanpur, Lucknow and Jhansi were the centres of revolt. They were subjugated one by one; Bahadur Shah was deported to Rangoon and his sons massacred. The leaders of the revolt were hung or shot.

Britain realized that the power and interests of the British in India were not safe in the hands of the East India Company. By an act of Parliament in 1858, the East India Company was dissolved, the administration of the country was directed by the British parliament and India became a vassal state of Britain, with Queen Victoria as its reigning monarch.

March to Freedom

The Indian Renaissance began in the nineteenth century, gathered increasing force and momentum, ultimately leading to withdrawal of British rule and the establishment of the independent republics of India and Pakistan in 1947.

It was the impact of the West on India and the introduction of western education in India which indirectly gave birth to this Renaissance. It opened the eyes of thinking Indians to the concepts of liberty, equality and fraternity, to the spirit of scientific inquiry which was the basis of progress in science, technology and industry. It also focused attention on the rot and decay within Indian society, to the casteism and inequality, the divisions and dissensions that permeated their social fabric, making India an easy prey to foreign domination and rule.

The Indian Renaissance started in Bengal and the father of the Renaissance was Raja Ram Mohan Roy. He was convinced that India could never break its shackles unless society was reformed, and that equality and fraternity replaced the evil social customs that went with caste and creed. The political organization that fought the battle for independence in India was the Indian National Congress. By a strange quirk of destiny it was founded by a retired British officer named Allan Octavian Hume in December 1885. The other founders included the great Dadabhai Naoroji and Pherozeshah Mehta. It is beyond the scope of this short introduction to trace the history of the independence movement. Many were the stalwarts who gave their all for freedom. The greatest of them all was Mohandas Karamchand Gandhi, revered in the country as Mahatma Gandhi. A Gujarati from Ahmedabad, he trained to be a barrister in London, went on to South Africa where he fought against the apartheid regime of that country through the method of civil disobedience. He returned to India in 1917, saw for himself the poverty in the country and launched the novel technique of *satyagraha* in the freedom struggle. Satyagraha meant resisting tyranny and injustice by non-violent means. He won many a victory with this novel method where the strength of the spirit triumphed over the force of physical might. The great British Empire capitulated before the spiritual force of this frail old man who organized the non-cooperation and the 'Quit India' movement against the rulers of India.

A counter to this non-violent approach to the freedom struggle was the armed revolt led by Subhas Chandra Bose, who organized the Indian National Army on foreign soil to fight the British. The emotional impact of this defiance on nationalists all over the country was immense.

Finally, mention must be made of Jawaharlal Nehru, a scion of a rich, aristocratic family of Allahabad who laid the foundations of modern secular India, and of Mohammed Ali Jinnah, who insisted that Pakistan be carved out of the old subcontinent so that it could be the home of the Muslims who desired to live within this new state.

Administrative System in India

The army, police, the Civil Service and the judiciary were the pillars of the British administration in India. The Civil Service was created by Lord Cornwallis in 1793. Appointees to the Civil Service were generally brilliant individuals selected through an extremely difficult competitive examination. Initially only Europeans were inducted into the service. For convenience of administration, the English divided their territorial possessions into districts. The chief officer of the district was the collector. The collection of revenue, the administration of justice and the maintenance of peace and order were his basic duties. The collectors were invariably honest, just individuals who spoke the local language and brought credit to the administration.

The modern concepts of justice and the rule of law were perhaps the greatest of all legacies left to India by the British. So also were the development of transport (both by road and rail), communications and postal services. The wireless telegraph was first introduced into India in 1853, linking major cities and centres to one another. The development of transport and communication was undertaken primarily to help govern the country. But better communication also had far-reaching effects on India by promoting easier contact between people living in distant places, thereby fostering a sense of closeness and unity among the people of the country.

The universities of Bombay, Bengal and Madras had been founded in 1857 as the acme of the East India Company's policy of fostering English education in India. The first graduates of these universities had their eyes opened to the philosophical, economic, scientific and technological changes and advances in the western world. The Indian educated elite, to start with, helped the British to govern India, emulating their British masters by seeking employment in the Indian Civil Service, legal service, medical service, journalism and education. In the years to come, many of those exposed to western thoughts and literature became the standard bearers of the fight for liberty and equality. Little did the British realize that it was the window to the West that was finally responsible for breaking the chains that bound India, setting it on the road to freedom.

A British legacy almost as great as the rule of law, was the practice of medicine. Started primarily to care for their own selves, it slowly evolved as the standard system of health care all over the country. It was the science behind the healing art that was given root in India. The medical service that they founded and administered, the hospitals and institutions they nourished, and the pioneering research that helped combat the scourge of disease, were enduring features of the impact of the West on India.

60 Medical Services of India

The best era of Indian medicine was contemporary with the rise of Buddhism (250 BC to AD 750). Buddhist princes established hospitals far and wide in every city and to these hospitals were attached medical schools. The works of Charaka and Susruta belong to this period. The system of medicine in that era may have had its idiosyncrasies, errors and even absurdities, yet it showed a far greater degree of progress in all branches of science. The practice of medicine, surgery, and the science of materia medica were equal to and in many instances superior to the west. The rise of Brahmanical Hinduism which replaced Buddhism as the main religious and cultural force in India saw the decline of medicine. The brahmins were averse to contact with blood or morbid matter; they withdrew from the practice of medicine leaving it in the hands of *vaidyas*—a lower caste. The *vaidyas* in turn were disinterested in medicine, so that the practice of the art and science of healing now rested in the hands of the village *kabiraj*. Medical services, ayurvedic in nature were comparatively primitive and varied in standards, depending on the wisdom and the knowledge of the practitioner.

The Muslim conquest of India brought with it a new school of physicians who derived their knowledge from Arabic texts and Arabic translations of ancient Sanskrit medical works and the works of ancient Greek physicians, notably Hippocrates and Galen. These Muslim doctors or *hakims* as mentioned in chapter 59, came to practise Unani medicine. They were chiefly patronized by the Muslim kings, princes and nobles of Mughal India, though their services were also available to all those who sought them.

Medical services were poorly organized immediately prior to the entry of the East India Company into the country. This trading company, if it had to survive in a foreign land and in a tropical climate, needed physicians and surgeons to care for the health and well-being of the Englishmen engaged in trade with India. From small beginnings they organized this service; yet it must be stressed again that the main purpose of their medical organization and service, and the research on the tropical problems that followed, was directed towards ensuring the survival of the company and later of the colonial rule of the British over India.

From the very beginning, the East India Company appointed British medical officers to care for the Englishmen within the company actively trading between England and India, and for the English in the factories and the settlements surrounding the factories. These doctors were chosen in England and the first surgeon-general to head this service was appointed in 1614. He was John Woodall, a qualified surgeon of experience and repute practising in London.

Consequent to the conflict between the French and English trading companies in the middle of the eighteenth century, the British used their surgeons not only for their factories and settlements but also had them accompany their troops in battles against the French. They were the first military surgeons in India. The need for military surgeons in Calcutta arose ten years later in the war waged by Clive against the Nawab of Bengal, after the latter had captured Calcutta from the British in 1756.

The names of their famous surgeons appear frequently in the records of the early days of English trade with India, commencing around 1608. They were Boughton, Hamilton and Holwell. There is also mention of John Fayrer, who served the company in India and Persia and was the author of an interesting volume of travel, published in 1698. Surgeon William Fullerton is recorded as the sole survivor of the Patna massacre of 5 October 1763. His life had been spared because he had rendered professional service to Mir Kasim, the Nawab of Bengal.

Indian Medical Service

The Bengal Medical Service was founded by orders passed in Fort William on 20 October 1763, to be effective from January 1764. The orders decreed that individual medical officers serving in the Bengal Presidency were to be combined into a regular medical establishment with fixed grades and rules for promotion from grade to grade.

The Madras and the Bombay Medical Services came into being at about the same time. Candidates for the Indian Medical Services possessed degrees or diplomas qualifying them to practise medicine or surgery. They were selected in England by a competitive examination. They then underwent a four-month training period and after passing a second examination joined the army in India. Except under special circumstances, they had to perform military duty for two years before being eligible for civil appointments.

Between 1780–84, the British Indian government found that the medical department was short of personnel. The first Maratha war (1780–1781), the Mysore war in 1781 and the campaign against the Raja of Benares in the same year strained the military medical service to breaking point. This prompted an increase in the local recruitment of surgeons employed by the East India Company and of subalterns or adventurers with some medical training. A few of these had practised medicine in their own country before seeking further fortune in India.

The first half of the nineteenth century was a period of great expansion and consolidation for the British power in India, which extended in the west to the Bombay Presidency, south to Mysore and Madras, east to Bengal, and north to Indore, Gwalior and Punjab. The medical services were expanded; selection was strict and stringent, requiring qualifications and a diploma from any one of the Colleges of Physicians or Surgeons of London, Edinburgh or Glasgow. A certain degree of experience in one of the large public hospitals in Britain was also mandatory.

In 1855, admission to the Indian Medical Service (IMS) was for the first time thrown open to all natural born subjects of her Majesty, through a competitive examination for all candidates. It is of interest that in the first competitive examination held in January 1855, the list of successful candidates was headed by S.C.G. Chuckerbutty, a Bengali student. He had served as an uncovenanted medical officer in Bengal from 1850–1853 before joining the Indian Medical Service. Almost all Indians entering the IMS served with great credit and distinction.

The three independent Indian Medical Services of Bengal, Madras and Bombay, after a separate existence of 133 years, ended their individual entities in 1896. From this period, all medical officers admitted to the Indian Medical Services were placed in one list and posted to four different commands of the Indian army; all however were liable to be posted to any command. With the changing political situation in the country, it was felt that the IMS should be increasingly Indianized with more jobs being given to trained and able Indian doctors. This was a political decision which took long to implement.

The officers of the IMS were well-qualified, well-trained and generally speaking, distinguished themselves. They had both civilian and military duties and could be switched from one to the other.

An IMS officer had multifarious duties. His hospital work sharpened his expertise both as physician and surgeon. His time was also occupied with post-mortems and medicolegal work, by supervision of jails, organization of vaccination campaigns and by administrative work in his office. He was a member of the district board and of the municipality and this further added to his responsibilities. He was therefore left with very little time for scientific work in relation to the prevention and treatment of endemic diseases in the country. It was only the specialists and those in charge of military duties who could find the time for research. Many of these officers carried out valuable research, some of their efforts being crowned with glorious success.

Besides the IMS, medical officers were also drawn from the civil and military assistant surgeons and the civil and military hospital assistants. Civil assistant surgeons formed the superior branch of the subordinate medical department. They were trained in medical colleges and possessed a university degree or diploma in medicine. They were then given charge of numerous minor hospitals and dispensaries, and filled subordinate posts in the large hospitals. Civil hospital assistants had lower medical qualifications and were employed in dispensaries and in a variety of subordinate posts. The military assistant surgeons were mostly Europeans or Eurasians. The military hospital assistants were usually drawn from the ranks of the native Indian population.

The chief of the civil medical department of British India was the Director-General of the IMS with the rank of a Surgeon-General. He took responsibility for the management of hospitals, dispensaries, lunatic asylums and jails. He was in charge of vital statistics, general sanitation, vaccination, the health of ports and shipping. Medicolegal affairs, bacteriology and scientific research also fell within his scope.

The winds of freedom began to blow stronger with the passage of time. The Indian Army Medical Corps was formed in 1943, during the Second World War. The dismemberment of the IMS had begun. On 15 August 1947, the Indian subcontinent was freed from its colonial masters and the IMS ceased to exist.

Medical Services After 1947

The post of Director-General of the IMS was abolished simultaneously with the dissolution of the Indian Medical Service. The supreme officer in charge of health was titled Director-General of Health Services. He became the principle adviser to the Union Government in both medical and public health matters.

Under the constitution of the Republic of India, the Central Government through the ministry of health took control of health at the national level. Postgraduate medical education, promotion of special studies in union territories, control over research institutions and over India's relationship with the World Health Organization and other foreign government bodies or agencies concerned with health care in India were the responsibilities of the central ministry of health

The various states of India have ministries of health headed by a minister of health. The technical organization is headed by the Director of Health Services, who is aided by the health secretariat of the state government led by a secretary. The basic unit of state administration is the district. There are more than 360 districts in India, the average population of which is over three million. Each district is provided with many primary health centres, which on paper are manned by medical and paramedical staff. For several reasons health care in India remains poor and it is an unforgivable tragedy that after fifty years of independence the country's poor continue to be ravaged by disease and continue to suffer from the effects of poor nutrition, poor sanitation and poor education.

61 Diseases and Discoveries

From time immemorial, perhaps extending as far back as the dawn of prehistory, epidemics of various diseases have decimated the population of India at frequent intervals. Cholera, plague, malaria and smallpox were the major killers. There were a number of other diseases that added to morbidity and mortality. It is not that the West was free of these diseases. All the diseases listed above also ravaged Europe from ancient times and were seen to persist right upto the end of the nineteenth century. India however, had very large pockets of diseases existing as endemic infections, and these strongly influenced public health in the country. Disease burst forth from these endemic pockets to rage as epidemics far and wide, sowing death and destruction at frequent intervals. It was in all probability the unhappy but close symbiosis between man, the environment and the 'seed' producing disease that led to a state of endemicity and that influenced the rapid spread of epidemics. The climate, the soil, the pitiable socio-economic state of the average man in the tropics, religious, social and cultural traditions and taboos were all instrumental in the perpetuation of disease and disaster in India.

The West made their initial foray into India around AD 1500 and for the next four centuries the British in particular, exerted an increasing dominance, which culminated in their imperial rule over the country. Epidemics of diseases raged with unabated fury even after AD 1500 and continued during the period of British ascendancy and rule.

Cholera

Prior to the last quarter of the eighteenth century only scattered reports of cholera epidemics are available. It is certain that widespread epidemics of cholera did occur, but were unrecognized, partly because of the unfamiliarity of the European and English physicians with the disease, and partly because no records were maintained.

After 1817, the organization that accompanied the growing paramountcy of British rule ensured a satisfactorily recorded history of death and disease. This record is dismal and depressing; it is lightened only by the pioneering research of great men in the field of tropical medicine. The names of these pioneering researchers will live in hallowed memory, forever enshrined in the history of man.

The earliest reports on cholera from AD 1500 onwards were from the Portuguese, who were the first to settle on the western coast of India. Gaspar Correa, a Portuguese, mentioned in his *Lendas da India* that during the spring of 1503, there was an epidemic that killed over 20,000 men in the army of the Zamorin in Calicut. The same author in 1543 witnessed and wrote about another cholera epidemic in Goa. The local people called the disease *moryxy;* the mortality was so great that it was with difficulty that the numerous dead could be buried.

The most vivid description of cholera was given in 1563 by the Portuguese Garcia da Orta, in his book titled *Colloquies on the Simples and Drugs in India*. This work was based on his experiences on cholera in Goa and Bombay. His description distinguished the severe form of cholera encountered in Asia from that in the West. He wrote of cholera in Goa: "The Arabs called it *hachaizia (haiza)*, the name it is known by throughout India to this day."

The Dutch who followed the Portuguese into India were also familiar with cholera, as were the Jesuits in the seventeenth and early eighteenth centuries. Father Martin, a Jesuit priest in Madurai gives a graphic description of the disease that nearly killed one of his cathechists. The Indians now called cholera *mordechien,* an abbreviation of the French term *morte de chien* (a dog's death). This rather picturesque name was given to the disease because it led to a violent and cruel death.

In 1781, cholera attacked a division of 5,000 Bengal troops under Colonel Pearce, marching through the district of Ganjam. It then spread to Calcutta, decimating the local Indian population. In the summer of 1782, cholera raged in an epidemic form at Trincomali and the British fleet anchored at the port was severely affected. M Sonneral in his *Travels in India,* mentions the presence of epidemic cholera along the Coromandel coast from 1772 to 1782.

The first full and accurate account of a cholera epidemic dates from the outbreak of the disease in the province of Bengal in 1817. It was so widespread and fatal that for a time it gave the impression of a new disease. The disease within three months spread like wildfire decimating the population of Bengal, hardly a village or town escaping its deadly effect. The epidemic spread upwards to the north along the river Ganges and even attacked the camp of the Marquis of Hastings in Bundlekhand. The camp took an appearance of a hospital; the dead lay unburied, the local or native troops deserted in flocks, the servant of the Marquis dropped dead and he himself was apprehensive of dying in the camp. He gave secret instructions that if his death transpired, he was to be buried in his tent.

Epidemics similar to those described above raged again and again through the whole of the nineteenth century. Two of these however deserve special mention—that of 1826–1834 and the epidemic of 1848–1853.

The epidemic of 1826 again struck in Bengal, spread north to Benares, Delhi, Agra, then to Hardwar, the North-West Frontier Province and along the Himalayas. In 1827, Bombay Presidency, Sind and the whole of Punjab were under its influence. In 1829, it reached Khiva and Herat via Kabul and by 1830, it had struck Tehran—the capital of Iran. The rich and the powerful left the city and retired to the mountains in the vicinity. The epidemic spread from Persia to Russia and Poland in 1830, to England in 1831–1832, to France in 1832, and to America in 1832, where it made its first appearance. It then travelled to Cuba and Mexico in 1833, again ravaged Europe in 1835–1837, and finally reached Africa in 1837. This was the first great world pandemic of which detailed records are available.

The cholera pandemic of 1833–1845, which started as an epidemic in India in 1833, was perhaps the worst of all. Starting in the north and the centre of the country, it soon involved the whole of India. It spread in 1840 from Calcutta to China through troops transported from Calcutta. From China it spread to Central Asia, Afghanistan, Persia and Turkey and reached Europe in 1847. The trail continued to Russia in 1847–1849, to western Europe, Holland and Scotland in 1848, to America in 1848–1849, to France in 1849, and to Mexico in 1850. This pandemic declined in 1851. This epidemic is probably the worst on record. The death toll in Russia alone exceeded one million; there were over 50,000 recorded deaths in England.

One more world pandemic occurred in 1848–1853, starting from Kanpur and Agra, enveloping the greater part of India and then spreading from 1851 onwards to Persia, Russia, England, Europe and even America.

There were three features noteworthy in cholera epidemics in India. The first was the endemicity within Bengal and the spread of epidemics originating from this province. This was unquestionably related to climatic conditions, the moist alluvial soil, the density of a closely-crowded population and the grossly unsanitary conditions prevailing in Calcutta and all over the province.

The second feature was the spread of disease along the great rivers of India, notably the Ganges. Contamination of the river waters and the density of the population living along the river banks were responsible for the spread.

Finally, religious gatherings and pilgrimages particularly at Hardwar and other religious sites such as the Kumbh Mela, provided an ideal scenario for the vicious spread of all water-borne infectious diseases. Millions of people conglomerated at these religious gatherings, facilitating the spread of epidemic diseases.

AETIOLOGY OF CHOLERA

It is of historical interest to briefly mention the conjectures and hypotheses made with reference to the cause of cholera before the brilliant discovery of Robert Koch in 1882. Koch reported the presence of vibrio cholera in the stools of cholera patients in Egypt, and maintained that these organisms were the cause of cholera.

The doctors of the Indian Medical Service (IMS) made a study of the first detailed reported epidemic of 1817–1823. They concluded that the disease 'was due to a pestilential virus acting on the stomach and intestines', and that it was spread by wind, particularly the East wind. They opined that it was not a contagious disease. In 1829, one of the leading physicians of India wrote extensively on the disequilibrium within the body of the recently discovered phenomenon of electricity as being responsible for disease.

While the IMS doctors in India were blaming air pollution as the cause of epidemics, physicians in England and Europe carried out investigations which led them to believe that polluted water was responsible for cholera.

The College of Physicians in London commenting on the epidemic of 1848–1849, added little to the wisdom of the day. They made an important observation that human interaction and gatherings were one factor in the spread of disease. Yet it was their considered belief that the main cause of spread from the sick to the healthy was by polluted wind. Notwithstanding this belief, during the cholera epidemic in London in 1853–1854, it was observed that the death rate of cholera varied from 37 per 1,000 in the Lambeth district which had a pure water supply, to 140 per 1,000 in areas where the drinking water was impure and uncared for. This confirmation of the water-borne theory led to the Metropolitan Water Supply Act, ensuring purified drinking water to the city. This made London perhaps the healthiest of the great cities of the world in that age.

It is of interest that Charles Morehead, professor of medicine at the J J Hospital, Bombay, studied 158 inmates ill with cholera in the 1848–54 epidemic. He believed in cleanliness, good ventilation and placing patients at wide distances. He also believed that the impurity of the atmosphere was the cause of the disease.

ROBERT KOCH AND CHOLERA

Robert Koch's discovery in 1857 in Egypt, of vibrio-like organisms as the cause of cholera, like all great discoveries was met with antagonism and even ridicule. In 1884, Koch requested permission to investigate cholera in Calcutta. His brilliant study left no doubt in discerning minds that cholera was an infectious and contagious disease caused by the vibrio-like organism he had discovered. His report of his scientific discovery is indeed a landmark in the history of science and medicine.

He studied twenty-two cholera cadavers and seventeen cholera patients, and with the aid of micro-special preparations, cultivation of organisms on gelatine media and on concave slides, he identified the comma-shaped, highly motile vibrio in every one of the above cases. His genius and technical virtuosity lay in his ability to focus on this causative organism and separate it from the large number of other bacteria present in the intestines of these patients.

As controls, Koch studied twenty-eight other cadavers, including eleven dead from dysentery, a healthy patient who had recovered from cholera, and also various animals which had died from different causes. He also examined polluted water in non-choleric areas. In not a single case, either in the alimentary tract, or in the evacuations, or in other fluids, rich as they were in bacteria, were cholera vibrio found. He concluded through this brilliant study that the vibrio were peculiar only to cholera. He noticed also that this organism multiplied markedly in moisture, particularly if the linen of cholera patients was kept in a moist state. He also noticed that acid destroyed this organism as did the presence of dry climatic conditions.

As mentioned above, his discovery met with ridicule, particularly with IMS officers in India. Interestingly enough, the British Cholera Commission sent to India to confirm or deny Koch's findings on cholera in 1884, also disbelieved his discovery and his views. Truth always prevails and it certainly triumphed over the prejudiced and unscientific views of a number of workers both in India and the West.

HAFFKINE'S WORK ON THE PROPHYLAXIS OF CHOLERA

While the IMS in India were busy debunking the work of Robert Koch, Waldemar Haffkine settled the issue by reporting that he had in his laboratory made an inoculum of dead cholera vibrio which could be safely injected into human beings. Two such injections at suitable intervals protected an individual from cholera even when exposed to the disease.

Haffkine, a young Russian Jew, was experimenting with the newly discovered cholera vibrio at the Pasteur Institute in Paris. He aimed at reducing their disease potential to such a degree that on injecting them, they would not cause disease but confer resistance or immunity when the individual was exposed to the natural form of disease. After growing the cholera vibrio in his laboratory, he exposed them to a blast of hot air and then injected them into rabbits. A few days later, he injected the rabbits with deadly cholera germs. The rabbits all survived. In July 1892, in the heroic tradition of scientists, he injected himself with this same cholera vaccine which contained live but markedly attenuated organisms. He had slight discomfort and fever, but that was all. His animal experiments and this self-experiment convinced him that he had developed a vaccine that was both safe and efficacious in the prevention of cholera. Later he inoculated a few of his Russian colleagues and further confirmed the safety of his vaccine.

An epidemic of cholera was raging in Calcutta and he asked permission of the British authorities to continue his research in that city. He arrived in India in March 1893 and plunged into work. He first proved that the cholera vibrio or the comma bacillus (so called because it was not straight as other bacteria, but curved like a comma) could be propagated in the laboratory by a series of cultures. With repeated passage through the peritoneal fluid of guinea pigs, the infectious properties of the bacillus could be exalted. A subcutaneous injection of such an 'exalted' strong vibrio culture produced severe necrosis of tissue in animals. Yet this property of causing severe necrosis could be destroyed if this strong vibrio was cultivated serially through a series of artificial cultures at a high temperature in a constantly renewed atmosphere. The vibrio at this stage was markedly attenuated or weak.

The principle of anti-cholera vaccination established by his experimental work, consisted of two separate inoculations given by a hypodermic injection under the skin of one or the other flank. The first was with the weakened or attenuated vibrio. It produced a slight local induration and fever which settled down in 24 hours. The induration disappeared in two days. The second inoculation, now with the 'strong' vibrio was done four to five days after the first, under the skin of the opposite flank; it caused the same symptoms as the first. Haffkine was convinced that his vaccine would afford protection against the natural infection of cholera.

Again Haffkine's work came under strong criticism, particularly from some of the rather bigoted IMS officers in India. His critics were however silenced when his work began to show results. Haffkine had personally taught this method of inoculation to many in the IMS. Inoculations on a large scale were thus put into effect all over India. The army, civilians, jail inmates, workers on tea gardens and bureaucrats in government service were all vaccinated. Fame now caught up with Waldemar Haffkine and he was invited to different provinces to help administer the vaccine. He travelled to Bengal, Assam, Uttar Pradesh, Delhi, Kashmir and the North-West Frontier Province, inoculating over 20,000 individuals in the first year, and 40,000 in the second year.

In August 1895, Haffkine returned to Europe for a few months to recover his health, which had been shattered by work, the rigours of travel and a disagreeable climate. He returned to Calcutta in March 1896 and again set to work, inoculating people in thousands. The mortality in cholera now fell from 80 per cent to 40 per cent. The scourge of the disease had been controlled and man looked forward to the day when it could be stamped out forever from the surface of the earth.

TREATMENT OF CHOLERA

The early years in the treatment of cholera were characterized by the practice of bleeding and blistering—methods that surely must have contributed to morbidity and mortality.

The credit of discovering the principles of treatment goes to Dr Leonard Rogers, an IMS officer. In a way he salvaged the reputation of this service, which had displayed ignorance and bigotry in its opposition to the pioneering work of Koch and Haffkine. Dr Rogers working in Calcutta Medical College in 1906, introduced the use of intravenous saline solution in the treatment of cholera. He estimated the quantity of saline necessary by determining the amount of chloride in the blood and in the rice water stools and by noting the change in the alkalinity of the blood. The use of large quantities of intravenous saline reduced mortality. Mortality was even further reduced in 1908, when Rogers raised the amount of sodium chloride from 60 g per pint of sterile water to 120 g per pint of sterile water. The use of this intravenous hypertonic saline resulted in a fall in mortality to 27 per cent. The next important clinical discovery was the role of acidosis in contributing to death in severe cholera. This lead Rogers and his teammates who included Dr S. C. Banerjee of the physiology department, to use intravenous sodium bicarbonate in addition to hypertonic saline in the management of the disease. The recovery rate in cholera now rose to over 80 per cent.

FURTHER RESEARCH ON THE CHOLERA VIBRIO

Further research on the bacteriology of the cholera vibrio consisted chiefly in elucidating their chemical and antigenic structures. The chemical structure consisted of two types of proteins and three types of carbohydrates. On this basis the vibrios were divided into six groups. Research on bacteriophages also contributed to the understanding of cholera. The prophylactic use of bacteriophage was tried in different parts of India with varying results.

Plague

The Black Death, as plague was universally named, was the most terrifying of all pestilences. It has existed in India since antiquity. Plague attacked the army of Muhammad Tughlak and followed the return of Timur from India. In 1443, a pestilence which was probably plague attacked the army of Sultan Ahmed I. A devastating epidemic of plague is believed to have hit Bihar in 1548, during the reign of Akbar. The great famine of 1590–1594 was followed by an epidemic which was probably plague. In the seventeenth century Bombay Presidency was twice ravaged by plague. One of these epidemics raged in 1618, then spread to Ahmedabad, and then up north into the Punjab and even to Kandahar and Kashmir.

The dreadful epidemic of plague in Gujarat from 1812 to 1821 is the first in India to be carefully documented. Dr D. V. Gilder, the civil surgeon of Ahmedabad who submitted a detailed report of this epidemic in February 1820 to George Ogilvy, secretary to the Medical Board, Bombay. It is of interest that this epidemic occurred three years subsequent to the dreadful famine which raged with such destructive fury in Gujarat and Kathiawar. Dr Gilder's descriptions of both bubonic plague and pneumonic plague are superlative and cannot be improved upon. They deserve a verbatim description in relation to bubonic plague. Dr Gilder described the "ghaut no rogue" to possess the following symptoms:

> Great and general uneasiness of the frame, pains in the head, lumbar regions and joints on the day of the attack; hard, knotty and highly painful swelling of the inguinal and axillary glands appear in some instances; the parotids are affected in four or five hours, fever supervenes; these symptoms go on increasing in violence attended by great thirst and delirium until the third day of the attack. when death closes the scene. Should the patient survive the third day, they begin to conceive hopes of his recovery. Suppuration of the glandular swellings occur on the fourth or fifth day; other symptoms gradually diminish in force, the fever assuming a milder aspect, and the patient regains his strength in 12 or 15 days; such favourable terminations are however rare.

Dr Gilder wrote thus with reference to pneumonic plague:

> The other form of the disease known to the natives by the names of "kogla" and "tao no rogue" and which at present prevails most, they describe as exhibiting the undermentioned symptoms. High fever attended with burning and excruciating pains about the scrobuculis cordis, skin intensely hot, and the patient feels as if the body within was on fire, hiccup with deep oppressive breathing ensue, he also feels a pricking sensation all over his body as if perforated with pins, considerable pains in the chest and joints and about the navel, delirium, great anxiety and thirst follow; at length the patient hawks up clots of blood, the difficulty of breathing increases and he generally dies on the second day of attack.

This pestilence was not limited to Gujarat—it spread to Rajputana, Kutch, and Central India and disappeared in 1821. It then broke out twice in Pali in Central India once in 1836 and again in 1837. There was a strong belief that the plague of 1837 was introduced at Pali and Rajputana from the Levant via the trading ports of Bhownagar and Surat.

Plague in an endemic form existed in the north of India particularly in the Kumaon and Garhwal districts of the Himalayas for centuries. This continued in the nineteenth century, the endemics often turning into epidemics and descending into the plains of northern India. Besides the spread of disease from within the country, health authorities were even more worried about the import of the disease from other epidemic and endemic areas of the world. The report of an epidemic of plague in Mesopotamia sent shivers through the health authorities of India. When plague was reported in Hong Kong in 1896, dread of its possible spread to Calcutta was genuine. The bustees of Calcutta, with their crowded mass of humanity and nonexistent sanitation lent themselves to utter annihilation if a virulent epidemic were to strike the city.

The dreaded spread of plague from outside to within India did indeed take place. The disease spread to both Bombay and Calcutta from Yunan, Canton, Swatow, Amoy, Hong Kong and other places in south China in 1896. On 18 September 1896, Dr Accacio Viegas diagnosed bubonic plague in a middle-aged woman and a young man in Mandvi. Both died within a day. He learnt of similar deaths in the neighbourhood and reported his findings to the Municipal Corporation of Bombay. To begin with the disease appeared to be confined to the merchants residing on the land near the docks. It then spread its tentacles all over the city, decimating the population of 800,000 and causing so fearful a panic that 400,000 fled the city. Public health measures were chiefly directed towards segregation and disinfection. The infected were taken to special plague hospitals and their relatives isolated in camps. Houses where plague was noticed were emptied and disinfected with carbolic acid. There was a tremendous dislocation of social life and the compulsory hospitalization of the sick led to great discomfort with many plague-infected victims hiding their disease and others fleeing the city only to spread the disease outside its confines. Plague thus spread as far as Poona, Dharwar and Karachi.

Bombay lived in the shadow of death, desolate, its shops closed, its houses abandoned, isolated from every port that had direct communication with it. As a result, trade was ruined and remained so for a long time. The mortality reached its peak towards the end of February 1897. It started to fall in June bringing some relief to its grief-stricken people, though the disease continued to occur even much later.

Waldemar Haffkine was in Purulia on the Bengal-Bihar border when news of the plague epidemic in Bombay reached him. He volunteered to come to Bombay and conduct research on the prevention and cure of the disease. Surgeon-General J. Cleghorn sent him a cable that he need not come as there was no plague in Bombay. However, on 29 September 1896, Surgeon-Major Dimmock identified the Pasteurella pestis, the causative organism of plague from the lymph nodes of one of the victims. Haffkine was summoned to help and he reached Bombay on 7 October 1896.

Waldemar Haffkine was born on 15 March 1860 at Odessa, a prosperous Black Sea port in the time of Tsarist Russia. He was the son of a schoolmaster named Aaron, a Jew. After finishing school where he studied German and Russian, he joined the faculty of natural science at Odessa. Here he learnt physics, mathematics and zoology and was awarded his degree of Candidate of Natural Science in 1882. He now joined the zoological museum of Odessa as its curator, working on the nutrition and hereditary characters of unicellular organisms. Being a Jew he faced both prejudice and persecution. After the assassination of Tsar Alexander, he was arrested on the pretext of being a member of the Jewish self-defence organization. It was only through the kindness of his well-known, famous teacher Professor Metchnikov, who appeared as a witness for his defence, that Waldemar Haffkine was released. He migrated to Switzerland and after working at the Geneva Medical School for a year went on to Paris in the hope of working with the great Louis Pasteur. It was here that he conducted his preliminary research on the cholera vaccine before coming to India.

From the day of his arrival in Bombay on 7 October 1896, he threw himself into his research on plague. He set up his laboratory in a small room at the Grant Medical College, and isolated colonies of Pasteurella pestis or the plague bacillus (identified in Hong Kong by Kitasato and Yersin in 1894) from seven live patients of plague, and from three who had succumbed to the disease. After isolating pure cultures of the plague bacillus, Haffkine heated the culture to 70°C so that the bacilli were killed and their toxin was inactivated. The heat-treated broth culture became the vaccine against plague. As with his cholera vaccine he first proved its efficacy against animals and then proved its safety by inoculating himself with the vaccine.

In January 1897, Dr N. F. Surveyor injected four times the dose of vaccine into Haffkine with no untoward effect. Volunteers now poured in for vaccination against the disease. Clinical trials of the efficacy of the vaccine were undertaken and proven on inmates of the Byculla Jail, the Umerkhadi Jail, among the Ismaili Muslims in Bombay and on people in Daman, Hubli, Gagad and Dharwar.

Despite the proven efficacy of his vaccine, the Bombay Plague Committee in 1898, ruled that Haffkine's vaccine was not sufficiently important to be included in the campaign against plague. The committee felt that the two-pronged efforts of segregation and disinfection sufficed. But the truth of a good discovery could not be hidden for long. International acclaim over Haffkine's work steadily grew. Official delegations from Germany and Austria visited Haffkine in 1897 to study the technique behind the making of his plague vaccine. Robert Koch headed the German delegation giving his approval after a year-long evaluation of the vaccine. In 1898, Joseph Lister, president of the Royal Society invited Haffkine to address the society and saluted his great work. The authorities in Bombay at last woke up to the fact that they had a brilliant scientist in their midst. Haffkine was appointed director of the Plague Research Laboratory at the old government house in Parel. The institute was inaugurated by Lord Sandhurst who paid tribute to Waldemar Haffkine on 10 August 1899. Haffkine took charge of the institute in February 1900.

After Haffkine retired from service in India, he settled in France, at Boulogne-sur-Seine. He had stopped active research though he wrote occasionally for medical journals. He felt a bit disappointed at the shabby treatment meted out by some of his colleagues in India and devoted his time to religious pursuits. He revisited Odessa in 1927, but was further disappointed with the state of his native country. He left Russia in 1928 and settled down in Lausanne, Switzerland. He died in Lausanne on 20 October 1930.

The Plague Research Institute, whose name was changed to the Bombay Bacteriological Laboratory in 1904, was renamed the Haffkine Institute in 1925 in honour of Waldemar Haffkine and in recognition of his pioneering research on cholera and plague. Haffkine was happy to hear this news when in retirement in France. He wrote:

> I am very greatly indebted to Col. Mackie for the name given to the Parel Laboratory and to you for the terms in which you have written to me . . . . The work at Bombay absorbed the best years of my life and I need not explain how much I feel everything connected therewith. I wish the institute prosperity as an active centre for work on behalf of the health organisation of the country and I send blessings to the whole of the staff.

Waldemar Haffkine was a Russian Jew. He did not belong to the ruling British regime of India. It could therefore be said with absolute certainty, that his motive for scientific inquiry into the scourges of cholera and plague in India did not include the preservation of the health of the ruling class of India so that their mission of colonial expansion could succeed. He was an unselfish hero in the history of medicine—we should endeavour to make the institute that bears his name reach greater heights of glory.

Malaria

Malaria was, and even today is, the pre-eminent tropical disease in the world. Current estimates place its clinical incidence to affect about 170 million people, the global death rate per year being close to one million people. The disease was rampant in India in the eighteenth and nineteenth centuries. The disease affected the greater part of the country from the foothills of the Himalayas up north to almost the tip of the continent down south. It also stretched itself across the width of the country from the Bombay Presidency in the west to Bengal in the east. Climate and mosquito ecology continue to determine the epidemiology of the disease today as it has from time immemorial.

In 1880, Dr Alphonse Laveran, a French army surgeon in Algeria found the parasitic organism in the blood of patients suffering from malaria. As mentioned in chapter 54, he rightly believed that these parasites were the cause of the disease. Five years later, Golgi of Pavia, discovered that there were three species of these parasites, each being responsible for a characteristic pattern in malarial fever. Laveran never accepted the view of different types of parasites.

The IMS doctors in India searched for the parasites described by Laveran in their malarial patients but failed to identify them. This was surely related to a lack of technical expertise. They therefore hypothesized that malaria was caused by 'spores' inhaled through the respiratory tract which gained access to the bloodstream, or through ingestion of infected water, in which case invasion took place through the intestinal vessels.

The breakthrough in the aetiology of malaria and an elucidation of the life cycle of the malarial parasite was pioneered by Ronald Ross. The gist of this great discovery has been given in an earlier section. The romance between man and medicine in relation to this great discovery of Ross is briefly touched upon below.

It was Patric Manson who demonstrated to Ross what malarial parasites looked like in the blood of malaria patients. This transpired when Ross consulted Manson on his return to London from India in 1894. It was Manson who showed Ross the path—mosquitoes he firmly believed were the vectors of the malarial parasite. On his return to India in 1895, Ross started his research on the subject. He wrote:

> I am only an army doctor, who found it difficult to obtain instruction or advice on any medical subject or even the necessary books. I worked almost solely by myself in my little regimental hospital in Secunderabad. Almost nothing was known about Indian mosquitoes and I was much laughed at for my pains. Not only so, but my colleagues seemed mostly to think that I was a kind of charlatan.

Ross bred mosquitoes and then let them bite patients who had malarial parasite 'crescents' in the blood. The patients were made to lie naked on a bed covered by a mosquito-net; the adult mosquitoes were released inside and not allowed to escape till they had fed. An assistant now collected these mosquitoes in test tubes. He later devised the simpler method of applying a test tube containing a single living mosquito to the skin of a malarial patient. The mosquitoes so collected were killed by a puff of tobacco smoke blown into the test tube. They were then dissected on glass slides with a pair of needles, the abdomen being separated from the thorax. The abdomen was transferred to a separate slide and the blood within squeezed out through the oesophageal end. Ross observed that the parasites in the mosquito blood were far greater in number than in the blood from a finger prick of the patient. In a mosquito killed fifteen minutes after it had imbibed blood the crescents had turned into spheres with oscillatory pigment. In those killed after thirty minutes the spheres were just masses of spent pigment, i.e., pigment left after the flagellae had escaped. In many instances he found scores of flagellate bodies in mosquitoes killed about twenty-five minutes after beginning to suck. He thus showed that within the mosquito, the malarial parasite

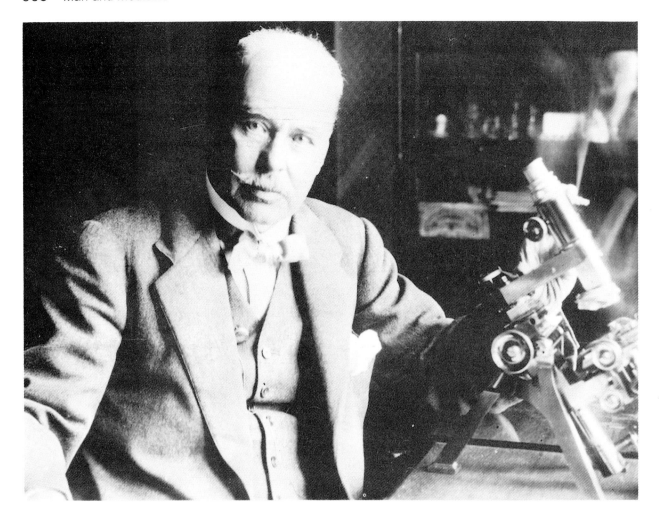

Fig. 61.1   Photograph of Ronald Ross with a microscope.

metamorphosed into flagellae. In his paper read at the meeting of the south Indian branch of the British Medical Association in December 1895, he maintained that the metamorphosis to flagellae was 'the first stage in the life of the malaria organism outside the human body'. He then went on to point out the great difficulty in tracing the further development and natural history of these flagellae. To quote his words:

> The flagella are, in fact, next door to being invisible and we are confronted with some such question as this—Trace the movements and metamorphosis of that which cannot be seen. Unless we call in the assistance of a theosophist or some such occult professor, it is difficult to know how the problem is to be attacked.

His next objective, around 1897, in Secunderabad was obviously to find out where the flagellae go in the body of the mosquito and what happens to them. He wrote: "The screws of my microscope were rusted from the sweat from my forehead and hands, and its last remaining eye-piece was cracked." On 16 August 1897 Mohammed Bux, an assistant, brought to him a dozen specimens of the anopheles mosquito. They were made to feed on malarial patients, each mosquito being then placed in a separate test-tube. Nine of these mosquitoes died and only three of the anopheles were left on the morning of 20 August 1897. One more died, leaving just two mosquitoes for dissection. He dissected the dead mosquito with no result. After finishing his morning rounds and his other routine work, he decided to dissect the remaining anopheles. It was 1 pm in the afternoon; he was hot and tired; and the eye-piece of his microscope was cracked. "Was it worth bothering about the last one? Better finish off the batch. Excellent copy-book maxim, but easier sometimes to say than to carry out."

Let me describe the romance of his discovery in his own words:

The dissection was excellent, and I went carefully through the tissues now familiar to me, searching every micron with the same passion and care as one would have in searching some vast ruined palace for a hidden treasure. Nothing. No, these new mosquitoes were also going to be a failure. There was something wrong with my theory. But the stomach tissue still remained to be examined—lying there empty and flaccid before me on the glass slide, a great vast expanse of cells like a large courtyard of flagstones each one of which must be scrutinised—half an hour's labour at least. I was tired and what was the use? I must have examined the stomachs of a thousand mosquitoes by this time. But the Angel of Fate fortunately laid his hand on my head; and I had an almost perfectly circular outline before me about 12 microns in diameter. The outline was much too sharp, the cell too small to be an ordinary stomach cell of a mosquito. I looked a little further, here was another and another exactly similar cell. That afternoon was very hot and overcast; and I remember opening the diaphragm of the substage condenser of the microscope to admit more light and then changing the focus. In each of these, there was a cluster of small granules, black as jet, and exactly like the black pigment granules of the plasmodium crescents.

He made notes and drawings of what he saw, and was elated beyond measure. The cells he saw indeed proved to be the malaria parasites growing in the spotted wing Anopheles mosquito. He now knew the appearance of these cells, their location and the probable species of mosquitoes concerned with the spread of the malarial parasite. On the night of the discovery he burst forth into poetic ecstasy when writing to his wife:

This day relenting God
Hath placed within my hand
A wondrous thing; and God
be praised. At his command.
Seeking His secret deeds
With tears and toiling breath,
I find thy cunning seeds,
O Million-murdering Death.
I know this little thing
A myriad men will slay.
O Death, where is thy sting?
Thy Victory O Grave?

For some inexplicable reason at this crucial stage in his research, Ross was transferred suddenly from Secunderabad to Kherwara in Rajasthan. Though he had reported his discovery to his chief in Madras Presidency, no one believed in the significance of his research. Fortunately, through the good offices of Manson (who had been informed by Ross of his findings), Ross was placed on special duty under the director general in Calcutta to continue his research on malaria.

The comparative scarcity of malarial patients in Calcutta, as well as the plague scare which caused many patients to refuse even a finger-prick for examination of blood, prompted Ross to investigate the lifecycle of the malarial parasite afflicting birds. He first discovered that the mosquito which carried the avian malarial parasite was the Culex fatigans. He correctly surmised that the life cycle of the parasite in avian malaria within the mosquito should be similar to that in man—only the species carrying avian malaria was different from that in human malaria. His further research proved that the 'pigmented cell' he had discovered grew in the outer wall of the mosquito's stomach and produced spores after a week. These spores were then extruded from the stomach wall into the general body cavity of the mosquito. They now worked their way into the salivary gland of the mosquito. The mosquito injected the parasites into the bloodstream of the human host (in human malaria) or the avian host (in avian malaria).

His discovery was complete. Here was the one doctor out of over a thousand British doctors in India, who had single-handedly at his own expense, pursued with dogged determination, research on the most frequent tropical disease in the world. He received no encouragement and often met with ridicule. His co-officers considered him a crank whose life revolved around buzzing mosquitoes. He was the last to be promoted and remained amongst the lowest on the salary scale. He was refused leave for his research while a fellow officer was granted leave for the training of race horses. When on the last lap of his malarial research in Calcutta, he was ordered to go to Assam to investigate *kala-azar*. He remarked, "Columbus having sighted America was ordered off to the North Pole."

His happiness at his great discovery must surely have been tinged with a little sadness. Though winning plaudits in England and Europe, his work was comparatively unrecognized for a long time in India. There also arose a bitter controversy on the priority of the discovery of the cause of malaria. Bignami of Italy claimed first credit for this discovery. This aspect has been briefly touched upon in an earlier section of the book. Sadly, the importance of Ross' discovery in relation to the control of malaria through the eradication of mosquitoes and their breeding grounds was ignored for over two decades. Ross pleaded his cause on behalf of the million and more people who died of malaria every year in India and the many other millions, mostly children, who suffered from it every year. His pleas fell on deaf ears.

Perhaps with a shade of bitterness he retired from the IMS in 1899, returned to England and took on the post of a lecturer at the School of Tropical Medicine and Hygiene at Liverpool. He subsequently became Professor of Tropical Medicine at the same school, was elected a Fellow of the Royal Society in 1901 and was awarded the Nobel Prize for Medicine in 1902. He was knighted in 1911. The Ross Institute was founded in his honour in 1922 and he was elected its first director and chief. He died on 16 September 1932.

Though great honours were heaped upon him by the world, no greater honour could exceed the unspoken gratitude of the millions of people in the world whose suffering his discovery helped to relieve.

Smallpox

Smallpox was known to India since ancient times. The disease left a trail of death and deformity every year. During the eighteenth century the disease was more prevalent in India than in other countries. The yearly death rate for example in London during the eighteenth century averaged 4000 per million. In Calcutta it averaged between ten to thirteen thousand per million and in the epidemic of 1865 it was 29,250 per million.

The prevalence of smallpox in the second half of the nineteenth century was as high as it was a century earlier. Terrible epidemics ravaged various parts of the country. It was estimated that seventy-five per cent of blindness in some parts of India during those years was due to smallpox.

Inoculation of material obtained from smallpox victims into healthy individuals with the idea of preventing or mitigating the severity of the natural form of the disease was practised from ancient times and continued well into the eighteenth and nineteenth centuries.

In 1798, Edward Jenner proved that cowpox vaccination protected the vaccinated individual from smallpox even after exposure to the disease. Vaccination as a preventive measure against smallpox was universally accepted in England, Europe, Russia and even America. Towards the end of 1799, Jenner had arranged to send a fair quantity of cowpox 'lymph' to India, on board the East India Company's ship, 'The Queen'. The ship was wrecked on the high seas and the 'lymph' did not reach India. It soon became known that the vaccinia virus could not retain its infective properties long enough to allow transport by sea to any port in India. Ultimately, the vaccine reached Bombay by an overland route through the good influence of Dr Jean de Carro in Vienna. The route from Vienna was via Constantinople, Baghdad and Basra. The lymph was still liquid in Basra. A child was now vaccinated in Basra and the lymph thus raised was sent in the ship, 'Recovery', to Bombay. Jean de Carro described his role in the introduction of vaccination to the East in a book titled *History of Vaccination in Turkey, Greece and East India* published in Vienna in 1804. In June 1802, Anna Dusthall, a three-year-old healthy girl in Bombay was vaccinated using the lymph that had arrived overland from Vienna. It has been recorded that "it was from this patient that the whole of the vaccinia virus now in use in India emanated".

Attempts to transport lymph for vaccination purposes in Bengal failed. Dr James Anderson, physician-general in Madras undertook the task ensuring success. He vaccinated a thirteen-year-old boy John Cresswell, and put him aboard the ship, 'Hunter'. From this boy, he used the lymph to vaccinate a female child; from her, a Malay boy and from this boy he vaccinated Charles Norton, a healthy boy of fifteen years of age who arrived in Calcutta on 17 November 1802 aboard the 'Hunter'. This became the source of lymph for vaccination in the province of Bengal.

Bengal showed its gratitude to Jenner for his life-saving discovery by presenting him £4,000 as a gift from the inhabitants of Calcutta. Bombay likewise presented a gift of £2,000 and Madras of £1,383.

The organization of vaccinating a huge population with differing cultural traditions was a formidable task. It slowly got under way, being spearheaded by the Bombay and Bengal Presidencies, but gradually involving all other provinces of India. Even up to the end of the nineteenth century the prejudice against the vaccine lymph taken from the cow persisted; however, slowly but surely these prejudices were steadily overcome and vaccination against smallpox became a national health policy. The number of cases of smallpox and the mortality rate from the disease progressively declined. The combined efforts of national and world bodies have today succeeded in erasing this scourge forever from the surface of the earth.

Tuberculosis

Tuberculosis was considered a comparatively rare disease among native Indians towards the end of the nineteenth century. A number of IMS officers with a large clinical experience believed that extrapulmonary tubercle was particularly uncommon. Charles Morehead, the professor of medicine at the J J Hospital however noted that during the six years from 1848–1853, tuberculosis constituted 1.7 per cent of hospital admissions and was responsible for 6.5 per cent of the total deaths during this period. In the European General Hospital in Bombay, tuberculosis formed 0.93 per cent of total hospital admissions and 6.1 per cent of total deaths for this period.

There is no doubt that tuberculosis by the beginning of the twentieth century was as prevalent among Indians as among the European population. The *Annual Report of the Health Officers* of Calcutta in 1902 showed that the mortality from tuberculosis was 6.4 per cent of the total deaths. Perhaps a correct estimate according to other authorities was 10 per cent of total deaths.

Whereas the incidence of tuberculosis in Europe showed a steady decline after the first quarter of the twentieth century, the enormity of the problem multiplied in India during the course of the twentieth century. The introduction of specific medicines against tuberculosis from the 1940s onwards has not helped even slightly in curbing the soaring incidence of the disease. Tuberculosis remains a premier raging public health problem in India today and as is explained in the next section will pose an even more formidable challenge in the years to come.

Leprosy

Leprosy existed in India as it did in the rest of the world from ancient times. The Dutch founded a *lazaretto* or leper hospital in 1728 at Cochin on the Malabar coast. The British established leper homes in different Presidencies but these were few and far between and inadequate to provide for the high prevalence rate of this disease. In Bombay, accommodation for lepers was provided in the Jamshedjee Jeejeebhoy Dharamsala; patients with exacerbations of the disease were given admission to a special ward at the J J Hospital.

The 1941 Report on leprosy and its control in India pointed out that there was a belt of high incidence which included the whole of the east coast and the south of the peninsula. This included Bengal, Bihar, Orissa, Madras, Travancore and Cochin. In Central India, the incidence tended to be lower, though there was a belt of moderate incidence along the foothills of the Himalayas, while in north-west India there was very little leprosy. The incidence in endemic areas was 2 per cent to 5 per cent of the population and in very highly endemic areas could reach 10 per cent to 20 per cent of the population.

The Bhore Committee Report in 1946 estimated that there were one million cases of leprosy in India. The lepromatous variety which was the more destructive and more infective form of the disease, constituted about 20 per cent of the total number of leprosy patients. In 1973, it was estimated that there were 3.2 millions cases of leprosy among a population of 37.2 million where the disease was endemic. Of these 3.2 million cases, 0.8 million were infectious.

The use of diamino-diphenyl sulphone and rifampicin taken in the correct dosage for the prescribed period of time should help to sharply reduce the incidence of the disease. The disease is slowly coming under control, but the belief that it will be stamped out in the next few years is wishful thinking.

The spectrum of diseases in India remains wide even today. Many diseases like cholera, plague and malaria were in the past common to Europe and to tropical countries such as India. These diseases are now extinct in western countries but still rear their ugly heads time and again in India. Typhoid and dysentery are at present rare in the west but remain frequent in India, sometimes occurring in epidemic form.

A disease peculiar and specific to India is *kala-azar*—*kala* meaning black and *azar* meaning sickness—a disease which causes black pigmentation. The first recorded outbreak was in 1824–1825 in Jessore, the disease being characterized by fever, marked hepatic and splenic enlargement, sometimes by ascites (fluid within the abdomen), increasing cachexia and death. This outbreak led to an appalling mortality, with more than 75,000 people dying in the district. The disease reached Burdwan town in 1866 and came to be known as 'Burdwan fever'. Death could occur during an acute bout of fever. If recovery ensued the disease lapsed into a chronic phase with frequent fever and increasing enlargement of the liver and spleen. Death in this phase was from intercurrent infections.

There was an epidemic of this disease in North Bengal in 1872. In Bihar it was known to have existed in 1882 and was known as the *kala-dukh*. The spread of the disease to Assam was probably consequent to the opening of road and steamer communication with Bengal. The disease spread along the newly-opened trunk road along the Brahmaputra river. The disease caused havoc in Assam towards the last quarter of the nineteenth century. It decimated the population, 25 per cent of the populace dying in some districts. By 1890, the epidemic had spread to Gauhati killing about one-third of the inhabitants. There was now a further extension of the disease to the Nowgong area. Over a year, the population in this area declined by over 30 per cent due to the ravages caused by the disease.

The cause of the disease for many years remained a puzzle. Leishman, an IMS officer was the first to report in 1900, the presence of peculiar bodies in the splenic pulp of a soldier who died of *kala-azar*. In 1903, Donovani reported the finding of similar bodies on puncturing, during life, the enlarged spleen of patients suffering from prolonged fever in Madras. Both Leishman and Donovani suggested that the organisms were trypanosomes and they could be dealing with cases of trypanosomiasis. Organisms similar to the Leishman-Donovani bodies were subsequently found by other workers in patients with *kala-azar* in India, in skin ulcerations in South and Central America and in ulcerations of the mucosa known as *espundia* in Peru. Leishman-Donovani bodies were thus established as the causative agents of *kala-azar* as well as of skin and mucosal sores called by various names.

The next step in research was to determine the method of transmission of the disease to man. This research was headed by L. E. Napier of the Calcutta School of Tropical Medicine and was carried out in Calcutta. It was soon discovered that sandflies made to feed on *kala-azar* patients developed a heavy flagellate infection in their mid-gut. It was further shown that the infection in the sandfly progressed towards its mouth so that when the fly again bit a human being it would contaminate the wound with the flagellates and thereby transmit infection. Experimental transmission of the disease to Chinese hamsters through bites of the sandfly *P. argentipes* was at first difficult, but with refinement in experimental techniques was proven beyond doubt. Research had thus conclusively demonstrated that the dreadful disease *kala-azar* was caused by Leishman-Donovani bodies and that the sandfly *P. argentipes* transmitted the disease to man.

Attention was now directed towards cure. Rogers in 1915 found that tartar emetic given intravenously could cure *kala-azar*. Cristinia and Caronia in Italy had used the same treatment in infantile *kala-azar* with beneficial results. Further work in Calcutta and Assam confirmed that the disease could be cured by two or more courses of antimony given in the form of tartar emetic.

Less toxic and more effective pentavalent antimony compounds were discovered by L. E. Napier and U. N. Brahmachari in the 1920s. Ninety per cent of *kala-azar* patients were cured within eight days of treatment. In 1922, U. N. Brahmachari prepared urea stibamine which was found to have a cure rate of 95 per cent. Finally, the introduction of aromatic diamidines formed an important landmark in the chemotherapy of the disease. This drug was found to be useful even in the treatment of antimony-resistant cases. The cure rate of *kala-azar* now stood close to 98 per cent. The disease remarkably enough had a mortality of 95 per cent before the advent of appropriate therapy.

There is one other important contribution to the therapeutic research on tropical disease that needs to be mentioned. This was the research on the treatment of amoebic abscess of the liver, a common ailment in the tropics with a death rate of over 60 per cent reported from Calcutta. Ipecacuanha was long noted for its efficacy in amoebic dysentery, a disease caused by the vegetative forms of entamoeba histolytica. Rogers had found emetine injections very effective in those cases of dysentery where ipecacuanha was of no avail. He now used emetine injections in the treatment of amoebic hepatitis and amoebic abscess of the liver with gratifying results. He also proved that open drainage of the abscess had a forbidding mortality, while mere aspiration of pus gave far better results. The mortality of this common tropical problem in India fell from 60 per cent to less than 3 per cent. In 1922, Rogers presented his work on liver abscesses in three Lettsomian lectures delivered before the Medical Society of London. He was awarded the Fothergillian Gold Medal for his research on amoebic disease.

62 Hospitals in India

The westerners after gaining entry into India built one hospital after another. It is a sad truth that to start with and for two centuries thereafter these hospitals were solely for Europeans. The natives did not matter. Health care was of paramount importance in all colonial conquests, for as mentioned in chapter 54, colonial missions could be only accomplished if those so engaged were physically fit and capable of performing the duties allotted to them.

The first European hospital was a Portuguese hospital; it was founded in 1510 by Albuquerque in Goa, on the western coast of India. In 1591 the administration of the hospital was given over to the Jesuits who made it one of the best managed hospitals of the world. A detailed account of this hospital was provided by a Frenchman Pyrard de Laval. Pyrard left France in 1601 and was cast away on the island of Maldives. He reached Calicut in 1607 and from there moved to the Portuguese fortress of Cochin, where he was arrested and imprisoned as he travelled without proper credentials. He was shipped to Goa in chains in 1608 and being ill, was admitted to the Portuguese Hospital for treatment. He found this hospital superior to the Hospital of the Holy Ghost in Rome and the Infirmary of the Knights of Malta, two of the best known hospitals in Europe. A few of his quotes bear testimony to the excellence of this hospital in Goa. Pyrard wrote: "Viewing it from outside we could hardly believe it was an hospital; it seemed to us a great palace, saving the inscription above the gate 'Hospital die Rey Nortro Seignoro'. The beds are beautifully shaped and lacquered with red varnish; the sacking is of cotton; the mattresses and coverlets are of the silk or cotton; adorned with different patterns . . . pillows of white calico."

Pyrard in his further description says, "There are physicians, surgeons and apothecaries, barbers and bleeders who do nothing else and are bound to visit each of the sick twice a day . . . . The sick are sometimes very numerous, as many as 1500, all of them either Portuguese soldiers or men of other Christian races of Europe, of every profession and quality. Indians are not taken in there."

The East India Trading Company needed hospitals to care for the White settlers working in factories, engaged in trade or living in the settlements around trading ports and factories—again, they were for the Whites; the natives could fend for themselves as they must have done before. These hospitals were set up in Bombay, Madras and Calcutta, the three burgeoning centres of power, trade and commerce in the seventeenth and eighteenth centuries, where the British populace was chiefly concentrated.

The first English hospital in the Madras Presidency was opened at Fort St George in 1664. It was only for the British. A second hospital was built in Madras between 1679 and 1688 by public subscription, at a cost of 838 pagodas (about Rs 3,000). The East India Company acquired this hospital and built their hospital in 1690; it stood in James Street in the Fort and was a handsome building in the Tuscan style costing 2,500 pagodas. It was almost after another one hundred years, in 1772, that the British built one more large hospital in Madras; this hospital became the Madras General Hospital, the entire building being reconstructed in 1859. It was through the enlightened efforts of assistant-surgeon John Underwood that a hospital for the care of the native poor was built at Pursawakkam, a suburb to the south of Madras, in 1799. It was called the Native Infirmary and came under the control and administration of the Medical Board. In the early part of the twentieth century, the Government took over the management of the Native Infirmary. A new hospital construction took place with 266 beds and an auditorium. The Native Infirmary was named the Stanley Hospital in 1940. It had a bed strength of a thousand and catered chiefly to the population of Madras and its suburbs.

The French were the colonial rivals of the British and had set up their headquarters in Pondicherry on the eastern coast of India. They established a hospital at Pondicherry in 1701 for the French soldiers, topas and other civilians employed by the French East India Company. La Haye and Jean Lafitte were two famous French surgeons of this hospital during the first half of the eighteenth century. Dupleix, the leader of the French was operated in 1742 in this hospital by La Haye for an anal fistula. This hospital continued well into the twentieth century and it is of historical interest that when the French left India, the Government of the Republic of India upgraded this hospital into the Jawaharlal Nehru Institute of Postgraduate Medical Education and Research.

Calcutta was not to be left behind. It was indeed the growing centre of British ascendancy and power from the eighteenth century onwards, even more so than Bombay or Madras. The first hospital in Calcutta was opened in Fort William in 1708. The second one was a temporary building erected inside the old fort on the recovery of Calcutta by the British under the leadership of Robert Clive. When the old fort in Calcutta was converted into a custom-house, it became imperative to build a new hospital. The third hospital was built in 1769 and was known as the Presidency General Hospital. All these hospitals were primarily intended for the Company's soldiers and sailors, but admitted all Europeans of all classes and all callings.

Almost 300 years after the entry of the West into India, the British thought it fit to build the first hospital for the native poor of the country. This hospital for the native poor was built in Calcutta between 1792 and 1793. It was the precursor of the later Medical College Hospital.

The Calcutta Medical College Hospital saw its early beginnings on 1 April 1838, when a small hospital with thirty beds and an outpatient department was opened to provide clinical instruction to the students of the new college. The foundation stone of the expanded Medical College Hospital was laid by the Governor General of India, Lord Dalhousie on 3 September 1848 and the hospital was completed at a cost of 20,000 pounds in 1853. The hospital contained 500 beds, accommodated within twenty-four wards. There was a ward for women and children, an obstetric ward as also an ophthalmic ward. This was the first hospital that admitted both Europeans and native Indian patients.

Bombay was a British stronghold second only to Calcutta. The first British hospital in Bombay was built in 1676 as judged from *The Surat Diaries* (1669–75) which contained instructions to this effect. By 1784, there existed three large hospitals in Bombay—one for Europeans within the gates of the Fort, another on the Esplanade for sepoys and a third for convalescents on the adjacent island.

The latter half of the nineteenth century witnessed the growth of a number of hospitals in Bombay. The foremost was the Jamshedjee Jeejeebhoy Hospital (J J Hospital) at Byculla, Bombay, erected through the munificent donation of Sir Jamshedjee Jeejeebhoy, an Indian practising the Zoroastrian faith. The foundation stone was laid by Sir James Barnes, secretary of the Medical Board on 3 January 1843. The building was completed in two years and the hospital was opened on

15 May 1845 by the Governor, Sir George Arthur Bart, in the presence of a distinguished gathering. The hospital building, to start with, had a ground floor with wings on either side. The central hall had an outpatient dispensary and an operation theatre. There was a marble tablet on the wall stating that the hospital was 'for the relief of the suffering poor', and that it was built through the generous donation of Sir Jamshedjee Jeejeebhoy and of the East India Company. The inscription on it was in four languages—English, Marathi, Urdu and Gujarati. Unfortunately, when the old building gave way to the new in the second half of the twentieth century, this tablet was removed and has been missing since then.

There stands even today in the main foyer of the hospital, the magnificent seated statue in bronze of Sir Jamshedjee Jeejeebhoy, resplendent in his Parsee attire. It was sculpted by the famous Italian sculptor Baron Marochetti. Every day innumerable candles burn at the foot of the statue of this great Parsee philanthropist—they are the offerings of the poorest of the poor in this country who bless this great soul for lightening their burden in life.

Affiliated to J J Hospital was the Grant Medical College. Both of these closely-linked, inseparable institutes came up together and started to function around the same time. They rose in unison to become in time to come the premier institute of medicine in the East. The history of the Grant Medical College is in truth the history of the vision and foresight of Sir Robert Grant (1780–1838), the Governor of Bombay in 1835. The Bombay Presidency was annexed to the British possessions in India in 1818. The state of medical practice was pathetic; quackery was rampant, and the poor sick were at the mercy of *vaids* and *hakeems,* whose practice was often based on dangerous and obsolete beliefs. In 1826, the government had started a medical school in Bombay which taught in the vernacular languages. The school functioned poorly and was closed within six years. The British Government in India had already started medical colleges, first in Calcutta and then in Madras on western lines. In 1835, Sir Robert Grant expressed his strong belief in the necessity of a medical school or college to impart scientific instruction in medicine to the natives of Bombay. This was both to help the spirit of scientific inquiry in medicine and to provide better patient care to the people of the Presidency through the training of medical practitioners skilled in their art, proficient in their knowledge and conscientious in their duties. It took two years to convince his colleagues on the justice and righteousness of his proposal which was finally minuted and sent on in the middle of 1838 for approval to Lord Auckland, the Governor-General of India. Sir Robert Grant died suddenly on 9 July 1838. A public meeting of the citizens of Bombay was held at the end of July 1838 to mourn the death of a great administrator, a kind, righteous man who had concentrated his efforts towards the upliftment of the native poor in the Presidency over which he ruled. A fund was started at this meeting for the public commemoration of Sir Robert Grant on the condition that the money so raised should go towards the founding of a medical college whose cause he had so zealously advocated. The college was to bear his name. The Government sanctioned this proposal and the foundation stone of the building was laid on 30 March 1843. The building was completed in October 1845, just five months after the J J Hospital was laid open to the poor sick of Bombay. The Grant Medical College and the J J Hospital thenceforth functioned as one great institute combining the pursuit of science with service and care towards the sick.

The college was fortunate in having as its head a brilliant pioneer in Dr Charles Morehead. He was the first superintendent and held this post for fifteen years. His brilliance as a physician, his ability as an administrator and his vision for the need of good medical education and medical services in India, laid the foundation of an institution which was to become the pride of the country. The torch of learning and of service that he lit has been kept aglow by a long line of his successors.

There seemed just one significant flaw in the Grant Medical College. All appointments on the faculty were British IMS officers. Perhaps the first Indian appointed was Captain Bhatia, who was appointed Professor of Physiology and Hygiene in 1920. From 1925 to 1937 as Major Bhatia, he served both as Professor of Physiology and the Dean of the College. In 1937, now as Lt. Col. Bhatia, he was appointed to the newly created combined administrative post of Principal of the Grant Medical College and Superintendent of the J J Hospital, a position which he held till 1941. He then became the Deputy Director-General of the Indian Medical Services with his headquarters in Simla. He retired with the rank of Major-General.

Numerous other hospitals came up in the city of Bombay after the J J Hospital was founded. The foundation stone of St George's Hospital was laid on 22 February 1889 on the site of old Fort George and the buildings were completed in 1892; the Bai Motlibai Wadia Obstetric hospital was founded on 9 March 1889.

The fact that there were no Indians on the teaching faculty of medicine in Bombay rankled with the increasing number of well-qualified Indian practitioners, a number of whom, by the 1920s had secured postgraduate degrees and diplomas in western countries. The Seth Gordhandas Sunderdas Medical College (GSMC) and the K E M Hospital arose almost as a counter to the British-managed, British-staffed Grant Medical College and J J Hospital. The GSMC owed its origin to the endowment in 1916, of fourteen-and-a-half lacs of rupees from the Seth Gordhandas Sunderdas Trust. The trustees offered the money to the Bombay Municipal Corporation for the founding of a medical college in association with the King Edward VII Memorial Hospital which the Corporation had already undertaken to build, equip and maintain. The most important condition for the endowment was that all members of all teaching faculties should be well-qualified Indians not in Government service. The college was opened in June 1925 and was affiliated to the Bombay University in 1926 for the MBBS degree. Its first dean was again a visionary—Dr Jivraj Mehta, a great administrator, an able physician and a staunch nationalist who within a few years raised the standard of medical teaching and patient care to a level comparable not only to the J J Hospital, but to the hospitals in the West.

In the early years of the twentieth century hospitals sprung into existence in various centres in central India—as in Hyderabad, and in north India, as in Delhi, Agra, and Indore. In 1912, there were 2,670 medical institutes in India in which 27,889,469 people were treated as outdoor patients and 453,900 as indoor patients. Surgical operations numbered more than a million operative procedures. It is of interest that the condition of the existing hospitals in India at the end of the nineteenth century and the beginning of the twentieth century was considerably better than in other countries in the East. This, for example, is how an English doctor in the service of the Egyptian Government described the Kasr-el-Ain Hospital, the best hospital in Egypt at that time. "The walls contained nests of living snakes, in holes, from which plaster crumbled away. . . The patients' wards, as now, were in the upper store rooms, but so closed in by doors and windows that there was an overpowering smell and practically no ventilation. . . The public in Cairo firmly believed that the hospital was merely a prelude to the cemetery and that the sick were beaten and robbed by the attendants and then poisoned by the doctors."

Medical Research Institutes of India

Medical research started late as compared to the West; it has unfortunately not made up for lost time. The lack of good infrastructure, the constraints of finance and also perhaps the lack of motivation to pursue scientific inquiry with a single-minded devotion have led to an unsatisfactory state of affairs.

The important state-funded research institutes include the Haffkine Institute, Bombay, which has already been commented upon in chapter 61, the Central Research Institute, Kasauli, the Pasteur Institutes in Coonoor and Shillong, the School of Tropical Medicine and Hygiene, Calcutta, the All India Institute of Hygiene and Public Health, Calcutta, the Malaria Institute of India, the All India Institute of Medical Sciences in Delhi and the Postgraduate Medical Institutes in Chandigarh and Pondicherry.

The Central Research Institute at Kasauli has carried out research in the epidemiology of malaria, typhus, cholera, kala-azar and other tropical problems. Its routine work consists of the large-scale manufacture of TAB vaccine, cholera vaccine, anti-rabies vaccine, anti-venom serum and sterilized surgical ligature material. It also constitutes a tertiary centre for laboratory diagnostic work. It has a fine record of research achievement over a period of nearly ninety years.

The Pasteur Institutes have a good record of research on tropical diseases. The work of the Institutes in the 1940s was organized in three sections—the rabies section, the laboratory diagnosis section and the vaccine-manufacturing section. The Tropical School of Medicine and Hygiene in Calcutta was designed on the pattern of the School in Liverpool. The research work undertaken covered tropical medicine, pharmacology, entomology, chemistry, pathology, bacteriology, protozoology, haematology, helminthology, leprosy, bowel diseases, indigenous drugs and nutrition. This school is one of the few institutes in India where excellent teaching and good research is carried out with the help of the wealth of clinical material available in the country.

The Nutritional Research Laboratories were established in 1925 in Coonoor. These research centres conducted research on nutritional problems and worked out the nutritive value of common Indian foodstuffs. From 1937, the laboratories were shifted to Hyderabad and named the National Institute of Nutrition. Its work in the field of nutrition is recognized all over the world.

The Malaria Institute of India established in 1938 was the successor to the Malaria Survey of India founded in 1926. This institute has carried out valuable research in all aspects of malaria—its epidemiology, the study of mosquitoes, anti-malarial and other preventive measures, clinical work on malaria, the effect of drugs in malaria. It has also assisted in affiliated research on other tropical problems like kala-azar, filariasis and dengue. The institute provides instruction courses on malariology to medical officers of the army, and to physicians in government service, spreads the knowledge of malaria throughout the country and stimulates malaria investigation and control in different centres of India.

The All India Institute of Medical Sciences was funded by the Union Government in 1956; this was followed within a few years by two other centrally-administered institutes—one in Chandigarh and the other in Pondicherry.

Numerous other medical schools attached to hospitals sprang into existence in different parts of India. It is outside the scope of this book to detail these. Mention must however be made of the Christian Medical College Vellore (CMC Vellore), a centre renowned for learning and good patient care. The CMC Vellore was founded through the vision and missionary zeal of Ida Scudder. As a young American girl, in the late 1800s, she reluctantly visited her medical missionary father, John Scudder at his post in South India. One fateful night, she was asked to help with three women in difficult childbirth. Ida could do nothing and custom prevented the families from accepting the help of a qualified male obstetrician. Ida was shocked to hear the next morning that all the three young girls had died. She went back to America, qualified as a doctor, and returned to India to open a one-bed clinic in Vellore in 1900. Two years later, she built a forty-bedded hospital and this grew over the years to the present 1,700-bedded medical centre. In 1909, she started the School of Nursing and in 1918, she opened a medical school for women. Her vision had been fulfilled; her missionary zeal has perpetuated a centre of excellence in the country.

Of the many illustrious individuals who worked as missionary doctors at the Christian Medical College and Hospital, Vellore, perhaps the most famous was the Englishman, Paul Brand. Born in south India in 1914 to missionary parents, he was professor of orthopaedics, combining orthopaedic surgery with an intensive programme of research and rehabilitation in leprosy. The reconstruction of the mangled hands of hundreds of patients with leprosy became the mission of his life.

William James Wanless was an internationally renowned Canadian medical missionary, who was born in Canada in 1865, and who came as a missionary doctor to India in 1889. Wanless started his work in the small township of Miraj in Maharashtra, his clinic being a single room—formerly a donkey's stable. Gradually, he introduced the latest medical technology and equipment to India and established a medical school, a leprosy hospital, the Mary Wanless Memorial Hospital and TB Sanatorium, named after his young wife who died of cholera. Today, hundreds of doctors, nurses and paramedicals are trained and thousands of patients treated each year at the medical centre established by him. These were some of the men and women who gave of themselves selflessly in the highest tradition of medicine. We must also pay tribute to others—some less known and many unknown, both Indian and from foreign lands, who toiled ceaselessly against death and disease to benefit the poor, the deprived and the downtrodden of this ancient country.

63

Thoughts and Afterthoughts

India was the jewel in the British crown and Britain surrendered this jewel in 1947. The surrender was inevitable which Britain graciously accepted. The scientific concepts of western medicine introduced into India by the British are rich legacies which have grown richer over the years. Where would medicine in India be if the British had not ventured into India in the seventeenth century and ruled over it till 1947? Would it have continued in the ancient strait-jacketed unchanging systems of ayurveda and unani medicine? Or is it possible that these old systems, through native talent, would have been shaken out of their apathy and torpor to blossom into a practice of medicine based on science and scientific research? Would such a freshly-evolving system have merged with the stream of western medicine, or would it have crystallized into a more holistic approach to disease that was even superior to western medicine? These questions can lead to endless debate without definite answers. It is certain that medicine could not have evolved in India in splendid isolation. There would have needed to be a total restructuring of society, a blossoming of thought bold enough to break through the narrow confines of tradition, a shattering of dogmas and old beliefs and a reaching out towards the truth in scientific inquiry for the benefit of its poor millions. A changing face of medicine for the better would have only been possible within a changing fabric of civilization.

Indian history has been chiefly written by her British masters. Many have made out that India in the seventeenth and eighteenth centuries was barbarous and that British rule was justified and righteous. Lord Curzon, an empire builder who had the good of India at heart said, "The message is carved in granite, it is hewn out of the rock of doom—our work is righteous and it shall endure." But India in this period of history was not barbarous; it was perhaps, far more civilized than the West. V. Astley has written that up to the end of the eighteenth century, "Indian methods of production and of industrial and commercial organization could stand comparison with those in vogue in any other part of the world." The difference between the East and West in this age was that the East was static, almost fossilized; the West was changing fast and reaching out to new horizons.

In summary, the West kick-started the East into the modern age. It introduced the East to fresh thoughts and ideas, new literature, philosophy, economics and above all to the tenets of universal law and to the practice of modern western medicine. On the debit side it enslaved and exploited India (and other eastern countries), filled its coffers with gold at the expense of the poor East. Worst of all, colonial rule left a dreadful scar on the psyche of the country that made the average Indian feel inferior. It is a scar which will take the efforts of generations to efface in its entirety. And did the West gain from its impact with the East? It probably gained more than it gave. The West was introduced to and learnt from the ancient philosophy and culture of the East. It recognized the supreme wisdom in the *Vedas* and *Upanishads,* the unequalled philosophy of the *Bhagwad Gita,* the brilliance of the works of Kalidasa, Aurobindo Ghose and Rabindranath Tagore. And in relation to medicine, it learnt that the ancient system of ayurveda had evolved when the greater part of the

Europe lived in barbaric savagery. It was a system that was equal in merit to the Hippocratic school from which western medicine originated and flourished.

There were a few great souls in India who abhorred the materialism of western countries, a sentiment now expressed by many leading thinkers of the world. One of them was the great Sufi poet, Mohammed Iqbal, who wrote beautifully in Persian and Urdu thus:

> The glitter of modern civilization dazzles the sight,
> But it is only a clever piecing together of false gems.
> The wisdom of science in which the wise ones of West took such pride
> Is but a warring sword in the bloody hand of greed and ambition.

The ugly westerner could only see the filth and disease in the East, and even today continues to see just that and nothing more. The discerning westerner saw the tranquility and beauty of the heart of India. Edwin Arnold in his beautiful translation of a verse from the *Bhagavad Gita* (The Song Celestial), writes:

> Never the spirit was born; the spirit shall cease to be never;
> Never was time it was not; End and Beginning are dreams!
> Birthless and deathless and changeless remaineth the spirit for ever;
> Death had not touched it at all, dead though the house of it seems!

These are just a few of the many mysterious whisperings that stirred the soul of the East long before the West discovered itself.

The number of great men in India who blossomed from the impact of the West and the East says, R. W. Frazer, "are no bastard bantlings of Western civilization; they were creative geniuses worthy to be reckoned in the history of India with such men of old as Kalidasa, Chaitanya, Jayadeva, Tulsidas and Shankaracharya, and destined in the future to shine clear as the fresh growing sparks sent out in the fiery furnace where new and old were fusing."

Contemporary Medicine

64 The Present Scenario

In the hands of the discoverer, medicine becomes a heroic art.

Ralph Waldo Emerson

It is difficult for a twentieth-century individual to write the history of Man and Medicine in this century because he lives in the midst of its turmoil. He is too close, too intimately related to the happenings in this world. He can only see bits and pieces; he cannot stand back and view the whole. He lacks a perspective because the perspective remains unfocused. Clarity will come only with time; only then will the relative importance of events, discoveries and individuals fall into place.

There is however no doubt that the twentieth century has produced far greater revolutionary changes in the affairs of man than those observed in the thousand years preceding it. Science and technology are the twin gods of this century, at whose altar man worships. These gods have altered man's economic and social state, enabled him to conquer time and space, ushered in a change of values and unleashed dangerous forces difficult to control. The face of medicine has also undergone a tremendous transformation. Based on science, but wedded to technology, inseparably linked to physics, chemistry, biology, bio-chemistry, as also to sociology and anthropology, it has evolved more in this century than it has ever done since Hippocratic times.

Today's world of medicine, broadly speaking, resembles an organized venture in the pursuit of new ideas and discoveries, where research through teamwork takes precedence over the individual efforts of solitary men however brilliant they be. Yet in this faceless panorama of medicine, time and again genius still shines forth with a luminosity that distinguishes him from other talented and dedicated men of science. Even so, the days of a Jenner or a Lister or a Pasteur seem past and over.

Inevitably there is a significant overlap in the events described in this chapter and in the previous section on Modern Medicine. The description of contemporary medicine that follows is chiefly limited to ideas, advances and discoveries. Fewer names will be mentioned than one would have desired. Future history will decide on the pride of place among those who have contributed to the benefit of man.

Political Background

The Treaty of Versailles which marked the end of the First World War (1914–1918) was a mere lull before the gathering storm. The early thirties saw the rise of Fascism in Spain and Italy and of the Nazi party in Germany. A civil war tore Spain apart with Fascism triumphant over the Republican forces. The Second World War erupted in 1939, ravaging Europe and Russia and engulfing the whole world in a cataclysmic catastrophe unprecedented in the history of man. Adolph Hitler, the evil star sought to establish German hegemony over the civilized West. Europe lay bleeding and prostrate under the savage Nazi heel. For a few glorious moments in history, Winston Churchill, leading Britain, stood alone with indomitable courage to defend the rights of man and the values of a civilized past. The combined might of the United States, Britain, France and their allies finally prevailed over Germany, Italy and Japan.

The discoveries of science and technology were harnessed for evil—for death and destruction, best exemplified by the atom bomb which annihilated Hiroshima and Nagasaki in Japan, bringing the conflagration of war to an end in 1944. It was then that the world discovered the horror of the ghastly concentration camps of Nazi Germany. It was at Auschwitz, Belsen and other similar death camps that the holocaust was perpetrated—an ethnic cleansing of millions of Jews, including women and children, tortured and gassed to death in specially devised ovens. There has been no greater act of savagery in the history of man.

The political map of the world now changed, for there started a collapse and dissolution of the great colonial empires that had evolved in the previous centuries. A number of independent nations, headed by the Republic of India were now born into the world.

The power and influence of victorious Britain and France declined and the sun eventually set over the British Empire. The world was now divided into two spheres of influence, one dominated by the United States espousing capitalism, and the other by the Union of the Soviet Socialist Republics advocating communism. The civil war in China ended with the triumph of Mao Tse Tung and communism. "Let China sleep, for when she awakes the world will tremble," Napoleon had warned. This great Asian giant was slowly and surely awakening from the torpor that had afflicted it for more than two centuries. She became a force that had to be increasingly reckoned with. Also emerging as a separate force in the second half of the twentieth century and playing a significant role in the balance of power, were the newly-born countries in the Middle East, Asia and Africa. They were the Third World countries, which had been exploited by the West; they were poor, with teeming populations often living in poverty and squalor and were way below the increasingly affluent West in science and technology.

The United States, Russia, China, Britain and France built for themselves a nuclear arsenal that had the potential to destroy our planet and erase mankind from history forever. The threat of such a catastrophe was in a way a deterrent, but the world still lives in fear of this possible calamity.

The last three decades of the century have seen a further transformation in the political map of our world. The ideological clash between communism represented by Russia, and capitalism represented by the United States of America, ended with the defeat of communism and the triumph of capitalism. The world now is dominated solely by the United States, which has taken upon herself the dubious role of policing our planet.

Local wars continue to plague mankind. The Palestinians in the Middle East are fighting for their homeland against Israel. Ethnic strifes in Africa have brought untold misery and disaster to the poor nations of this continent. The recent carnage in Kosovo is a further witness to man's inhumanity to man. Terrorism is a new form of violence, which is ugly and faceless and which respects no frontiers. The clash of nations which reverberated in earlier centuries, may well be replaced by the clash of civilizations in the decades to come—Islam versus the West, so reminiscent of a similar clash in the Medieval Age.

Economics

Western economy shattered by the Second World War was rebuilt with the help of the United States. Today, both the social and economic fields stand transformed. Gigantic corporations now control finance and industry. Trade unions struggling for existence at the turn of the century are now both powerful and wealthy. Women stand emancipated. The prejudice, the economic and social restrictions against the non-whites of the world are steadily crumbling. Yet the world is now divided between the rich and the poor. The North–South divide can indeed have ominous consequences if this gulf is left unabridged and allowed to grow. A great name in the field of economics is that of John Maynard Keynes. The Keynsian theory that governments should spend money they did not have, may have saved capitalism in its clash with communism. His economic theories probably influenced the twentieth century world as much as Adam Smith's *Wealth of Nations* did in 1776.

Natural Sciences

The pioneering discoveries of geniuses like Albert Einstein, Max Planck, Niels Bohr and Ernest Rutherford in the first quarter of the twentieth century have already been mentioned. In 1930, C. V. Raman was awarded the Nobel Prize for his discovery of the 'Raman Effect'. H. J. Bhabha pioneered atomic physics in India around the middle of the twentieth century. The other great men who delved into the secrets of the unknown include W. Heisenberg, who formulated matrix quantum mechanics, E. Schrodinger, who discovered wave mechanics, and W. Pauli, who predicted the existence of the neutrino two decades before it was discovered. Perhaps the greatest physicist of the mid-twentieth century was Richard Feynman, who researched in quantum mechanics, converting it into a practical mechanical tool. He wrote his famous and brilliant *Feynman Lectures* on physics and the erudite and entertaining. *Surely, You're Joking, Mr Feynman*. A great atomic physicist of the century was Enrico Fermi, who in his paper on beta decay in 1932, introduced the last of the four basic forces known in nature (gravity, electromagnetism and within the nucleus of the atom, the strong force and Fermi's 'weak force'). He invented the nuclear reactor working at the Colombia university and achieved the first man-made nuclear chain reaction at the university of Chicago in 1942. This was the precursor to the manufacture of the atom bomb. Fermi argued, strongly against the development of the hydrogen bomb. He died of cancer of the stomach in 1954. Atomic physics provided a source of power that reduced man's dependence on combustible fuel supplies.

The discovery of electronic and computer chips ushered in the computer age giving birth to increasingly sophisticated and powerful computers, which could compute with far greater speed, dexterity and accuracy than was ever deemed possible.

The astrophysicists made startling discoveries on the genesis of the universe. They described the universe as expanding and debated whether it was born in a single explosion (the Big Bang) of a universal atom or was renewed constantly through continuous creation. It was Edwin Hubble who proved that the universe extends far beyond the margins of the Milky Way and found the first hints that its genesis was from a 'Big Bang'. A. Eddington and S. Chandrashekhar were the two other distinguished astrophysicists of the twentieth century contributing to the study of stellar structure, stellar dynamics and to 'black holes' in outer space.

The advances in chemistry were nearly as great as in physics. Man's dependence on natural or animal sources was freed by the discovery of synthetic fabrics, which could replace cotton and wool. The discovery of plastics revolutionized numerous facets of industry.

Basic Medical Sciences

The discipline of molecular biology and genetics became the frontiers of science in this century. Physiologists, biologists, biophysicists, and biochemists joined forces to delve into the mysteries of the living cell, the workings of its metabolic cycles. They discovered genes and their structure, and sought to determine how genetic information was transferred. Virologists opened up an increasingly fascinating avenue of research on these smallest of living particles.

Physiologists and pathologists studied enzymes, metabolites, hormones and the interrelation between organ systems. Their study has become increasingly directed towards the molecular biology of cells, the cytokines secreted in health and disease, and their interrelation and interaction. Their researches have revealed the ever-increasing complexity of nature, which is yet to be fathomed.

Technology

Technology rules the twentieth century world. It is a part of man's every day existence. It has enabled man to wield an incredible control over his environment. The pioneering effort of the Wright brothers in the early part of the twentieth century fulfilled Leonardo da Vinci's dream of flying. Today, with the discovery of the jet engine man can fly faster than the speed of sound. In the second half of this century, science and technology helped man to orbit vehicles around the earth, shoot rockets containing humans into outer space, land humans on the moon returning them safely to earth and set up manned satellite stations in outer space. The science fiction of Jules Verne, H.G. Wells and several others has come alive; fantasy and fiction have been incredibly transformed into stark reality.

The last three decades of this century should aptly be termed the 'Information Age' because of the rapid strides in information technology. Television, computers, fax machines, and the internet have revolutionized information technology, altering the concept of time and space and with it the affairs of man.

Philosophy

The speculative philosophy of past centuries gave place to the mathematical logic developed by Alfred North Whitehead and Bertrand Russell. They both wrote the *Principia Mathematica* (1910–1913), elaborating on their philosophical concepts. Bertrand Russell was an ardent pacifist and led the movement for nuclear disarmament. He was awarded the Nobel Prize for literature in 1980. Ludwig Wittgenstein became the protégé of Bertrand Russell and wrote his *Tractatus Logico-philosophicus* in 1922, in which he claimed to have brought philosophy to an end by solving once and for all its key problems. He later recanted, claimed that he was mistaken and wrote his *Philosophical Investigations* for posthumous publication, in 1953.

The discoveries in science and technology shook man's traditional faith in God, religion and in the very concept of life. It led him into a search for new beliefs, as in the Oriental philosophy of Zen Buddhism or in the practice of yoga or in accepting the cult of 'Krishna'. The German existentialist school of Karl Jaspers advocated the 'phenomenologic' system, preaching an introspective guidance to behaviour on the basis of experience. The atheist existentialist doctrine of man living in a meaningless, godless, irrational world as though it had meaning, was first propounded by Martin Heidegger and then developed and popularized by the famous French philosopher Jean Paul Sartre, after the Second World War.

A great historian of the twentieth century was Arnold Toynbee. His philosophical and holistic view of history was a significant departure from the usual narrative style of earlier historians.

Culture

Culture in relation to music and art reflected the change in the world brought about by the dominance of science and technology, and by the loss of traditional faith, beliefs and values. Music divorced itself from its old romantic moorings to evolve into the twelve-tone system and dissonances, first introduced by Schonberg. Musicians used electronic devices and oscillations to create a weird cacophony of sounds reflecting the confusion caused by conflicting interests and ideas in the affairs of the world.

Artists, poets and authors were the collective conscience of the age. They saw through the hollowness of many western values and felt that scientific progress was an illusion, and that the capitalist system ushered in by the Industrial Revolution was self-destructive. They had lost faith in a society torn by cruelty, violence and war. Modern art and modern sculpture grew out of these philosophical and artistic ruminations. Pablo Picasso (1881–1973) was the colossus of modern art. His 'Guernica' expressed symbolically the savagery of war and of man who perpetrated war. Kandinsky and Mondrian sought the more spiritual in art, 'an art of inner necessity'. They termed this movement Abstract Art and Abstract Expressionism. Dadaism expressed its revulsion to the First World War and Surrealism championed by Salvador Dali and Marc Chagall obliterated the conscious outside world to inhabit and express the Freudian realm of the unconscious and the surreal world of fantasy and dreams.

Jackson Pollock of America, Lucian Freud and Francis Bacon of Britain, Raza, Souza and Hussein of India and several other modern artists and great sculptors like Rodin, Henry Moore and Giacometti reflected in their work the change in man's concept of his own image. They expressed his isolation in the world by creating an art of universal nature, again through the exploration of the unconscious.

Architecture reflected the technological era, showing a greater awareness of light, space and air. Open constructions with large windows and terraces, whose overall effect was to blend with the natural environment became important considerations in the architecture of Le Corbusier and Frank Lloyd Wright. Frank Ghery who designed the Guggenheim Museum in Bilbao, Spain, I.M. Pei who designed the glass pyramid at the entrance of the Louvre in Paris, and Charles Correa, who conceived the Art Centre in Bhopal, India, give us a foretaste of the futuristic architecture of the twenty-first century.

The eastern half of the world has been strongly influenced by the West. Western mores and western culture have permeated traditional strongholds, particularly in the cities of the East. Science and technology have vastly improved in countries such as India. But the East labours at a great disadvantage. It has to catch up with lost time, lost centuries. It could do so if science stood still. But science continues to advance at an exponential rate. Again most countries in the East remain handicapped by a strained economy, by poor infrastructure, by internal dissensions and political instability. To level with the West and at the same time to reach out to the skies to keep abreast of the western world is a formidable challenge that may take decades to realize.

The change in medicine, its content, discoveries and advances, and above all its ethics and philosophy only can be understood in the context of the altered fabric of human society and civilization in the twentieth century. Science and technology were undoubtedly of immediate practical value to medicine. They provided, to cite just a few examples, the diagnostic tools derived from advances in the natural sciences—radioactive isotopes, electrophoresis, micro-spectrophotometry, electrocardiography, electroencephalography, electromyography and the various techniques of imaging different parts of the human body. The electron microscope opened up avenues of research in molecular biology, on the basic structure of cells, bacteria and viruses and on the pathology of several diseases. But the technological advances in medicine have been countered by an inescapable change in the philosophy of medicine and ethical values which lie at the very core of the ancient art and science of healing.

65 The Discovery of Penicillin—The Era of Drugs

Louis Pasteur and Paul Ehrlich had spear-headed the fight against infection—Pasteur through the use of vaccines made of killed or attenuated organisms and Ehrlich through the use of chemical agents. As early as 1877, Pasteur had made the observation that whilst anthrax bacilli rapidly multiplied in sterile urine, their growth was arrested by the addition of 'common bacteria' to the urine. Paul Vuillemin (1861–1932) was the first to use the term 'antibiotic' for the condition in which 'one creature destroys the life of another to preserve its own'. It was Selman Waksman (1888–1973) who introduced the term antibiotic into medicine. The first antibiotic to be discovered was penicillin, a by-product from the mould of the genus penicillium. This epoch-making discovery was made by Alexander Fleming (1888–1955), a Scottish bacteriologist at St Mary's Hospital in London.

Alexander Fleming was a brilliant student who wished to become a surgeon. However in 1906, with the intention of staying in the hospital rifle-shooting squad, he took a temporary job in the inoculation department headed by the famous scientist Almroth Wright, at St Mary's Hospital, London. This was a quirk of destiny for Fleming and for the world. He took up bacteriology, discovered penicillin in 1928 and stayed on at St Mary's for forty-nine years.

During the First World War, Fleming worked on wounds, infection in wounds and resistance to infection. He noted that chemical agents used to clean wounds damaged the natural defences, failing to kill the bacteria responsible for infection. His first important discovery was the discovery of an enzyme present in tears and mucous fluids. He called this enzyme 'lysozyme' because of its ability to lyse organisms contaminating a culture of nasal mucous. He regarded lysozyme as part of the natural defences of the body against infection.

In 1928, Fleming started his work on the bacteriology of staphylococci, dangerous pus-forming organisms often contaminating wounds and frequently responsible for abscesses, fatal sepsis and septicaemia. Returning from a three-week holiday, he noted that one of the petri dishes growing staphylococci had been contaminated by mould spores and that the bacteria near that mould had been destroyed. The mould spores could have come in through an open window, though it is more probable that they floated up the stairs from a laboratory below, where a researcher was investigating fungi. Fleming could have just thrown the petri dish away as 'contaminated'. He did not; he was intrigued, and he researched further, identifying the mould as penicillium. He made the discovery that a powerful antibiotic substance had seeped out of the penicillium and killed the staphylococci. He called this antibiotic 'penicillin'. He believed that the mould responsible for secreting penicillin was Penicillium rubrum. In fact it was later shown to be Penicillium notatum. His further work proved that penicillin was effective against gram-positive cocci, like streptococci, pneumococci, meningococci, gonococci, and staphylococci, but not against gram-negative organisms. He also noted that the antibiotic did not adversely affect healthy tissues or

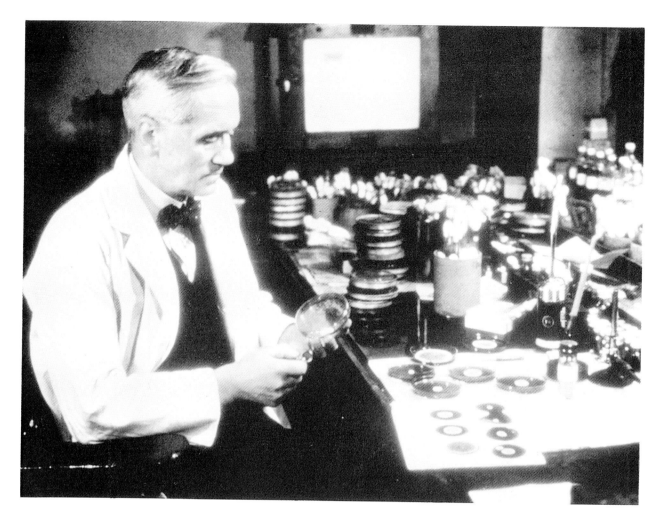

Fig. 65.1   Sir Alexander Fleming in his laboratory.

leucocyte function. Fleming and the scientific world now forgot about this discovery. He failed to take the next obvious step of using penicillin in animals deliberately inoculated with gram-positive pathogenic bacteria. This lapse is amazing and was probably due to his observation that when penicillin was mixed with blood in a laboratory, it lost its efficacy. He failed to realize that what happens in a test-tube in a laboratory could not necessarily be equated with what happens in a human body. In 1929, Fleming published his work on the discovery of penicillin and turned his attention to other research.

The discovery of penicillin would have remained buried in the archives of medical journals had it not been for a brilliant Australian pathologist, Howard Florey. Howard Florey headed the Dunn School of Pathology at Oxford at the young age of thirty-seven. In 1935, he hired biochemist Ernst Chain, a German Jew who had just escaped from the Nazis. The two teamed up and began a search for a powerful antibacterial substance. After going through over 200 papers they came across the work of Fleming. Florey and Chain grew Penicillium notatum, but encountered great difficulties in isolating the active ingredient from the liquid produced by the mould. Only one part in two million was pure penicillin. Perhaps they might have given up, had it not been for Norman Heatley, another biochemist in the team. Heatley devised techniques to improve the yield of penicillin and of purifying it.

The Second World War had commenced, but this work went on despite lack of funds and equipment as well as the risk of German air raids. On Saturday 25 May 1940, Florey and his colleagues inoculated eight mice with lethal doses of streptococci; four were then given penicillin. By 1:45 am the next morning, the mice that had not received the drug had died, but the four who had received the penicillin were alive and well. Florey exulted, 'It looks like a miracle.'

The three scientists realized the great potential of penicillin for treating infections and in particular war wounds. Florey converted his whole department into a manufacturing plant and funnily enough Heatley found that the best receptacle for growing penicillin was a bedpan! At last they thought they had just enough of the drug to try it on a human patient, a policeman, Albert Alexander, who developed staphylococcal septicaemia and multiple abscesses all over his body following a scratch sustained while pruning his roses. There was so little drug available that on the first day of treatment, the patient's urine was collected to recover as much penicillin from it as possible. This was given on the third day. The patient improved on the fourth day, but now the drug ran out and he died.

Florey and his colleagues tried out the drug successfully in four other patients but were convinced that their laboratory in Oxford could not produce sufficient quantities of the drug for a proper clinical trial. British pharmaceutical companies when approached were too busy to attempt the manufacture of penicillin. Florey and Heatley in July 1941 therefore went to the United States to enlist help in the production of the drug. Research on penicillin in the United States was centred at the Northern Regional Research Laboratory at Illinois. Heatley worked with Andrew J Moyer (1899–1959) at this laboratory for several weeks. Moyer extracted as much information from Heatley as possible, but did not share his own findings. Moyer succeeded in increasing the yield of penicillin thirty-four times. America by now had entered the war, and both the Government and the US pharmaceutical companies gave top priority to the manufacture of the drug.

In 1942, Fleming asked for some penicillin to save a friend dying of acute infection. His friend recovered and the report of this miraculous recovery appeared in the *Times*. It was then that Almroth Wright wrote a letter ascribing the discovery of penicillin to his protégé—Fleming. The hall of fame now opened its doors to Alexander Fleming.

In 1943, British drug companies had also begun to produce penicillin in bulk. Florey went over to the war zone in North Africa and proved the successful use of the drug on battle wounds. The drug was also found extremely useful in the treatment of gonorrhea, a disease afflicting several soldiers in the war. By D-Day, 6 June 1944, penicillin was freely available to treat all Allied servicemen. The Germans, Italians and Japanese never discovered the secret of penicillin; in a way the drug helped the Allies to win the war.

In 1945, Alexander Fleming, Howard Florey and Ernst Chain shared the Nobel Prize for the discovery of penicillin. It is a sad travesty of fate that Norman Heatley received nothing. Andrew Moyer had written and published his research on penicillin in his name alone, even though it was Heatley's work that was its basis. In 1945, Moyer took out a British patent in the production of penicillin and became a millionaire. It was as late as October 1990 that Norman Heatley's work was finally acknowledged, when he was awarded an honorary doctorate of medicine from the university of Oxford.

Penicillin became the wonder drug in medicine for several decades bringing down the morbidity and mortality in numerous infections, including diphtheria, syphilis and anthrax. It had a wide range of activity, was strongly bactericidal and other than the occasional rare anaphylactic reaction (which could prove fatal), was remarkably free of side-effects.

Research in the antibacterial effects of several fungi and moulds continued unabated. In 1940, Selman Waksman (1888–1973), a Russian who had migrated to the United States and had become a soil microbiologist, isolated an antibiotic actinomycin. Though very effective against bacteria, it was too toxic for clinical use. In 1942, he discovered another species of this fungus, later named Streptomyces griseus. He isolated the antibiotic streptomycin from this fungus; and this antibiotic was found to be effective against the tubercle bacillus. Unfortunately the use of the drug soon led to the multiplication of resistant strains.

There now followed a quick succession   of two further drugs in the treatment of tuberculosis. The impetus to discovery was partly due to the fact that the tubercle bacillus quickly became resistant to the use of a single drug regime. The discovery of para-amino-salicylic acid (PAS) was followed in 1950 by the discovery of isoniazid. Excellent clinical trials in the United Kingdom showed that the combined use of streptomycin, PAS and isoniazid would almost always cure tuberculosis, provided the drugs were taken regularly and for the prescribed period of time. Strains of resistant tubercle bacilli however occurred when patient compliance was poor. The next four decades saw tremendous research on other drugs to counter the growing menace of tuberculosis. Numerous drugs have come into use, but other than rifampicin, none of these drugs in use can match the efficacy of isoniazid and streptomycin.

The last half of this century has truly been the age of proliferating drugs and pills. They continue to multiply, converting most parts of the civilized world into a 'pill-popping' society. For example, there have come into existence sedatives, tranquillizers, vitamins, numerous antibiotics, anti-hypertensives, anti-convulsants, anti-depressants, anti-arrhythmics, diuretics, hormone replacements, antacids, bronchodilators, ionotropes to stimulate the heart muscle, drugs against parkinsonism, cytotoxic drugs against cancer, corticosteroids, the non-steroidal anti-inflammatory drugs and drugs against metabolic disorders.

One of the most commonly used drugs is cortisone, discovered at the Mayo Clinic in the 1930s. The drug was initially used with unequalled success in the treatment of rheumatoid arthritis. It was however soon realized that cortisone gave relief but was no cure, and that it had numerous dangerous side-effects. Nevertheless, corticosteroids have helped in the management of a wide spectrum of diverse medical diseases.

Safety requirements for the use of drugs in clinical medicine came into strict force after the 1960s. These requirements are indeed imperative for preventing disasters that could otherwise occur. An example of such a disaster was the introduction of thalidomide as a safe sleeping tablet. This drug when administered to pregnant women caused the most ghastly foetal defects in over 5,000 babies before it was banned.

In the fight against disease, the greatest benefit to man has been conferred by the development of effective vaccines against smallpox, measles, rubella, whooping cough, typhoid, cholera, tetanus, plague, yellow fever and poliomyelitis. The old adage that prevention is better than cure has been amply borne out by modern medicine. The microbe hunters of the nineteenth century blazed a trail, raising hopes that mass victory over infectious diseases would not be just a utopian dream but would soon be a happy reality. But this was not to be and in the foreseeable future it never will be. There is an ecological balance between man and other living creatures, big and small on our planet. Man can upset this ecological balance only at his peril. We cannot kill all the microorganisms in the world because they will adapt in order to survive and in the process of adaptation will pose new threats and fresh challenges to mankind.

66 Medicine in the Present Day

Medicine has stood to gain a great deal from the new developments in research and from discoveries in different fields, which tend to cross-fertilize each other. Each organ system has stood to gain; more and more is now known of even small esoteric aspects of the structure and function of various parts of the human body. To recount all that has transpired in medicine and its allied branches in this century would fill volumes and is outside the scope of this book. A few selected features in certain branches of medicine are briefly touched upon to illustrate the current advances and the vibrancy of contemporary medicine.

Neurology and Psychiatry

Neurology has seen far-reaching developments in the twentieth century, some of which have been briefly outlined in chapter 51. Electrophysiology elucidated the nature of the nerve impulse. Keith Lucas (1879–1916) pioneered this study, followed by Lord Adrian (1889–1977) and others. Electrical recordings from individual nerve fibres and brain cells were made possible using micromethods, valve amplifiers, cathode ray tubes and other sophisticated instrumentation. Lord Adrian demonstrated that a constant external stimulus to an area on the skin caused immediate excitation of the sense organs as evinced by an impulse travelling up the nerve supplying this sense organ. However, even if the stimulus continued, the excitation of the end-organ diminished. This decremental result of a constantly applied external stimulus probably enables us to sense our environment without being overwhelmed and confused by numerous and conflicting sensory inputs.

Electromyography, a study of nerve muscle function is today an invaluable aid in the study of neurological diseases involving nerve roots, the peripheral nerves, the myoneural junction and the muscles. Electroencephalography (EEG) is a study of the electrical discharges from the cerebral cortex. These discharges are recorded as waves and evaluate important aspects of cerebral function. The EEG relates to the brain in much the same manner as the ECG relates to the heart. The EEG is however more complex, being the resultant of a number of 'electrical generators' distributed over the head, all sensitive to subtle influences, attention and consciousness. The EEG is particularly useful in the diagnosis of epilepsy, in certain metabolic disturbances producing a loss of consciousness and in disturbance of cerebral function produced by neurological disease.

Advances in pharmacology have contributed significantly to the science of clinical neurology. Pharmacology has provided both the means to investigate nervous function and effective treatment for conditions such as epilepsy, parkinsonism and myasthenia. In a similar way, biochemistry has unravelled the existence and identity of chemical neuro-transmitters in the nervous system, and also provided tests for the diagnosis of a number of diseases. Important chemical neurotransmitters and their enzymes discovered in contemporary medicine are dopamine, noradrenaline, acetyl-choline and γ-aminobutyric acid (GABA). Parkinson's disease is now related to the significant loss of the neurotransmitter dopamine in the striatum and substantia nigra, both of which show extensive cell loss, atrophy and glial scarring.

New diseases have come to the fore in the last twenty years of this century. A rare group of diseases which could assume greater significance in the years to come, is the group of *prion* diseases, which are neuro-degenerative conditions affecting both humans and animals. They were previously termed as spongiform encephalopathies, slow virus diseases or transmissable dementias. The transmissable agent in these diseases is a *prion*—unique in many ways. Though a rare disease in our age and time, patterns of diseases have been known to change. The recent epidemic of *prion disease* among the cattle in the United Kingdom (mad cow disease) has aroused renewed research in view of the potential health hazard to man.

Perhaps the greatest advance in neurology in the second half of the twentieth century is in the use of highly sophisticated diagnostic procedures. These include the use of computerized scanning techniques, magnetic resonance imaging, cerebral angiography and digital subtraction angiography. Even more recent are the use of radioactive isotope scans as with the single proton emission computed tomography (SPECT) and positron emission tomography (PET). The conventional CT scan and MRI scan define structural details, while the SPECT and PET scans attempt to determine function and metabolism of nerve tissue.

With an increasing number of people surviving beyond their sixties, the incidence of cerebrovascular accidents has increased. The use of thrombolytic agents under appropriate indications and interventional methods to dilate stenosed cerebral vessels through angioplastic procedures (using balloon catheters) are being currently assessed.

Neurosurgery has made immense strides since the pioneering work of Harvey Cushing. Hydrocephalus, Parkinson's disease, vascular anomalies and large aneurysms are all amenable to surgical treatment. The gamma knife is a recent invention, allowing access to areas of the brain which were unapproachable through the use of conventional methods.

The functions of the brain, the ability to think, conceive and the spontaneous flowering of an untutored mathematical genius of the nature of a Ramanujan form the subjects of intense research. In spite of what we know, there is a great deal more that we do not know. The human brain may resemble a computer, but as yet it has features that a computer does not have. A rather unusual but fascinating concept on the working of the brain was enunciated recently by Gerard Maurice Edelman, who as an immunologist won the Nobel Prize for unravelling the chemical structure of γ-globulin, but who then concentrated his research activities on neuroscience. "The brain in its working," Edelman postulated, "is a selective system, more like evolution than computation." He theorized that brain function and activity are characterized by a selective process among neurones, akin to the selective mechanism among the species competing in the struggle to exist and evolve in nature.

Though neurology in all its aspects is an increasingly fascinating subject, the fruits of research, unfortunately have not significantly affected patient care. Most neurological diseases, barring a few important exceptions, run their natural course without being influenced by the practice of medicine.

Psychiatry in the twentieth century saw two revolutions. The first was the Freudian revolution of psychoanalysis. Freud and his views reigned supreme by the 1950s. But then came the counter-revolution—a pharmacological approach to the treatment of the mentally unbalanced. Today psychiatry is in a state of flux with greater weightage being given to the use of drugs than to psychoanalysis.

The first psychotropic drug used in the treatment of manic-depressive psychosis was lithium in 1949. Other drugs followed in quick pursuit, notably the phenothiazines and imipramine. Psychiatry according to a number of practising psychiatrists was at last liberated from the Freudian clutch. Psychopharmacology opened the door to quick results without hospital admission and was far more cost-effective than the interminable sessions necessitated in Freudian psychoanalysis. Of interest was the shift in emphasis from the major psychotic disorders to minor deviations from the norm, so frequently observed in the community at large. It would appear that the more 'advanced' a society, the greater were these minor aberrations. Thus on an average, one in ten individuals in the United States seeks the help and guidance of a psychiatrist. Drugs for the treatment of anxiety states and other aberrations have multiplied and a pill-popping society willingly pops tranquillizers and sedatives to temporarily relieve these aberrations. During the sixties, the tranquillizer diazepam, was the most widely prescribed drug in the world. Numerous other drugs with similar properties flooded the market and the sale of drugs acting on the central nervous system in America was a quarter of all drug sales.

The problems to be addressed by modern psychiatry are however not just in the management of the overall ill psychotics or of individuals with minor deviations from the accepted norm. There are an increasing number of psychosomatic diseases, where emotional stress and conflict can cause or aggravate organic disease. They rarely need deep psychoanalysis, they do not need sophisticated expensive investigations; they need understanding and the wisdom of an experienced, caring physician who is prepared to spend time listening and talking to patients. After all, the psyche influences all human activity, all aspects of living. This basic concept had been responsible for the development of child psychology, industrial psychology, group sessions, family therapy and psychiatric and social help to the community. A third revolution in psychiatry is overdue. It should include the evolution of a new and different system of care, which reduces pill-popping to the minimum and should resort to Freudian psychoanalysis only under special circumstances. Perhaps molecular biology, biochemistry and a greater elucidation of the working of the brain might form the scientific basis for this long-awaited approach.

THE VACCINE AGAINST POLIOMYELITIS

Perhaps the greatest benefit to man pertaining to neurology in contemporary medicine was the discovery of vaccination against poliomyelitis. Violent epidemics of poliomyelitis engulfed the western world, particularly the United States, in the 1940s and 1950s. Poliomyelitis also struck the poor, developing nations causing crippling deformities in children and young adults, but its incidence was difficult to compute.

John Enders, Thomas Weller and Frederick Robbins had by 1949, succeeded in growing the polio virus on human and animal tissues, for which they were awarded the Nobel Prize in 1954. The US National Foundation for Infantile Paralysis (NFIP) funded a huge research project to classify the different strains of the polio virus. The research project succeeded in identifying three strains of the polio virus, opening the way for research on the polio vaccine.

THE SALK VACCINE

Jonas Salk (1914–1995) during the Second World War had researched on and developed an inactivated influenza vaccine. He now started his research on a formalin–killed polio vaccine against all three strains. There were many scientists of renown in the race to prepare this vaccine. Salk won the race and was soon ready to test his vaccine on a group of children, including his three sons. The results were encouraging and the NFIP now tested his vaccine in the United States on close to 1.8

million children, at a cost of 7.5 million dollars. It was found to be 90 per cent or more effective against polio type II and type III, and only 60 to 70 per cent effective against type I. By May 1955, four million doses of the vaccine had been dispensed in America, and the Center for Disease Control in Atlanta was able to confirm that the decline in the attack rate of paralytic poliomyelitis was two to five times greater among vaccinated children than among the unvaccinated.

THE SABIN VACCINE

The Russian born virologist Albert Sabin (1906–1993), working at the University of Cincinnati, believed that a vaccine made from live virus which had been rendered avirulent would be effective against all strains, even when given orally. Sabin was a contrast to the urbane and charming Salk, and found it difficult to get financial and other encouragement from the NFIP. When he and his team threatened to resign, the NFIP relented and the Sabin oral vaccine was tested in many parts of the world, but not in the United States. It took three years of mass trials to prove the greater efficacy of this oral vaccine which has today largely replaced the Salk vaccine.

Salk and Sabin were men of contrasts. Both were heroes of science. Perhaps Sabin was the better scientist, yet Salk fitted better into the operational style of contemporary medicine, where institutions did research and required funds to do so. His career is marked by the sheer speed with which he out-raced the others in the field and the honours he failed to receive for doing so!

Superspecialities in Medicine

Medicine in the contemporary world has been fragmented not only into specialities, but into ever-increasing superspecialities. Thus for example, a specialist in blood disorders (haematologist) may superspecialize and deal solely with leukaemias (a form of blood cancer); a cardiologist might decide to confine his professional expertise only to opening up blocked coronary arteries; an orthopaedic surgeon may just perform knee or hip replacement. There is some advantage to super-specialization, but the great disadvantage is the loss of the holistic view of medicine, the over-concentration on 'bits' and 'pieces' of human anatomy and physiology at the expense of treating the patient as a whole.

An important speciality today is critical care medicine. It implies the special and intensive care devoted to patients suffering from acute life-threatening illnesses which have the potential for recovery. Critical care was perhaps born 130 years ago in the post-operative recovery room (adjacent to the operation theatre), where operated patients were carefully looked after till their condition was stable enough to allow transfer to the wards. Florence Nightingale wrote in 1863: "It is not uncommon in small country hospitals to have a recess or small room leading into the operation theatre in which the patients remain until they have recovered, or at least recover from the immediate effects of operation."

The 1952 epidemic of poliomyelitis in Denmark caused respiratory paralysis in many patients. They were managed by endotracheal intubation and manual bag ventilation round the clock, and by nurses and students who took turns to sustain respiration and keep the patient alive till recovery from paralysis ensued. This catastrophic epidemic spurred the formation of special units with the medical, nursing and technical expertise to care for critically ill patients. Critical care as defined above came into its own in North America and the West in the early 1960s. It took root in India in the middle sixties and was established in Bombay by the late sixties and early seventies.

Critical care units have salvaged many lives all over the world. Even so, they have raised difficult economic issues and ethical dilemmas. They constitute great hazards in inexperienced or uncaring hands and have been responsible for an increasing incidence of life-threatening iatrogenic problems.

Cardiology

Advances in technology and in basic science have contributed to making cardiology a high-profile speciality, particularly in the second half of the twentieth century. The advances in the diagnosis of heart disease have been incredibly swift. After Scipione Riva-Roccis' (1863–1937) discovery of the sphygmomanometer to measure arterial blood pressure, the next most important diagnostic aid came from Williem Einthoven's (1860–1927) discovery of the electrocardiographic (ECG) machine, which consisted of a specialized type of galvanometer that recorded the electrical current generated by the heart prior to the physical contraction of its chambers. The electrocardiograph was further improved by the studies of Sir Thomas Lewis, who had amongst his assistants Dr M. D. Gilder, an Indian medical student from Bombay. Disturbances in rhythm, delay in impulse conduction and changes in thickness of the ventricular walls were among the features that could be recognized by the electrocardiograph of the early formative years.

In 1929, Werner Forssmann, a resident surgeon at Eberswalde, Germany, inserted a catheter from a cut-down in his left ante-cubital vein, pushing the catheter into the right atrium, aided by self-fluoroscopy and a mirror. Cournand in 1940 made extensive use of the catheter to study cardiovascular physiology. Within a few more years cardiac catheterization was used in many centres of the West, and even in the East, in the diagnosis of congenital and certain acquired heart diseases. Cardiac catheterization was soon supplemented by the use of angiocardiography and angiography, which enabled a visualization (through the injection of radio-opaque dye) of the chambers of the heart and the blood vessels opacified by the dye. Finally in 1958, Sones developed a safe and reliable method for coronary angiography, opening the field for coronary artery bypass surgery.

Numerous non-invasive diagnostic tests for evaluating the heart include stress testing, thallium stress test (both evaluating the adequacy of blood supply to the heart muscle), holter monitoring (which records the ECG tracing for 24 hours), and echocardiography (an ultrasound mode of visualizing cardiac valves and chambers).

Hypertension and ischaemic heart disease became the high-profile diseases of the second half of this century. Atherosclerosis or thickening of the arteries due to deposition of fat beneath the intima of the arteries, became and continues to be the subject of intense research. Research on risk factors for coronary artery narrowing, ischaemic heart disease and myocardial infarction revealed the contributory role played by smoking, genetic background, hypertension, diabetes, hyperchole-sterolaemia, lack of physical activity and to a lesser extent, obesity. Acute myocardial infarction was first described clinically ante-mortem by a Chicago physician, James Herrick in 1905. It is a lesson in medical history that a disease first described with accuracy in the early years of the twentieth century should become one of the major killers of man within fifty to sixty years. The impression that myocardial infarction is rare in the East is false. In India as also in other eastern countries, it is increasingly common and can affect the poor almost with as much frequency as the affluent.

The management of heart disease improved in the second half of the twentieth century. Diuretics helped to alleviate salt and water retention in heart failure. Numerous anti-hypertensives were discovered to control hypertension and cholesterol-lowering drugs together with a diet low in saturated or animal fats helped reduce cholesterol and fatty acids in the blood. The advent of betablockers which blocked the beta-receptors of the sympathetic nervous system was of value in hypertension, angina and supraventricular arrhythmias. Numerous anti-arrhythmic drugs were developed to control disturbances in the rhythm of the heart. Electronic pacemakers could be implanted under the skin to pace hearts whose rhythm was dangerously slow due to heart block. Implantable defibrillators can now sense fibrillation of the ventricles (a catastrophic event, causing death) and can 'shock' the heart into a stable rhythm.

Blood thinning drugs with clot-resolving properties were developed and were extremely useful. Streptokinase, developed in the 1960s, when given within a few hours of a heart attack, and followed by the use of heparin (a blood-thinning drug), produced a significant fall in mortality from myocardial infarction. Aspirin was shown to be cheap and extremely effective in the prevention of both heart attacks and strokes.

Coronary angiography not only opened the way for coronary artery bypass surgery but also opened the field for interventional cardiology. Blocked arteries under certain indications could be opened up by balloon catheters. Currently the use of stents made of special material helps to keep the 'angioplasted' vessel patent, with a reduction in the closure rate of the vessel from 30 per cent to 15 per cent. Interventional cardiology can also open up stenosed valves, again under specified conditions, obviating the need for open heart surgery.

It is of interest that none of the recent advances in management can offer a radical cure for the diseases against which they are used. They can palliate, control and perhaps reduce the tempo of the natural history of disease. The crucial importance of prevention even in contemporary medicine is evident. There has been a clear decline in the incidence of ischaemic heart disease between 1970 and 1990 in a number of western countries, particularly the United States. This is not due to modern medicine but to a change in lifestyle which has helped eliminate or control, as far as possible, the risk factors mentioned above.

New Diseases and the Resurgence of the Old

The summer of 1981 saw the beginnings of a new scourge that was soon to threaten the safety of the whole world. The Centre for Disease Control (CDC) in Atlanta reported the presence of a mysterious illness in five patients in San Francisco, diagnosed as suffering from pneumocystis carinii pneumonia. This is a rare pneumonia that had previously been reported only in individuals severely immunocompromised by drugs or certain diseases. All five patients were homosexuals, and the CDC report speculated that their way of life and their sexual preference and proclivities could have a connection with this disease. Very soon, similar findings were reported by doctors working in San Francisco, New York and Los Angeles. The underlying feature characterizing all these reports was the breakdown of the body immune system, laying it open to invasion by the usual pathogenic organisms and more importantly by opportunistic organisms, notably the pneumocystis carinii. The predominance of homosexuals contracting the disease was noteworthy and the disease initially acquired the term 'Gay Related Immune Disease'. It was soon apparent that other groups at risk for this disease were drug abusers, haemophiliacs and blood transfusion recipients. Studies on larger population groups proved its occurrence in individuals of all ages, in both sexes and with any and every sexual preference. It was thus reported in heterosexuals, particularly in those who had sexual contact with many partners, the disease being transmitted through infected seminal fluid and vaginal and anal secretions. In fact, in Africa, India and many Third World countries where the disease quickly spread, this new scourge was most frequently transmitted by heterosexual contact. The disease was now named the Acquired Immuno-Deficiency Syndrome (AIDS). Clinical description showed that AIDS had protean manifestations, which could involve every system in the body. The disease has a 100 per cent mortality, with death occurring within a few months to a few years.

From the beginning scientists felt that AIDS was due to a virus that spread from person to person, chiefly through sexual contact. The increasing spread of the disease in different countries of the world prompted intense research to identify the causative agent. In 1984, a French research team successfully identified the cause as a retrovirus. An unseemly dispute now arose between the Frenchman Luc Montagnier and the American Robert Gallo, as to the priority for the discovery of the AIDS virus. The first credit almost certainly should go to Luc Montagnier and his team at the Pasteur Institute in Paris. The virus was soon called 'Human Immuno-Deficiency Virus' (HIV). When another HIV virus was discovered, the one causing AIDS was termed HIV Type I.

Research on the HIV virus showed that after entry into the body, it was incorporated within the nuclear structure of the infected cell; it then reproduced virions, which after extrusion from the cell infected other cells. The virus destroyed the immune system, particularly affecting a subpopulation of lymphocytes termed CD4 cells, which are the 'helper cells' in the immune response to infection. A destruction of the immune response leads to a loss of the integrity of the body, leaving it open to various ordinary infections and also to extraordinary opportunistic infections—for example the pneumocystis carinii, viruses, mycobacteria and fungi. A loss of appropriate immune response also predisposes these individuals to malignant disease, chiefly to non-Hodgkin's lymphoma.

French and American researchers soon devised a test to indicate the presence of the virus within the body, even before symptoms appeared. It was apparent that the virus could remain in the body for several years before it resulted in AIDS. This latency stretched on an average from three to ten years; in rare instances it could extend to as long as fifteen to twenty years. The risk of spread to others through sexual contact or through blood donations, even when the virus was latent, remained unchanged and was an important factor in the ever-increasing incidence of the disease all over the world.

HIV infection spread by the nineties like wildfire through Africa, the Middle East, India and the Far-Eastern countries. Zaire and the adjacent areas of Central Africa were well-nigh decimated with AIDS. More than 50 per cent of the population in Zaire became HIV-positive. Many of the young able-bodied men and women died of AIDS. Young mothers with AIDS gave birth to children who developed AIDS. Ghost villages dotted the provinces of Central Africa, being inhabited by elderly people and by the very young, who had no one to care for them. Death, starvation, famine were the legacies left by this disease.

The incidence of HIV infection in India, particularly in the large cities of Bombay, Delhi, Calcutta and Madras, is rising exponentially. By one estimate, close to 50 per cent of the prostitutes in the 'red light' area of Bombay are HIV-positive, and each prostitute entertains on an average six to eight customers a day. India now accounts for more than one in four Asian HIV-infected individuals. The WHO estimated that in India there were 2.3 million HIV-positive and 1.79 million patients with AIDS in 1996. We are sitting on a time bomb, which on explosion could rain disaster on a country still struggling against poverty and disease.

World authorities in combination with local authorities in different countries have tried their best to control AIDS through preventive measures. These measures include wide publicity through television, radio and through every possible source of information on the nature of AIDS, its method of spread and the way to prevent it. The HIV screening of blood donors and the heat treatment of blood products became a standard practice in many countries, though only after thousands of cases of infection by these routes had already occurred. The term 'safe sex' came into being. This included greater care over the choice of sexual partners and the use of condoms as prophylactics. The danger of the sharing of needles among drug abusers was also repeatedly stressed. Psycho-social factors could only be influenced for the better over a longer period of time through intensive educational programmes.

In the meanwhile, the search for a cure remains frantic and unrewarding. Researchers all over the world are trying desperately to prepare a vaccine against the disease. They soon realized that the AIDS virus mutates frequently, changing its face a thousand times faster than most influenza viruses. How could a vaccine be developed against a constantly changing target? Even today, the cure seems remote and we have to rely on preventive measures to halt this scourge from wreaking havoc, particularly in the vulnerable poor countries of the world.

How did the HIV virus causing AIDS strike an unprepared, ignorant, defenceless world? Is it a new virus that has mutated from one which existed for long but which lacked invasive properties? Or has the HIV virus existed, perhaps in isolated pockets of Central Africa, away from the prying eyes of civilization? Was this virus confined to animals, such as monkeys, and could it have gained access to man through rituals and practices by which contaminated animal blood reached human beings, thereby forming a reservoir of potential spread? Perhaps the opening up of isolated areas to colonial and economic exploitation, and the migration of people for several reasons could have allowed this virus to reach and infect civilized society, thus initiating a pandemic that continues to prove a serious danger to the world. Further research in epidemiology, genetics, immunology and anthropology may provide an answer to these questions in the future.

HIV infection may well be an example of the danger the world is exposed to when the ecological balance between man and his microscopic fellow creatures is seriously disturbed. It is a warning to remember, for the future may well bring with it even more cataclysmic 'new diseases' that have the potential to annihilate humankind.

The other comparatively new viral diseases with a high morbidity and mortality include the Lassa, Marburg, and Rift Valley fevers in Africa, and the Bolivian haemorrhagic fever in South America. These viral diseases have animal reservoirs, are highly infectious and are characterized by haemorrhagic manifestations, multiple organ failure and death. In 1976, an unknown disease caused by a new virus (later identified as the Ebola virus) broke out in Nzara, a town in southern Sudan. The Ebola virus disease was even more fulminant and infectious than the Marburg and Lassa fevers. It led to external and internal bleeding, multiple organ failure, shock and death. The disease spread to a hospital nearby claiming 300 victims, half of whom died. Two months later, it erupted in the Ebola river region of Zaire, again causing death among patients and the staff looking after infected patients. The epidemic died out in 1976. However two further localized epidemics again struck Africa in 1979, one in Sudan and the other in Zaire. The mortality was again very high. The risk of these or similar viruses reaching thickly-populated areas of Africa and other Third World countries, or reaching the West or the United States is genuine. The catastrophe that befell the world with AIDS may well be a forerunner of catastrophes to come.

The two viruses which have contributed a great deal to morbidity and mortality in the contemporary world, and will do so increasingly in future, are the hepatitis B and hepatitis C viruses. There are over 300 million carriers of the hepatitis B virus in the world, and an undetermined but perhaps equally large number of the patients infected with hepatitis C virus. Chronic hepatitis leading to progressive cirrhosis of the liver and liver cancer are the two possible sequels of this infection. If even a small fraction of these carriers were to develop chronic progressive hepatitis or hepatic cancer, or both, the death toll would perhaps be even more horrendous than that caused by the HIV virus.

TUBERCULOSIS

An example of the resurgence of an old disease is tuberculosis. Tuberculosis is a disease of antiquity. It has played an important role in world history and it is necessary to take a brief glance at its past, so that we can better understand the present and the future. The disease is caused by acid-fast mycobacteria of which the most important are M. tuberculosis and M. bovis. M. bovis caused disease in animals, chiefly cattle, even before the advent of man. M. tuberculosis and M. bovis should be regarded as subspecies than distinct species. The extreme degree of DNA homology and the immunological properties shared between the two have prompted the suggestion that M. tuberculosis evolved in the human organism from M. bovis after the domestication of cattle, that is between 10,000 and 4000 BC. There is good historical, biological and circumstantial evidence to support this suggestion.

Origin and Spread

It has been mentioned earlier that both Neolithic skeletons and skeletons in very ancient Egypt had changes suggestive of tuberculosis of the spine. Modern paleopathologists feel that though this diagnosis is very probable, it cannot be assumed to be certain, as various fungal infections of the spine and rheumatoid disease involving the spine cannot be excluded with absolute surety. With this caveat in mind, the oldest such skeleton is dated 5000 BC. Between 4000 and 1000 BC, evidence of skeletal tuberculosis has been found not only in Egypt, but in Jordan, Italy, France and even Denmark. Current historical, paleopathological and archaeological research suggests that cases before 1000 BC were due to M. bovis as the likely pathogen. The present data does not offer definite evidence that M. tuberculosis was encountered in human disease before 1000 BC. Yet the lack of evidence should not be construed as evidence of absence. The issue should remain open as DNA studies are continuing and may well alter our present concepts.

The original source of human tuberculosis due to mycobacterium tuberculosis and the spread of this disease has come in for a great deal of research. The prevailing view is that M. tuberculosis evolved from M. bovis among the milk-drinking Indo-European or Aryan race who then spread the disease during their invasions and migration into India, West Asia, Greece and Western Europe. These invasions and migrations date around 1500 BC. With the establishment of large cities, migration of populations and increase in trade and commerce, pulmonary tuberculosis spread quickly and widely. Medical writings in the last several centuries of the first millenium BC prove that pulmonary tuberculosis by then had spread all over the world. The *Atharva-veda* (circa 400 BC) from India advises the physician thus:

> The physician who values his future should not undertake to take care of a patient who has three great symptoms: fever, cough and bloody sputum. If however the patient has a good appetite and digests well the food and the disease is in its infancy a cure may be possible.

Recent medical, archaeological and paleopathological data further suggest that tuberculosis spread through Europe and Asia into the Americas by the first millenium AD, well before the discovery of America by Columbus.

Early Clinical Observations

Widespread knowledge of the clinical features of pulmonary tuberculosis were recognized in the first half of the first millenium BC. Both Greek and Indian medical texts give an apt clinical description of the disease. Perhaps the earliest record on clinical features is on a clay tablet inscription from the library of the Assyrian King, Assurbamipal (668 to 626 BC).

> The patient coughs frequently, his sputum is thick and sometimes contains blood. His breathing is like a flute. His skin is cold, but his feet are hot. He sweats greatly and his heart is much disturbed.

The disease went by different names in different ages and in different parts of the world. The Indians called the disease *sosha* (cough) or *jayakshma* (wasting). The Greeks named it *pthisis* (to waste), and the Romans used the word *tabes* (wasting). The English-speaking world spoke of *consumption* (from the Latin *consumere*, to consume or to waste away).

The contagiousness of the disease was suspected from very early times. Aristotle (384–322 BC) correctly guessed the infectious nature of pulmonary tuberculosis when in his *Problems* he questioned thus:

> Why, when one comes near consumptives or people with ophthalmia or the itch does one contract the disease, while one does not contract dropsy, apoplexy, fever or many ills?

He answered:

> With the phthisic, the reason is that the breath is bad and heavy. . . In approaching the consumptive, one breathes this pernicious air. One takes the disease because there is in the air something disease-producing.

Aristotle's answer besides pointing to the infectiousness of tuberculosis came close to postulating the germ theory of disease elaborated by Girolamo Fracastoro in the Renaissance. It was however only in the latter half of the nineteenth century, with Robert Koch's discovery of the tubercle bacillus that the contagiouness of pulmonary tuberculosis was conclusively proven.

Epidemiology

Infectious diseases like smallpox, diphtheria, typhus, typhoid and plague (to quote a few examples), have burst forth into epidemics that reached a peak and died away within a few years. Epidemics of these infections occurred in repeated cycles of varying duration over centuries. Tuberculosis has behaved differently. The epidemic of tuberculosis has continued unabated for several centuries. Historical records suggest that this epidemic had very nearly reached its peak in Greece and Western Europe at the time of Hippocrates and remained so for centuries. It then slowly but progressively declined in Europe and in North America after the first quarter of the twentieth century, to persist in the sixties and seventies of the twentieth century at a low prevalence rate. The epidemic in the West had thus abated but had not died. Interestingly enough this slow progressive decline was observed well before specific antituberculosis drugs were available. The anti-tuberculosis drugs undoubtedly helped this decline in incidence, but were not solely responsible for it. In India and the Third World countries, there has as yet been no decline in the incidence of the disease which has continued at 'peak level'. Poverty, poor sanitation, poor nutrition, overcrowding and poor education have been responsible for this unfortunate state of affairs.

A terrifying feature since the 1980s is a sudden resurgence of tuberculosis in the whole world. The most important reason for this is the advent of AIDS. Tuberculosis which was at a low ebb in the United States and the West, has again raised its ugly head, particularly in the inner cities of New York and Los Angeles, where crowding and deprivation in the black ghettos are as bad as the slums in Third World countries. With AIDS destroying the immune system, tuberculosis has become a frequent complication of the disease. It is caused by a reactivation of an old quiet focus within the body or a fresh infection which the body cannot resist because of its poor immune defence. What is worse is that the incidence of multiple drug-resistant tuberculosis has increased. This form of tuberculosis is invariably fatal within a year or two. Between 1984–1991, the incidence of tuberculosis rose by 12 per cent in the United States and by 30 per cent in Europe. In Africa, the increase in incidence during this period was 300 per cent. A major cause of this worldwide incidence is the coexistence of AIDS, which predisposes to tuberculosis. Tuberculosis now kills three million people every year—95 per cent of these are from the poor Third World countries.

The increased incidence of tuberculosis and in particular multiple drug resistant tuberculosis in India is ominous and of grave concern. Of the current population of over 900 million people in India, over 300 million are infected with Mycobacterium tuberculosis. About 13 million have active disease and a quarter of these are sputum-positive. A recent WHO report estimated that the loss to the Indian economy from tuberculosis is around 400 million dollars every year. By a conservative estimate, 500 thousand people die annually of tuberculosis. The further spread of AIDS, which brings tuberculosis in its wake could turn into a holocaust for India and other Third World countries. In 1995, about 9 per cent of patients admitted for chest problems to the tuberculosis wards of a large public hospital in Bombay were HIV-positive. The incidence of tuberculosis in patients with AIDS was 500 times greater than in the general population. Tuberculosis and AIDS form a lethal combination that has the potential to decimate the population of the poor countries.

Another great killer that is resurgent is malaria. The Anopheles mosquito is becoming increasingly resistant to the disinfectants in common use and the plasmodium falciparum parasite which causes a malignant and often fatal infection is becoming increasingly resistant to chloroquine. Resistance first reported in Thailand, has now spread to other Asian countries, including India. Three million people die of malaria every year; even today, millions of human beings in Africa and Asia continue to be infected by this disease. The immensity of the problem of resistant malaria is staggering, particularly if the parasites in time to come also develop resistance against quinine.

Cholera is one more disease which except for small, localized outbreaks in Third World countries remained under surveillance and check. In 1961 Indonesia was struck by an epidemic of the El Tor strain of cholera. The epidemic turned into a pandemic, spreading through Asia and reaching Africa in the early seventies. It persisted for another thirty years, constituting the largest ever pandemic in the world. The pandemic now reached Peru in 1991, probably carried by a cargo ship from Asia. The ship is believed to have flushed the contaminated water from its ballast tanks into the sea. The disease broke out in Lima after the inhabitants had eaten raw fish infected by the vibrio cholera. Poor hygiene and inadequate, antiquated methods of sewage disposal led to a terrifying epidemic involving nearly 200,000 people. The disease spread from Peru to Chile, Colombia, Equador, Bolivia, Brazil, Argentina and Guatemala. The greater part of the South American continent was in the grip of this disease which infected over 700,000 South Americans and killed around 400,000.

With all our advances in science and medicine, diseases and in particular infections continue to stalk the world. It is an irony that the cutting edge of medicine spends its energy and fortune in saving individuals for a short while with heart and lung transplants, when vast populations of the world suffer and may well be decimated by killer diseases that as yet have no cure.

67 Immunology

The science of immunology has seen spectacular advances in the twentieth century, particularly during the last four decades. From early times, bacteriology had given pre-eminence to the study of specific acquired resistance to invading micro-organisms as a means of conferring protection. Vaccines and antisera against major infections, like typhoid, cholera, plague, yellow fever and diphtheria, were the major effective measures that medicine could offer against disease in the early years of this century. Antigenic stimulation and antibody production came initially to be understood in relation to infectious diseases and the production of immunity to these diseases. Immunization and immunology are terms that arose from these origins.

Immunization through antigenic stimulation of dead or attenuated micro-organisms afforded specific protection, yet it could be shown that an equally specific increased clinical reactivity towards apparently similar antigenic material could also be readily induced. The explanation for these apparently antithetical results was first proposed by a Viennese paediatrician, Clemens von Pirquet (1874–1929), and this marked the birth of modern immunology. Pirquet postulated that in both cases the individual had developed after exposure to the antigen, a changed reactivity—in one case recognized as immunity and in the other as hypersensitivity. Pirquet termed this change in reactivity 'allergy'. His concept was a fundamental one because it recognized that a common biological process of specific sensitization was the underlying factor in all immune responses, irrespective of the clinical outcome.

The earliest explanation of antigen-antibody reaction was given by Ehrlich's side-chain chemical theory, which has already been described in chapter 48. Karl Landsteiner (1868–1943) in Vienna, proposed a physico-chemical explanation for the antigen-antibody reaction. Landsteiner's major contribution was the discovery of antigens on the surface of red blood cells. He labelled these antigen A (Group A), antigen B (Group B), and antigen AB (Group AB). He labelled cells with no antigen O (Group O). The discovery of blood groups, at last permitted the safe use of blood transfusions in medicine. The disasters observed with transfusions in earlier centuries could now be avoided by ensuring that the donor's blood matched the recipient's blood with respect to the blood groups discovered by Landsteiner. Transfusions of incompatible blood (i.e., blood of a different group) would induce antibody reaction to the antigens in the red blood cells of the donor's blood, causing severe haemolysis of red blood cells and even death. Landsteiner won the Nobel Prize in 1930 for his work on blood groups.

Another major discovery to the credit of Landsteiner was the finding of one or more antigens on the surface of red blood cells, which he called the 'Rhesus factor'. This factor was so called because it was also present on the surface of red blood cells of rhesus monkeys. The above discovery helped elucidate the mechanism underlying haemolytic disease of the newborn. Thus if a Rh-negative mother conceived a foetus which was Rh-positive (this could happen if the father was Rh-positive), maternal antibodies produced against the Rh antigen on the foetal red blood cells could cause haemolysis of foetal blood, leading either to stillbirth, or if the foetus was born alive, to erythroblastosis foetalis (haemolytic disease of the newborn). This discovery led to tests for the Rh antigen and also to the use of appropriate treatment for the newborns afflicted with the above disease.

Various aspects of immunology now came under close scrutiny. The functions of granulocytes, phagocytes, lymphocytes and mononuclear cells became better known. There has evolved over the last forty years, an integrated well-organized immune system within the body. Antibody production was shown to reside within the B-lymphocytes (originating in the bone marrow), which recognized antigen through their surface antibody receptors. The B-lymphocytes were found to be the precursors of the antibody secreting plasma cells. The progeny or clone of this B-lymphocyte retains the same commitment and the antibody secreted uses the same variable genes. The 'clonal theory' of antibody production was an important advance in the science of immunology.

Antibody production represents merely the humoral immune response to antigenic stimulation. An equally important response is the cell-mediated immune response through the T-lymphocytes. Research on T-cell lymphocytes showed that they could be divided into the helper (Th) cells which carry the CD4 glycoprotein and cytotoxic (CTL) cells which carry the CD8 glycoprotein. Some researchers believe that there is yet another subgroup of T-lymphocytes termed suppressor cells.

The thymus has been shown to play a crucial role in the immune system of the body. Newborn mice when thymectomized, failed to produce antibodies, became ill and died. A congenital absence of the thymus in newborn's babies was associated with severe crippling immune deficiencies (di Georgi syndrome). The T-cells were proven to be thymus-derived, in contrast to B-cell lymphocytes which were derived from the bone marrow. Recent work has shown other accessory cells in the immune response—these include antigen-presenting cells, mast cells, natural killer cells and macrophages.

The humoral and cellular responses of the immune system do not work in isolated compartments. There is in fact a close correlation and interaction and even inter-dependence, between these two main branches. An important aspect of modern immunology is the ability of the immune system to recognize the 'self'. The antigenic proteins within one's own self do not ordinarily cause either a humoral or cell-mediated response—they are recognized as part of one's self; as 'allies' in contrast to a foreign protein, which is recognized as such and 'attacked' by the immune system. Research has further shown that the immune system also has a 'memory', in that it remembers its earlier encounter with an antigen, if this antigen is reintroduced within the body. Such memory or recognition ability is stored in special lymphocytes.

In 1984, Dr Cesal Milstein and his team at Cambridge University won the Nobel Prize for their work on monoclonal antibodies. It is now possible to make antibodies to exact specifications to target a specific antigen on the surface of a cell or on a group of similar cells. The possible benefits that could arise from the successful use of monoclonal antibodies in medicine is immense. As yet this remains a dream that the future may well realize.

Current research in immunology is increasingly focused on anomalies of the immune process, which are harmful and can lead to disease. For example, a failure to recognize the 'self' can lead to devastating autoimmune disease, where antibodies are directed to specific tissues or organ systems within the body. This has been briefly touched upon in the previous chapter. There are many diseases in medicine today which are grouped as 'autoimmune' or related to an immunological basis. It is believed that even in normal circumstances, cells within the body mutate, assuming the features of cancerous cells. These are promptly recognized by the immune system and destroyed.

Failure to do so may allow such cells to proliferate. Finally, the purpose of the immune system is to protect the body from insults from within and without. This does not always happen. Recent work in sepsis and in other non-infectious insults to the human system has shown that the immune response in some instances is unorchestrated and bizarre, so that it harms the organ systems of the body instead of protecting them. The role of cytokines, secreted by various effector cells of the immune system has gained increasing significance in this unorchestrated response.

In summary, immunology today is not just concerned with response to infection. It encompasses research into the immune mechanisms which maintain the integrity and harmonious working of the human body. It also involves a study of the problems and diseases faced in clinical medicine due to an unusual response or bizarre functioning of the immune system. Immunology is the meeting ground for biochemistry, biology, molecular biology, genetics, physiology, pathology and clinical medicine. It is the science of the future.

68 The Frontiers of Medicine—The Structure of Life

Genetics aided by molecular biology and immunology are the frontiers of medicine—they form the cutting edge of science and have already begun to influence the practice of medicine.

Modern genetics began with hybridization experiments of the monk Gregor Mendel with the common garden pea at a monastery in Bohemia. Charles Darwin had earlier enunciated his radical revolutionary theory in his work, *On the Origin of Species*. However, the causes of the changes that occur in species which are then inherited to enable the species to survive remained unknown. The riddle was to be solved in 1953, though much preliminary research was needed before this great discovery could take place.

In clinical medicine, the earliest scientific contribution to inherited disease was made by Archibald Garrod in 1897. He studied alkaptonuria, characterized by black urine and progressive arthritis chiefly involving the spine. He noticed that in unaffected parents who produced alkaptonuric offspring, there was a high incidence of consanguinity. He coined the term 'inborn errors of metabolism' and considered these errors as congenital. His theories were ignored. Scientific proof that some diseases could be hereditary came in the middle of the twentieth century. Sickle-cell anaemia was thus shown to be a hereditary disease in 1923. Linus Pauling (1901–1994) showed that the haemoglobin molecule in patients with sickle-cell disease was abnormal, the abnormality residing in the globulin part of the molecule. The hereditary nature of Down's syndrome, characterized by mongoloid features and retarded physical and mental growth, was ultimately proved as late as 1989 to be related to an extra chromosome (chromosome 21).

The ultimate unravelling of the structure of life, the biochemistry of inheritance, was suprisingly not solved by researchers in the field of medicine. In 1869, the Swiss biochemist Friedrich Miescher discovered that an identical substance was present in the nucleus of every living cell. He called this 'nuclein'—later changed to 'nucleic acid'. At the beginning of the century, biochemists had determined that the nucleic acid molecule contained five chemical bases—guanine (G), adenine (A), cytosine (C), thymine (T) and uracil (U). By the 1920s, two forms of nucleic acid were identified—DNA (desoxyribonucleic acid) and RNA (ribonucleic acid). The belief among basic scientists at this time was that the DNA structure was simple and repetitive and thus could not transmit information. It was Edwin Schrodinger, a pioneer in quantum physics who disputed this view. In 1944, in a little book titled *What is life?*, he described the unit responsible for heredity in purely molecular terms. He likened it to an 'aperiodic crystal', a structure obeying fundamental laws of physics but not repetitive, so that it was capable of holding a huge amount of coded information. This description promptly attracted a number of physicists who till then had not researched on living matter. Maurice Wilkins, Francis Crick and James Watson took up the challenge to discover the exact biochemistry of existence.

Maurice Wilkins was an assistant director in the Medical Research Council (MRC), Bio-physics Unit, at King's College, London. He was given a sample of pure DNA and using a hurriedly assembled X-ray diffraction equipment, he obtained pictures of the spotted patterns produced when the DNA was pulled out to form a thin fibre. The spotted pattern suggested a helix but he lacked the expertise to interpret this X-ray finding. This was provided by Rosalind Franklin (1920–1958), who having worked on the structure of coal, joined the team at King's College on the understanding that she would take over the study of DNA from Wilkins. Wilkins, however continued, treated Franklin as a junior, causing bitterness and acrimony not conducive to successful research.

In 1949, Francis Crick (1916–   ) a physicist joined the MRC's unit at Cambridge University as a research student. He was joined two years later by James Watson (1928–   ), a brilliant American physicist and a famous child prodigy who had entered Chicago University at the age of fifteen. Neither knew much biochemistry, but both realized that no DNA research was possible without X-ray diffraction data. Crick knew that this work was being carried out at King's College. Crick and Watson established a rapport with Wilkins of King's College, who discussed his work on the DNA with them.

Watson and Crick built their first model of the DNA. based on the theory of Linus Pauling that the structure comprised a triple helix. Wilkins brought Franklin to see this model and she showed that the idea of a triple helix was totally incompatible with her X-ray data. Disappointed, Watson and Crick stopped their research on DNA for nearly six months.

In January 1953, two events spurred the researchers on once again. Peter Pauling showed Watson a paper his father was about to publish regarding the structure of the DNA as a triple helix with phosphate backbones inside. Watson and Crick knew from their own previous mistake that this had to be wrong. It would take six weeks for Pauling's paper to be published—the two young researchers gave themselves this span of time to come up with the right answers. Fate was now kind to them. Wilkins gave Watson (without Franklin's permission) a print of one of Franklin's best X-ray photographs of the DNA. This print told Watson that the structure of the DNA was a double helix. They hurriedly began another model in which they placed the backbones on the inside with the bases sticking out. They realized their mistake when they compared this model to Franklin's X-ray print and changed their model so that the backbones were on the outside and the bases on the inside. The final model resembles a twisted ladder with the bases as the rungs. It took another week for them to assemble the bases in the correct order. Watson and Crick completed the final correct model on 7 March 1953, and the results of their discovery were published in a short paper in *Nature* on 25 April 1953. Rosalind Franklin never realized how much Watson and Cricks' discovery was due to her data because she was unaware that they had seen her X-ray photograph of DNA prior to the construction of the correct model. In 1962, Watson, Crick and Wilkins were awarded the Nobel Prize for physiology and medicine. Rosalind Franklin had died of cancer in 1958.

The biochemistry of life was solved and it was accepted that a complicated genetic code could be contained in the DNA. The field of genetics was now wide open. In the 1980s it became possible to chemically read the genetic code, to isolate genes and to duplicate (i.e., clone) them. Through the study of amniotic fluid (amniocentesis), it now became possible to screen a foetus in utero for genetic defects, so that a number of congenital disorders could be diagnosed before birth. The isolation of a gene responsible for a particular disease, either because it does not produce a specific gene product or produces an abnormal product holds great attraction both in the theory and practice of medicine. Perhaps herein lies the future of medicine.

A revolution in gene discovery is currently afoot. The human genome project, initiated in 1990, aims to determine the complete sequence of the human genome, including the estimated 100,000 genes by the year 2005. The project appears to be ahead of time. The question arises as to how does one determine whether the hereditary susceptibility to a particular disorder is related to alteration in one particular gene out of the 100,000 genes. A credible answer to this question may well determine the future course of medicine.

69 The History of Birth Control and the Contemporary Science of Reproduction

Attempts at birth control probably commenced from the era of antiquity, perhaps even from prehistoric times. They took the form of chemical compounds and mechanical devices used to prevent pregnancy. In ancient Egypt, in the third millennium BC, women inserted pessaries of honey and crocodile dung into the vagina as contraceptives. Arab women used crushed pomegranate, alum and rock salt for the same effect. Aristotle of Greece, believed in the contraceptive power of a concoction of frankincense, cedar and olive oil, when inserted in the vagina. Perhaps these methods worked to an extent by increasing the acidity within the vagina, thereby destroying or inactivating sperm.

It was Gabriele Falloppia in the sixteenth century who first invented the linen condom. His interest was primarily directed towards the prevention of syphilis, which was ravaging Europe in that era and not for birth control. The condom thus for the next four centuries was associated more with prostitution and prevention of sexually-transmitted diseases than with contraception.

In Europe the style of the condom changed, linen being replaced by the gut of a sheep, chemically treated, softened and dried. In the East, as in Japan, condoms were made of tortoise shell horn or leather. Remarkably enough, in the west each country dubbed the condom with a foreign name. Thus in France, it became known as the 'English Cap' and in England, it was called the 'French letter'. Casanova of Italy dubbed it the 'English overcoat'! The design all over the world changed to rubber, and later to latex; amusingly enough, the 'French letter' in England was decorated by a portrait of Queen Victoria, who had been blessed with nine children!

The first rubber contraceptive for women was devised by a German, Adolphe Wilde, in 1838, in the form of a cervical cap which plugged the cervix. Another German doctor named Heinse, under the pseudonym of 'Mensinga' devised the rubber diaphragm, which remains popular to this day. Current medicine advocates the use of a copper loop which when inserted into the cervical canal offers good protection against pregnancy.

The acceptance of contraceptives for birth control was slow. Perhaps the acceptance was triggered by the work of Thomas Malthus (1766–1834), who proposed the Malthusian theory that the world's population would soon outstrip the food supply with disastrous consequences. This was seized upon by eugenists who founded the Malthusian League in Britain, France, Germany and Holland. The world's first birth control clinic was opened in the Netherlands in1882 by Dr Aletta Jacobs, a member of the Malthusian group. Dr Jacobs advocated the use of the diaphragm as the safest contraceptive for women—it thus became nicknamed the 'Dutch cap'.

The greatest advance in contemporary medicine in relation to birth control was the discovery of the contraceptive pill. In the early 1940s Russell Marker, working in a laboratory, was able to isolate the female hormone progesterone from a yam that grew wild near the jungles of Veracruz, Mexico. Marker formed a company, Syntex, in Mexico City to exploit his discovery. He for some obscure reason suddenly lost interest, abandoned chemistry and his company, and took to making replicas of European silver antiques till his death in 1984. Other scientists in Syntex continued the work on progesterone and finally succeeded in modifying it to form a compound, norethisterone or norethindrone, which was more active than human progesterone taken orally. This new compound was sent to Gregory Pincus, a biologist at the Worcester foundation in Massachusetts, who found that it inhibited ovulation. At around the same time, in 1953, Frank Colton of Searle pharmaceutical company filed a patent for norethynodrel, a compound similar to norethisterone.

Pincus and his colleagues with the aid of a large grant now commenced research on hormonal birth control. Contraception was to remain illegal in Massachusetts till 1967. The 'hormonal trial' in 1953 was therefore carried out among the poor in Puerto Rico. Pincus being a consultant to Searle used the Searle product norethynodrel in preference to norethisterone. The result of this successful trial was published in the *Science Journal* in 1956. In 1957 norethynodrel was accepted as a hormone regulator and in the following year, as an oral contraceptive.

The eugenic implications of an easily available oral contraceptive in the teeming, multiplying populations of the poor Third World countries was evident to all the workers in the field. Searle now removed impurities from their product, but the pure progesterone caused breakthrough bleeding and even allowed occasional unwanted pregnancies. Researchers now realized that the original compound contained over 1 per cent of an oestrogen-type substance called mestranol which they reinserted into the pills. The efficacy of the oestrogen–progesterone combination was thus discovered fortuitously.

The oral contraceptive pill was considered to 'liberate' modern women—it certainly led to a laxity of moral values and to a sexual precocity that had obvious dangers to individuals and to society. Its mass use in poor countries had many difficulties and failed to curb the population growth in India and other Third World countries. In 1961, dangerous side-effects now came to be reported. These included thrombophlebitis, thromboembolism, migraine and jaundice. There was also a higher incidence of strokes and heart attacks among women on the pill. The UK committee of safety of medicine, in 1969, advised that the pill should contain no more than fifty micrograms of oestrogen, as higher doses were responsible for the dangerous complications mentioned above.

Birth control is one end of the human reproductive spectrum. The other end of the spectrum is infertility and the attempts of science and medicine to correct or circumvent it. There has been a measure of spectacular success in this field, but this has been seriously marred by the ethical dilemmas and quandaries that the contemporary science of reproduction has raised.

An important cause of female infertility is blocked fallopian tubes which prevents an ovum from travelling via the fallopian tube into the uterus. Patrick Steptoe (1913–1988) theorized that if an ovum (egg) was removed from the ovary laparoscopically and fertilized *in vitro* by a sperm, the fertilized ovum could then be placed into the uterus and could conceivably grow into a baby. This was the concept of a 'test tube baby', though the *in vitro* fertilization was done in a petri dish and not a test-tube.

Steptoe now worked with Robert Edwards, a Cambridge physiologist, on the *in vitro* fertilization of human ova and reported in 1969 that they had fertilized thirteen out of fifty-six ova outside the body. Their research met with crowning success nine years later when in 1978, Louise Brown was born as the first test tube baby in the world, at the Oldham District Hospital. The success rate of the technique of *in vitro* fertilization was low—no more than one in ten treatments produced live babies.

Ethical and philosophical quandaries were expressed by numerous people all over the world—from the Pope in the Vatican to renowned scientists and Nobel laureates. All *in vitro* fertilized ova had a right to live; should all be implanted? What became of those that remained unimplanted—was it ethical to destroy them, and was it ethical to store them and to research on them? The ethics of permitting growth of a fertilized ovum in an external environment gave rise to furious debates. The dilemmas worsened when artificial insemination by a donor was used to fertilize an egg, and when the fertilized egg was implanted into the womb of a surrogate mother who agreed to carry the pregnancy to term. The legitimacy of parenthood, particularly of surrogate motherhood came into question and dispute.

In the United Kingdom, a committee chaired by the philosopher Mary Warnock, considered *in vitro* fertilization (IVF) legitimate for infertile women. The committee decreed that extra-uterine development of the fertilized ovum should not exceed two weeks, by which time the fertilized egg should be implanted in the womb. It was advised that fertilized ova should not be implanted into the womb for purposes of research either in humans or in other species.

Ethical approaches however varied in different countries. The Vatican banned IVF; surrogate mothers were unacceptable in several countries. In the meanwhile, the limits of contemporary medicine in reproduction were stretched when a fifty-nine year old Italian woman was reported pregnant through the implantation of a donor egg fertilized *in vitro* by her husband's sperm. In 1997, a sixty-three year old woman gave birth to a healthy child after an *in vitro* fertilization. When and where is this going to end? Is it ethical to hire wombs? Is it not dreadfully immoral to sell and accept the sale of organs like the kidney for transplants as is the unfortunate custom in poor countries? Science and technology are now ever so often pitted against ethics and morality, raising issues which the future might find difficult to solve.

70 Cancer

Cancer is one of mankind's most dreaded, ruthless and mortal enemies. Cancer can arise in any organ or tissue within the body and has two basic features. These are anaplasia and autonomy. Anaplasia is the loss of the normal appearance of cells under the microscope. Cancerous cells therefore vary in size and shape, appear disarranged, with a cytoplasm and nucleus unlike that observed in the normal cells of the tissue or organ in which the cancer arises. Autonomy is the loss of inhibition or control over cell growth, resulting in their independent behaviour and function. Cancer cells are cells gone berserk. They often multiply chaotically to form increasingly large tumors or masses destroying or invading adjacent tissue and breaking off to be carried through lymphatics and blood vessels to form distant islands of cancerous cells, termed metastasis.

Unless successfully treated, cancer kills—slowly, relentlessly, inexorably, often causing great discomfort and pain. It is the deadliness and frequency of cancer that arouses a universal dread and fear of this disease in man.

In many countries of the West, cancer is second only to heart disease as a cause of death. More than one million new cases of cancer and 500,000 deaths occur every year in the United States. The four common cancers are lung cancer, colorectal cancer, breast cancer and prostate cancer. These four cancers account for 56 per cent of the incidence and 55 per cent of deaths in cancer. The incidence of cancer in Third World countries is on the increase. In India cancer has become one of the major causes of death.

There is however a great deal of variation in the incidence of cancer afflicting different organs in different countries. There is thus a very high incidence of oesophageal cancer in China and Iran, of the oral cavity in India, liver cancer in parts of Africa and Asia, Burkitt's lymphoma in Africa, and urinary bladder cancer in the areas endemic for bilharziasis. The epidemiological significance of these variations has stimulated a great deal of research.

Historical Background

Cancer is a disease of ancient times and has existed before written history. Recent evidence suggests that it probably afflicted animals long before man first appeared on the earth. Malignant neoplasms in man have been described in Egyptian mummies dating from the third to the fifth dynasties 5,000 years ago, as also among the mummies of pre-Columbian Incas of Peru 2,600 years ago. The Egyptian papyruses which are among the oldest written records of the history of man give descriptions pointing to the occurrence of both benign and malignant tumors.

Hippocrates and his school unquestionably knew cancer, particularly of the breast, uterus, stomach, skin and mouth. Indeed, it was he who termed the disease *karcinos* (Greek for crab). He could not do much for the disease and applied to it his cardinal principle, *primum non nocere,* (first, do not harm). One of his aphorisms states, "It is better not to apply treatment in case of occult cancer, for if treated the patients die quickly; but if not treated, they may live for a long time." Hippocrates proposed the theory of disequilibrium of the four humors as the cause of disease. The accumulation of black bile or melanchole or atrabilis was considered the cause of cancer. This theory prevailed for over 2,000 years. Celsus of Rome, Araetus of Cappadocia and Galen all echoed the views of Hippocrates. For external cancers, they advocated the application of caustics and occasionally the use of the knife and the cautery.

The period of history from AD 500 to the Renaissance was one of scientific hibernation and slumber. Then Vesalius revolutionized anatomy and Paré revolutionized surgery. Harvey discovered the circulation of blood and Gaspari Asseli (1585–1621) of Milan discovered the lymphatic vessels. With these discoveries the cause of cancer was related to obstruction to lymph flow and to abnormalities in lymph. John Hunter in the eighteenth century elevated surgery from a craft to a science. The diagnosis and treatment of cancer improved but the end result remained bleak. Percival Pott described the frequent occurrence of scrotal cancers in chimmney-sweeps, the first occupational and environmental cancer to be described in man.

The nineteenth century was a century of discoveries and the birth of the biomedical sciences. In 1837, Johannes Muller ushered in the histological, study of oncology when he looked at cancerous tissue through an achromatic microscope. The introduction of anaesthesia in 1846 and of antisepsis in 1867 saw a great leap in the scope and craft of surgery. Surgeons soon innovated operative techniques for cancers within the body. Theodor Billroth, about whom we have written in the section on Modern Medicine was a pioneer in the surgical treatment of cancer of the internal organs. His surgical triumphs included resection of the oesophagus in 1871, complete excision of the larynx in 1873, partial gastrectomy in 1881 and gastro-jejunotomy in 1885. He performed numerous intestinal resections, mastectomies and pelvic operations. He was a great teacher, and among his many pupils were Mikulicz, Czerny, Wolfler and Kocher. Alexander von Winiwarter of Belgium, who was one of his assistants reviewed the end results of 548 patients with cancers treated at Billroth's clinic between 1867 and 1876. He reported that 40 per cent of the 170 patients with cancer of the breast were alive and well three years or more later. This was the first statistical review in cancer surgery.

William Halsted's operation in 1891 for radical mastectomy, as mentioned earlier remained unchallenged for half a century. This procedure increased the survival rate from under 20 per cent to nearly 40 per cent over a three-year follow-up. In the nineteenth century, research directed towards understanding the complexity of cancer was poor and laborious. Virchow with his revolutionary cellular theory believed that tumors arose from immature cells. Homologous tumors arose from cells already present and were benign. Heterologous tumors arose from cells that changed their character and were malignant. He believed that malignant tumors arose from connective tissue. It was Robert Remak (1815–1865), an embryologist, Carl Thiersch (1822–1895), a surgeon, and Wilhelm Waldeyer (1837–1921), an anatomist, who proved that carcinomas arose from epithelial tissue. Waldeyer also observed that cancer metastasis arose from embolization of tumor cells via lymphatic and blood vessels.

Twentieth-century Contemporary Medicine

The twentieth century saw the birth of oncology (the study of tumors) as a special scientific discipline. Hitherto, the discoveries in basic science and in biomedicine had been applied to the problem of cancer. They continue to do so, but more importantly oncology now began to make its own contribution to biology and to biomedicine. Contemporary medicine has concentrated its research on the cause and cure of cancer. Some of the best brains in the world, with the support of billions of dollars in grants and funds are engaged in this struggle. As yet the goal seems distant, but the struggle continues. It is beyond the scope of this book to give more than the barest outline of what man and medicine have achieved in this century against this disease. Molecular biology, genetics, virology, and immunology have all combined in a common effort to try and unearth the cause of carcinogenesis.

The genetic make-up of an individual influences all physiological and pathological processes. Heredity therefore must have an obvious role in cancer. It is the degree of genetic control for different kinds of cancers that requires specification. There are several pre-neoplastic and neoplastic conditions that have proved Mendelian inheritance. Most of these are inherited as autosomal dominants; at least one, Xeroderma pigmentosa, is inherited as an autosomal recessive. This is a pre-cancerous skin condition in which extreme sensitivity to actinic rays causes cancerous changes to occur in the skin.

Theodor Boveri (1862–1918), professor of zoology at Wurzberg, in Germany, first enunciated the concept of genes in the science of genetics in the early years of the twentieth century. He proposed the somatic mutation theory, believing that cancer was caused by abnormal chromosomes. The somatic mutation theory was a rival to the oncogenic viral theory of cancer espoused by Amedeé Borrel (1867–1936), who was professor of bacteriology and hygiene at the university of Strasbourg. Borrel postulated the viral theory of cancer well before cell-free filtrates were shown to transmit cancer in animal experiments. It was in 1910 that Peyton Rous (1879–1970), a young investigator at the Rockefeller Institute of New York, began his studies on chicken sarcomas. He passed the tumor material through filters impermeable to cells and bacteria and proved that the filtrate injected into chicken produced sarcomas. The viral theory of cancer now had experimental backing. Other oncogenic (tumor-producing) viruses were soon discovered. Rous received the Nobel Prize for medicine in 1966 for his research.

It is of interest that at the beginning of the twentieth century, cancer could also be experimentally produced in animals by various chemical and physical agents. These included coal tar, ultraviolet light, exposure to X-rays, radium and uranium. The carcinogenic substances in coal tar were soon discovered to be polycyclic hydrocarbons.

The discovery of the structure of the DNA molecule in 1953 by Watson and Crick was a great advance in molecular biology. This science came of use in fathoming the genetic mechanism of cancer and other diseases and to study the interaction between these mechanisms and environmental stimuli. In fact a revolution is taking place in the field of cancer research. The traditional avenues of research were in animal tumor systems. The ability to successfully grow cancer cells in tissue culture was a notable landmark in cancer research. Advances in molecular biology have now permitted the identification of genes that can cause cancer—oncogenes. The first oncogenes were studied in cancer-producing retroviruses. Human oncogenes have now been detected by DNA transfection or gene transfer. They have also been detected through the recognition of non-random chromosomal abnormalities. Recent research has also identified the presence of tumor-suppressor genes or recessive oncogenes. Many human leukaemias and lymphomas appear to be due to specific chromosomal translocations, while solid tumors often involve multiple mutations in oncogenes, loss of recessor or suppressor genes and/or chromosomal rearrangements. Cancer is characterized by genome instability and immortality. The current hypothesis is that cancer could be due to the mutation of one or more genes responsible for the stability of the genome.

There exist today, notwithstanding subtle variations, two main theories in the causation and nature of cancer. These are the protovirus theory of Howard Temin and David Baltimore, and the oncogenic concept of Robert Huebner and George Todaro. In a way they are the restatements of the virus infestation proposed by Borrel and chromosomal changes suggested by Boveri in 1903. Remarkably enough, these theories are not mutually exclusive.

Temin and Baltimore postulated in the 1960s that when a tumor-producing virus enters a cell, the RNA of the virus through the enzyme reverse transcriptase makes DNA copies of itself, causing the host cell to become cancerous.

The oncogenic theory does not exclude an associated viral aetiology. It suggests that in the course of evolution a type RNA virus becomes incorporated into the genome and exists as a silent infection at birth. The oncogene can be activated by many exogenous factors causing cancer. The loss of suppressor oncogenes further favours the likelihood of cancer.

A study of the immunology of cancer has thrown further light on carcinogenesis. The immune system probably destroys 'rogue cells' or cells gone 'berserk' no sooner or very soon, after the transformation takes place. An inability to recognize and destroy these cells allows the cancer to grow.

There is now evidence that cancer cells have specific antigens that can elicit a cancer-destructive immune response. It has also been shown that tumor viruses can impart antigen to the surface of the cells they render cancerous, rendering them immunologically foreign and subject to immunological attack. G. I. Abelev, of the Gamaleya Institute of Epidemiology and Microbiology in Moscow, discovered that antigens like the fetoproteins, normally evident only in the embryo, can reappear in certain forms of cancer. This discovery has been put to clinical use particularly in the diagnosis of cancer of the colon, where the fetoproteins may be raised, or of the ovary, where the C125 levels are high.

Robert J. Huebner proved that viral antigens may persist in animal cancers from which the causative virus can no longer be recovered. Werner and Gertrud Henle of the Children Hospital, Philadelphia, through their brilliant immunological research, demonstrated the relation of the Epstein-Barr herpes virus to cancer of the nasopharynx and to Burkitt's lymphoma. Recent work has substantiated the association between active hepatitis B and hepatitis C infection with the occurrence of cancer of the liver, and of the human papilloma virus to cancer of the cervix. The causative role of the HIV virus in the production of lymphomas and other rare cancers has also been established.

Cesar Milstein and George Kohler developed monoclonal antibodies. These were antibodies specific against only one particular antigen. Monoclonal antibodies thus targeted on to their specific antigen attached to the cell wall, destroying it or nullifying its effect. Tagged with radioactive material, monoclonal antibodies were used for diagnosis to recognize cancer cells, or for treatment to destroy them. The hopes raised by these new techniques have unfortunately not been fulfilled in clinical practice.

The early diagnosis of cancer was of paramount importance as treatment at an early stage afforded better chances of long-term survival. George Nicholas Papanicolaou (1883–1962) at the Cornell Medical College in New York, and his clinical collaborator Herbert Frederick Traut (1894–1963) showed that studies on vaginal cytology could help in the pre-clinical diagnosis of cancer of the uterine cervix. The simplicity of this method has permitted an examination of the 'pap smear' te be introduced all over the world as a clinical and public health measure. Diagnosis of cervical cancer before it has become invasive reduced the mortality from cervical cancer. An extremely useful screening procedure for cancer of the breast is mammography and palpation of the breast to detect small, silent cancers within it. Field studies showed that there was a significant reduction in the mortality from breast cancer (through early detection and treatment) in a large study group after five years of follow-up. New methods of diagnosis have resulted through studies in genetics, molecular biology and immunology. These include the detection of tumor markers within the blood, the use of special histopathological techniques and of newer techniques in immunohistochemistry.

Modern research in the treatment of cancer has made only a small dent in its morbidity and mortality. To start with, surgery was the sheet anchor of treatment. Ernest Wertheim (1864–1920) of Vienna, in 1898, carried out his first radical hysterectomy for cervix cancer publishing his experience on 500 patients in 1911.

H. Morriston Davies (1879–1965) of London in 1912, performed the first lobectomy for cancer of the lung. The patient died of empyema (pus in the pleural space). The first successful pneumonectomy for lung cancer was performed by Evarts Ambrose Graham (1883–1957) of St Louis, United States. Surgery for cancer reached its apogee after the Second World War, when extensive radical resection of cancer involving internal organs with spread to adjacent tissue was vigorously pursued. Problems of rehabilitation became increasingly difficult and important in the retraining of salvaged cancer patients. Halsted's operation of radical mastectomy was further extended (making it supraradical!) to include the removal of the chain of internal mammary lymph glands in cancers medial to the nipple. Statistical support for such massive resections when compared to limited surgery were however not forthcoming. In 1948, Robert McWhirter, a radiotherapist at Edinburgh, reported that the results of simple mastectomy plus radiotherapy were equal to those of radical mastectomy. His work was the forerunner to a more sensible surgical approach in the management of cancer and with the advent of chemotherapy, new directions employing combined treatment were quickly established. Today most breast cancers are treated by 'lumpectomy' (removal of the tumor), a resection of axillary lymph glands, followed by chemotherapy, radiotherapy or both, with good results and with minimal physical and psychological trauma to the patient.

The nonsurgical treatment of cancers includes radiotherapy and chemotherapy. It was Leopold Freund, who a hundred years ago founded the new scientific discipline of radiotherapy. Freund provided the first scientific proof of the effectiveness of radiation therapy when he successfully treated with X-rays, a five-year old girl with a large-hairy nevus on her back. Today radiotherapy and radiation oncology contribute to nearly one-half of all cancer cures. This has been made possible by remarkable developments in technology. Thus the introduction of Cobalt-60 units and linear accelerators in the 1950s allowed for treatment of deep-seated tumors without the skin, bone and other complications met with in conventional deep X-ray therapy. Specialized treatments, such as automated after-loading brachytherapy, total body irradiation, stereotaxic radiosurgery and computerized 3D planning to improve dose distribution have improved results in some cancers.

Alkylating agents like nitrogen mustard and their analogues were the first chemotherapeutic drugs used against cancer. Nitrogen mustard was first prepared for possible use as a chemical weapon in the First World War. It proved to be a cytotoxic agent and was tried out for its effect against cancer. Like every other chemotherapeutic agent that followed it, the drug besides destroying cancer cells also destroyed or damaged other normal living cells. Remissions with a temporary reprieve followed by recurrence and death has been the story of chemotherapy. There is however one important exception to this bleak statement and that is the successful use of appropriate chemotherapy in childhood leukaemia. Acute lymphatic leukaemia in children which had a 100 per cent mortality, can now be offered a cure in over 90 per cent of patients. Acute myeloid leukaemia has a cure rate of over 50 per cent. The prognosis of acute leukaemia in adults is unfortunately poor, but even so there is a significant cure rate of 50 per cent in acute lymphatic leukaemia, and of 30 per cent in acute myeloid leukaemia. The group of various lymphomas has also shown a better prognosis with modern chemotherapy.

The science of molecular biology has discovered the presence of a number of 'cytokines', secreted by normal and abnormal cells. Some of these have been used recently against cancer. They include the use of interferon, interleukins and of immunity-boosting LAK cells and interleukin-2. Hopes were raised inordinately and often unfairly, only to be followed by renewed despondency and despair. The adverse side-effects, the unpleasantness and discomfort of many chemotherapeutic regimes by far outweigh the short reprieve they occasionally provide. Sufferers from cancer more often than not suffer even more through the over-zealous efforts of doctors who have forgotten the cardinal Hippocratic doctrine of *Primum non nocere*.

Most countries in the world today have one or more special hospitals devoted specially to the research and treatment of cancer. The first such hospital was built in Rheims, France in 1740, from funds donated by the Canon of the Cathedral at Rheims, who felt that cancer was contagious and patients needed to be isolated. The cancer ward at the Middlesex Hospital, London, donated by the brewer Samuel Whitbread in 1791, has been mentioned in chapter 42. In 1827, William Marsden started a dispensary for the poor in London which ultimately became the Royal Free and Cancer Hospital. The word 'Free' meant that unlike the rule in other hospitals, a letter of recommendation was not necessary for admission.

The idea of establishing a research institute on cancer was espoused by Sir Henry Morris (1844–1920), a leading surgeon of London, who headed the cancer department at the Middlesex Hospital. The Cancer Research Fund was founded in 1902 through private funds but was controlled by the Royal Colleges. The title 'Imperial' was added when royal patronage was extended to this effort. Similar associations for cancer research were launched in France, Germany and the United States. The Memorial Sloan Kettering Institute in New York was established in the 1930s. The Tata Memorial Hospital was established in Bombay in 1941 and remains a landmark in India's fight against cancer. It was founded by the Dorabji Tata Trust; in 1962, the management was transferred to the atomic energy department of the Government of India. It has modernized its facilities and doubled its bed strength to cope with the heavy demands on its resources. The hospital has a well-equipped and a very active research centre associated with it.

Research on the epidemiology of cancers has yielded fruitful results. Environmental and occupational causes of cancer are on the increase. They include exposure to asbestos which can lead to cancer of the lung and malignant diseases of the pleura. Cancer of the skin was observed in those handling arsenic; miners in cobalt, nickel, and uranium mines had a high incidence of lung cancer. The aftermath of the atomic explosions at Hiroshima and Nagasaki saw a high incidence of genetic defects and of blood cancer (leukaemia) in those who survived the horrific destruction. Unquestionably, the most important carcinogen to man today is cigarette smoke. It was the pioneering work of Austin Bradford Hill (1897–1991) and Richard Doll, published in 1961, that statistically proved the relation between cigarette-smoking and lung cancer. The incidence of cancer of the lung in heavy smokers (20 or more cigarettes daily) was forty times higher than in non-smokers. Very recent studies have shown that continued cigarette-smoking throughout adult life doubles age-specific mortality, nearly trebling mortality rates in late middle age. Passive smoking (inhalation of cigarette smoke by non-smokers) is also associated with an increased incidence of cancer of the lung, and women who smoke during pregnancy can induce damage to the unborn foetus. In 1956, Doll and Hill in a study on smoking in the medical profession, showed that the mortality from cancer of the lung fell in individuals who stopped smoking. The adage of prevention being far superior to cure could now be applicable to one of the common forms of cancer afflicting man. Yet the tobacco industry has a powerful lobby with a great deal of money at its disposal. The pernicious habit of smoking persists in all parts of the world and in fact is increasing among women in the West. The epidemiological trend of an increasing incidence of cancer of the lung in women is now already apparent. Perhaps more research directed towards the preventive aspects of cancer would yield far better results than concentration on discovering a cure. Epidemiological studies in India have shown that oral cancer (the commonest form of cancer in the country) can be prevented by stopping the use of *supari* and chewable tobacco, kept as a 'bolus' against the buccal mucosa. Unnecessary exposure to X-rays is a further source of cancer, as is exposure to ionizing radiation. The potential carcinogenecity of pesticides, fertilizers and of chemical effluents discharged into the rivers and seas of our world may well play an important role in the rising incidence of cancer. The ecological change, damage and disruption wrought by man may one day prove to be an increasingly important cause of disease and death in the world.

71 World Health and Medicine

The West had begun to colonize the rest of the world by the seventeenth century, but the health hazards and problems of the colonies for the next two centuries were in the main different from those of the increasingly industrialized West. The twentieth century saw a progressively interdependent world. The rise and fall of empires, world wars, the rise of capitalism and the influence of multinational companies, the speed of transport and communication, and the migrations of populations on a vast scale were all in a way responsible for events in one corner of the world to reverberate and influence distant countries. Disease did not necessarily respect boundaries and this was illustrated by the great pandemic of influenza starting in 1918 and then sweeping across the world with a fury not witnessed since the days of the Black Death. Influenza killed twenty-five million people in a record time of six months—this was greater than all the casualties of the First World War. It was followed by a wave of encephalitis lethargica and then again in 1920 by a renewed wave of lethal influenza.

The idea of an international body to monitor health and control disease in a world where countries were certain to become increasingly interlinked was now born. The treaty of Versailles after the First World War saw the birth of the League of Nations, whose purpose was to maintain harmony and peace among the countries of the world. A subdivision of this body was the Health Organization of the League of Nations. The international health activities initiated by this organization included a Malaria Commission and a Cancer Commission. These commissions reported on malnutrition, typhus, leprosy, medical education and public health.

In 1939, the Second World War erupted with the invasion of Poland by Germany. The League of Nations which had watched the march of events that led to this war with helplessness, collapsed, and with it also collapsed the Health Organization. After the end of the Second World War, the World Health Organization (WHO) was established under the aegis of a political body called the United Nations. It was determined by those who founded and established the WHO that its survival should not be dependent on its parent body—the United Nations. The WHO established a separate secretariat in Geneva and had fifty-five national signatories approving its charter and objectives. The objective proclaimed by the WHO was to achieve 'a state of complete physical, mental and social well-being and not merely the absence of disease or infirmity'. There were two other allied organizations set up to work in coordination with the WHO. They were again under the aegis of the United Nations. The first was the United Nations International Children's Emergency Fund (UNICEF), which directed funds for the supply of food, drugs and equipment. The UNICEF came under the supervision of the United Nations Educational, Scientific and Cultural Organization (UNESCO).

The WHO initially directed its attention to immunization against six killer infectious diseases chiefly afflicting the Third World countries. These were tetanus, measles, whooping cough, diphtheria, poliomyelitis and tuberculosis. A major function of WHO was the collection of statistics of disease, particularly in Third World countries (where statistics were nonexistent or poorly recorded), improving cooperation in the control and fight against disease, intervening in crisis situations and helping to develop and financially assist better health plans in the poor Third World countries. Financial aid was of essence, and this largesse was decided upon by the World Health body. Financial aid to poor countries was not only directed towards the promotion of health, but also to industrial and agricultural development, medical education and educational public health programmes. The United States remains in the forefront as the chief aid-giver, providing health assistance to more than sixty countries.

The greatest success scored by the WHO so far has been the eradication of small-pox from the world. In 1966, about fifteen million people in thirty-three countries of the world caught small-pox and two million died. The WHO embarked on a ten-year vaccination programme to eradicate the disease. The project was headed by an American, Dr Donald Henderson, who had working with him a large team of fifty full-time and six hundred part-time workers. Dedication, organizational skill, finance and Jenner's great discovery in the seventeenth century joined hands to stamp out the disease in Africa, the Middle East and South America. India and Pakistan held out, but ultimately the disease was conquered. The victory was complete in 1974 when Bangladesh reported that the country was free from small-pox.

The danger of doctors and technicians working with the small-pox virus and those in the immediate vicinity of these research laboratories was illustrated when in 1978, Janet Parker died of the disease in Birmingham. She was a photographer who worked on the floor immediately above a research laboratory when the virus escaped through the ventilation system to infect and kill her. This so far has been the last fatality in the world from smallpox. The virus is now known to exist in just two laboratories in the world—one at the Centre for Disease Control in Atlanta and the other in Moscow. The stocks of virus in research laboratories all over the world have on purpose been destroyed. At least one hopes that this is true and that samples have not been hidden for possible use as biological weapons by monster nations.

The WHO is now directing its technical, financial and medical resources to eradicating poliomyelitis, diphtheria, measles and whooping cough—killer diseases responsible for millions of deaths in Africa, Asia and the poor South American countries. This is a difficult task and the immediate prospects of preventing and eradicating these diseases appear remote. The exponential increase in the birth rate in India and the lack of proper infrastructure render immunization programmes against these diseases to be only partially effective. With over twenty-five million children born in the country each year, India can manage to immunize just about half of them. China, which curbed its population more effectively, has succeeded in immunizing close to 90 per cent of its susceptible population.

72 Imaging the Body

After the discovery of X-rays by Wilhelm Roentgen, the basic principles, concepts and technology behind medical radiography were established within a few years. Though refinements in technique helped to improve the quality of X-ray pictures, the next imaging technique was introduced in the fifties through the use of ultrasound. The principles of medical ultrasound were developed by Ian Donald (1910–1987), professor of midwifery in Glasgow. These principles were based on the wartime discovery and use of the naval echo-sounding technique known as SONAR (Sound Navigation and Ranging). Certain crystals when subjected to an electric charge, emit sound waves at very high frequencies which cannot be heard by the human ear. When these ultrasonic waves travelling through water encounter a solid object, they send back echoes. The time lapse for the return of echoes allows the distance to be calculated. Donald showed that solids with different densities gave different echoes and was able to diagnose different kinds of abdominal tumours. In 1957, he was using the ultrasound technique, first to diagnose foetal disorders and then in the diagnosis of pregnancy itself. It was proven quite conclusively that unlike X-rays, ultrasound had no harmful effect on the developing foetus.

The more extensive use of ultrasound scanning, not just in obstetrics alone but in medicine and its allied branches, came into existence with the new generation of ultra-sound machines and scanners in the late sixties. There now followed the discovery of one other imaging technique—the X-ray computerized axial tomography (CAT scan), which revolutionized diagnostic imaging of the human body.

These new imaging techniques have one common feature—a scanner that scans. Each scanner, whether rudimentary or sophisticated, examines any part of the human anatomy bit by bit, taking a number of complicated mathematical measurements from which images are generated by the technique of mathematical reconstruction. The earlier computers were slow as they relied on analogue components to achieve practicable speed. The improvements in scanning techniques in the 1980s and 1990s are largely due to extremely sophisticated computers, which compute with great speed.

The Scope of Present Day Ultrasound (USG)

The present-day USG machines and scanners can produce two-dimensional information at high speed, so that they are capable of tracking moving structures, for example the valves within the heart. The scanner can recognize and record changes in the density of the tissue that they scan and simultaneously map in colour, the flow of blood over the whole field of the moving image.

Ultrasound transducers have been designed and constructed in many special forms for external scanning of different organs and for insertion into body cavities. Probes as minute as 1 mm have now been mounted on catheters to be used in conjunction with endoscopes and surgical instruments. They are small enough to negotiate the coronary arteries within the heart, helping to map irregularities in the arterial wall and narrowing of the lumen. The rapid sophistication of ultrasound techniques has been of immense diagnostic help in almost every field of medicine. The use of portable machines has taken imaging power to the bedside and to the operation theatre. The incorporation of Doppler scanning records the rate of blood flow within a vessel, picking up areas of narrowing or blockage within the vessels—an immense help to the vascular surgeon. Ultrasonography of the abdomen is now a routine screening procedure in many centres and can often recognize and record silent pathology within the abdominal organs.

In 1967, Godfrey Hounsfield designed a scanning system to build a three-dimensional body image. He was a scientist, an engineer and a computer expert, working with the British company, EMI. The method which he established and which became operational in the 1970s was computerized axial tomography (CAT), wherein transmission of X-rays through the patient were made to produce detailed cross-sections, which were then computer-processed to produce a three-dimensional picture. The latest machines employ continuously rotating gentries and table movements, scan in a spiral fashion and sweep an X-ray beam through a volume of tissue to produce high-resolution images of thirty cross-sections in thirty seconds. This high speed of scanning allows the mapping of an injected contrast agent through blood vessels and into organs and tumors within organs. The CT scan has made diagnosis easier. It is non-invasive, yet the radiation hazards of repeated scans though small, cannot be ignored. It allows interventional procedures like drainage of a deep-seated abscess, biopsy of tissues, embolization of bleeding vessels—all minimally invasive techniques, causing minimal trauma to the human body.

The CT scanner was soon followed by the positron emission transaxial tomography (PETT) scanner. This technique dispensed with X-rays and relied on radioactive emissions that help study brain activity. Patients are injected with radioactive glucose, which is taken up differentially in different parts of the brain, depending on the function and activity level of different areas of the brain. An analysis of different patterns of uptake gives an index of function rather than structure. Diagnosis of functional changes in psychiatric disorders, strokes and other neurological problems has become easier, and these problems are now better understood.

A recent novel technique is the magnetic resonance imaging (MRI) technique, which examines a patient with special sequences of radio pulses in a strong magnetic field. This provides images of the distribution of water and the chemical environment within the area scanned. The strong magnetic fields necessary for this imaging technique are provided by superconducting magnets of enormous size and power. MRI scans are of great use for the diagnosis of problems within the brain, spinal cord, as also of pathologies in the spine, joints and the musculo-skeletal system.

There is an unfortunate aspect to the newer technologies of imaging. They have become a status symbol for every hospital—as though a hospital that does not have a CT scan or MRI machine ceases to be a hospital. These glittering machines of the late twentieth century have unfortunately become the altars at which the newer generations of doctors are taught to worship.

73 Advances in Surgery

The advances in surgery in the twentieth century, particularly in its last sixty years have been phenomenal. Today, the surgeon reigns supreme. The operation theatre is the temple of medicine, the surgeon the high priest who presides over the rituals and the drama that go on within. There is no diseased organ or organ system within the body inaccessible to the surgeon's skill.

The day of the general surgeon is drawing to a close; it is the specialist surgeon who dominates the field. Urogenital surgery, abdominal and gastrointestinal surgery, cancer surgery, thoracic surgery, vascular surgery, cardiac surgery, neurosurgery, orthopaedic surgery and plastic surgery are some of the special fields into which surgery has ramified. To trace the history of advances in each of these special fields is outside the scope of this book. A few great landmarks in some chosen fields will be touched upon.

The breakthrough in thoracic surgery was difficult. In the early third of the twentieth century, tuberculosis was rampant in the West and there were many who felt that the best way to defeat pulmonary tuberculosis was to cut it out with a knife. Carlo Forlanini (1847–1918) of Pavia, attempted the first artificially-induced pneumothorax in a patient with cavitative tuberculosis in 1888. The rationale was to 'relax' the cavity by partially collapsing the diseased lung. 'Resting' the lung could promote healing of the cavity and of tuberculosis. A more radical surgical approach termed thoracoplasty was to remove the posterior portions of the second to the seventh ribs, thus enabling partial collapse of the lung on the affected side. This again promoted healing of cavities in tuberculosis. Ferdinand Sauerbuch (1875–1951), professor at Berlin's Charité Hospital, pioneered experimental work on thoracic surgery. In 1904, he devised a negative pressure chamber, which could hold an operation table, the patient and the surgical team. The purpose of the negative chamber was to prevent the lung from collapsing when the chest was opened at surgery. By 1920, with new techniques and improved anaesthesia, thoracoplasty came into vogue, the surgery being performed in the usual operation theatre. The apparatus for artificial pneumothorax (the instillation of air between two pleural surfaces), which was cumbersome to start with, was also simplified and the procedure could now be easily performed at the bedside by a physician.

The next advance in thoracic surgery was resection of part or the whole of the lung. The pioneer was Evarts Graham (1883–1957), in Washington, who first performed resections for lung cancer. Increasing skill and practice allowed not only lobectomies (removal of a lobe of the lung), but also pneumonectomies (removal of the whole lung) and segmental resections (removal of a segment of a lobe) to be performed. Thoracic surgery came of use not only in lung cancer, but also in other lung tumours, in tuberculosis and in suppurative lung diseases. However the earlier optimism of effecting a cure in tuberculosis and cancer through surgery gave way to increasing disillusionment; neither tuberculosis nor cancer would allow an easy conquest.

Perhaps the greatest success story of surgery in the twentieth century was in the domain of cardiovascular disease, a domain that seemed to offer insurmountable obstacles to a successful surgical approach. The heart was the last bastion that held out against the surgeon, the only unconquered terrain that the surgeon as yet had not trod upon. A pioneer in reconstructive vascular surgery was Alexis Carrel (1877–1948), a surgeon from Lyons, in France. He perfected the finesse of his surgical skills by taking lessons from a lacemaker. Carrel replaced a piece of the aortic wall (of an aneurysm) with a fragment from another artery or vein. In 1910, he demonstrated the technique of transplanting an entire vessel, joining the cut ends to the recipient vessel with sutures that did not impinge on the inner lining of the vessel wall. The lethal complication of thrombosis within the lumen of the vessel was thus prevented. His work in the anastomosis of vessel walls laid the foundation for transplant surgery in the years to come. Alexis Carrel also made the crucial observation that animals grafted with their own organs survived; donor grafts of other animals were rejected. This led to intense research into the cause of rejection and into the means by which rejection could be overcome. Alexis Carrel thus paved the way for transplant surgery.

Heart surgery advanced slowly but surely. The two World Wars gave surgeons a great deal of experience in the suturing of stab wounds in the heart. The mortality was formidable, but was reduced significantly during the Second World War, with the advent of better anaesthesia and the use of sulpha drugs and penicillin to fight infection. The major impetus to heart surgery as mentioned in chapter 66, was through the discovery of catheterization of the heart, pioneered by Werner Forssmann in 1929 and by André Cournand in 1940.

The first acquired valvular defect that was surgically corrected was mitral stenosis, an important sequel to rheumatic fever. In mitral stenosis there is a narrowing of the valve between the left atrium and the left ventricle, causing a back pressure to be built up within the pulmonary circulation. Breathlessness, cough, haemoptysis and increasing tiredness are features of mitral stenosis. In 1925, Henry Souttar (1875–1964) reported an operation on a patient who had been diagnosed as suffering from mitral stenosis. Though his diagnosis proved wrong, he observed that he could insert a finger through the mitral valve and suggested that this technique could be used to widen a narrowed mitral orifice. Twenty-three years later in 1948, a Boston surgeon Dwight Harken, dilated a stenosed mitral valve with his finger and with a small knife attached to his finger. Increasingly refined techniques came into being, culminating in the open commissurotomy of the stenosed mitral valve, with the patient on by-pass. Simultaneously, valvular stenosis of the other valves of the heart came under successful attack.

The most significant landmark in cardiovascular surgery was the correction of congenital cyanotic heart disease. Most 'blue babies' (so called because of their cyanosis), died in infancy or at a very young age, the cyanosis being due to congenital defects within the chambers of the heart and the vessels arising from them, so that venous blood mixed with arterial blood. The commonest and most important congenital cyanotic heart disease was the Tetralogy of Fallot, described in 1888 by Etienne-Louis Fallot, professor of anatomical pathology at Marseilles, France. The Tetralogy of Fallot had four major defects—a tightly narrowed pulmonary valve, a thickened (hypertrophied) right ventricular wall which had to pump blood through this narrow orifice, a 'hole' between the left and right ventricle, and an 'over-riding' aorta, which was so displaced that it received blood from both the right ventricle and the left ventricle. The net result of these defects was the circulation of very poorly oxygenated blood to the tissues and the presence of a bluish tinge to the skin and mucosa (cyanosis). Death occurred at an early age.

It took the vision of a physician and the skill and daring of a surgeon to help solve this problem. The physician was Helen Taussig (1898–1986). As she was a woman, she was refused entry to the Harvard and Boston universities; and so she joined John Hopkins Medical School in 1921. She became a paediatric cardiologist, a speciality in its infancy. Taussig visited Maude Abbot of Canada's McGill University, who was a world authority on congenital heart disease and who on the basis of 1,000 dissections had published a classic, *Congenital Cardiac Diseases*. Helen Taussig became an expert in the diagnosis of congenital heart disease. She made the important observation that patients with the Tetralogy of Fallot, who also had a persistent patent ductus arteriosus (a vessel connecting the aorta to the pulmonary artery in foetal life, but which normally closes soon after birth), did better than the usual patients with just the Tetralogy of Fallot. The ductus allowed blood to bypass the narrowed pulmonary valve and allowed better blood flow to the lungs. Taussig believed that the answer to the usual patient with Tetralogy of Fallot was to create an artificial ductus between the aorta and the pulmonary artery.

The skill and daring for the surgical procedure came from Alfred Blalock (1899–1964), chairman of the John Hopkins department of surgery. Blalock's assistant was a black man, Vivian Thomas, who carried out 200 animal experiments, establishing a method of attaching the subclavian artery to the pulmonary artery. Blalock had assisted at only a few of these experiments. The day of judgement dawned on 29 November 1944. Fifteen month old Eilen Saxon weighing just 9.2 lb and suffering from the Tetralogy of Fallot was wheeled into the theatre. She was blue, feeble and near death. A true to life drama was now enacted, with Blalock operating, Thomas close at hand to advise and Taussig looking anxiously and hoping that her views would pass the test of practicality. The child hovered between life and death for two weeks, her lungs repeatedly going into oedema because of the extra blood that suddenly began to flow through them. She slowly improved and was discharged on 25 January 1945.

Blalock operated on two other children and in February 1945, Blalock and Taussig published their pioneering results in the *Journal of the American Medical Association*. By 1950, Blalock and his co-workers performed over a thousand such operations with a mortality of just 5 per cent. Other centres in the world followed suit. The Blalock-Taussig operation saved thousands of children from certain death till the advent of open-heart surgery, when a total correction of the defects in the heart became possible.

Blalock was now feted all over the world, but Taussig had to wait another fourteen years before being appointed professor at John Hopkins Hospital. She became the first woman president of the American Heart Association and was elected to the National Academy of Sciences. Her text, *Congenital Malformations of the Heart* remains a classic to this very day. In 1967, Helen Taussig undertook investigations into the horrendous congenital deformities caused by the drug thalidomide in Germany. She was instrumental in having the drug banned for all time. Helen Taussig continued her research into congenital heart disease till three days before her eighty-eighth birthday, when she was killed in a road accident.

The correction of Fallot's Tetralogy was followed by the correction of even more complex congenital abnormalities within the heart. The trail-blazing triumph in this field was due to a combination of technology and science which saw the birth of the heart-lung machine, surgical skill, improved anaesthesia and improved post-operative care. An important adjunct to anaesthesia in heart surgery was the use of hypothermia. Cooling the core temperature of the body reduced the oxygen needs of tissues, particularly the brain, which otherwise could not withstand oxygen deprivation for more than three or four minutes without death to the brain cells. Hypothermia thus allowed greater time to the surgeon to correct deformities within the heart. Yet hypothermia was not enough for lengthy operative procedures to correct complex abnormalities within the heart. John Gibbon (1903–1970) in Philadelphia, solved this problem in 1950 by devising a heart-lung machine. This machine would do the work of the heart and lungs, pumping oxygenated blood through the circulation while bypassing the heart, so that the surgeon could operate on the heart at leisure for a much longer period of time. Now came the era of open-heart surgery. After many animal experiments, John Gibbon operated in 1952, on his first human patient, a fifteen-month old baby who unfortunately died. On 5 May 1953, he operated on an eighteen-year old girl with a hole in her heart (a septal defect), connecting her to the heart-lung machine for forty-five minutes. The operation was successful and the patient survived. Open-heart surgery soon became a rage all over the West and spread to other parts of the world, including India and the Far East.

The surgeons now addressed their skills to replacing diseased heart valves. In 1952, Charles A. Hufnagel (1916–1989) inserted a plastic valve to replace a diseased aortic valve. Soon prosthetic valves of different shapes and mechanisms were devised to replace not only the aortic valve, but also the mitral and even the tricuspid valves. Patients with prosthetic valves needed to take anticoagulants for life—else the blood would clot on the valves. This led to experiments with biografts—valves from human cadavers and from pericardial tissue. Biografts were successfully used as valves, though their life span was significantly shorter than prosthetic valves.

In 1967, René Favaloro (born 1923), a cardiovascular surgeon at the Cleveland Clinic, Ohio, bypassed for the first time a blocked coronary artery using a venous graft from the leg vein. One end of the graft was sutured to an opening in the aorta and the other to the coronary artery distal to the block. Coronary artery bypass surgery now became the rage, first in America, then in Europe and finally all over the world. The enthusiasm of the early years is now tempered with both circumspection and disappointment. It has been realized by most discerning physicians that coronary artery bypass surgery is at best a plumbing job. Though arterial grafts (the internal mammary artery is the one most commonly used today) remain patent for over twelve years, bypass surgery provides symptomatic relief from angina and in selected cases prolongs life. It cannot alter the natural history of coronary artery disease, which seems inbuilt within each patient afflicted with the problem. Unfortunately, the rash of coronary artery bypass surgeries continues unabated all over the world, including India. Not uncommonly, for several reasons, these surgeries are performed even in situations where the patient is best managed on medical lines. Surgery can only bring disrepute on itself if this attitude stands uncorrected.

Vascular surgery progressed side by side with cardiac surgery. Diseased vessels which were either blocked or were abnormally dilated (aneurysmal) were excised and replaced by dacron grafts, which restored the integrity of the vessel and established good blood flow. Limbs threatened with gangrene could thus be saved. Michael DeBakey of Houston, Texas, was one of the pioneers of both cardiac and vascular surgery. He devised techniques for the surgical approach and management of dissecting aneurysm of the aorta. This catastrophe, characterized by a spreading tear in the aortic wall, almost always caused death without appropriate surgical intervention. DeBakey, still active in his late eighties, is an outstanding example of a thinking surgeon who has pushed back the frontiers of cardiovascular surgery.

Surgery usually brings to mind the image of a scalpel and of the nimble use of fingers to cut and excise. But there is an equally important aspect of surgery which broke new ground and gained great recognition in the twentieth century. This new speciality was reconstructive surgery.

Reconstructive surgery or plastic surgery finds mention in ancient Chinese medicine and in the works of the great surgeon Susruta, in the ayurvedic system of Indian medicine. Reconstructive surgery can take many forms. It includes, for example, the correction of congenital defects like hare-lip and cleft palate, replacement of extensive skin loss in burns, reconstructing the face after facial trauma, or following the ravages of diseases like leprosy. Reconstructive surgery is of essence after mutilating surgical procedures in cancer, particularly those involving the head, face and neck. Cosmetic surgery for aesthetic purposes has a great market in the West and is becoming increasingly popular all over the world.

Skin transplants have been used since ancient times. Jacques Reverdin (1842–1908) in Geneva, laid thin slivers of skin on the surface of a large wound. These slivers formed fresh islands of skin which at places merged together to cover the wound. It was however the horrors of the First World War which advanced the cause of reconstructive surgery and the use of skin transplants to treat facial wounds. Harold Gillies (1882–1960) was the hero of this battle and a pioneering plastic surgeon; he set up a plastic surgery unit in Aldershot, South England. He recognized the importance of reconstructing deformities caused by burns and wounds to restore a patient's appearance to as normal as possible. After the battle of the Somme in 1916, he personally dealt with over 2,000 soldiers with dreadful facial injuries and damage. His war work brought him no recognition, but he suddenly came into prominence when he was rushed to Copenhagen to treat over two dozen seamen who had been burned in an accident.

In 1932, Gillies hired McIndoe as his assistant; a distant cousin who had trained at Mayo Clinic in Rochester. McIndoe learnt his art, craft and science from Gillies, and in 1936 replaced Gillies as the consultant in plastic surgery to the Royal Air Force. McIndoe shortly before the outbreak of the Second World War, founded a unit at Queen Victoria Hospital in East Grinstead, in Sussex. The war erupted; the Battle of Britain in 1940 brought in over 4,000 casualties with ghastly burns and injuries, chiefly produced by ignited high octane fuel. McIndoe felt that 'plastic surgery' did not fully depict the basic objective in the treatment of such injuries, which required years and often dozens of operative procedures to rectify. He therefore coined the term 'reconstructive surgery'. For serious facial injuries, he used Gillies' tubed pedicle graft—a large piece of skin from the donor site which remains attached by a stalk to ensure a blood supply till a new one establishes itself. This was a laborious, time-consuming procedure. On one occasion, a nosocomial streptococcal infection swept the ward; the pedicle grafts were found to be very susceptible to infection and did not serve their purpose. McIndoe who was a rather artistic surgeon, changed to the cutting and use of free skin grafts, which took more easily and quickly. Undoubtedly it was not just his technical skill but his approach to surgery and the attitude towards his patients that stamped him as a great surgeon. He communicated with them and won them over to apply the procedures he contemplated. His ward had the radio and the loudspeaker on at full blast to take the men's minds off their injuries and to drown out the groans of those having their dressings changed in salt baths.

In 1942, those who had been through McIndoe's ward decided to form a society club. They called themselves the Maxillonians, since the unit was officially a maxillo-facial unit. A few months later, a badly burnt RAF pilot, waiting for one of his innumerable reconstructive operations was heard to murmur, "We are not fliers any more; we are nothing but a plastic surgeon's guinea pigs." The Society now named itself 'McIndoe's Guinea Pigs' and there were 600 such 'guinea pigs', belonging to sixteen different nationalities. McIndoe was voted president for life of this club, which continued to meet long after the war ended.

After successful skin transplants, the next objective was organ transplants. Organs such as the kidneys, tissues such as skin and bone marrow may be removed from an animal and replaced in the same body, though not necessarily in the correct anatomical position—these are auto-transplants or replants. Alternatively, they may be taken from one animal and transplanted into another animal of the same species—these are homo-transplants. When taken from one animal and transplanted into another of a different species—they constitute hetero-transplants. Experimental work was concentrated on homo-transplants. The pioneers of modern transplant surgery in the twentieth century were surgeon Alexis Carrel and physiologist Charles Guthrie. Carrel's new suturing technique permitted vascular anastomosis without the danger of thrombus formation at the site of anastomosis. This was the prime requisite and the springboard of all future transplant surgeries. Carrel and Guthrie were able to show that technically, transplants of organs, tissues and limbs were possible. Remarkably enough, these transplants could function even if there were no nervous connections. Carrel received recognition and fame for his work; unfortunately Guthrie's contribution received little attention. Though Carrel successfully transplanted kidneys, heart and other organs like the spleen, after a very brief period the transplant would die. It was as if the recipient body sensed the transplant as an invading alien and 'rejected' it. The first three decades of the twentieth century were frustrating and unpleasant for transplant surgery. Yet there were glimpses of hope. In 1905, Eduard Zirm in Olmutz, Moravia, performed the first successful corneal transplant. The technique was forgotten for fifty years before it was revived and practised all over the world. In 1912, Guthrie grafted the head of a puppy to the neck of an adult dog, which lived for several hours after surgery. The Russian surgeon Vladimir Demikhov repeated the experiment after 35 years, the puppy's head now remaining alive for four weeks. These feats of technical bravado did not solve the basic problem of incompatibility between the tissues and organs of animals of the same species and the rejection of these organs by the recipient of the transplant.

An understanding of the mechanism of the rejection of transplants was provided in the 1940s by Professor McFarlane Burnet, from Melbourne, Australia, and Peter Medawar (1915–1987), London University's professor of zoology, working at the Natural Institute for Medical Research in London. Burnet proposed that the body's immune system was formed *in utero,* when as a developing foetus it 'learns' to produce on demand a very wide range of antibodies. Antibody production is stimulated when the need arises; also as mentioned earlier, each body has a recognition of its own self, but regards any tissue, even of the same species as an 'alien'. The immune system is activated and 'rejects' this alien tissue.

Peter Medawar working with skin grafts, showed that if an animal received more than one graft from the same donor, the second graft was destroyed far more quickly than the first. He also showed that if the recipient was injected with white blood cells from a prospective donor before grafting, the survival time of the graft was markedly shortened. The skin and leucocytes shared common antigens and the prior injection of leucocytes had stimulated antibodies within the recipient with a quicker destruction of the graft.

This basic understanding of the rejection phenomenon now led to attempts to combat it. In 1951, Medawar tried the use of cortisone, an immunosuppressive drug, in the hope of suppressing the host's immune response. Cortisone was found to be partially effective. In 1959, a new drug, azathioprine was found to be a better immunosuppressant. It was as late as the 1970s that cyclosporin was discovered—this ranks as the best immunosuppressant to date and it paved the way for increasingly successful transplant surgery.

The concentration of medical science was initially devoted to the transplantation of the kidney. Chronic renal disease with renal failure was common, invariably progressive, leading to a poor quality of life and to death. The human body was endowed with two kidneys, so that a live donor could donate one kidney, without prejudice to health. Also, a kidney was easy to remove from a donor and the technique of transplanting this organ into the recipient did not possess formidable difficulties.

Before kidney transplants came into being, Williem Kolff in the Netherlands in 1944, devised the first 'artificial kidney' or the dialysis machine to be successfully used on humans. In essence this machine consisted of a special dialysing membrane through which blood from a large artery of the patient was made to pass. The dialysing membrane was bathed in a liquid dialysate. The waste products within the blood passed through the dialysing membrane and the purified blood was returned to the patient. Initially the dialysis machine was used for patients with acute renal failure to buy time, hoping for the kidneys to start functioning again. By the 1960s, modifications within the dialysis machine by Belding Scribner allowed patients with chronic renal failure to go on long-term dialysis.

Human kidney transplants were tried in the United States since 1951, but failed again and again. There were two reasons for this. The first was the need for the tissue compatibility of the donor to match that of the recipient. Technically speaking, the chances of rejection were significantly reduced if the histocompatibility group of the donor was the same as that of the recipient. It was not enough for the blood group to match; it was equally necessary for the histocompatibility groups to match. It was only when this fact was realized that successful transplants became possible. The second reason for failure was that in the early fifties, potent immunosuppressant drugs capable of suppressing the host's immune response had yet to be discovered. Even so, the first successful human kidney transplant was performed on identical twins in December 1954, in Boston, by J. Harrison and Joseph Murray. The donor kidney was transplanted into a twenty-four year old man who was dying of terminal chronic renal disease. The healthy donor kidney was donated by his identical twin brother, so that immunological problems of rejection did not arise. Murray was awarded the Nobel Prize for this technical feat.

There was now literally a competition in organ transplantation. In 1963, James Hardy performed the first human lung transplant. The donor lung came from a patient who had died of a heart attack; the recipient was a middle-aged man dying of lung cancer. The transplant functioned for 18 days—the patient ultimately dying of renal failure.

The ultimate in transplant surgery in the sixties was a heart transplant. Experimental research in the United States proceeded at a furious pace. Technical difficulties apart, a major hurdle was that the tissues of the heart deteriorated within minutes of death, so that the organ had to be removed and transplanted with great speed, with no time for tissue typing. Norman Shumway of Stanford University, California, was a pioneer in the experimental work on heart transplants. His major break-through in 1961 was to devise an improved surgical technique to help nourish the heart more efficiently. After surgery, Shumway used a machine to keep the recipient's circulation going till the new heart became slowly accustomed to take over. His experimental dogs with heart transplants lived as long as twenty-one days, during which period they functioned normally. Death was ultimately due to rejection of the transplant.

James Hardy, of lung transplant fame, attempted the first human heart transplant on 23 January 1964 at the Mississippi Medical Centre in the United States. A sixty-eight year old man was admitted to the medical centre with advanced heart failure. Hardy put him on a heart-lung machine in preparation for the transplant. The donor was to be a young man suffering from irreversible brain damage. The plan went awry, for the prospective donor hung on to life and the prospective recipient's heart suddenly failed. Hardy was not to be outdone; ethical considerations apart, he transplanted a chimpanzee's heart, which was too small to take on the circulatory load, and the patient died. Four more years went by before the world witnessed the first successful human heart transplant surgery. The event took place in South Africa at the Groote Schuur Hospital in

Capetown, on 3 December 1967, and the star was the forty-five year old surgeon Christian Barnard. He had worked at Shumway's laboratory at Stanford and was witness to the pioneering experimental heart transplant work directed by Shumway, before returning to the Groote Schuur Hospital in Capetown. The donor heart was from a young woman Denise Darvall, who was certified brain dead after a car accident. The recipient was Barnard's patient Louis Washkansky, who had suffered several heart attacks, was hopelessly incapacitated and had perhaps a few weeks to live. The donor heart functioned well; Louis Washkansky improved to start with, but died of pneumonia eighteen days after surgery.

The next heart transplant was expectedly by Norman Shumway at Stanford University, California in January 1968, followed by Denton Cooley at Houston, Texas, in May 1968. Ambition, fame and fortune combined to produce a rash of heart transplant operations, first in America and then in many centres in Europe. The mortality and morbidity was forbidding to start with. However, by the mid-eighties; 75 per cent of heart transplant patients lived for a year and nearly two-thirds survived for five years. Lung transplants and heart transplants were now followed by heart–lung transplants where the heart and lungs were transplanted into the same patient. Severe bilateral lung diseases in the form of end-stage pulmonary fibrosis, severe emphysema and cystic fibrosis were prime indications for heart-lung transplants. Liver transplants for inoperable hepatic tumours, acute fulminant hepatitis or severe progressive liver cell dysfunction as in advanced cirrhosis of the liver, required great technical expertise and after-care, and are now performed in large numbers at various centres in the world.

A few surgeons ran amuck—transplants of many different organs in the same patient were attempted, sometimes prolonging life but at a terrific cost of human suffering. To many it became obvious that it was not always patient care that mattered most; it was more the gratification of an overweening ambition to display surgical prowess and to win acclaim from a world increasingly wedded to technology than to humanity.

Microsurgery (surgery performed with the use of an operating microscope) came into its own in the sixties. The magnification thus achieved allowed delicate surgery on fine structures, impossibly difficult without a microscope. The first successful replantation of a severed limb took place in Boston in 1962. A twelve-year old boy lost an arm below the shoulder in an accident. The boy and the arm were taken to the Massachusetts General Hospital; the arm was packed in a solution of ice and salt and then grafted successfully on to the boy. A few months later, surgeons reconstructed the nerves to the limb. Within two years the boy recovered full use of the limb, including the hand and could even lift weights with it.

A far less glamorous, much less costly but of far greater benefit to man than the organ transplants described above was surgery for replacement of the hip, developed in the 1960s by John Charnley(1911–1982), at the Manchester Royal Infirmary. Severe hip joint disease can cause crippling, unbearable pain, particularly on walking. Attempts at hip replacement in severely diseased joints commenced at the turn of the twentieth century, but were soon abandoned. With the advent of acrylics, plastic and biologically inert material before the Second World War, the idea of hip replacement became increasingly feasible. However problems of materials, fixation and design of prosthesis thwarted the ingenuity of all surgeons. It was John Charnley who came up with a solution, announcing his operative technique for low-friction arthroplasty in the Lancet in 1961. Charnley was both an engineer and an orthopaedic surgeon. His low-friction arthroplasty involved using different materials for the femoral head and the acetabular cap. Friction between the two ould be kept to a minimum if one material was hard and the other soft and smooth. For the femoral head he used stainless steel which could withstand the load the femur has to bear; for the acetabular cap he used polytetrafluoroethylene or teflon. Teflon is a low-friction plastic, but Charnley noted that it wore off easily and did not last long. In 1962, he developed a high-density polythene which caused more friction but lasted much longer than teflon. Charnley bonded both the cap and the shaft of the prosthesis into position using acrylic cement. This produced an efficient bond between the prosthesis and the patient's own bone, preventing loosening of the artificial joint.

Infection was a common cause of failure in the early years of hip replacement surgery. Scrupulous asepsis, the prophylactic use of antibiotics at surgery and a few days after surgery reduced the infection rate drastically. Thousands of patients all over the world have benefited for many years with hip replacement surgery, their crippling pain completely relieved and the quality of life vastly improved.

In the 1980s, a new form of surgery termed minimally invasive surgery came into being. It was the combination of technology and technical and surgical skill which allowed the practice of surgery to be less invasive to the human body. There were two advances that made this surgery possible. The first was the refinement in diagnostic techniques through the use of the ultrasound, CT scan and magnetic resonance imaging (MRI). The other was the introduction of endoscopes, with associated gadgetry and instruments, including the use of laser energy to replace the surgical scalpel. The historical use of the endoscope dates back to 1853 with the development of a rigid instrument to visualize the urethra and the urinary bladder. For more than a century, endoscopes were inserted through the natural body orifices—the mouth, anus and vagina. A great advance was the introduction of flexible fibreoptic endoscopes which increased both manoeuverability and vision. Extra channels were now introduced into the instruments, providing means to inflate an organ with air or carbon dioxide to ensure better vision, and to flush and irrigate the area under vision. Working channels were also created to allow instruments, snares and coagulation devices to arrest bleeding, and fibre sources to allow the use of laser energy for the removal of tumors or for treating atherosclerotic lesions.

Percutaneous procedures for transluminal coronary angioplasty (PTCA), through the use of balloon-tipped catheters, have already been mentioned earlier. Steel or plastic tubes of varying sizes can also be inserted under angioscopic guidance, as mentioned earlier, to prevent the collapse of vessels. Blocked ducts, as for example in the biliary system, can be stented and kept open through endoscopic guidance. Self-expanding stents, or even vascular prosthesis can now be introduced under specific indications through the skin or through minimal surgical intervention. Drainage of deep-seated abscesses and cysts, and biopsy of pathologies within an abdominal organ can be done non-invasively with the help of accurate localization through ultrasound techniques and other imaging procedures.

Extracorporeal shock wave lithotripsy (ESWL) was introduced in the early 1980s to treat urinary stones. Shock waves are beamed at these stones from outside the body, causing them to disintegrate into very small pieces that can be easily passed through the urine. Under certain indications, a similar technique has been tried to disintegrate biliary stones and even pancreatic calculi.

The scope of endoscopic surgery of the upper and lower GI tract has increased immensely Palliative relief of obstruction to the bile duct and to the pancreatic duct from malignant tumor through the introduction of stents is a commonplace technique in many centres of the world.

Even more recent has been the introduction of laparoscopic surgery—again a triumph o technology and surgical skill. An operating laparoscope is introduced through holes within the abdomen, the inside of which is viewed on a video screen. Removal of the gall bladder through the laparoscope—laparoscopic cholecystectomy, is now performed in all good centres of the world. Video-assisted thoracoscopy has enabled the surgeons to perform major thoracic operations, like for example, removal of a localised tumor or even the lobe of a lung, without having to open the thorax. The laparoscope in gynaecology, has extended diagnostic facilities and allowed gynaecological work through minimally invasive surgery, such as in the operative management of endometriosis or in the removal of benign tumors. Besides laparoscopic cholecystectomy, removal of a spleen, kidney or stomach and repair of a hiatus hernia are all done through a laparoscope in special centres of laparoscopic surgery. The advantages of laparoscopic surgery are—less pain, a shorter stay in hospital, a quicker return to work and less trauma to the patient. There are some who consider this form of surgery the next best achievement after anaesthesia and asepsis. There are many who feel that this is an exaggeration. We are too close to these events to judge their significance in history. Time and experience will remain the arbiters of better judgement.

74 A Perspective of Contemporary Medicine

No one should approach the temple of science with the soul of a money changer.

Sir Thomas Browne

Medicine was born with the awakening of consciousness in the magic-governed shamans of the primitive world and in the struggle between priest-physicians and demons of disease in ancient Sumer and Egypt. Over 5,000 years of history, medicine evolved with man—strengthened by observation, experience and judgement, influenced by religion, faith, philosophy and economics, and enriched above all by science. The advance of science and technology has been stupendous. Over the last one hundred years, science has changed the world and changed medicine with it. Immunology, genetics and molecular biology, which are the frontiers of contemporary medicine owe their success largely to the advances in the natural sciences and to technology.

Medicine and surgery are today capable of performing mind-boggling feats deemed incredible half a century ago. Many a life has been saved, many marvels performed and many indeed must have reaped the benefits from the knowledge and power that a revolutionized medical science has to offer. Yet paradoxically, Man and Medicine stand together on the threshold of the twenty-first century, sharing an uncertain future. There is a seething discontent against medicine and the medical profession among lay people—a discontent which is also shared by many within the profession. And why should this be so? The mechanization of medicine has robbed it of its essence, its humanism. All through the ages—from Imhotep, Hippocrates, Charaka and Susruta of antiquity to Paré, Jenner, Hunter, Lister, Pasteur, Osler and several others—medicine meant care, compassion and a special empathy for the patient. Whatever garb medicine assumed, whatever philosophy it followed, whatever its blemishes and faults, human qualities lay entrenched at its very core, central to its being and existence. The essence of these human qualities expressed in a single word is humanity. Humanity is the sensibility which enables a physician to feel for the distress and suffering of a patient, prompting him to provide relief. True humanity in a physician is a fount of sympathy and care. The advent of machines, sophisticated gadgets and increasing technology has depersonalized medicine, lessened its humanity and adversely affected the doctor–patient relationship. Patients today are often made to relate to machines than to human beings and doctors relate more to sophisticated gadgetry than to patients.

A companion-in-arms of increasing mechanization is increasing super-specialization. A super-specialist is of unquestionable importance in certain well-defined situations and can be an invaluable asset to modern medicine. But an over-enthusiastic encouragement of super-specialities is self-defeating, for it negates the holistic aspect of medicine. Medicine cannot be compartmentalized. No organ functions in splendid isolation, for the human system is a mysterious, yet integrated whole. A poorly trained or self-proclaimed specialist (and there are many such in India), or the one who lacks the necessary background and experience in general medicine and surgery ignores this basic concept. He tends to view medicine with myopic eyes, loses his perspective and his sense of priorities, and can thereby discredit medicine. Contemporary medicine often presents the tragicomic scene of a critically ill individual being looked after by a number of super-specialists, aided and abetted by the trappings of technology and science. Each specialist concentrates solely on his small exclusive field of expertise; the overall aspect of disease and of the patient as a human being suffering from disease is then easily lost.

To the mechanization of medicine is added the sin of commercialization. Money is increasingly a driving force in today's medicine. Its acquisition through the charging of unreasonable fees, even from the poor and unaffording goes against its basic tenets. The healing art in many parts of the world is more a business than a profession. Even worse, it is a business that has become increasingly corrupt. What is more corrupt than the practice of doctors who on purpose refer unsuspecting, vulnerable patients from one specialist to another for no reason other than profit? Or what is more corrupt than the nefarious practice of commissions demanded by general practitioners from a specialist to whom a patient is referred? Corrupt practices such as these are commonplace in the larger cities of India and perhaps occur with varying frequency and in various guises in other parts of the world.

One other major drawback of contemporary medicine is its crippling expense in relation to investigations, treatment and the cost of hospitalization. This is partly due to the fact that the physician of today has forgotten the art of medicine and remains deeply immersed in its science. His rapport is with machines and not with patients; it is technology that dictates his course of action and not his clinical judgement. History-taking becomes a neglected art; he forgets to use his senses—his eyes, ears and hands, but remembers numbers, equations and formulae. Expensive investigations and expensive modes of treatment often result when simple tests and simpler measures would have easily sufficed.

In the West, the escalating cost of medicine has prompted the state or insurance companies to exert a control over its practice. This is unfortunate for several reasons. The control over medicine should come from within; it would hurt the practice of medicine if it is forced from without. In the poor countries of the world, where the state has by and large abjured its responsibilities for patient care and where insurance for illnesses is meagre and unsatisfactory, the financial burden often falls directly on the patient and his relatives. This is a cruel burden that can reduce a family to penury and despair.

A seething antagonism against contemporary medicine has led both to increasing litigation against doctors and a search for relief through 'alternative medicine'. Homoeopathy, ayurvedic medicine, acupuncture, herbal and folk medicine, spiritual healing, a new form of the 'laying of hands' called Reiki, all have an increasing demand today. Special centres both in the West and the East, have been set up to scientifically assess the value of some of these alternative methods of medicine. The modern physician in his love for science and technology, has forgotten to appreciate that faith and nature are two of the greatest healing forces that can mend and restore the mind and body. He also needs to be reminded that ancient systems of medicine like Ayurveda, herbal and folk medicine have stood the test of time and are still effectively used by millions all over the world.

Institutionalized medicine has also contributed to malpractices. It is a matter of prestige for every hospital in the poorer countries of the world to be equipped with the latest in western technology and science. Yet rapid advances in medicine render most machines obsolete within five to at the most ten years. If an institution or hospital is to profit after spending a fortune on machines, it has to feed the machines. Patients become the fodder for these machines. If an audit were carried out on the cost-effectiveness of modern day investigations in medicine, the result would be shocking.

Perhaps the underlying explanation for the decline in the ethics of contemporary medicine is a change in the sense of values in our world. A burning desire for material gain and wealth at any cost dominates life today. It is indeed difficult for any profession to remain an island of high-mindedness and virtue when surrounded by a sea of filth and corruption. The island is first eroded and then swamped. But the medical profession has an ancient heritage to cherish and maintain. This is being slowly but increasingly realized all over the world and there is now a growing force imbued with a determination to uproot the canker eating into the heart of medicine.

Let us now examine the content of contemporary medicine. To an extent, it can claim credit for the eradication or near-extinction of many infectious diseases that prevailed at the outset of the industrial age in the West. Plague, cholera, smallpox, diphtheria, typhoid, tetanus, scarlet fever and poliomyelitis are some of the scourges that have been rendered practically extinct. Yet, victory over these diseases in the West has been more through effective preventive measures, rather than through drugs or the use of sophisticated gadgetry and technology. It is clean drinking water, good nutrition, improved housing, sanitation, hygiene, education and thriving economies that have led to the conquest of infectious diseases. Man was on the road to the conquest of age-old infections well before modern technology captured medicine. Perhaps the greatest gift of medicine to mankind is the discovery of vaccines to prevent disease. Outstanding among these discoveries is that of Edward Jenner in the prevention of smallpox.

It is of interest that tuberculosis was as much a scourge in Europe and in the United States in the nineteenth century as it is in India and other poor countries of the world today. Modern anti-tuberculosis drugs are effective and have reduced the incidence and mortality of tuberculosis. But the maximum decline in the disease occurred well before the introduction of anti-tuberculosis drugs, and even well before the first sanatorium opened to isolate patients with tuberculosis. That drugs alone are not enough is seen in the increasing incidence, morbidity and mortality of tuberculosis in India and Africa. These countries can never wipe out tuberculosis and numerous other infections without an improvement in their economies, their public health and education.

The above discussion should not detract from the merit of newly discovered drugs, effective antibiotics and the use of various medical and surgical procedures that have saved human lives, which would otherwise have been surely lost. Acute meningitis, infections of heart valves and acute septicaemia from fulminant organisms are just a few examples of diseases which had a universal mortality till the discoveries of modern medicine came into use. Transplant surgery, surgery on the heart for congenital and acquired diseases, thoracic surgery, neurosurgery and plastic surgery are all landmarks in the progress of medicine, science and technology, that evoke our unstinted admiration.

The world today, the West in particular, faces the 'modern epidemics' of coronary heart disease, chronic bronchitis, emphysema, hypertension, cancer, diabetes and an increasing incidence of mental disorders. Medicine does not know why many of these diseases occur; it offers relief but has no cure. Contemporary medicine has also no answer to the occurrence of the deadly new infections such as AIDS, or the deadly haemorrhagic viral infections, fortunately localized to a few parts of the world. It has also to contend with the recrudescence of old infections, such as tuberculosis and malaria.

The progress of medicine from ancient times to the present era is evident in the earlier chapters of this book. But there is a 'seamier' side to present-day progress, which has been eloquently stressed by Ivan Illich in his book, *Limits to Medicine*. Illich contends 'that the medical establishment has become a major threat to health'. To my mind, this is an overstatement, an exaggeration that is a travesty of truth. Yet his contention that the 'medicalization of life' has three major disadvantages does carry a germ of truth within it and needs careful consideration.

The first disadvantage is the production of 'clinical iatrogenesis' (*iatros* in Greek means 'physician'; *genesis* means 'to make'). Iatrogenic diseases in medicine are those produced by physicians either through treatment or investigations, or by the hospitals in which the patients are treated. But then, iatrogenic disease is as old as medicine. It has been an inseparable companion of medicine since antiquity. The pharmacopoeias up to the nineteenth century contained substances which must have done far more harm than good. As mentioned in earlier chapters, the frequent practice of blood-letting almost always hastened a patient's demise. The only excuse for iatrogenic disease in the earlier ages is that medicine then did not know that it could inflict harm. But today, we do know the potential iatrogenesis of medicine. Unfortunately, our awareness has not helped.

Contemporary medicine has indeed produced an epidemic of iatrogenesis, because the more potent the drug, the more sophisticated the gadgetry and the more invasive the procedures used in the diagnosis or management, the greater the risk of harm to patients. Yet, it will be impossible in the foreseeable future to separate the art and science of medicine completely from iatrogenesis. There is no drug worth the name which is totally free of side-effects. Yet dreadful illnesses often demand risky procedures or potent drugs with inherent toxicity to the human system. The practice of medicine forces a physician to take a balanced risk if a critically ill patient is to be salvaged. It is not just a knowledge of the science of medicine that determines this risk; it is also determined by experience, judgement and wisdom—it involves in equal measure, the art that constitutes medicine even today.

The second disadvantage of contemporary medicine is the production of 'social iatrogenesis', by which is meant the creation of an environment which no longer has the ability to allow people in society to look after themselves. People are thus hopelessly dependent on the medical system and the medical system functions in a manner to ensure that this remains so. The medicalization of life would prompt people to consume medicine and seek hospitalization or medical treatment for inadequate reasons. An encouragement to take recourse to institutionalized medicine perpetuates the stranglehold of the medical profession and medical institutions over society. This to an extent, is indeed true. It is being increasingly recognized both by the medical profession and by society at large. Almost certainly, the excessive dependence of society on institutionalized medicine is a passing phase and will be tempered by better judgement and by an increasing awareness of the need for a healthier relationship between the two. It must be remembered that the link between man and medicine is impossible to sever. Both are dependent on each other; it is important that neither takes advantage of the other.

The third disadvantage of contemporary medicine according to Illich, is the encouragement of a 'cultural iatrogenesis', whereby institutionalized medicine has sapped the ability of people to face the reality of suffering in life and the inevitability of death. This may be partly true in the West, but it is not so in India and in many other eastern countries. A patient's and for that matter a doctor's attitude to suffering, pain, approaching death and death itself is conditioned by socio-cultural and religious factors. Most people in the East accept that life cannot be divorced from pain and suffering, that we live within their midst, and that each is apportioned his or her share of pain and suffering in life. It is being increasingly recognized today, that modern medicine with its powerful technology should relieve all forms of suffering, but should refrain from prolonging the act of dying. Above all, it should prevent death from being lonely, gruesome, obscene, dehumanized and ruinous to the patient and his family.

The attitudes of contemporary medicine require a change, yet it must be remembered that it is society which has conditioned some of these attitudes. A great deal more is expected of medicine today than it can offer. The stupendous advances in medical science and the glamour and excitement of so-called miracle cures flashed across the world by the information media, have led people to believe that contemporary medicine is all-knowing, all-powerful and all-successful. This is unfortunately far from the truth. There are limits to medicine—today and in the foreseeable future. If one takes the sum total of all diseases, there are just a few which medicine can completely cure, though there are many which it can alleviate. Therefore the great expectations from medicine are unreal and unfulfilled. When people experience this fact personally, and also encounter the unseemly aspects of medicine with its escalating costs, it arouses disappointment, distrust and anger. The doctor–patient relationship which is the essence of medicine, stands inevitably poisoned.

The decline of values today is not restricted to medicine and the medical profession. It afflicts all professions and the whole of society, perhaps even to a greater extent than that observed in medicine. The frustration of patients and relatives is often translated into litigation and a demand for compensation. Not uncommonly this demand is motivated more by a greed for money than by a true sense of injured justice. To protect himself, the doctor falls back on defensive medicine. He over-investigates to ensure that he is not sued for missing out on rare disorders; he uses the more powerful weapons of medicine and science involving greater risks of iatrogenicity, when simpler ones would have sufficed. When faced with a life-threatening emergency, he would rather let the patient die than take the risk of doing a procedure or offering treatment, which though inherently risky constitutes the only hope to salvage life. He progressively divorces himself from all that really matters in medicine. This is not to excuse even in the slightest manner, malpractice, incompetence, callousness, or disregard for patient welfare, even in the presence of utmost provocation. These are infirmities, pock-marks that need to be wiped off the face of medicine. Yet it must be admitted that a healthy interaction and interrelation between medicine and society is a two-way, reciprocal affair. Both need to look at each other with fresh eyes, both need to communicate with each other if this indeed is to transpire.

In most countries of the world, disputes between doctors and patients are decided by duly constituted professional bodies or by courts of law. In India, the doctor is more often brought before a 'consumer court' for any alleged incompetence or offence. This is because the highest court of justice in the country has decreed that the practice of medicine is similar to a consumer industry and the service rendered by a doctor to a patient is akin to a 'consumer product'. Nothing in my opinion, could be further from the truth. It is patently absurd to equate the years of study, the knowledge, expertise, experience, wisdom and above all, the care lavished on a patient with a 'consumer product'. The doubts, anxieties, uncertainties, the sleepless nights, the anguish that goes into an irrevocable life or death decision are surely different from the gift-wrap paper and the consumer product enclosed within, however expensive this product may be. After all, is it not the human values of good medicine that distinguish it from a business or industry?

Sadly, the reason for this predicament, at least in India, lies chiefly with the medical profession. The crisis has arisen because of the attitudinal changes in modern-day medicine, described earlier in this chapter. It has been further accentuated by a lack of internal audit within the profession. The medical bodies that should adjudicate and mete out justice to both patients and doctors are seen by many to have not lived up to their responsibilities. Lacking internal control, a control is sought to be established from without. But in doing so, the courts in India have done a disservice to the profession and in the long run, to society, whose rights they are keen to protect. Their decision has lent legal sanctity to the concept of medicine being considered a business and the service of a doctor being akin to a consumer product. It has only served to freeze and perpetuate the unsatisfactory state of affairs and not improve them.

Contemporary medicine faces a special challenge in India and other Third World countries, as health problems in these countries are significantly different from those in the West. Infection and infectious diseases (with the sole exception of smallpox) are still as prevalent in these poor countries as they were in the West more than a hundred years ago. Poor nutrition and poverty form the backdrop against which many common diseases unfold. Unfortunately, India has the dubious distinction of also facing the 'new epidemics' prevalent today in the West—coronary heart disease, chronic bronchitis, cancer and diabetes, to name just a few. It is not that the science and technology incorporated in contemporary western medicine should be abandoned in the poor countries of the world. Their use must be viewed in a balanced perspective. Far greater attention must be paid to the preventive aspects of medicine. Far more money should be allocated to providing clean water, good nutrition, sanitation, housing, education, with special emphasis on female education, population control and the use of preventive vaccines, than to the purchase of glittering machines and to the building of five-star hospitals in the urban centres of these countries. Medical education in a country such as India should be oriented to the problems facing this country and not those facing the West. Ethics should be taught more by example and precept than by oft-repeated platitudes. An equitable distribution of the meagre resources, with a focused attention on the problems afflicting 70 per cent of the population residing in the villages of India, may well be rewarded by greater benefits to greater numbers of people.

The implementation of health measures in poor countries does not require the adoption of expensive western methods of health delivery. Villagers locally recruited and trained have been shown to impart basic health care efficiently and at an infinitely smaller cost. A growing economy, increasing education, honest and efficient governance and self-reliance are the basic necessities that can effectively curb disease and promote health care in the poor countries of the world.

In conclusion, contemporary medicine reflects the virtues and shortcomings, the strengths and weaknesses of our contemporary world. From an overall perspective, medicine today has benefited mankind more than ever before. Those who mock it and see no good within it are often the first to seek its protection when the need arises. It is sheer cant and bigotry to believe with Ivan Illich that the medical establishment is a hazard to health. Even so, we must recognize and admit its faults and blemishes. The crisis in contemporary medicine is paradoxically related to the crisis caused by over-rapid progress and to shattered expectations. Its basic drawback stems from the overpowering dominance of its science, which has robbed it of its humanity and submerged its art. Science divorced from humanity and art; science which is allowed to dictate and command rather than to serve and obey will be a tragedy for both medicine and man. The medicine of today and the future must recognize this fact. Contemporary medicine needs to recapture the spirit of humanism and to re-establish the special empathy in a doctor–patient relationship, if it is to restore its pristine image and meet the universal respect and approval of man. It can only do so if it divorces itself from the lure of money, raises its ethical standards and places the welfare and care of patients above all else.

75 The Future

Science cannot solve the ultimate mystery of nature. And that is because, in the last analysis, we ourselves are part of nature and therefore part of the mystery we are trying to solve.

Max Planck

The future is already upon us. The writing is on the wall—it is there for all to see. Medical science will battle in the twenty-first century to discover the secret of our origin and the mystery of our mortality. The twenty-first century will be the century of biotechnology—genetics and molecular biology will dominate research in medicine and strongly influence its practice. The seeds of future discoveries in these fields were planted in our present era when Watson and Crick, in 1953, unravelled the detailed structure and the self-copying code of the DNA molecule. Today we are just a few years away from one of the most important discoveries and landmarks in the history of science—the deciphering of the human genome.

For those unfamiliar with biology or medicine, a brief explanation of what medical science is on the threshold of achieving is necessary. The human body contains 75 trillion cells. The nucleus of each cell contains forty-six chromosomes arranged in twenty-three pairs. Each chromosome is a wadded-up strand of DNA. Unfolded and stretched the DNA strand would measure about three to nine feet in length and twenty atoms across. Genes are segments of DNA that contain the instructions to make proteins—the building blocks of life. The DNA molecule has hundreds of millions of base-pairs. The sum of the DNA in all forty-six chromosomes is the human genome. The Human Genome Project, initiated in 1990, aims to determine the complete sequence of the

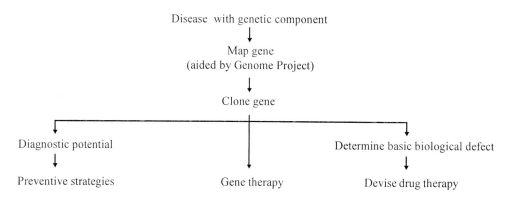

Fig. 75.1   Future scope of molecular medicine. A diseased gene will need to be mapped and cloned. The time needed to do this in the future (based on maps and improved technologies) will shorten. After gene cloning, diagnostic capabilities become possible, allowing preventive strategies. Drug therapy and gene therapy also become possible though the time-line for these to evolve cannot be predicted.

human genome, including the estimated 100,000 genes by the year 2005. The project is ahead of time and is expected to be completed by 2003. The science of medicine will thus soon have access to the 'book of life'—the precise biochemical code of each of these genes, which by and large, determines every physical characteristic within the human body. Genomic science in the near future should then determine how each gene functions and more importantly, how a malfunctioning gene can produce or influence specific disease. A number of diseases are genetic in origin while others have a genetic component. If a gene responsible for a disease is once localized and mapped, it can be cloned through bioengineering techniques. The future potential for medicine is immense and is briefly summarized in Fig. 75.1. The disease-producing cloned gene, could as explained in the figure be used for diagnostic purposes, and this in some instances could initiate preventive strategies. An example is the indication for colonoscopy in individuals at genetically high risk for colonic cancer. The cloned disease-producing gene could also enable us to understand the basic biological defect in the disease. Genes sometimes produce proteins linked to the disease. Researchers call these genes and proteins 'targets'. Drugs could target the gene or target the abnormal disease-related protein produced by the gene, thereby altering its action. Finally, medical science is heading towards the future prospect of effective gene therapy. An abnormal gene responsible for a particular malfunction or disease could theoretically be countered by introducing into the body or the organ involved the appropriate normal functioning gene. This would restore normal function and thereby reverse disease.

The diagnostic consequences of gene discovery (prediction of susceptibility to disease) will almost certainly be available in the near future. But the time sequence in the development of simple and cost-effective curative therapies (either drugs or gene therapy) will be unquestionably longer and is difficult to predict.

Future medicine will attempt to contain the 'new epidemics' of cancer, hypertension, diabetes, coronary heart disease, cerebro-vascular disease, chronic bronchitis, mental disorders and disorders affecting an increasingly ageing population. There is no true cure visible on the horizon for any of these afflictions. Cancer will continue to have the maximum funding for research. Molecular pathology may perhaps revolutionize the diagnosis and treatment of cancer. A tumor's molecular fingerprints will determine how it behaves. Most researchers believe that the future holds no single magic bullet against cancer, because 'there are probably a million cancers, may be as there are patients with cancers'. However, emerging research from molecular pathology laboratories holds out a promise for specific tools for early detection, and for choosing treatment that is far more appropriate in a given situation than exists today. The identification of genes which can induce the synthesis of growth-control molecules has stimulated a search for specific anti-cancer drugs that can change the activity of selected genes, so that the synthesis of RNA from a DNA template is selectively inhibited.

The future also holds promise in its ability to modify the genetic basis of immunity—the technique of immunomodulation. When genes controlling the synthesis of cytokines are introduced into cancer cells and lymphocytes, they trigger a cytotoxic response that results in death of the cancer cells and other diseased cells. Unfortunately, cytokines are not sufficiently selective and cause unwanted side-effects through damage and death of healthy cells. Methods to improve selectivity include the use of chemically modified anti-cancer drugs which remain nontoxic till they reach their target site. Once in place they are activated by light (photoactivation), or by monoclonal antibodies exerting a selective distinctive action on cancer cells.

Monoclonal antibodies unfortunately have not lived up to expectations. Even so, the theoretical concept underlying their use is attractive; research on their therapeutic application is certain to continue. A possible future for monoclonal antibodies is in the treatment of multiple sclerosis, an autoimmune disease in which the lymphocytes instead of performing their usual protective role, attack and injure the brain and spinal cord. Research is being directed to finding the appropriate monoclonal antibodies which latch on to a feature of lymphocytes, which will prevent them from injuring the central nervous system. This is not beyond the realm of possibility. Scientists are also attempting to attach drugs to monoclonal antibodies to ensure that the drugs reach exactly the desired target, thereby producing the expected results with little or no side-effects.

Genetic Science and the Future

Gene-based drug therapy, gene therapy and the increasing use of recombinant DNA vaccines in the prevention of disease are the obvious happy non-controversial benefits that should result from our increasing mastery over genetic science. However the potential of genetic engineering and of advances in biotechnology could conceivably produce incredible revolutionary changes in mankind. These could include new sources of organs and tissues for transplants, methods to halt the ageing process, cloning of human beings, producing of 'designer babies', and perhaps modifying the human genome in an attempt to improve upon the several million years of Darwinian selection.

Let us first briefly recapitulate what genetic science has achieved today so that we have a base that enables us to imagine the exciting yet terrifying future. It was in 1986 that the FDA approved the first genetically-engineered hepatitis B vaccine for use in humans. As mentioned earlier, the International Human Genome Project was launched in 1990 under the leadership of James Watson. The three billion dollar project is to map and sequence all human DNA and should be complete by 2003. The American geneticist, W. French Anderson performed in 1990, the first gene therapy on a four-year-old girl afflicted with a congenital immune deficiency disease. American and British scientists in 1992 devised techniques to test human embryos for genetic defects such as cystic fibrosis and haemophilia. In 1993, researchers at George Washington University cloned human embryos and nurtured them in petri dishes for several days drawing great criticism from many sources. The world stood astounded and a trifle aghast, when on 27 February 1997, embryologist Ian Wilmut, heading a research team at Scotland's Roslin Institute reported in *Nature* the cloning of a sheep named Dolly—from the cell of an adult ewe. This was followed in 1998 by researchers at Hawaii University cloning a mouse, creating dozens of copies and three generations of cloned clones! In Japan scientists at Kinki University have cloned eight identical calves from a single adult cow. The Oregon Regional Primate Research Centre in Beaverton, United States has reported the birth of two successfully cloned rhesus monkeys. The successful cloning of animals has sent shock waves throughout the world raising both ethical issues and moral dilemmas.

Research on the controlled development of embryonic stem cells also holds promise for the future. In the human being, the only time cells possess the potential to develop into any or all body parts is in early pregnancy when the stem cells have not begun to differentiate. In the autumn of 1998, scientists at the Wisconsin University finally managed to isolate embryonic stem cells and induced them to grow into neural, gut, muscle and bone cells. The research is in its infancy and may perhaps have its limitations. If however, stem cell growth and differentiation to any desired tissue is achieved, medicine would be revolutionized. Doctors would be able to replace injured and dead tissues of disease with healthy tissue. Perhaps organs like the liver, heart and kidney could also be grown in the laboratory, making transplant surgery available to all.

Cloning holds a similar potential. As in the case of Dolly the sheep, cloning involves the use of a developed somatic cell and reactivating the genome within, so that its instruction to develop is reset to the earliest pristine state. Once this transpires the cell develops into a full-fledged animal, genetically identical to the parent. The cloning technique used above is best termed the 'somatic cell nuclear transfer'. In Dolly's case the somatic cell was taken from the udder of an adult ewe; the nuclear transfer was effected by inserting the genomic material into an oocyte which had been earlier ennucleated, i.e., had its nucleus removed.

As with the development of stem cells, cloning could in the future also help to develop organs for transplants, or healthy tissues to replace diseased tissues. In the not too distant future, organs and tissues for transplants may well be up for sale in the shopping centres of many large cities of the world! If animals can be cloned, the cloning of humans, though technically more difficult, will almost certainly come about one day. The emotional, ethical and legal problems that the future world would then face may well be insurmountable.

The frightening aspect of genetic science is the prospect of the possible results of the insertion of functional genetic material into the human germ cells—sperm or ovum. This could well change the course of our future evolution, could affect nature's process of natural selection and in the centuries or perhaps in the millennia to come, create a new form of living species that would be unrecognizable to humans inhabiting the world today. Though no government wishes to take steps to initiate or sanction this research, the demand to move in the above direction in the years to come may be irresistible. Today in the advanced centres of fertility and reproduction in the West, parents can choose a child's sex and screen for genetic illness. Gene therapy to correct genetic illness in embryos is however still a few years away. As yet, the genes responsible for most of the physical and mental attributes have not been identified. Perhaps in a decade or two, these would be known, so that it will be possible to screen embryos and foetuses for different physical and mental characteristics. If gene therapy lives up to its potential, parents may not only want the undesirable traits of their unborn child weeded out, they would perhaps insist on inserting genes they desire. It sends a shudder to think that the new millenium after some decades may well open into an era of 'designer babies'. The overall prospect is awesome and frightening. It may read as science fiction today, but we must remember that much of science fiction in the past has come to be true in the present. Will the future see medical science and technology change man into an unrecognizable species?

Infections of the Future

The poor countries of the world including India, will continue to grapple against infections for several decades. The infections that will dominate the first decades of the next century in countries like India and Africa will be tuberculosis and AIDS. These two diseases will also continue to take a toll of human life in the West. India in particular, is heading for an explosive increase in HIV infection. It is estimated that about 40 million Indians will be infected by the HIV virus by the first two decades of the twenty-first century. The danger from tuberculosis in developing countries is even worse. In 1993, the WHO declared TB a 'global emergency'. In 1995, there were more deaths from tuberculosis than in any other year. The years 1990–1999 saw 90 million new cases and close to 30 million deaths. The horrendous present incidence of tuberculosis in India has been detailed in chapter 61. This ancient disease is today the largest cause of death from a single pathogen. In the global context it is responsible for twice the number of deaths that are caused by AIDS, diarrhoea and all other parasitic diseases put together.

Tuberculosis and AIDS are companions-in-arms; they aid and abet each other. The increasing incidence of HIV infection and AIDS in many poor countries of the world in the next century will bring in its wake a six to ten fold increase in the incidence of tuberculosis. It has been aptly stated that 'TB has been a time bomb, AIDS has shortened its fuse'. Like the horsemen of the Apocalypse, these two diseases promise a savage destruction of humanity in India and Africa in the twenty-first century. The problem in the future will be further compounded by the rising incidence of multiple drug resistant (MDR) tuberculosis. Data on the incidence of MDR tuberculosis in India is sparse, but one large survey showed an incidence as high as 44 per cent. If even half this incidence is representative of the country, it forecasts the death of many more millions in the first few years of the next millenium. The WHO has advocated the DOTS (directly observed therapy) regime to help in the conquest of tuberculosis, pointing to its success in reducing very significantly the incidence of the disease, and in preventing MDR TB, as judged from studies carried out in New York, Tanzania and China. But these are small studies carried out by motivated medical and social workers. It is impossible in my opinion, to significantly alter the high incidence of tuberculosis and for that matter any other widely prevalent infection by drugs alone in a country such as India. The size of the country, the inaccessibility of so many areas within the country, the corruption, dishonesty and lack of motivation at all levels, and above all, the poverty, ignorance, overcrowding, lack of sanitation and hygiene, coupled with poor nutrition, are great impediments to the successful implementation of DOTS.

René Dubois wrote in 1952: "Tuberculosis is the ultimate social disease! A disease that medicine never cured, wealth never warded off." The road to its conquest is the road to socio-economic emancipation. Till then, we can at best hope to stage a holding action against tuberculosis and other infections which plague the poor countries of the world.

It is inconceivable to visualize even a distant future in which man and medicine have banished all infections. There is a remarkable ecological balance between man and his microscopic fellow creatures. It is impossible to destroy all the pathogenic organisms with powerful antibiotics, for nature breeds resistant strains that continue to cause disease. Resistant pneumococci, staphylococci, and resistant gram-negative organisms particularly those belonging to the enterobacter species pose grave dangers today in many parts of the world. The indiscriminate use of antibiotics disrupts the ecological balance between man and micro-organisms, and is perilous to the safety of man.

In fact, it is more than likely that the future world will witness new diseases and new infections. New disease could result from changes in social and environmental conditions. Microorganisms and in particular viruses can mutate for known and unknown reasons. They can then produce new infections and diseases never encountered earlier in the history of man. The HIV is an example of a virus which has probably mutated several times before it struck our contemporary world.

Health problems in the future world will be accentuated by the anticipated population explosion in the poor countries. A recent UN report projected that the world population could reach 9.4 billion by 2050. A statistical study identifies 28 countries (20 of them in Africa) where the fertility rate increased during the past decade. Malthus' gloomy forecast embodied in *An Essay on the Principle Population as it Affects the Future Improvement of the Society,* may still, at least in part, come true. Feeding the world's masses even with continuing advances in the science of agriculture, may prove to be a problem which may be insoluble in times of war and natural disasters. Just as dangerous will be the uncontrolled consumption of non-renewable resources, the irreversible destruction of habitats and species, the pollution of the air, rivers and seas, and many other dangers of an exploding human population.

The Future World

Future medicine will reflect the future world. Quantum science of the twentieth century gave birth to the biomolecular and computer age, ushering in revolutions that have changed the world and will continue to do so in an exponential manner in the next century. We have given a brief glimpse of the future potential of the biomolecular and biotechnical revolutions. The computer revolution has also strongly influenced both man and medicine and will increasingly do so in the years to come. It is the computer which has spawned information technology, introduced the world to the Internet, abolished our age-old concept of time and space and promises in the future to knit the world in a tighter, closer embrace.

Michio Kaku, an internationally known theoretical physicist and the Henry Sernat professor at The City University of New York, is of the opinion that the quantum theory will, in the near future give us nanotechnology—the ability to make machines the size of atoms, thereby ushering in another industrial revolution. Professor Kaku forecasts the possibility of a tiny computer, the size of atoms, inserted into our bloodstream, giving us continuous data on our health and at the same time, correcting any deviations from health that may arise within us. He contends that by 2020, according to Moore's law, computer chips will cost next to nothing—perhaps less than a scrap of paper. All appliances will be computerized. Prototypes already exist—the internet watch: one talks to it and it talks back assessing the whole database on the internet; the intelligent tie-clasp, which has the combined power of a laptop and the cell-phone; the Geo-positioning earring, which will access the Geo-positioning Satellites in orbit and give the wearer his or her location within twenty feet; smart spectacles, which will video-image a medical conference in the wearer's eyeglasses; smart clothes and toilet—the clothes will monitor the wearer's health and in case of a heart attack, will automatically call the ambulance to the exact location. Professor Kaku mentions that the Japanese are already marketing a smart toilet, which automatically analyses one's body fluids.

The dream of scientists is to create true artificial intelligence. Is a computer brain possible? Raymond Ruszweil, author of *The Age of Spiritual Machines* contends that scientists have already replicated input-output characteristics of clusters of hundreds of neurones. Is there a possibility of scaling up from hundreds of neurones to billions of neurones, like the human brain contains, and of computing more than 500 trillion bytes per second, as our human brain does? Even if this becomes possible in the distant future, there are certain human qualities which a machine, however intelligent, can never possess—for these are qualities which are not directly related or linked to intelligence. How can a machine ever possess imagination, experience, wisdom, or intuition, and above all, how can it blossom into a spirituality which was the essence of great prophets such as Zoroaster, Buddha, Mahavir and Christ, or on a lesser plane, of great human beings such as Hippocrates, Charaka and Susruta, or Martin Luther King, Mahatma Gandhi and Mother Theresa?

Many an eminent scientist believes that 'consciousness' and 'intelligence' are not the same. Sir John Eccles, a famous scientist and a Nobel laureate, in his Gifford lectures, writes that 'consciousness' is distinct from 'thinking' or 'intelligence'. 'The Unity of conscious experience is provided by the self-conscious mind and not by the neuronal machinery of the liaison areas of the cerebral hemispheres.' And what is the self-conscious mind? How has it come about? This indeed is the mystery of life, a mystery that may well be beyond the grasp of future science. Eccles considers the self-conscious mind a self-subsistent entity which integrates the multifarious activities of the neuronal machinery to give the unity of conscious existence, from moment to moment.

Science, Medicine, God

The future holds the prospect of science and medicine questioning the need for religion and the existence of God. If the mysteries of birth and life, of health and disease, come to be increasingly unravelled, if human beings in the future are cloned, science may well exclaim, "Does God exist!" Darwin's theory of evolution explains the genesis of man. After a delay at the stage of unicellular organisms for billions of years, there commenced a slow evolution of increasingly complex living organisms, culminating in the appearance of man on earth. Our evolutionary path has been long, unpredictable and beset by many hazards. Medical science claims that this evolutionary path was governed solely by chance and necessity. I believe this to be the apparent truth but not the whole truth. I believe that there is Providence, or a Divine Force operating over and above and guiding the visible happenings of biological evolution. 'Evidence-based medicine' (an unfortunate slogan of contemporary medicine) would undoubtedly scoff at this unscientific 'evidence-lacking' concept. But then, truth does not necessarily cease to be so because it cannot be proven. On a lesser plane, this is applicable to some of the unpredictable and impossible to prove responses of man to disease and his equally unpredictable interaction with the art and science of medicine. On a higher plane this concept embraces some of the mysteries of the universe and of the existence of man as a conscious, thinking, experiencing, creating individual, who comes into being at birth, but apparently ceases to be at death. It would be a profound tragedy for man and medicine if science were to refute this religious vision of the universe or if scientific dogma were to negate the innate spirituality within man.

Ethical Questions

Future medicine will pose grave moral and ethical questions. The pace of development   in the science of genetics in relation to reproduction and procreation has far outstripped the pace at which ethical questions are being resolved. Bioethics is an unchartered sea, and we need to map and charter this sea if humanity is not to be wrecked on its shoals and reefs. It is not within the scope of this book to discuss at length the ethical and moral issues raised by medical science now and in the future. The future will need to ensure the freedom of scientific research and yet, safeguard the respect for fundamental human rights; it will need to strike a balance between science and humanity for the benefit of man and medicine. The General Conference of Unesco in November 1997 discussed these issues and adopted the 'Declaration on the Human Genome and Human Rights'. The Declaration considered the explosion in genetic engineering techniques, their application in medicine and the fundamental rights of man to exercise choice. The Declaration states that freedom of research is part of freedom of thought and is necessary for the progress of knowledge. It maintains that the application of research in genetics, biology and medicine, concerning the human genome must be directed to the relief of suffering and improving the health of individuals and of humankind.

It is impossible to ban or curb freedom of thought or the research that goes with the freedom of thought. Yet, should the science of genetics on the pretext of reducing human suffering be permitted to extinguish any life that is doomed to disease at its very genesis? It would be unethical and immoral to allow the application of scientific research on the human genome to prevail over the respect for fundamental human rights, freedom and dignity. It would in my opinion be dangerous to trespass into the future and use the power of science to ensure that only good genes prevail and that 'bad' or 'not so good' genes are eliminated. If man and medicine were to counter nature and the process of natural selection, would the world have seen Homer, Toulouse Lautrec, Hellen Keller or Stephen Hawkins? To consider every genetic defect in the human genome as a tragedy that needs to be extinguished at its very origin violates human dignity and rights. Genetic engineering to cure diseases such as cystic fibrosis or defects such as muscular dystrophy is welcome and is to be encouraged. But again to trespass into the future and use the science of genetics to alter our DNA and genome radically with a view to encode our vanities, change our attributes, or what is even more sinister, quickly evolve into new life-forms or into a new super-race, is wrong and fraught with danger. We must tread carefully if our world in the future is not to become a stage for a true-to-life Greek tragedy.

The moral philosophy that many scientists today consider worth following is that of Immanuel Kant, the moralist and philosopher of the nineteenth century. Kant considered each human being an individual and an end but not as a means to an end. Under this moral precept, human cloning stands condemned as unethical and undesirable. There is always the possibility of science being reduced to depravity and made to clone Frankensteins. Even otherwise, human clones will be means to an end; they will not be valued as individuals in their own right but as 'copies' of others we respected or loved.

Ethical questions in the near future will also be increasingly centred on the problem of active euthanasia, which under certain conditions and safeguards has already been legalized in the Netherlands and Australia. Many in the West are increasingly concerned with maintaining a good quality of life and putting an end to unbearable suffering in incurable disease. But who is to judge the basic minimum in the quality of life? And is it ever possible to quantitate suffering? Is not suffering often a state of mind and cannot the state of mind be subject to changing social pressures and social mores?

As mentioned in chapter 74, pain and suffering are an integral part of life and living. Each one of us has to accept the cross he or she is ordained to bear. What is more, modern medicine has both the art and science of relieving suffering. Should doctors of the future take on the role of gods and decide who lives and who dies? If that be so, the future world could be a witness to the horrendous prospect of special institutions meant to do away with perhaps thousands who are deemed to have a poor quality of life, or profess their inability to withstand suffering. It would be a holocaust that would put to shame the Nazi extermination camps of the Second World War.

The dangers of legalizing euthanasia in a poor country such as India would be even more immense. The poverty, corruption and the exploitation of loopholes in the legal system would open the floodgates to murder.

Active euthanasia can never be a solution to the relief of human suffering or to the poor quality of life so many of us are condemned to live. Yet there should be a tacit pact between Man and Medicine that all forms of suffering be relieved, and that the act of dying be smooth, humane and in no way prolonged. This pact would guarantee the protection of human rights and human dignity.

Quo Vadis Medicine

Where is medicine heading, which road will it follow and what is its destination? In the final analysis, the future of Man and Medicine will be linked as in the past with the concepts, philosophies, morals, ethics, economics and attitudes to life and living prevailing in the centuries to come. If science captures medicine in its entirety, medicine will become increasingly cold, uncaring and even inhumane. In the not too distant past, all that the physician had to combat disease with was courage, common sense, compassion and just a few specific cures. Now that he has the awesome power of science and technology to back him, his human qualities are on the ebb. Is it not likely that the high-powered physician of tomorrow will be embarrassed to hold the hand of a dying man, or tarry with him a while to ease his passage into the unknown? The terrifying futuristic prospect of machines, computers and robots ministering to the sick and suffering is matched by the even more terrifying concept of future man evolving as an appendage to a machine, or evolving into half-machine half-man. Hopefully, this will not come to pass, as mankind will reject such medicine as unworthy of its trust.

Science can be both powerful and beautiful, yet it is cold and impersonal; machines may work wonders but they are incapable of care and compassion. Medicine without care and compassion, however powerful and beautiful will be unacceptable to humankind because a human being who is truly ill craves for compassion and care. Also each human being is a separate, unique individual, a law unto himself. Unlike a machine, he is unpredictable in his functions and his reactions. He has feelings, emotions, dreams, desires and ambitions which colour his symptoms and condition his response to disease, as well as to the treatment of disease. He not uncommonly defies the mathematical laws of statistics, for he may live when expected to die and die when one is sure that he should have lived. Therein lies the art of medicine, an art that will endure till mankind survives. If medicine in the future strays from its true path, it will be the suffering and the sick who will correct and redirect its course, so that it combines within itself the best of science with an equal measure of art.

Medicine from early centuries was built around changing 'models'. Whereas Morgagni took the gross changes in the structure of an organ as the model for disease, Bichat took changes in tissues as his model. Virchow looked at the cell as his model; contemporary and future medicine will make the molecule its model. This too will change in the not too distant future, for the history of science from the beginning of time is a chronicle of change. Medicine will hopefully in the future, embrace the holistic model of the mind–body complex in which man is an integral part of nature. This will transpire when science proves that organs 'talk' to each other, communicate with and influence one another, to ensure that the human organism works as an integrated harmonious whole, to vibrate in unison with nature. It will transpire when science realizes that 'consciousness' is a mysterious feature, distinct from and unexplained by the anatomy and physiology of the billions of neurones that constitute the human brain. The control of the mind over the myriad functions of the body will then be elucidated, as will the importance and use of biofeedback mechanisms to influence the course of disease.

The future of man and medicine rests with Man. He should not be blinded by the dazzling light of science, nor bewitched by its power and beauty so as to be servile to it. He should channelize it for the benefit of mankind, subjecting it to ethical and moral constraints. If he does so, man and medicine in the distant future may usher in a brave new world. If not, mankind will once again be plunged into 'a new Dark Age made more sinister and perhaps more protracted by the lights of perverted science'.

Bibliography

Ackernecht, E.H., *A Short History of Medicine*, New York: Ronald Press, 1955.

Octave, A., *Napoleon*, London: Paul Hamlyn Ltd., 1961.

Brieger, G.H., 'The Historiography of Medicine', in W.F. Bynum and Roy Porter (eds.), *Companion Encyclopaedia of the History of Medicine*, London: Routledge, 1993, pp. 24–44.

Cambridge Ancient History, 13 Vols, New York: Cambridge University Press, 1902–12.

Cambridge Modern History, 12 Vols, New York: Cambridge University Press, 1923–51.

Carmichael, A.G., and Richard M.R., *Medicine a Treasury of Art and Literature*, Beaux Arts Editions, 1991.

Cassedy, J.H., *Medicine in America: A Short History*, Baltimore: John Hopkins University Press, 1991.

Castiglioni, A.A., *History of Medicine*, E.B. Krumbhaar tr, New York: Knopf, 1947.

Christopher, H.J., *The Age of Napoleon*, London: Weidenfeld and Nicholson, 1963.

Clark, K., *Civilization*, London: British Broadcasting Corporation, 1969.

Durant, W., and Ariel, *The Story of Civilization*, Vols I–XI, New York: Simon and Schuster, 1975.

Duin, N.A., *History of Medicine: From Prehistory to the Year 2020*, London and New York: Simon and Schuster, 1992.

Gibbons, *The Decline and Fall of the Roman Empire*, (abr.) 3 Vols, D.M. Low (abr.), New York: Washington Square Press, Inc., 1962.

Kiple, K.F. (ed.), *The Cambridge World History of Human Disease*, Cambridge: Cambridge University Press, 1993.

Kiple, K.F., 'The Ecology of Disease', in W.F. Bynum and Roy Porter (eds.), *Companion Encyclopaedia of the History of Medicine*, London: Routledge, 1993, pp. 357–81.

Marti–Ibanez, F., Ariel, *Essays on the Arts and the History of Philosophy of Medicine*, New York: M.D. Publications, 1962.

Marti–Ibanez, F., *A Prelude to Medical History*, New York: M.D. Publications, 1961.

Marti–Ibanez, F. (eds.), *A Pictorial History of Medicine*, London: Spring Books, 1965.

Margotta, R., *An Illustrated History of Medicine*, Paul Lewis (ed.), Middlesex: the Hamlyn Publishing Group, 1967.

McGrew, R.E., *Encyclopaedia of Medical History*, New York: Mc Graw Hill, 1985.

Porter, R. (ed.), *The Cambridge Illustrated History of Medicine*, Cambridge: Cambridge University Press, 1996.

Porter, R., *The Greatest Benefit to Mankind*, London: Harper Collins, 1997.

Sigerist, H.E., *Civilization and Disease*, Ithaca: Cornell University Press, 1943, reprinted ed, Phoenix: University of Chicago Press, 1962.

Sigerist, H.E., *A History of Medicine*, 3 Vols, New York: Oxford University Press, 1955.

Toynbee, A., *Mankind and Mother Earth*, New York and London: Oxford University Press, 1976.

Toynbee, A., *A Study of History,* London: Oxford University Press with Thames and Hudson, 1972.

Toynbee, A. (ed.), *Cities of Destiny,* New York: Mc Graw Hill Book Company, 1973.

Toynbee, A. (ed.), *Half the World,* London: Thames and Hudson, 1973.

Walton, J., Jenemial, A. Barondess and Stephen Lock (eds), *The Oxford Medical Companion,* Oxford: Oxford University Press, 1994.

Wells, H.G., *Outline of History,* Great Britain: Cessel and Company Ltd., 1932.

Prelude

Brothwell, D., and Sandison, A.T., *Diseases in Antiquity,* Springfield, Illinois: Charles C. Thomas, 1967.

Eliade, M., and Shamanism, A., *Techniques of Ecstasy,* translated from the French by Williard R. Trask, London: Routledge and Kegan Paul, 1964.

Rivers, W.H.R., *Medicine, Magic and Religion,* the Fitzpatrick lectures delivered before the Royal College of Physicians of London, 1915, 1916, London: Kegan Paul, Trench Trubner and Co. Ltd., 1924.

Mesopotamia and Egypt

Casson, L., *Great Ages of Man—Ancient Egypt,* Time–Life International, 1969.

Reeves, C., *Egyptian Medicine,* Princes Risborough, Bucks: Shire Publications, 1992.

Margotta, R., *An Illustrated History of Medicine,* Middlesex: Hamlyn Publishing Group, 1968.

Marti-Ibanez, F., *A Pictorial History of Medicine,* London: Spring Books, 1965.

Sigerist, H.E., *A History of Medicine,* Vol. I: Primitive and Archaic Medicine, New York: Oxford University Press, 1951.

Medicine in Ancient Persia

Boyce, M., *Zoroastrians—Their Religious Beliefs and Practices,* London: Routledge and Kegan Paul, 1979.

Cambridge Ancient History, Vol. IV: The Persian Empire and the West, Cambridge, 1926.

Dabu, K.S., *Message of Zarathushtra,* Bombay: The New Book Company Pvt. Ltd., 1959.

Darmesteter, J., and Mills L.N., *Sacred Books of the East,* F. Max Muller (ed.), Oxford, 1880–87.

Sigerist, H., *A History of Medicine,* Vol. II: Early Greek, Hindu and Persian Medicine, New York and Oxford: Oxford University Press, 1961.

Taraporewala, I.J.S., *The Religion of Zarathushtra,* The Bombay Chronicle Press, 1965.

Vendidad

Zend Avesta

Indian Medicine

Charaka, *Agnivesa's Charaka Samhita,* Ram Kumar Sharma and Vaidya Bhagwan Das tr., Varanasi, India: Chawkhamba Sanskrit Series Office, 1976.

Gallagher, N.E., 'Islamic and Indian Medicine', in Kenneth F. Kiple (ed.), *The Cambridge World History of Human Disease*, Cambridge: Cambridge University Press, 1993.

Jaggi, O.P., *History of Science and Technology in India*, Vol. 4: *Indian System of Medicine*, Delhi: Atmaram and Sons, 1973.

Kutumbiah, P., *Ancient Indian Medicine*, Madras: Orient Longman, 1962.

Kutumbiah, P., 'Medicine in Medieval India', *Indian Journal of History of Medicine*, 7.1.1, 1962.

Kutumbiah, P., 'Pulse in Indian Medicine', *Indian Journal of History of Medicine*, 12.1.11, 1967.

Ramchandra Rao, S.K., *Encyclopaedia of Indian Medicine*, 6 Vols, Bombay: Popular Prakashan Pvt. Ltd., 1985.

Ray, P., Gupta, H. and Mira R., *Susruta Samhita: A Scientific Synopsis*, New Delhi: Indian Science Academy, 1980.

Sharma, P.V., *History of Medicine in India (from Antiquity to 1000 AD)*, New Delhi: Indian National Science Academy, 1992.

Vakil, R.J., 'Early Contributions to the Study of Pulse', *Indian Journal of History of Medicine*, 1.22.22, 1956.

Wujastyk, D., 'Indian Medicine', in W.F. Bynum and Roy Porter (eds), *Companion Encyclopaedia of the History of Medicine*, London: Routledge, 1993.

Wujastyk, D., *The Roots of Ayurveda*, New Delhi: Penguin Books India (P) Ltd., 1998.

Chinese Medicine

Bray, F., 'Chinese Medicine', in W.F. Bynum and Roy Porter (eds), *Companion Encyclopaedia of the History of Medicine*, London: Routledge, 1993.

Hoizey, D., *A History of Chinese Medicine*, Edinburgh: Edinburgh University Press, 1993.

McNamara, and Dr Song Xuan Ke, *Traditional Chinese Medicine*, Hamish Hamilton Ltd., Penguin Group, 1995.

Reid, D.P., *Chinese Herbal Medicine*, Boston Mass: Shambhala Publications, Inc., 1996.

Sivin, N. (ed.), *Traditional Medicine in Contemporary China*, Ann Arbor, MI: University of Michigan Press, 1987.

Unschuld, P.U., 'History of Chinese Medicine', in Kenneth F. Kiple (ed.), *The Cambridge World History of Human Disease*, Cambridge: Cambridge University Press, 1993.

Wong, K.C. and Wu L., *History of Chinese Medicine*, (second ed.), Shanghai: National Quarantine Service, 1936.

Medicine in the Classical Age of Greece

Barker, E. (ed.), *Greek Medicine*, London and Toronto: J.M. Dert and Sons Ltd., 1929.

Bowra, C.M., *Great Ages of Man—Classical Greece*, Time–Life International, 1968.

Durant, W., *The Life of Greece*, New York: Simon and Schuster, 1929.

Durant, W. and Durant, A., *The Story of Civilization*, vol. 2: The Life of Greece, New York: Simon and Schuster, 1975.

Lloyd, G. (ed.), *Hippocratic Writings*, Harmondsworth: Penguin, 1978.

Longrigg, J.N., The Plague of Athens, *History of Science*, XVIII, 1980.

Marti-Ibanez, F. (ed.), *A Pictorial History of Medicine*, London: Spring Books, 1965.

Nutton, V., 'Humoralism', in W.F. Bynum and Roy Porter (eds.), *Companion Encyclopaedia of the History of Medicine*, London: Routledge, 1993, pp. 281–91.

Philips, E.D., *Greek Medicine*, London: Thames and Hudson, 1973.

Porter, R., *The Greatest Benefit to Mankind*, London: Harper Collins Publishers, 1997.

Sigerist, H.E., *A History of Medicine*, Vol. 2: Early Greek, Hindu and Persian Medicine. New York: Oxford University Press, 1961.

Roman Medicine

Brian, P., *Galen on Bloodletting*, New York: Cambridge University Press, 1986.

Durant, W. and Durant, A., *The Story of Civilization*, Vol. 3: Caesar and Christ, New York: Simon and Schuster, 1975.

Gibbons, *The Decline and Fall of the Roman Empire*, abr. by D.M. Low in 3 Vols, New York: Washington Square Press Inc., 1962.

Hadas, M., *Great Ages of Man, Imperial Rome*, Time–Life International, 1966.

Margotta, R., *An Illustrated History of Medicine*, Paul Lewis (ed.), Paul Hamlyn, 1968.

Marti-Ibanez, F. (ed.), *A Pictorial History of Medicine*, London: Spring Books, 1965.

Nutton, V. (ed.), *Galen: Problems and Prospects*, London: Wellcome Institute for the History of Medicine, 1981.

Temkin, O., *Galenism*: *Rise and Decline of a Medical Philosophy*, Ithaca, NY: Cornell University Press, 1973.

Medicine in the Dark Ages

Conred, L.I., 'Arab–Islamic Medicine' in W.F. Bynum and Roy Porter (eds.), *Companion Encyclopaedia of the History of Medicine*, London, Routledge, 1993.

Dols, M.W., 'Diseases of the Islamic World', in Kenneth F. Kiple (ed.), *The Cambridge World History of Human Disease*, Cambridge: Cambridge University Press, 1993.

Gallagher, N.E., '*Islamic and Indian Medicine*', in Kenneth F. Kiple (ed.), *The Cambridge World History of Human Disease*, Cambridge: Cambridge University Press, 1993.

Gibbons, *The Decline and Fall of the Roman Empire*, 3 Vols, D.M. Low (abr), New York: Washington Square Press Inc., 1962.

Khan, M.S., *Islamic Medicine*, London: Routledge and Kegan Paul, 1986.

Margotta, R., *An Illustrated History of Medicine*, Paul Lewis (ed.), Middlesex, Paul Hamlyn: The Hamlyn Publishing Group, 1967.

Miller, T.S., *The Birth of the Hospital in the Byzantine Empire*, Baltimore: John Hopkins University Press, 1985.

Park, K., 'Black Death', in Kenneth F. Kiple (ed.), *The Cambridge World History of Human Disease*, Cambridge: Cambridge University Press, 1993.

Porter, R., *The Greatest Benefit to Mankind*, London: Harper Collin Publishers, 1997.

Siraisi, N.G., *Medieval and Early Renaissance Medicine: An Introduction to Knowledge and Practice*, Chicago: Chicago University Press, 1990.

Renaissance Medicine

Arrizabalaga, J., Henderson, J. and French, R., *The Great Pox: The French Disease in Renaissance Europe*, New Haven: Yale University Press, 1997.

Carmichael, A.G., *Plague and the Poor in Renaissance Florence*, Cambridge and New York: Cambridge University Press, 1986.

Durant, W. and Durant A., *The Story of Civilization*, Vol. 5: The Renaissance, New York: Simon and Schuster, 1975.

French, R., 'The Anatomical Tradition', in W.F. Bynum and Roy Porter (eds), *Companion Encyclopaedia of the History of Medicine*, London: Routledge, 1993.

Hale, J.R., *Great Ages of Man—Renaissance*, Time–Life International, 1966.

O'Malley, C.D. and de. J.B, Saunders, C.M. (eds), *Leonardo da Vinci on the Human Body*, New York: Schuman, 1952.

O'Malley, C.D., *Andreas Vesalius of Brussels 1514–1564*, California: University of California Press, 1964.

Ambroise Paré, *Ten Books of Surgery*, Linker, R.W. and Womack Tr., N., Athens, GA: University of Georgia Press, 1969.

Wear, A., French R. and Lonia, I. (eds), *The Medical Renaissance of the Sixteenth Century*, Cambridge: Cambridge University Press, 1995.

Medicine in the Baroque Period (17th Century)

Dewhurst, K. (ed.), *Dr. Thomas Sydenham (1624–1689): His Life and Original Writings*, Berkeley, CA: University of California Press, 1966.

Frank, R.G., *Harvey and the Oxford Physiologists: Scientific Ideas and Social Interaction*, Berkeley, CA: University of California Press, 1980.

French, R. and Wear A. (eds), *The Medical Revolution of the Seventeenth Century*, Cambridge and New York: Cambridge University Press, 1989.

Harvey, W., *An Anatomical Disputation Concerning the Movement of the Heart and Blood in Living Creatures*, Tr. by Whitteridge G., Oxford: Blackwell Scientific, 1976.

Webster, C., *From Paracelsus to Newton, Magic and the Making of Modern Science*, Cambridge: Cambridge University Press, 1982.

Medicine in the Age of Enlightenment and Reason (18th Century)

Bynum, W.F., and Porter R. (eds), *William Hunter and the Eighteenth Century Medical World*, Cambridge: Cambridge University Press, 1985.

Fisher, R.B., *Edward Jenner, 1749–1823*, London: Andre Deutsch, 1991.

Porter, R. (ed.), *Medicine in the Enlightenment*, Amsterdam: Rodopi, 1995.

Porter, R., *The Greatest Benefit to Mankind*, London: Harper Collins, 1997.

Modern Medicine (19th Century)

Ackerknecht, E.H., *Rudolf Virchow: Doctor, Statesman, Anthropologist*, Madison, WI: University of Wisconsin Press, 1953.

Akroyd, W.R., *Conquest of Deficiency Diseases,* Geneva: World Health Organization, 1972.

Arnold, D., 'Medicine and Colonialism', in W.F. Bynum and Roy Porter (eds), *Companion Encyclopaedia of the History of Medicine,* London: Routledge, 1993.

Baly, M.E., *Florence Nightingale and the Nursing Legacy,* London: Routledge, 1988.

Berrios, G.E., and Porter, R. (eds), *A History of Clinical Psychiatry: The Origin and History of Psychiatric Disorders,* London: Athlone, 1995.

Bliss, M., *The Discovery of Insulin,* Edinburgh: Paul Harris, 1983.

Boyd, B.A., *Rudolf Virchow: The Scientist as Citizen,* New York: Garland, 1991.

Brock, W.H., 'The Biochemical Tradition', in W.F. Bynum and Roy Porter (eds), *Companion Encyclopaedia of the History of Medicine,* London: Routledge, 1993.

Brock, W.H., *Justus van Liebig: The Chemical Gatekeeper,* Cambridge: Cambridge University Press, 1997.

Brock, T.D., and Koch R., *A Life in Medicine and Bacteriology,* Madison, Wisc: Science Tech. Publishers, 1988.

Bynum, W.F., *Science and the Practice of Medicine in the Nineteenth Century,* New York: Cambridge University Press, 1994.

Carmichael, A.G., and Richard, M.R. (eds), *Medicine a Treasury of Art and Literature,* Beaux Arts Edition, 1991.

Carpenter. K.J., 'Nutritional Disease', in W.F. Bynum and Roy Porter (eds), *Companion Encyclopaedia of the History of Medicine,* London: Routledge, 1993.

Crowe, S.J., *Halsted of John Hopkins: The Man and his Men,* Springfield Il: Charles C. Thomas, 1957.

Cushing, H., *The Life of Sir William Osler,* 2 Vols, Clarendon Press, 1925.

Farley, J.B., *A History of Imperial Tropical Medicine,* Cambridge and New York: Cambridge University Press, 1991.

Fisher, R.B., *Joseph Lister 1827–1912,* London: Macdonald and Janes, 1977.

Geison, G.L., *The Private Science of Louis Pasteur,* Princeton University Press, 1995.

Granshaw, L., 'The Hospital', in W.F. Bynum and Roy Porter (eds), *Companion Encyclopaedia of the History of Medicine,* London: Routledge, 1993.

Holmes, F.L., *Claude Bernard and Animal Chemistry: The Emergence of a Scientist,* Cambridge: Mass Harvard University Press, 1974.

Lasky, E., *The Vienna Medical School of the Nineteenth Century,* tr. from German by L. Williams and J.S. Levij, Baltimore and London: John Hopkins University Press, 1965.

Le, Fanu, J., *The Rise and Fall of Medicine,* Little Brown and Company, 1999.

Loudon, I., *Death in Childbirth: An International Study of Maternal Care and Maternal Mortality 1800–1950,* Oxford: Clarendon Press, 1992.

Lyons, A.S., and Petrucelli II, R.J., *Medicine: An Illustrated History,* New York: Harry N. Abrams Inc., 1978.

Manson, P.H., *Manson's Tropical Diseases: A Manual of the Diseases of Warm Climates,* (thirteenth ed.), Sir Philip H. Manson–Bahr (ed.), Cassel and Company Ltd., 1951.

Margotta, R., *An Illustrated History of Medicine,* Paul Lewis (ed.), Middlesex: Paul Hamlyn, 1968.

Maulitz, R.C., 'The Pathological Tradition', in W.F. Bynum and Roy Porter (eds), *Companion Encyclopaedia of the History of Medicine,* London: Routledge, 1993.

Maryinez, L., *The Colonial Disease: A Social History of Sleeping Sickness in North Zaire 1900–1940,* Cambridge and New York: Cambridge University Press, 1992.

Osler, Sir W., *Aequanimitas*, (3rd ed.), The Blakiston Division, Mc Graw Hill Book Company Inc., 1906.

Porter, R., *The Greatest Benefit to Mankind*, Harper Collins, 1997.

Shorter, E., *A History of Psychiatry*, New York: Free Press, 1997.

Tauber, A.I., and Leone C., *Metchnikoff and the Origins of Immunology*, New York: Oxford University Press, 1991.

Thorwold, J., *The Triumph of Surgery*, tr. from German by Richard and Clara Winston, London: Pan Books Ltd., 1962.

Wintrobe, M.M., *Hematology, The Blossoming of a Science: A Story of Inspiration and Effort*, Philadelphia: Lee and Febiger, 1985.

Worboys, M., 'Tropical Diseases', in W.F. Bynum and Roy Porter (eds), *Companion Encyclopaedia of the History of Medicine*, London: Routledge, 1993.

Young, A., *The Men Who Made Surgery*, New York: Hillman Books, published by Bartholomew House Inc., 1961.

Western Medicine in India

Boxer, C.R., *Two Pioneers of Tropical Medicine: Garcie d' Orte and Nicolas Monardes*, lecture series no. 1, Wellcome Historical Medical Library, London, 1963.

de Cunha, J.G., 'The Origin of Bombay', *Journal of the Bombay Branch of the Royal Asiatic Society*, Vol. 20, Extra Number, Kraus Reprint, Nendeln/Leichtenstein, 1969.

de Orta, G., *Colloquies on the Simples and Drugs of India*, Sir Clements Markham tr., London: Henry Sotheran and Co., 1913.

Garrison, F.H., *An Introduction to the History of Medicine*, (4th ed.), Philadelphia: W.B. Saunders Co., 1967.

Haffkine, W.M., 'The Plague Prophylactic', *Indian Medical Gazette*, 32, 201, 1897.

Hance, Lt. Gen. Sir B., 'The Development and Goal of Western Medicine in the Indian Subcontinent', Sir Gerald Birdwood Memorial Lecture, *Journal of the Royal Society of Arts*, pp. 296–318, 25 March 1949.

Jaggi, O.P., *History of Science and Technology in India*, Vol. 8: Medicine in Medical India, Delhi: Atmaram and Sons, 1981.

Jaggi, O.P., *History of Science and Technology in India*, Vol. 12: Western Medicine in India: Epidemics and Other Tropical Diseases, Delhi: Atmaram and Sons, 1979.

Jaggi, O.P., *History of Science and Technology in India*, Vol. 13: Western Medicine in India: Medical Education and Research, Delhi: Atmaram and Sons, 1979.

Jaggi, O.P., *History of Science and Technology in India*, Vol. 14: Western Medicine in India: Public Health and its Administration, Delhi: Atmaram and Sons, 1979.

Jaggi, O.P., *History of Science and Technology in India*, Vol. 15: Western Medicine in India: Social Impact, Scientists of Ancient India and their Achievements, Delhi: Atmaram and Sons, 1980.

Langer, W.L., 'Immunization Against Smallpox Before Jenner', *Scientific American*, 234, pp. 112–117, 1976.

Montenegro, J.V., *Bubonic Plague: Its Course and Symptoms and Means of Prevention and Treatment According to the Latest Scientific Discoveries Including Notes on Cases in Oporto*, London: Bailliere, Tindall and Cox, 1900.

Morehead, C., *Clinical Researches on Diseases in India*, (2nd ed.), London: Longman and Roberts, 1860.

Napier, L.E., 'The Transmission of Kala-Azar in India', *Indian Medical Gazette*, 70, 269, 1935.

Pandya, S.K., 'Major Epidemics in Bombay—A Brief Historical Review', lecture delivered in August 1986, published by the Bombay Local History Society, 1986, Sokhey, Sohib Singh. The Passing of the Present Plague Pandemic and India. (Haffkine Institute Diamond Jubilee Souvenir 1899–1959, Bombay, 1959.

Talwalkar, N.G., *Men and Memorabilia of Grant Medical College and J.J. Group of Hospitals*, Bombay: United Printer, 1995.

Contemporary Medicine

Aird, R.B., *Foundation of Modern Neurology: A Century of Progress*, New York: Raven Press, 1993.

Christian, B., *One Life*, Harrop, 1970.

Berris, G.E., Porter, R. (eds), *A History of Clinical Psychiatry: The Origin and History of Psychiatric Disorders*, London: Athlone, 1993.

Bodmer, W., Mckie, R., *The Book of Man*, Little Brown, 1994.

Bradford, H., *A Statistical Method in Clinical and Preventive Medicine*, E and S Livingstone, 1962.

Burnet, F.M., and White, D.O., *The Natural History of Infectious Disease*, (4th ed.), New York: Cambridge University Press, 1972.

Canton, D., 'Cortisone and the Politics of Drama, 1949–1955', Pickstone (ed.), in John V., *Medical Innovations in Historical Perspective*, Macmillan, 1992.

Churchill, W., *Second World War*, Vols 1–12, London: Cessell and Co., 1948.

de Vita, V., Helloman, S., Rosenberg, S.A. (eds), *Cancer: Principles and Practice of Oncology*, Philadelphia: J.B. Lippincott Company, 1993.

Devor, E.J., 'Genetic Disease', in Kenneth F. Kiple (ed.), *Cambridge World History of Human Disease*, Cambridge University Press, 1993.

Duin, N., Sutcliffe, J.A., *History of Medicine from Prehistory to the Year 2020*, London: Simon and Schusler, 1992.

Fleming, P.A., *History of Cardiology*, Amsterdam: Rodopi, 1997.

Gibbon, J.H., 'The Development of Heart–Lung Apparatus', *American Journal of Surgery*, 135: 608–619, 1978.

Hare, R., *The Birth of Penicillin*, London: George Allen and Unwin, 1970.

Johnson, S.L., *The History of Cardiac Surgery 1896–1955*, Baltimore, MD: John Hopkins University Press, 1970.

Kandinsky, W., *Concerning the Spiritual in Art*, tr. by M.T.H. Sadler, New York: Dover Publication Inc., 1977.

Lau, W.Y., 'History of Endoscopic and Laparoscopic Surgery', *World Journal of Surgery*, 21: 444–453, 1997.

Levay, D., *The History of Orthopedics*, Carnforth: Panthenon, 1990.

Macfarlane, G., *Howard Florry: The Making of a Great Scientist*, Oxford: Oxford University Press, 1979.

Macfarlane, G., *Alexander Fleming: The Man and the Myth*, New York: Oxford University Press, 1979.

Rom, W.N., Garay, S., *Tuberculosis*, (first ed.), Little Brown and Company Inc., 1996.

Sande, M.A., and Volberding, P.A., *The Medical Management of AIDS*, W.B. Saunders Co., 1997.

Shimkin, M.B., *Contrary to Nature*, U.S. Department of Health, Education and Welfare, Public Health Service, National Institute of Health, 1977, reprinted 1979, London: Castle House Publication Ltd.

Shumacker, H.B., *The Evolution of Cardiac Surgery*, Bloomington, IN: Indiana University Press, 1992.

Snellen, H.A., *History and Perspective of Cardiology*, Leiden: Leiden University Press, 1981.

Stark, T., *Knife to the Heart: The Story of Transplant Surgery*, Macmillan, 1996.

'The Century's Greatest Minds', *Time Magazine*, 29 March 1999.

Waksman, S.A., *The Role of Antibiotics in Nature. Perspective in Biology and Medicine*, Spring, 1961.

Watson, J.D., and Crick, F.H.C., 'Molecular Structure of Nucleic Acids: A Structure for Deoxyribose Nucleic Acid', *Nature*, 171: 737, 1953.

Watson, J.D., and Crick, F.H.C., 'Genetic Implications of the Structure of DNA', *Nature*, 171: 964–966, 1953.

Watson, J.D., *The Double Helix*, Weidenfeld and Nicholson, 1997.

Waugh, W., *John Chernley: The Man and the Hip*, Berlin: Springer Verlag, 1990.

Weatherall, D., *The New Genetics and Clinical Practice*, Oxford: Oxford University Press, 1991.

Weatherall, D., *Science and the Quiet Art*, Oxford: Oxford University Press, 1993.

Weatherall, M., *In Search of a Cure*, Oxford: Oxford University Press, 1990.

Wilkie, T., *Perilous Knowledge: The Human Genome Project and its Implications*, Berkley: University of California Press, 1993.

World Health Organization, *The Global Eradication of Smallpox*, Geneva: World Health Organization, 1980.

The Future

Bodner, W., and Mc Kie, R., *The Book of Man*, Little Brown, 1994.

Eccles, J., *The Human Mystery*, the Gifford Lectures, University of Edinburgh, 1977–78, Springer International, 1979.

Edwards, R. and Steptoe, P.A., *Matter of Life*, Sphere, 1981.

Horrobin, D.F., *Medical Hubris—A Reply to Ivan Illich*, Churchill Livingstone, Medical Division of Longman Group Ltd., 1978.

Illich, I., *Limits to Medicine: Expropriation of Health*, Harmondsworth: Penguin, 1977.

Kurzwell, R., *The Age of Spiritual Machines*, Viking, 1999.

Medvei, V.C., *The History of Medical Endocrinology*, Carnforth: Pantheon, 1993.

Nelkin, D., and Lindee, M.S., *The DNA Mystique: The Gene as a Cultural Icon*, New York: W.H. Freeman, 1995.

O'Dowd, M.J., and Philipp, E.E., *A History of Obstetrics and Gynecology*, Carnforth: Panthenon, 1994.

Taylor, R., *Medicine Out of Control—The Anatomy of a Malignant Technology*, Melbourne: Sun Books, 1979.

'The Future of Medicine', *Time Magazine*, 22 March 1999.

Udwadia, F.E., *Ethics in Terminal Care, Including Euthanasia*, World Congress of Anaesthesiology, The Hague, Netherlands, 1984.

Weatherall, D., *Science and the Quiet Art,* Oxford: Oxford University Press, 1993.

Wilber, K. (ed.), *Quantum Questions: Mystical Writings of the World's Great Physicists,* Boston and London: Shambhala Publications Inc., New Science Library 1985.

Wyke, A., *21st Century Miracle Medicine: Robo-Surgery Wonder Cures and the Quest for Immortality,* New York: Plenum, 1997.

Index

Donatello 165
dopamine 396–7
Doppler scanning records 427
Dorians, Greece 74
Dover's powder 235
Down's syndrome 411
Drake, Daniel 342
Dreyfus 257
drinking water, clean 440
    and epidemics 245
dropsy 235–6
drugs 19, 31, 35, 196
dualism, concept of 192, 222
Dubois, René 448
Du Bois-Reymond 270
Duchenne, Guillaume 312
Duchenne's disease 312
Dulaurent 174
Dumas, Alexander 256
Dunant, Henri 300–1
dungeons, reform of 248
Dupleix 376
Dupuytren, Guillaume 155, 263, 332
Dutch school of painting 189
dyes, use of 298
dysentery 204, 372, 374

East India Company 352–4, 356, 371
Ebers papyrus 19
Ebola virus 403
Eccles, John 449
echocardiography 400
'Electics' 94
Eddington, A. 387
Edelman, Maurice 397
Edinburgh Infirmary 282
Edinburgh medical school 232
Edinburgh pharmacopoeia 236
Edinburgh Royal College of Surgeons 233
Edison, Thomas Alva 259
Editio Princeps 110
Edward II 148
Edward VII 335
Edward, the Confessor 155
Edwards, Robert 415
Edwin Smith papyrus 19
Egypt 9, 15, 31, 438
    decline of 23
    civilization of 16, 120

medicine in 92
    religion in 16
    society in 15
Ehrlich, Paul 296, 298–9, 330, 391, 408
Eijkman, Christiaan 324
1871 Commune 323
Einstein, Albert 259, 308, 387
Einthoven, Williem 400
El Tor strain, of cholera 406
Electra complex 317
electric lamp, discovery of 259
electricity, discovery of 258
electrocardiograph (ECG) 396, 400
electroencephalogram 313
electroencephalography (EEG) 396
electromagnetism 258
electromyography 396
electron microscope 290, 308, 390
electronic pacemaker 401
electrophysiology 225, 39
electrostatic machines 234
electrotherapy 234
Elementa Physiologiae Corporis Humani 224
elements, symbolic, in Chinese philosophy 64–5
elephantiasis 327
11 Principe 161
Elliotson, John 273
EMI 427
embolism 272
embroynic stem cells, research on 446
embryology 94, 270
Emerson, Ralph Waldo 385
emetine injection 374
Empedocles 83
emphysema 440
empirical medicine 31
empiricism 94
Encyclopaedia 219
encyclopaedists 107–8
Enders, John 398
endocrinology 265, 319–22
endoscopic surgery 436
endotracheal tubes 278
England, medieval 148–9
    rise of 187
    see also Britain
Enlightenment 217, 233
Ephedra 67
epidemics 203–4
    BlackDeath and 151–3